Essentials of

APPLIED
MICROBIOLOGY

for BSc Nursing Students

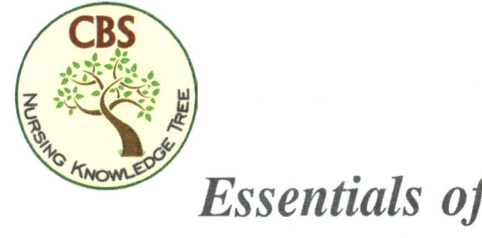

Essentials of

APPLIED
MICROBIOLOGY

for BSc Nursing Students

(As per the New Revised INC Syllabus for Nursing Students)

—— **Second Edition** ——

D R Arora MD PhD MNAMS

Ex-Professor and Head, Department of Microbiology
Postgraduate Institute of Medical Sciences, Rohtak, Haryana, and
Maharaja Agarsen Medical College, Agroha, Haryana

Ex-Professor and Head, Department of Microbiology
Medical Superintendent and Dean, Faculty of Allied Health Sciences
SGT University, Gurugram, Haryana

Ex-WHO Fellow and Visiting Professor, University of Mauritius

Lead Assessor and Member, Accreditation Committee
National Accreditation Board for Testing and Calibration Laboratories (NABL)
Gurugram, Haryana

Principal Assessor, National Accreditation Board for Hospitals and
Healthcare Providers (NABH), New Delhi

Assessor, National Accreditation Board for
Education and Training (NABET), New Delhi

Late Brij Bala Arora MD

Ex-Senior Professor and Head, Department of Pathology
Postgraduate Institute of Medical Sciences, Rohtak, Haryana

Ex-Director-Principal and Senior Professor and Head
Department of Pathology, SGT Medical College, Budhera
Gurugram, Haryana

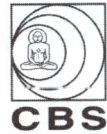

CBS
Dedicated to Education

CBS Publishers & Distributors Pvt Ltd

• New Delhi • Bengaluru • Chennai • Kochi • Kolkata • Mumbai
• Hyderabad • Nagpur • Patna • Pune • Vijayawada

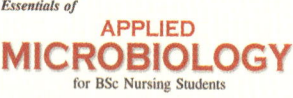

Essentials of
APPLIED
MICROBIOLOGY
for BSc Nursing Students

ISBN: 978-81-945234-4-4

Second Edition: 2020-2021

First Edition: 2017

Published by **Satish Kumar Jain** and produced by **Varun Jain** for

CBS Publishers & Distributors Pvt Ltd

4819/XI Prahlad Street, 24 Ansari Road, Daryaganj, New Delhi 110 002, India.
Ph: +91-11-23289259, 23266861, 23266867 . Website: www.cbspd.com
Fax: 011-23243014
e-mail: delhi@cbspd.com; cbspubs@airtelmail.in.

Corporate Office: 204 FIE, Industrial Area, Patparganj, Delhi 110 092
Ph: +91-11-4934 4934 Fax: 4934 4935
e-mail: feedback@cbspd.com; bhupesharora@cbspd.com

Branches

- **Bengaluru:** Seema House 2975, 17th Cross, K.R. Road, Banasankari 2nd Stage, Bengaluru 560 070, Karnataka
  Ph: +91-80-26771678/79 Fax: +91-80-26771680 e-mail: bangalore@cbspd.com
- **Chennai:** 7, Subbaraya Street, Shenoy Nagar, Chennai 600 030, Tamil Nadu
  Ph: +91-44-26680620, 26681266 Fax: +91-44-42032115 e-mail: chennai@cbspd.com
- **Kochi:** 68/1534, 35, 36-Power House Road, Opp. KSEB, Cochin-682018, Kochi, Kerala
  Ph: +91-484-4059061-65 Fax: +91-484-4059065 e-mail: kochi@cbspd.com
- **Kolkata:** 6/B, Ground Floor, Rameswar Shaw Road, Kolkata-700 014, West Bengal
  Ph: +91-33-22891126, 22891127, 22891128 e-mail: kolkata@cbspd.com
- **Mumbai:** 83-C, Dr E Moses Road, Worli, Mumbai-400018, Maharashtra
  Ph: +91-22-24902340/41 Fax: +91-22-24902342 e-mail: mumbai@cbspd.com

Representatives

- **Hyderabad** +91-9885175004
- **Pune** +91-9623451994
- **Patna** +91-9334159340
- **Vijayawada** +91-9000660880

Printed at: Goyal Offset Work Pvt Ltd.

Dedicated to the Sweet Memories of
our Loving Daughter

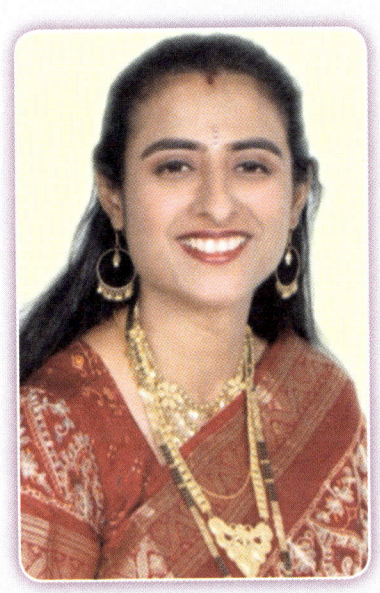

Dr Hina Arora

BDS, IDES 2001
09-04-1976 to 02-11-2009

Preface to the Second Edition

Infectious diseases account for 26% of the total diseases in the world and this percentage is much higher in the developing world. A sound knowledge of microbes that cause these diseases is vital in the understanding of their epidemiology, pathogenesis, diagnosis, management and prevention. The emergence of new microbes and the diseases caused by them, due to changing environment and ecology, and genetic engineering by terrorists, is a challenge. The world is now facing a serious pandemic of COVID-19. The persistent problem of hospital-acquired infections (HAIs) of immunocompromised patients nowadays and the difficulty of their management and non-availability of new anti-microbial molecules is a problem faced by the medical faculty. Microbiology is central to these problems. Nurses play a significant role in the prevention of HAIs. The second edition of this book is thoroughly revised fully colored edition. The book is divided into 9 sections: Introduction, General Characteristics of Microbes, Infection Control and Safety, Pathogenic Organisms-I Bacteria, Pathogenic Organisms-II Viruses, Pathogenic Organisms-III Fungi, Pathogenic Organisms-IV Parasites and Medically Important Arthropods, Immunity and Miscellaneous. All chapters have been written and arranged as per the latest Indian Nursing Council (INC) syllabus. The text has been presented in a lucid manner for the students to help them thoroughly imbibe the basics of the subject. A picture speaks more than a thousand words. Keeping this fact in mind, all the diagrams have been redrawn and a number of colored photographs have been given wherever relevant to enhance the reading experience of the students. The text has been interspersed with boxes that highlight the important information given in the text. Each chapter ends with key points that enlist the highly important points of the chapter for quick revision. Assess Yourself section given at the end of chapter contains Long and Short Answer Questions and MCQs to reinforce the subject and prepare students for examination.

I am thankful to Dr PS Gill Professor of Microbiology, Postgraduate Institute of Medical Sciences, for drawing the figures.

I am grateful to **Mr Bhupesh Arora** (Vice President – Publishing & Marketing, PGMEE & Nursing Division) for his valuable professional help and support; and Ms Nitasha Arora (Production Head & Content Strategist), CBS Publishers and Distributors Pvt Ltd, New Delhi. I honestly acknowledge the sincere and dedicated support of Mr Phool Kumar (Sr InDesing Operator). Thanks are also due to Mr Ashutosh Pathak (Senior Proof Reader) for thorough and careful proof reading.

This book will be highly useful to BSc (N) and BSc (N) Post Basic students. It is also hoped that it will serve as a useful resource for the teachers of Microbiology. The readers are requested to send suggestions for improvement of the book which will be incorporated in the subsequent editions. Shortcomings, if any, may please be communicated at draroradr@rediffmail.com.

D R Arora

Preface to the First Edition

Microbiology is a valuable and useful discipline that offers an exhaustive view of an invisible world. One has only to pick up a newspaper to be struck by daily reminders of the impact microbiology has on the world around us, whether it be emerging diseases, the roles of viruses in cancer, the development of new vaccines, drugs, etc. As we look back over these past few years, one idea that sounds even truer than ever is an observation made by the renowned microbiologist Louis Pasteur, about 120 years ago:

Life would not long remain possible in the absence of microbes

With the revision of syllabus recently by the Indian Nursing Council, we felt a need to develop a textbook for nursing students that adheres to the syllabus thoroughly and can develop their interest in the subject as well. Every relevant development in the field of microbiology has been added in the chapters to keep the students abreast of the latest advancements. The text has been presented in a simple and lucid manner. Every chapter has been well illustrated with relevant fully colored diagrams, clinical photographs and photomicrographs to enhance the understanding of the students. All the important information in the chapters has been highlighted in separate boxes. Key points given at the end of each chapter summarise the most important points discussed in the chapter. *Assess Yourself* section that includes long and short answer questions as well as multiple choice questions has been given for quick review and recapitulation.

The primary goals of this textbook are to:

1. Involve you in the relevance and excitement of microbiology.
2. Help you understand the natural roles, structure, and functions of microorganisms.
3. Keep building your knowledge and facilitating your ability to apply the subject matter.

It is sincerely hoped that this textbook will be able to fulfill its goals and justify its name by bringing the Essentials of the subject to the doorstep of every nursing student. The readers are requested to send suggestions for the improvement of the book at draroradr@rediffmail.com. The suggestions and changes will be incorporated in subsequent editions.

We hope you enjoy reading this book, as much as we enjoyed writing it!

D R Arora

Syllabus

Applied Microbiology

Unit	Time (Hrs) Th.	Time (Hrs) Pr.	Learning Objectives	Content	Teaching Learning Activities	Assessment Methods
I	3		Explain concepts and principles of microbiology and its importance in nursing	**Introduction:** • Importance and relevance to nursing • Historical perspective • Concepts and terminology • Principles of microbiology	• Lecture cum discussion	• Short answer questions • Objective type
II	10	10 (L/E)	Describe structure, classification morphology and growth of bacteria	**General characteristics of microbes:** • Structure and classification of microbes • Morphological types • Size and form of bacteria • Motility • Colonization • Growth and nutrition of microbes • Temperature • Moisture • Blood and body fluids	• Lecture cum discussion • Demonstration • Experiential Learning through visual	• Short answer questions • Objective type
			Identify microorganisms	• Laboratory methods for Identification of microorganisms • Types of staining—simple, differential (Gram's, AFB), special—capsular staining (negative), spore, LPCB, KOH mount. • Culture and media preparation—solid and liquid. Types of media—semi synthetic, synthetic, enriched, enrichment, selective and differential media. Pure culture techniques – tube dilution, pour, spread, streak plate. Anaerobic cultivation of bacteria		
III	4	6 (L/E)	Describe the different disease producing organisms	**Pathogenic organisms** • Microorganisms - Cocci—Gram-positive and Gram-negative; Bacilli—Gram-positive and Gram-negative • Viruses • Fungi—superficial and deep mycoses • Parasites • Rodents & vectors • Characteristics, source, portal of entry, transmission of infection, Identification of disease producing microorganisms	• Lecture cum discussion • Demonstration • Experiential learning through visual	• Short answer • Objective type

Contd...

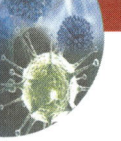

Unit	Time (Hrs) Th.	Time (Hrs) Pr.	Learning Objectives	Content	Teaching Learning Activities	Assessment Methods
IV	3	4 (L/E)	Explain the concepts of immunity, hypersensitivity and immunization	**Immunity** • Immunity—types, classification • Antigen and antibody reaction • Hypersensitivity reactions • Serological tests • Immunoglobulins—structure, types and properties • Vaccines—types and classification, storage and handling, cold chain, Immunization for various diseases • Immunization schedule	• Lecture • Discussion • Demonstration • Visit to observe vaccine storage • Clinical practice	• Short answers • Objective type • Visit report

Infection Control and Safety

Unit	Time (Hrs) Th.	Time (Hrs) Pr.	Learning Objectives	Content	Teaching Learning Activities	Assessment Methods
i	2	2(E)	Summarize the evidence-based and effective patient care practices for the prevention of common healthcare associated infections in the healthcare setting	**HAI (Hospital Acquired Infection)** • Hospital acquired infection • Bundle approach ▪ Prevention of Urinary Tract Infection (UTI) ▪ Prevention of Surgical Site Infection (SSI) ▪ Prevention of Ventilator Associated Events (VAE) ▪ Prevention of Central Line Associated Blood Stream Infection (CLABSI) • Surveillance of HAI—Infection control team and Infection control committee	• Lecture and discussion • Experiential learning	• Knowledge assessment-MCQ, Short answer type
II	3	4 (L/E)	Demonstrate appropriate use of different types of PPEs and the critical use of risk assessment	**Isolation Precautions and use of Personal Protective Equipment (PPE)** • Types of isolation system, standard precaution and transmission-based precautions (Direct Contact, Droplet, Indirect) • Epidemiology and Infection prevention – CDC guidelines • Effective use of PPE	• Lecture • Demonstration and Redemonstration	• Performance assessment
III	1	2 (L)	Demonstrate the hand hygiene practice and its effectiveness on infection control	**Hand Hygiene** • Types of Hand hygiene. • Hand washing and use of alcohol hand rub • Moments of Hand Hygiene • WHO hand hygiene promotion	• Lecture • Demonstration and Redemonstration	• Performance assessment
IV	1	2 (E)	Illustrates disinfection and sterilization in the healthcare setting	**Disinfection and sterilization** • Definitions • Types of disinfection and sterilization • Environment cleaning • Equipment cleaning • Guides on use of disinfectants • Spaulding's principle	• Lecture discussion • Experiential learning through visit	• Short answers • Objective type

Contd...

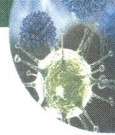

Unit	Time (Hrs) Th.	Time (Hrs) Pr.	Learning Objectives	Content	Teaching Learning Activities	Assessment Methods
V	1		Illustrate on what, when, how, why specimens are collected to optimize the diagnosis for treatment and management.	**Specimen Collection (Review)** • Principle of specimen collection • Types of specimens • Collection techniques and special considerations • Appropriate containers • Transportation of the sample • Staff precautions in handling specimens	• Discussion	• Knowledge evaluation- Quiz and Performance assessment - Checklist
VI	2	2 (E)	Explain on Biomedical waste management and laundry management	**BMW (Biomedical Waste Management)** *Laundry management process and infection control and prevention* • Waste management process and infection prevention • Staff precautions • Laundry management • Country ordinance and BMW National guidelines 2017: Segration of wastes, Colour coded waste containers, waste collection and storage, Packaging and labeling, Transportation	• Discussion Demonstration • Experiential learning through visit	• Knowledge assessment by short answers, objective type • Performance assessment
VII	2		Explain in detail about Antibiotic stewardship, AMR Describe MRSA/MDRO and its prevention	**Antibiotic stewardship** • Importance of Antibiotic Stewardship • Anti Microbial Resistance • Prevention of MRSA, MDRO in healthcare setting	Lecture and Discussion • Written assignment- Recent AMR guidelines	Short answers, Objective type • Assessment of assignment
VIII	2	4 (L/E)	Enlist the patient safety indicators followed in a healthcare organization and the role of nurse in the patient safety audit process	**Patient Safety Indicators** • Care of Vulnerable patients • Prevention of Iatrogenic injury • Care of lines, drains and tubing's • Restrain policy and care—Physical and Chemical • Blood and blood transfusion policy • Prevention of IV complication • Prevention of fall • Prevention of DVT • Shifting and transporting of patients • Surgical safety • Care coordination event related to medication reconciliation and administration • Prevention of communication errors • Prevention of HAI • Documentation	• Lecture • Demonstration • Experiential learning	• Knowledge assessment • Checklist
IX	1	1 (E)	Captures and analyzes incidents and events for quality improvement	**Incidents and adverse events** • Capturing of incidents • RCA • CAPA • Report writing	• Lecture • Role-play • Inquiry-based learning	• Knowledge assessment— short answers, objective type

Contd...

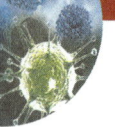

Unit	Time (Hrs)		Learning Objectives	Content	Teaching Learning Activities	Assessment Methods
	Th.	Pr.				
X	1		Enumerate IPSG and application of the goals in the patient care settings	**IPSG (International Patient Safety Goals)** • Identify patient correctly • Improve effective communication • Improve safety of high alert medication • Ensure safe surgery • Reduce the risk of healthcare associated infection • Reduce the risk of patient harm resulting from falls • Reduce the harm associated with clinical alarm system	• Lecture • Role play	• Objective type

XI	2	3 (L/E)	Enumerate the various safety protocols and its applications	**Safety protocol**
				• 5S
				• Radiation safety
				• Laser safety
				• Fire safety
				  ▪ Types and classification of fire
				  ▪ Fire alarms
				  ▪ Fire fighting equipment
				• HAZMAT safety
				  ▪ Types of spill
				  ▪ Spillage management
				  ▪ MSDS
				• Environmental safety
				  ▪ Risk assessment
				  ▪ Aspect impact analysis
				  ▪ Maintenance of Temperature and Humidity (Department-wise)
				  ▪ Audits
				• Emergency Codes
				• Role of nurse in times of disaster
					• Lecture
					• Demonstration/ Experiential learning
						• Mock drills
						• Post tests
						• Checklist

XII	1		Explain importance of employee safety indicators	**Employee Safety Indicators** • Vaccination • NSI prevention • Fall prevention • Radiation safety • Annual health check	• Lecture • Discussion	• Knowledge assessment by short answers, objective type
XIII	1		Identify risk of occupational hazards, prevention and post exposure prophylaxis.	**Healthcare Worker Immunization Program and Management of Occupational Exposure** • Occupational health ordinance • Vaccination program for healthcare staff • Needle stick injuries and prevention • Post-exposure prophylaxis	• Lecture method • Journal review	• Short answer

Special Features of the Book

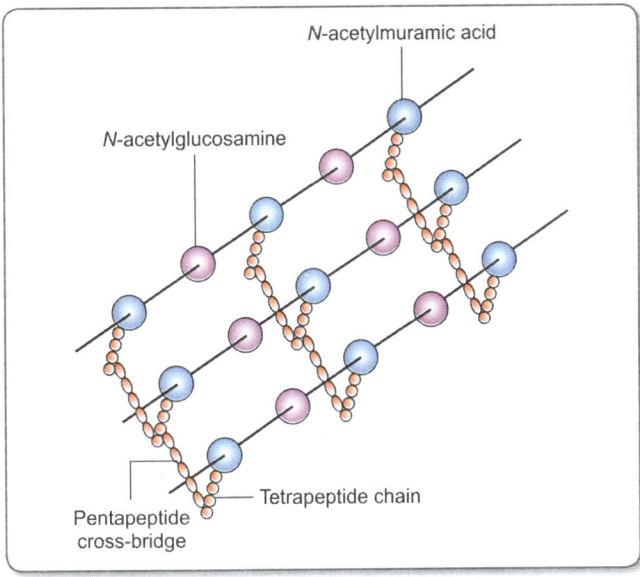

Fig. 2.4: Chemical structure of peptidoglycan.

N-acetylmuramic acid

N-acetylglucosamine

Tetrapeptide chain

Pentapeptide cross-bridge

Numerous Tables are used to supplement the text, for ease to understand the concept

TABLE 8.2: Suggested infection control committee members

Hospital Director/Dean/Principal	Chairman
Microbiologist/Epidemiologist	Infection Control Officer
Chief of medical services	Member
Quality control/assurance officer	Member
Heads of various clinical departments	Members
Head of pharmacy	Member
Head of support services	Member
Chief nurse	Member
Infection control nurses	Members

Supplemented with 200 + fully colored images and illustrations for easy and quick grasp of the relevant topic.

Additional information Boxes have been incorporated throughout the text

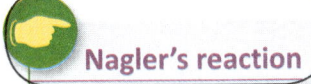

Nagler's reaction

A culture plate containing 6% agar, 5% peptic digest of sheep blood and 20% human serum or 5% egg yolk is prepared. The plate is dried. On one half of the plate, 2–3 drops of *C. perfringens* antitoxin are spread and allowed to dry. The plate is then inoculated with the test organisms or the exudate under study and incubated anaerobically at 37°C for 18 hours. On the section containing no antitoxin, *C. perfringens* colonies show surrounding zone of opalescence, i.e. Nagler's reaction whereas colonies of the remainder half of the plate show no change (Fig. 15.2).

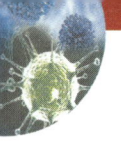

> **Important key terms used in the chapter are presented to familiarize the readers with the important terminologies.**

🔑 Key Points

- *Hospital-acquired infection may be defined as an infection occurring in a patient in a hospital or other healthcare facility in whom the infection was not present or incubating at the time of admission. This includes infections acquired in the hospital but appearing after discharge, and also occupational infections among staff of the facility.*
- **Factors influencing nosocomial infection** include hospital environment, injudicious use of antibiotics, hospitalized patients with pre-existing diseases such as diabetes, immunosuppression and patients with prosthetic implants, diagnostic or therapeutic intervention and blood and blood products used for transfusion.
- **Routes of transmission of infection** in hospital include contact spread, airborne spread, oral route, parenteral route and self infection.
- *Every hospital should have* **antibiotic policy, disinfection policy** *and* **infection control committee.** *The functions of the latter include surveillance and control of infection and monitoring of hygiene practices.*

> **Assess Yourself section at the last of every chapter will help for self-evaluation and analysis**

❓ ASSESS YOURSELF

LONG AND SHORT ANSWER QUESTIONS

1. Discuss the pathogenesis of anthrax.
2. Discuss laboratory diagnosis of anthrax.
3. Write short notes on:
   - (a) Malignant pustule
   - (b) Prophylaxis of anthrax

MULTIPLE CHOICE QUESTIONS

1. Koch's postulates were satisfied for the first time with:
   - (a) *Bacillus anthracis*
   - (b) *Clostridium tetani*
   - (c) *Corynebacterium diphtheriae*
   - (d) *Salmonella* Typhi
2. 'Medusa head' appearance of the colonies is characteristic of:
   - (a) *Proteus mirabilis*
   - (b) *Clostridium tetani*
   - (c) *Bacillus anthracis*
   - (d) *Pseudomonas aeruginosa*
3. Malignant pustule is characteristic of:
   - (a) cutaneous anthrax
   - (b) pulmonary anthrax
   - (c) intestinal anthrax
   - (d) All of the above
4. An organism that can cause cutaneous infection and can be transmitted by spores is:
   - (a) *Staphylococcus aureus*
   - (b) *Streptococcus pyogenes*
   - (c) *Yersinia pestis*
   - (d) *Bacillus anthracis*

ANSWERS TO MCQs

1. a   **2.** c   **3.** a   **4.** d

Contents

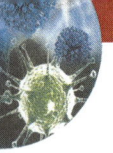

Section 5 · Pathogenic Organisms-II Viruses · 185–223

Section 6 · Pathogenic Organisms-III Fungi · 225–237

Section 7 · Pathogenic Organisms-IV Parasites and Medically Important Arthropods · 239–275

Section 8 · Immunity · 277–314

Section 9 · Miscellaneous · 315–319

Section

I

Introduction

Chapter 1

Introduction to Microbiology: History of Development

INTRODUCTION

Microbiology is the study of living organisms of microscopic size. This term was introduced by French chemist Louis Pasteur (1822–1895), who demonstrated that fermentation was caused by the growth of bacteria and yeasts. Medical microbiology deals with the causative agents of infectious diseases of man, the response generated by him against them and various methods of diagnosis, treatment and prevention. The term **microbe** was first used by Sedillot in 1878, but it has now been replaced by **microorganism**.

HISTORICAL PERSPECTIVE

Ancient man had thought the infectious diseases to be because of divine wrath and supernatural powers. Later, concepts like bodily constitution, faulty diet and the influence of environment were proposed. From very early times, there have been many suggestions that these diseases result from invasion of body by external agents. In summarizing the history of bacteriology, it is customary, at least, in relation to medicine, to refer to the concept advanced by Fracastorius of Verona in 1546 of a *Contagium vivum* as the cause of infective disease, and to the view suggested by von Plenciz (1762) on the specificity of disease, based on a belief in its microbial origin.

Antonie van Leeuwenhoek (1632–1723)

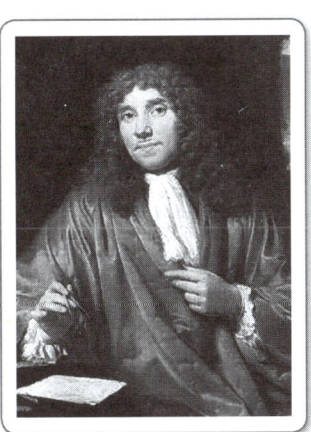

The construction and use of the compound microscope was an essential prerequisite to study the microbial forms. To Antonie van Leeuwenhoek must be ascribed the credit of placing the science of microbiology on the firm basis of direct observation. This Dutch maker of lenses from Holland devised an apparatus and technique which enabled him to observe and describe various microbial forms with accuracy and care. He observed, drew and measured a large number of minute living organisms including bacteria and protozoa and communicated them to Royal Society of London in 1683.

Antonie van Leeuwenhoek first accurately described the different shapes of bacteria (coccal, bacillary and spiral) and pictured their arrangement in infected material (1683).

Louis Pastuer (1822–1895)

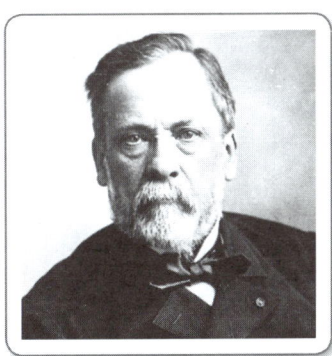

In 1856, Louis Pasteur was commissioned by an industrialist of Lille to investigate the problem which had arisen in manufacture of alcohol. The beet juice, from which alcohol was derived, was contaminated with a grey material which interfered with alcohol production. During the course of investigation his attention was abruptly focused on the role of microorganisms in alcohol fermentation and spoilage. Undesirable forms of life could be destroyed at temperatures of 50–60°C in a short period of time. Subsequently, this modified process of heating came to be known as pasteurization. Pasteur established that different types of fermentations were due to the activity of different kinds of microbes. In the course of studies, Pasteur introduced the techniques of sterilization and developed steam sterilizer, hot air oven and autoclave.

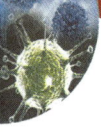

Joseph Lister (1827–1912)

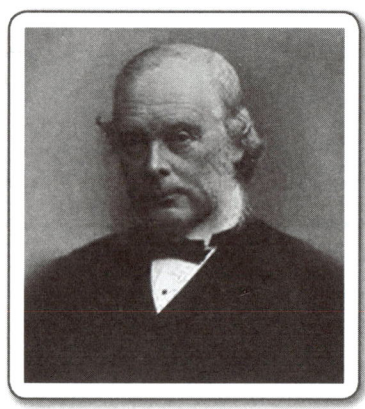

Joseph Lister (1827–1912), an English surgeon and contemporary of Pasteur, was among the first to appreciate the ramifications of the emerging germ theory of disease. He attributed the frequent disastrous consequences following repair of compound fractures to invasions by airborne microorganisms. Lister advocated the use of carbolic acid as an aerosol during surgery and for impregnation of dressings to reduce the risk of postsurgical infections. He established the guiding principle of antisepsis for good surgical practice upon which the present day specialists depend. For this work he is known as 'father of antiseptic surgery'.

Robert Koch (1843–1910)

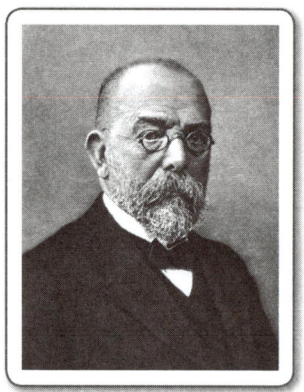

Robert Koch (1843–1910), a German physician, perfected the bacteriological techniques, staining procedures and methods of obtaining bacteria in pure culture using solid media during his studies on the culture and characters of anthrax bacillus.

The causative agents of various diseases were reported rapidly by different investigators. Robert Koch discovered the bacillus of anthrax (1876), bacillus of tuberculosis (1882) and cholera vibrio (1883); Hansen described the leprosy bacillus in 1874; Neisser discovered the gonococcus in the pus discharge from urethra in 1879; Alexander Ogston in 1880 described the staphylococci in abscesses and suppurative lesions; Eberth observed the typhoid bacillus in 1880; Klebs (1883) and Loeffler (1884) observed and described the diphtheria bacillus; Rosenbach (1886) demonstrated the tetanus bacillus with round terminal spore; Weichselbaum (1887) described and isolated the meningococcus from the spinal fluid of a patient; Bruce (1887) identified the causative agent of malta fever in 1905 and Schaudinn and Hoffmann described the spirochaete of syphilis.

As the agents were being reported in such profusion it became necessary to introduce criteria for proving the claims that a microorganism isolated from a disease was indeed causally related to it. Henle indicated such criteria but were enunciated by Koch which consisted of guidelines for the association of particular microorganisms with specific infectious diseases. A microorganism can be accepted as the causative agent of an infectious disease only if following postulates, known as Koch's postulates, are satisfied:

- The organism must be present in the lesions in every case of the infectious disease.
- It should be possible to isolate the organism in pure culture from the lesions.
- Inoculation of the pure culture into suitable laboratory animals should produce a similar disease.
- It should again be possible to reisolate the organism in pure culture from the lesions produced in the experimental animals (Fig. 1.1).

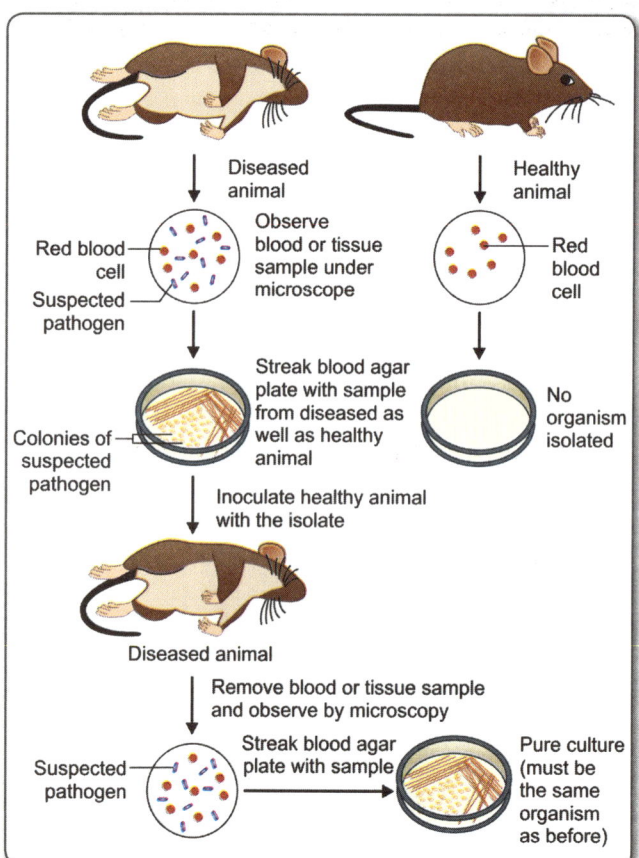

Fig. 1.1: Koch's postulates.

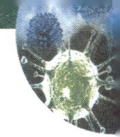

A fifth criterion introduced subsequently states that specific antibodies to the organism should be demonstrable in the serum of the patient suffering from the disease. These postulates have proved extremely useful in confirming the authenticity of doubtful claims made regarding the causative agents of infectious diseases.

Exceptions to Koch's Postulates

Koch's postulates have remained a mainstay of microbiology; however, many microorganisms that do not meet the criteria of Koch's postulates have been shown to cause disease. For example:

- *Treponema pallidum* and *Mycobacterium leprae*, causative agents of syphilis and leprosy respectively, cannot be grown *in vitro*; however, there are animal models of infection with these agents.
- In another example, *Neisseria gonorrhoeae*, which causes gonorrhoea, there is no animal model even though the bacteria can readily be cultured *in vitro*.

The Beginning of Virology

For many years the term virus was used to describe any poison or microbial agent capable of causing an infection. In a large number of diseases such as smallpox, chickenpox, measles, influenza, poliomyelitis and the common cold, no bacterial cause could be established. Pasteur had suspected that rabies in dogs could be caused by a microbe too small to be seen under the microscope.

The first man to describe a filtered extract capable of causing disease in plants was Dmitri Iwanowski (1864–1920), a Russian scientist, who started his studies on diseases of tobacco while he was still a student. He reproduced mosaic disease in tobacco plant by applying juice from diseased plants to healthy leaves from which all bacteria had been removed by passage through fine filters (1892). In 1898, Martinus Beijerinck, unaware of Iwanowski's work, attributed the cause of tobacco-mosaic disease to *Contagium vivum fluidum*, a living liquid virus.

In 1898, Loeffler and Paul Frosch from Germany reported that the causative agent of foot-and-mouth disease in cattle would pass through a bacterial filter. Walter Reed (1902) in Cuba proved that the causative agent of yellow fever was not only a filterable virus but also transmitted through the bite of infected mosquitoes. The term 'filterable' was dropped in time and the tiny infectious agents were merely called viruses. Larger viruses could be seen under light microscope after appropriate staining but their detailed morphology could only be studied by electron microscope introduced by Ruska (1934). The technique of growing them on chick embryos developed by Goodpasture in 1930s and the application of tissue culture in virology expanded the scope of virological techniques considerably.

Ellerman and Bang (1908) suggested the possibility that virus infection could lead to malignancy. Peyton Rous (1911) isolated a virus causing sarcoma in fowls. Several viruses have been blamed to cause natural and experimental tumours in birds and animals. Experimentally, viruses can cause malignant transformation of infected cells in tissue cultures. The discovery of viral and cellular oncogenes have put forth the possible mechanisms of viral oncogenesis.

IMPORTANCE OF MICROBIOLOGY TO NURSING

Laboratory diagnosis of microbial infections can be divided into pre-examination processes, examination processes and post-examination processes. Nurses play an important role in the pre-examination processes. This includes collection of primary samples, labelling of primary samples, safe disposal of materials used in collection and transportation of the samples to the laboratory such that they are transported:

- Within a time frame appropriate to the nature of requested examinations;
- Maintaining cold chain; and
- In a manner that ensures safety of the carrier.

Quality of examinations is improved if proper precautions are taken during pre-examination processes.

Hospital-associated infections (HAI) or nosocomial infections are increasingly becoming a major concern all over the world. The source of infecting organisms may be exogenous from another patient or a member of the staff including nursing staff or from inanimate objects in the hospital like medical equipment (endoscopes, cystoscopes, catheters, needles, etc.), bed pans, food, water, hospital air and surfaces contaminated by the patients' secretions, excretions, blood and body fluids. It may be endogenous from patient's own flora which at the time of infection may invade the patient's tissues spontaneously or be introduced into them by surgical operation, instrumental manipulation or nursing procedures. Nurses can help in prevention of HAI by:

- The provision of sterile instruments, dressings, surgical gloves, face masks, theatre clothing and fluids; and
- Thorough hand washing after any procedure involving nursing care or close contact with the patient.
- Infection control nurses are important members of infection control committee which meets regularly, at least once in a month and as often as required to discuss measures to control infection in a hospital. Nurses play an important role in biomedical waste management.

CONTRIBUTIONS OF VARIOUS SCIENTISTS IN THE FIELD OF MICROBIOLOGY

A large number of scientists has contributed in the field of microbiology. Principal contributions of some of them are given below.

Louis Pasteur

Louis Pasteur (1822–1895) was born in the village of Dole, France on December 27, 1822, the son of humble parents. His father was

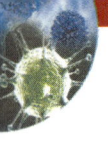

a tanner. He was originally trained as a chemist, but his studies on fermentation led him to take interest in microorganisms. His discoveries revolutionized medical practice, although he never studied medicine.

1. The term **microbiology**, as the study of living organisms of microscopic size, was coined by Pasteur.
2. He also coined the term **vaccine**.
3. He used various forms of nutrient fluid to grow micro-organisms.
4. He showed that some organisms were not destroyed by boiling. For the sterilization of fluids he advocated heating to 120°C under pressure and for glassware the use of dry heat at 170°C. He showed that cotton plugs (a primitive air-filtration device) could prevent microbes from reaching otherwise air-exposed sterile broths.
5. In 1860–61, he disapproved the **theory of spontaneous generation**. In a series of classic experiments, Pasteur proved conclusively that all forms of life, even microbes, arose only from their alike and not *de novo*.
6. In 1860–64, he gave experimental evidence that fermentation and putrefaction are effects of microbial growth.
7. In 1863–65, he devised the process of destroying bacteria, known as **pasteurization**.
8. In 1877, Koch and Pasteur demonstrated that anthrax is caused by bacteria. Pasteur grew the organisms in sterilized yeast water and kept them in the laboratory for several months, transferring them frequently to new culture fluid, in which they multiplied readily, and showed that these cultures would always cause anthrax when inoculated into healthy animals.
9. In 1880, he prevented chicken cholera by injection of live attenuated culture. He found that pure cultures of the germ of this disease which had been kept in the laboratory for some time would not kill his animals as fresh cultures did, but would merely cause a passing illness from which the chickens recovered. Then he discovered that the animals that had recovered from a previous inoculation of weakened germs were immune, and did not succumb to the disease. Pasteur immediately perceived that it might be possible to make individuals resistant by inoculating them with the weakened (and therefore harmless) germs of a particular disease.
10. In 1880, he first cultured staphylococci in liquid medium and produced abscesses by inoculating them into rabbits.
11. In 1881, he developed **live attenuated anthrax vaccine**.
12. In 1881, pneumococci were first noticed by Pasteur and Sternberg independently.
13. The crowning achievement of Pasteur was the successful application of the principle of vaccination to the prevention of rabies, or hydrophobia, in human beings and developed **Pasteur rabies vaccine** in 1885. He obtained fixed rabies virus by serial intracerebral passage in rabbits. The rabies vaccine was prepared by drying pieces of spinal cord from rabbits infected with fixed virus. Rabies vaccine prevented the development of this fatal disease if the inoculations are given soon after the bite of the rabid animal. He gave the first treatment for rabies in 1885 to a young boy bitten by a rabid dog.
14. In 1887, Pasteur and Joubert first described *Clostridium septicum* and called it *Vibrion septique*.

In 1888, in recognition of his incomparable achievements, the Pasteur Institute of Paris was built by public contribution during his lifetime for investigations of infectious diseases and preparation of vaccines. Acclaimed the world over for his epoch making discoveries, Pasteur died in Paris on September 28, 1895. His body lies in Pasteur Institute of Paris. Today the Pasteur Institute is a thriving research centre—an appropriate memorial to its founder.

Robert Koch

Contributions of Robert Koch, to microbiology, are variegated and enormous.

1. In 1876, Robert Koch reported the isolation of anthrax bacillus in pure culture, formation and germination of its spores and the proof of its infectiousness. This agent as the sole cause of anthrax was confirmed by Pasteur.
2. In 1877, he introduced the method of making smears of bacteria on glass slides, and of staining them with the aniline dyes.
3. In 1881, he described means of cultivating bacteria on solid media, thus making it possible to obtain pure cultures by transferring material from a single colony.
4. The **hanging-drop method** of studying bacteria as used today is a product of his genius.
5. In 1882, Koch startled the world by announcing his discovery of **tubercle bacillus** (*Mycobacterium tuberculosis*), the causative agent of tuberculosis. He described a special staining method for detection of this organism and grew it in pure cultures in the laboratory.
6. In 1883, he discovered the causative agents of cholera (*Vibrio cholerae*), Egyptian ophthalmia (pink eye) and Koch Weeks bacillus.
7. In 1884, Koch expounded the postulates or laws by which an organism may be proved to be the cause of a particular disease. These are known as **Koch's postulates**.
8. Koch continued his work on tuberculosis and in 1890–91 he showed how a normal guinea pig and an already infected guinea pig behaved differently to an infection with tubercle bacillus. This is known as **Koch's phenomenon** (*see* Chapter 17).

In 1905, he was awarded the **Nobel Prize in Medicine**' for his work on tuberculosis. Together with Louis Pasteur, he laid the foundations of modern bacteriology.

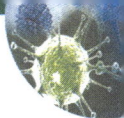

Antonie van Leeuwenhoek

Antonie van Leeuwenhoek was expert in the grinding of simple magnifying lenses. He made these lenses of same bits of glass, polished them very carefully, and mounted each separately between two brass, copper, silver, or gold plates, to which he fastened an adjustable holder for the object to be examined. He constructed many of these 'microscopes' each containing a single lens ground by himself. The best of lenses magnified about 200 times. He observed, drew and measured a large number of living organisms including bacteria and protozoa in materials such as rain water, pond and well water, and saliva and the intestinal contents of healthy subjects and communicated them to the Royal Society of London in 1683. He was the first to accurately describe different shapes of bacteria (coccal, bacillary and spiral) and picture their arrangement in infected material.

Leeuwenhoek observed that very large numbers of bacteria appeared in watery infusions of animals or vegetable matter which were left to stand for a week or two at room temperature. He believed that these huge populations were the progeny of a few parental organisms, or seeds, that were originally present in the materials of the infusion or had entered it from the air. The significance of these observations was not realized then and to Leeuwenhoek the world of '*little animalcules*' represented only a curiosity of nature. Their importance in medicine and other areas of biology came to be recognized two centuries later.

Edward Jenner (1749–1823)

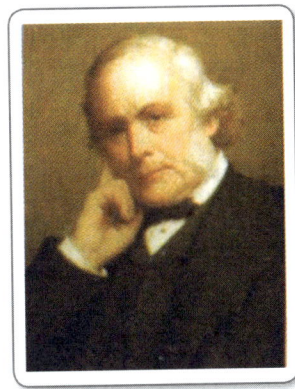

Edward Jenner *introduced the modern method of vaccination to prevent smallpox*. He observed that milkmaids who contracted cowpox or vaccinia while milking were subsequently immune to smallpox. On May 14, 1796, he devised a brave experiment. He performed a vaccination against smallpox by transferring material from a cowpox pustule on the hand of a milkmaid, Sarah Nelmes, to the arm of a small boy named James Phipps, his gardener's son. 6 weeks later the boy was inoculated with smallpox. He failed to develop the disease. *The terms vaccine and vaccination were first used by Pasteur out of deference to Jenner.*

In 1967, the World Health Organization masterminded a final global plan to eradicate smallpox. Success was announced in 1980 with the declaration: Smallpox is dead. Thanks to Jenner. Edward Jenner's discovery has now been developed into one of the most important parts of modern medicine—**immunology**.

Paul Ehrlich (1854–1915)

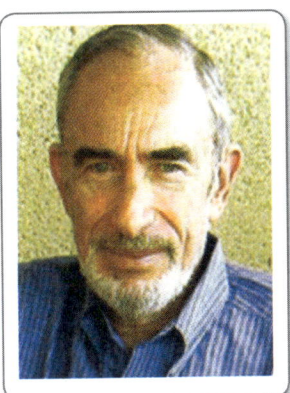

1. In 1882, he reported the *acid-fastness* of tubercle bacillus.
2. From 1890 to 1900, he did important research in immunology. He soon found that the specific effect of immune serum could be demonstrated *in vivo* and *in vitro* and introduced methods of standardizing toxin and antitoxin. To him goes the credit of *minimum lethal dose*.
3. In 1898, he proposed *side chain theory of antibody production*.
4. In 1909, he introduced salvarsan, an arsenical compound, sometimes called the '*magic bullet*'. It was capable of destroying the spirochaete of syphilis with only moderate toxic effects. He continued his experimentation until 1912 when he announced the discovery of neosalvarsan. Thus he created a new branch of medicine known as *chemotherapy*.

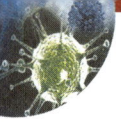

Essentials of Applied Microbiology for BSc Nursing

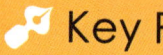

Key Points

- Microbiology is the biology of *microscopic organisms*, its subjects being microorganisms.
- Microorganism is an organism that *cannot be seen without the use of a microscope.*
- *Medical microbiology* deals with those *organisms which are responsible for infectious diseases of humans.*
- A microorganism is generally accepted as the causative agent of an infectious disease if it satisfies *Koch's postulates.*
- *Treponema pallidum*, *Mycobacterium leprae* and *Neisseria gonorrhoeae* do not fulfil all the criteria of Koch's postulates; the first two *cannot be grown in vitro* and for the third there is *no animal model.*

? ASSESS YOURSELF

SHORT ANSWER QUESTION

1. Write short notes on:
   - (a) Koch's postulates
   - (b) Contributions of Robert Koch in microbiology
   - (c) Contributions of Antonie van Leeuwenhoek in microbiology
   - (d) Contributions of Louis Paster in microbiology

MULTIPLE CHOICE QUESTIONS

1. Which of the following organisms **does not** meet all the criteria of Koch's Postulates?
   - (a) *Streptococcus pneumoniae*
   - (b) *Treponema pallidum*
   - (c) *Leptospira interrogans*
   - (d) *Mycobacterium scrofulaceum*

2. The techniques of sterilization were introduced by:
   - (a) Louis Pasteur
   - (b) Robert Koch
   - (c) Ferdinand Cohn
   - (d) John Needham

3. Bacillus of tuberculosis was discovered by:
   - (a) Hansen
   - (b) Loeffler
   - (c) Robert Koch
   - (d) Bruce

4. The term microbiology, as the study of living organisms of microscopic size, was coined by:
   - (a) Antonie van Leeuwenhoek
   - (b) Robert Koch
   - (c) Louis Pasteur
   - (d) Edward Jenner

5. Which of the following is **not** a condition of Koch's postulates?
   - (a) Isolate the causative agent of a disease
   - (b) Cultivate the microbe in the laboratory
   - (c) Inoculate a test animal to observe the disease
   - (d) Produce a vaccine

ANSWERS TO MCQs

1. b   **2.** a   **3.** c   **4.** c   **5.** d

General Characteristics of Microbes

Chapter 2

Morphology and Classification of Bacteria

BACTERIA

Bacteria are free-living, microscopic, unicellular organisms capable of performing all the essential functions of life, e.g. growth, metabolism and reproduction. They possess both deoxyribonucleic acid (DNA) and ribonucleic acid (RNA) and lack chlorophyll. Bacteria have been placed in a kingdom separate from the animal and plant kingdoms, **Monera**.

Cells that have a well-defined nucleus are called **eukaryotes**, whereas cells that lack a well-defined nucleus are called **prokaryotes**. Bacteria are prokaryotes, while fungi, algae, protozoa, plant and animal cells are eukaryotes. In general, the interior organization of eukaryotic cells is more complex than that of prokaryotic cells. The comparison of prokaryotes and eukaryotes is given in Table 2.1.

Bacteria do not contain a membrane-bound nucleus. Their DNA consists of a single circular chromosome, which is attached to a mesosome, a saclike structure in the cell membrane. Bacterial ribosomes are found free in the cytoplasm and attached to the cytoplasmic membrane. They are 70S in size and dissociate into two subunits, 50S and 30S in size. The cell envelope, in bacteria, consists of cytoplasmic (cell) membrane and cell wall. Some species also produce capsules and slime layers.

Size of Bacteria

Bacteria are very small in size. The unit of measurement of bacteria is called micrometre (μm). One μm is a thousandth part of a millimetre (mm). One nanometre (nm) is a thousandth part of a μm and one Angstrom unit (Å) is one tenth of a nanometre.

TABLE 2.1: **Comparison of prokaryotes and eukaryotes**

Characterisitics	Prokaryote	Eukaryote
Genetic material		
Location	Free in the cytoplasm attached to a structure called a mesosome located in the cell membrane	Contained within a membrane-bound nucleus inside the cell
Form	A single circular piece of DNA	Multiple chromosomes, which are surrounded by basic proteins called histones
Nucleolus	Absent	Present
Replication	By binary fission	By mitosis and meiosis
Extrachromosomal DNA	Plasmids, small circular pieces of DNA containing accessory information, present in the cytoplasm	In mitochondria
Protein production site	No endoplasmic reticulum; ribosomes –free in the cytoplasm or attached to the cell membrane	Rough endoplasmic reticulum, a membrane covered with ribosomes, where protein is made
		Smooth endoplasmic reticulum or Golgi complex, where secreted proteins are packaged and transported to the cell surface
Ribosomes	70S in size, consisting of a 50S and 30S subunit	80S in size, consisting of a 60S and 40S subunit
Energy production site	Electron transport chain located in the cell membrane; no mitochondria present	Within membrane-bound mitochondria
Intracellular organelles (lysosomes)	Absent	Present, contain hydrolytic enzymes
Plasma membrane	Lipoprotein membrane; regulates transport	Lipoprotein membrane; regulates transport
Cell wall	Present; imparts rigidity	Usually absent except in fungi, which contain chitin in the cell wall

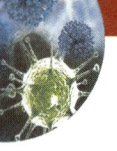

The diameter of the smallest body that can be resolved and seen clearly with naked eye is about 200 µm. Medically important bacteria generally measure 0.2–1.5 µm in diameter and 3–5 µm in length. Therefore, to visualize most bacteria one must use the higher powers of magnification of a good light microscope and enlarge them about 1000 times. To visualize their surfaces distinctly, it is usually necessary to stain them. Electron microscopy is essential for clear visualization of internal structures of the bacteria.

Shape of Bacteria

Bacteria exist in different shapes as under (Fig. 2.1):

- **Cocci** (from *kokkos* meaning berry) are round or oval cells.
- **Bacilli** (from *baculus* meaning rod) are rod or stick-shaped. In some of the bacilli the length of the cells may be equal to width. Such bacillary forms are known as **coccobacilli**. The latter have to be carefully differentiated from cocci.
- **Vibrios** are curved or comma-shaped rods.
- **Spirilla** are non-flexuous spiral forms with one to three fixed curves in their rigid bodies.
- **Spirochaetes** (from *spira* meaning coil and *chaite* meaning hair) are slender and flexuous spiral forms.

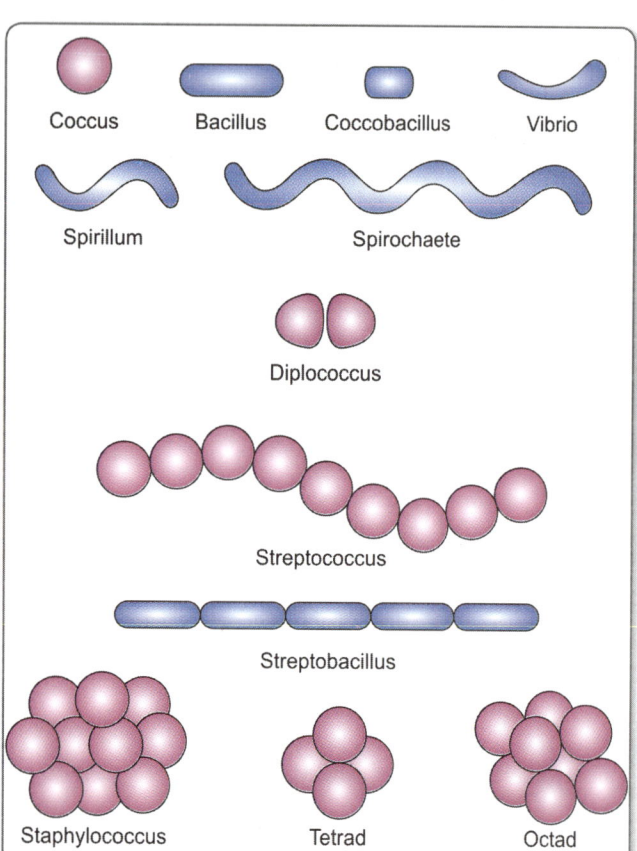

Fig. 2.1: Shapes and group patterns of bacteria.

- **Mycoplasmas** are cell wall deficient organisms. Therefore, they do not possess stable morphology. They occur as round or oval bodies or as interlacing filaments.

Group Patterns

The most frequent method of reproduction among bacteria is asexual binary fission, that is each cell splits in half, forming two new cells. As they increase in number they form distinct groups. Cocci that split along one plane only tend to arrange themselves in pairs (**diplococci**) or in chains (**streptococci**). When the division occurs alternatively in each of two planes, groups of four (**tetrads**) or eight (**octads**) are formed. Haphazard splitting in several planes results in the formation of clusters of cocci (Fig. 2.1).

Bacilli split only across their short axes, therefore, the patterns formed by them are limited. They may appear as end-to-end pairs (**diplobacilli**), or chains (**streptobacilli**) (Fig. 2.1). In some instances, there occurs incomplete separation of the daughter cells after binary fission. The bacilli remain attached to each other at various angles, resembling the letters V or L. This is called **Chinese letter arrangement** and is characteristic of *Corynebacterium diphtheriae*.

MICROSCOPY

A microscope is used to visualize the forms of life that are beyond the perception of naked eye. Microscopy is done to:

- magnify an object;
- increase the resolution; and
- optimise the contrast between structures, organisms and background.

Parts of a Microscope (Fig. 2.2)

- **Eyepiece lens:** The lens at the top through which visualization is done. These are usually of 10× or 15× power.
- **Tube**: Connects the eyepiece to the objective lenses.
- **Arm**: Supports the tube and connects it to the base.
- **Base**: The bottom of the microscope, used for support.
- **Illuminator:** A light source used in place of a mirror. If the microscope has a mirror, it is used to reflect light from an external light source up through the bottom of the stage.
- **Stage:** The flat platform to place the slides. Stage clips hold the slides in place.
- **Revolving nosepiece or turret**: This is the part that holds two or more objective lenses and can be rotated to easily change power.
- **Objective lenses**: Three or four objective lenses (4×, 10×, 40× and 100×) in a microscope. When examined with a 10× (most common) eyepiece lens, we get total magnifications of 40×, 100×, 400× and 1000×, respectively.
- **Rack stop**: This is an adjustment that determines how close the objective lens can get to the slide.

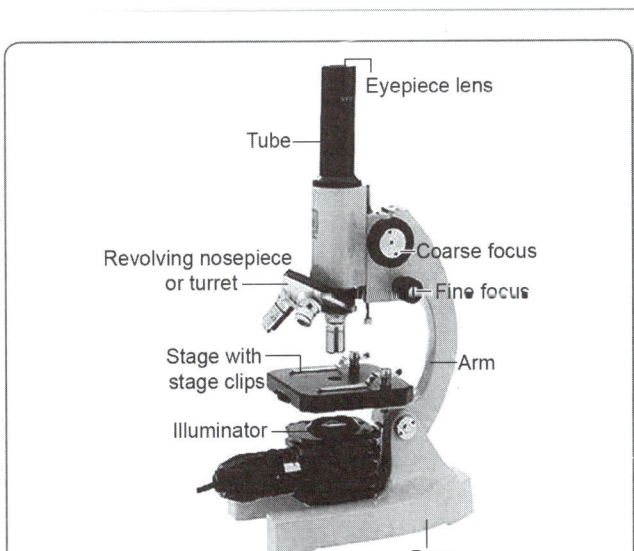

Fig. 2.2: Parts of a Microscope.

- **Condenser lens:** The purpose of the condenser is to focus the light onto the specimen. Condenser is most useful at the higher powers (400× and above).
- **Diaphragm or iris:** Many microscopes have a rotating disk under the stage. This diaphragm has different sized holes and is used to vary the intensity and size of the cone of light that is projected upward to the slide.

ANATOMY OF A BACTERIAL CELL

The principal structure of a bacterial cell is shown in Figure 2.3. The interior of the cell, the protoplast, is differentiated into cytoplasm and nuclear material. Cytoplasm is bounded by a thin, elastic and semipermeable cytoplasmic membrane. Outside this lies cell wall, which gives the bacterium its shape and rigidity. Cell wall, in many bacteria, is enclosed by a protective gelatinous covering layer called capsule. Many bacteria also possess flagella which are the organelles of motility and some species have fimbriae (pili) too.

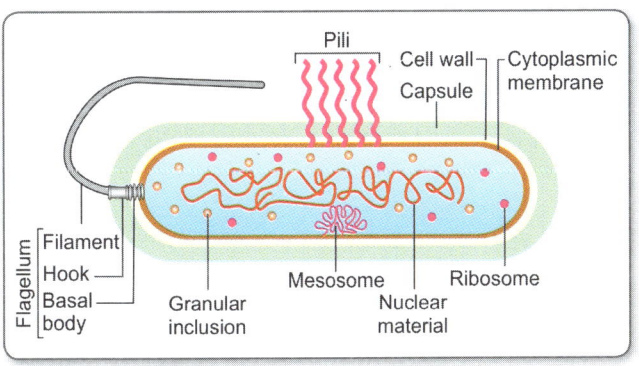

Fig. 2.3: Anatomy of a bacterial cell.

Bacterial Cell Wall

- It is a complex rigid structure which gives bacteria their definite shape.
- It is permeable to passage of liquid nutrient material into the cell and to outward passage of substances produced within the cell.
- It is about 10–20 nm in thickness and constitutes 20–30% of dry weight of the cell. The cell walls of Gram-positive bacteria are generally thicker than those of Gram-negative bacteria.
- The strength of the bacterial cell wall is due to the presence in it of a substance referred to as peptidoglycan, muco-peptide or murein.

Peptidoglycan consists of three parts—a backbone, composed of alternating N-acetylglucosamine and N-acetylmuramic acid; a set of identical tetrapeptide side chains attached to N-acetylmuramic acid and a set of identical pentapeptide cross-bridges (Fig. 2.4). In all bacterial species the backbone is the same, however, tetra-peptide side chains and pentapeptide cross-bridges vary from species to species.

Differences between cell walls of Gram-positive and Gram-negative bacteria are given in Table 2.2.

Cytoplasmic Membrane

Bacterial cytoplasmic membrane, also called cell membrane, limits the bacterial protoplast externally. It is thin (5–10 nm), elastic and consists of a phospholipid bilayer in which various constituent proteins are embedded. With the exception of *Mycoplasma*, bacterial cytoplasmic membrane lacks sterols. **It acts as a semipermeable membrane controlling the inflow and outflow of metabolites to and from the protoplasm.** It permits

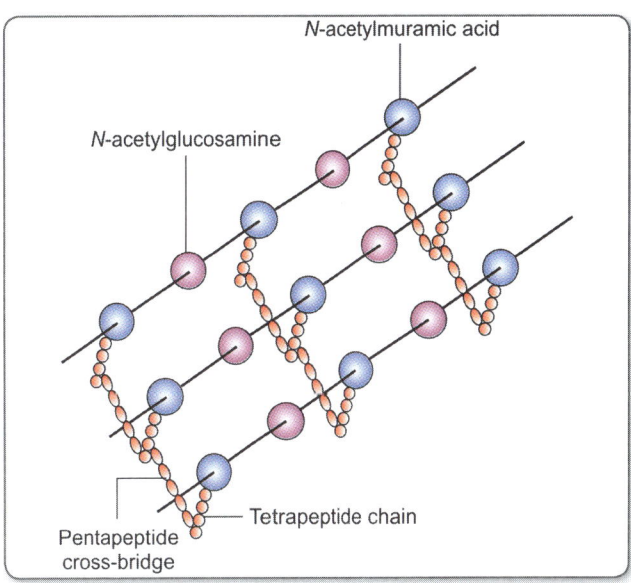

Fig. 2.4: Chemical structure of peptidoglycan.

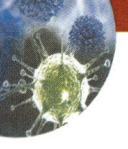

SECTION II • GENERAL CHARACTERISTICS OF MICROBES

TABLE 2.2: Differences between cell walls of Gram-positive and Gram-negative bacteria

Character	Gram-positive cell wall	Gram-negative cell wall
Thickness	Thicker	Thinner
Peptidoglycan	Thick layer (16-80 nm)	Thin layer (2 nm)
Lipid content	2–5%	15–20%
Techoic acid	Absent	Present
Porin proteins	Absent	Present
Variety of amino acids	Few	Several
Periplasmic space	Absent	Present
Endotoxic activity	Absent	Present

the passive diffusion inward and outward of water and other small molecular substances, but it actively effects the selective transport of specific nutrients into the cell and that of waste products out of it. This is mediated through specific enzymes (permeases) present in the cytoplasmic membrane.

Cytoplasm

Cytoplasm of the bacterial cell is a viscous watery solution of soft gel, containing a variety of organic and inorganic solutes. It contains all biosynthetic components required by the bacterium for the growth and cell division, together with genetic material. The cytoplasm of bacteria differs from that of higher eukaryotic organisms in not containing endoplasmic reticulum, Golgi apparatus, mitochondria, lysosomes and in not showing signs of internal mobility, e.g. cytoplasmic streaming, the formation, migration and disappearance of vacuoles and amoeboid movement. Cytoplasm contains ribosomes, mesosomes and intracytoplasmic inclusion bodies (Fig. 2.3).

Bacterial Nucleus

The genetic information of a bacterial cell is contained in a single, circular, double-stranded molecule of DNA. It is often accompanied by a smaller extrachromosomal DNA known as **plasmid**. It is 1000 μm or more in length, about 1000 times the length of the cell. Therefore, it occurs tightly coiled like a skein of woollen thread. Since it is not bound to proteins, therefore, it does not stain like a eukaryotic chromosome. **Bacterial nucleus does not possess nuclear membrane, nucleolus, deoxyribonucleoprotein and does not divide by mitosis.**

Capsule or Slime Layer

Cell wall in many bacteria is enclosed by a protective gelatinous covering layer. If it is easily washed off and does not appear to be

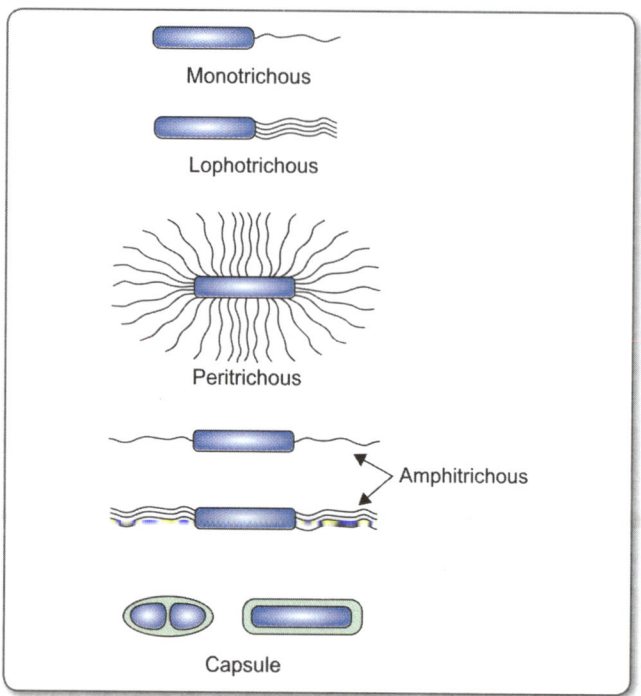

Fig. 2.5: Arrangement of flagella and capsule.

associated with the cell in any definite fashion it is referred to as a **slime layer**, on the other hand if it appears as discrete, thickened gel around each cell, it is called a **capsule** (Fig. 2.5). If capsule is too thin to be seen with light microscope, it is called **microcapsule**. In most species it is made up of a complex polysaccharide (e.g. pneumococcus), though in some species its main constituent is polypeptide (e.g. anthrax bacillus). When slime forming bacteria are grown on a solid culture medium, the slime remains around the bacteria as a matrix in which they are embedded and its presence confers on growth a **mucoid character**.

Demonstration of Capsule

- Capsule cannot be stained with ordinary stains like Gram staining.
- It can be visualized by suspending the organisms in India ink and observing microscopically the exclusion of the colloidal ink particles from the area around the cell that is occupied by the capsule.
- It may also be visualized by reaction with specific antibody which causes a characteristic swelling of the capsule. It is known as **Quellung reaction**.

Functions

- Capsules protect the bacteria from antibacterial agents such as lytic enzymes found in nature.
- They inhibit phagocytosis thus contributing to the virulence of the bacteria.

Loss of capsule by mutation may render the bacterium avirulent. Bacteria tend to lose capsules on repeated subcultures *in vitro*.

Flagella

A large number of bacteria including a few coccal forms, about one half of bacilli and almost all of the spirilla and vibrios are motile by means of flagella. Flagella are long, hollow, helical filaments usually several times the length of the cell. They are 10–20 nm in diameter, 3–20 μm in length and are found on both Gram-positive and Gram-negative bacteria.

Arrangement

There are four types of arrangement of flagella (Fig. 2.5):
- **Monotrichous:** These organisms have a single polar flagellum.
- **Lophotrichous:** They have a tuft of flagella at one pole.
- **Amphitrichous:** They have single polar flagellum or tuft of flagella at both poles.
- **Peritrichous:** Flagella are distributed all round the cell.

The motility in spirochaetes is due to one or more pairs of axial filaments which run between **outer membrane and peptidoglycan layer and are anchored by knobs at both poles**.

Flagella consist mainly of a protein called flagellin which belongs to the same chemical group as myosin – the contractile protein of muscle. Though flagella of different genera of bacteria have the same chemical composition, they are antigenically different. Flagellar antigens induce specific antibodies in high titres. These antibodies are not protective but are useful in serodiagnosis.

Structure of Flagellum

The flagellum consists of three parts—the **filament**, the **hook** and the **basal body**. The basal body, anchored in the cytoplasmic membrane, comprises a rod and two or more sets of encircling rings. In Gram-negative bacteria four types of rings (M, S, P and L) are seen. Through ring M it attaches to the cytoplasmic membrane, ring S is located just above cytoplasmic membrane and through rings P and L it is attached to peptidoglycan and outer lipopolysaccharide membrane respectively (Fig. 2.6). Rings P and L are absent in Gram-positive bacteria.

Demonstration of Flagella

Because of their extreme thinness, flagella are best demonstrated with electron microscope. Flagella can also be demonstrated by the light microscope using special staining methods such as Hugh-Leifson's method. To make possible their resolution, the flagella must be thickened at least ten-fold by superficial deposition of stain. Indirect method of demonstration of flagella include demonstration of motility of the bacteria by (a) dark-ground microscopy, (b) hanging-drop method, or (c) observing spreading type growth in semisolid media.

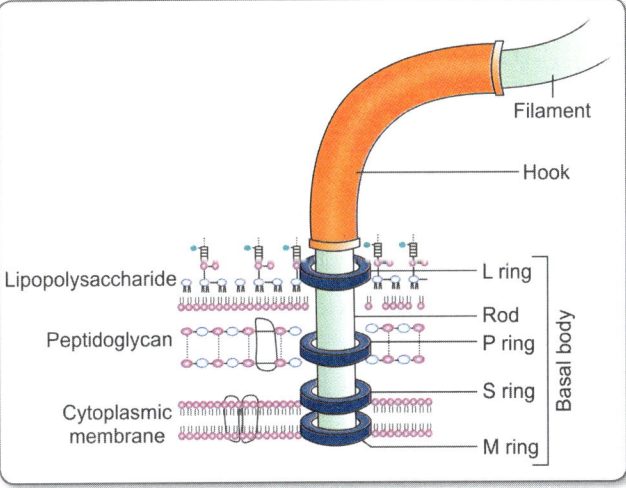

Fig. 2.6: Structure of flagellum.

Hanging-drop method: It is frequently used for the demonstration of motility:
- Take a glass slide having a circular concavity in the centre.
- Spread a ring of petroleum jelly around the concavity.
- With a wire loop place a loopful of the bacterial culture in the centre of a coverslip laid on the bench.
- Invert the slide over the coverslip, allowing the coverslip to adhere to the jelly, and quickly turn round the slide so that the coverslip is uppermost. The drop should then be 'hanging' from the coverslip in the centre of the concavity.
- Place the slide on the microscope, rack down the condenser slightly and partially close the iris diaphragm because excessive illumination renders the organisms invisible.
- With the low-power objective, focus the edge of the drop so that it appears across the centre of the field.
- Turn the high-power lens into position and focus the edge of the drop. Obtain the best illumination by lowering or raising the condenser, and secure sharp definition by reducing the aperture of the iris diaphragm.

Motile bacteria are seen swimming in different directions across the field, with a darting, wriggling or tumbling movement. True motility must be distinguished from Brownian movement, which is a rapid oscillation of each bacterium within a very limited area due to bombardment by the water molecules.

Fimbriae or Pili

They are hair-like microfibrils 1–1.5 μm in length and 4–8 nm in diameter. They are straighter, thinner and shorter than flagella (Fig. 2.3). They are present on many Gram-negative cells and provide a means for adherence to other cells, either bacterial or animal. They are an example of a class of surface structures termed **adhesins** that allow attachment of bacterial cell-to-cell surfaces (organelles of adhesion). Therefore, they are very important for bacterial survival in an animal host. They occur in both flagellated and non-flagellated bacteria and are far more

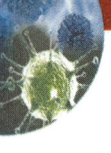

numerous than flagella. Each bacterium possesses 100–500 peritrichously-borne fimbriae. They can be seen by electron microscopy. They originate in the cytoplasmic membrane and are composed of self-aggregating protein monomers.

Bacterial Spore

Some species particularly those of genera *Bacillus* and *Clostridium* are capable of forming spores inside original cell. Each bacterium forms one spore which on germination forms a single vegetative cell. Sporulation in bacteria, therefore, is a method of preservation and not of reproduction.

Spores are small, highly resistant, metabolically dormant structures which develop as a response to starvation. They are not formed as long as conditions continue to favour maximal vegetative growth. Formation of spores occurs over a period of 4–8 hours after the cells stop growing upon depletion of their carbohydrate supply.

Sporulation

It develops from a portion of protoplasm near one end of the cell. This part of the bacterial cell is known as **forespore** and the remaining part as **sporangium** (Fig. 2.7). Bacterial DNA replicates and partitions into two halves and one of them, which is equivalent to one genome of the cell, is incorporated into forespore. A transverse septum derived from the cytoplasmic membrane is then formed by a process of invagination which divides forespore and sporangium. The forespore is subsequently completely encircled by dividing septum as a double layered membrane.

The two spore membranes now engage in active synthesis of various layers of the spore. The inner layer becomes the **inner membrane**. Between the two layers is laid **spore cortex** and outer layer is transformed into **spore coat** which consists of several layers. In some species from outer layer also develops **exosporium** which bears ridges and folds (Fig. 2.8). Finally, exosporium disintegrates and the spore is freed. Mesosomes appear to play a role in the development of spore and may be involved in the compartmentation of the spore's share of the nuclear material.

Shape and Position

The spores may be round, oval or elongated occupying a terminal, subterminal or central position. They may be narrower than the width of the bacilli or broader and bulging (Fig. 2.9).

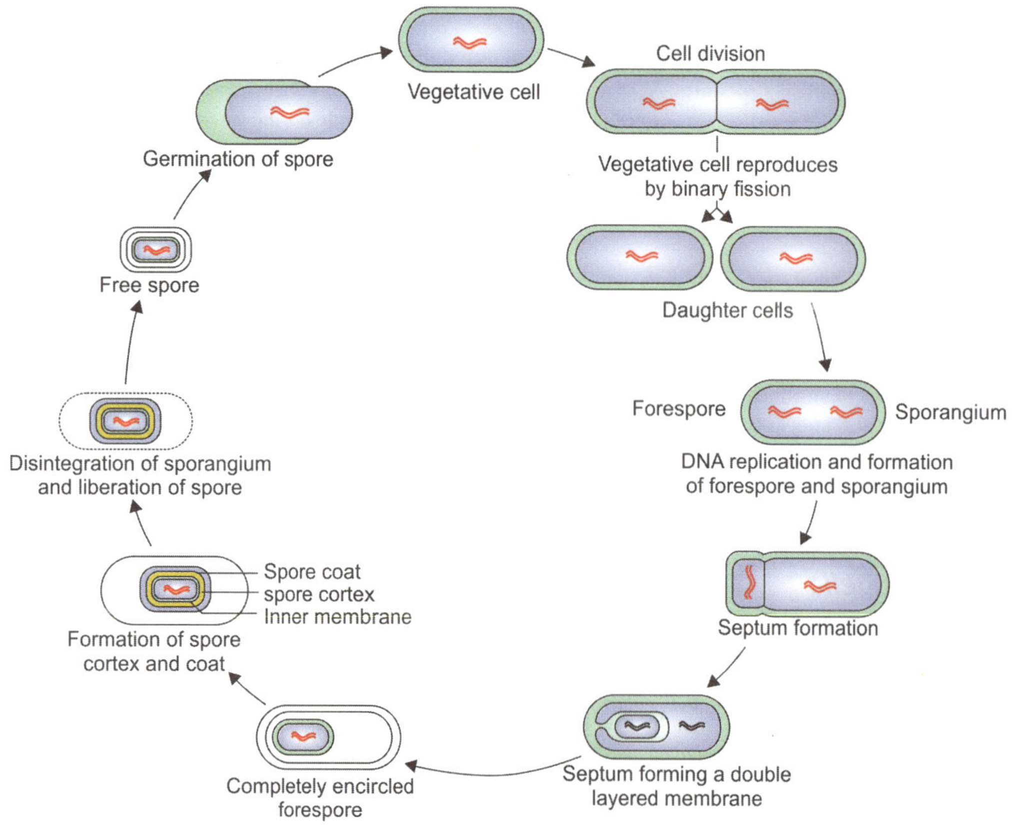

Fig. 2.7: Morphological events in sporulation.

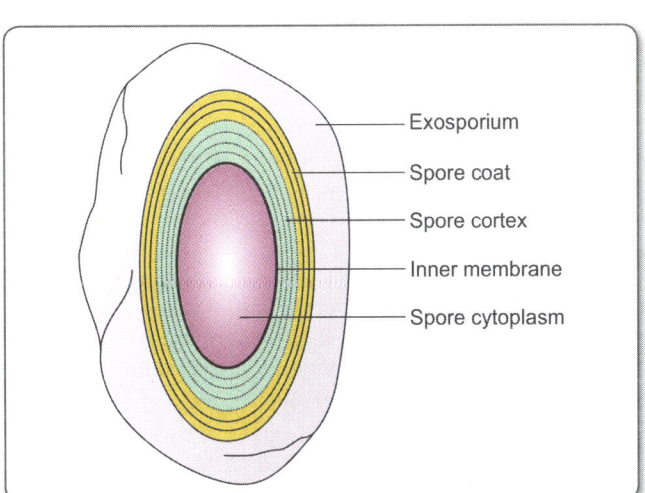

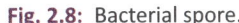

Fig. 2.8: Bacterial spore.

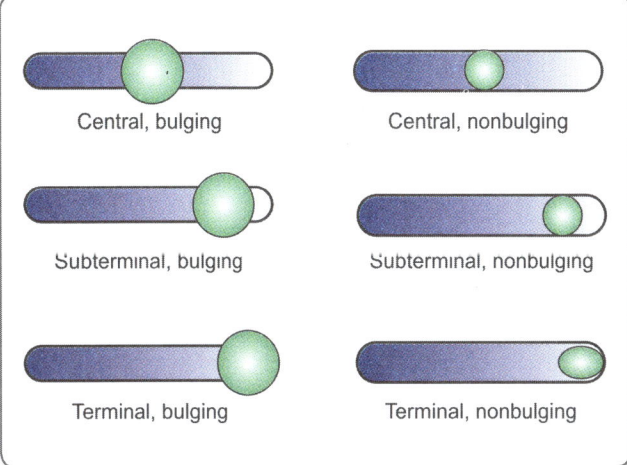

Fig. 2.9: Types of spores.

Resistance

Spores can remain dormant for many years. They are extremely resistant to chemical and physical agents. Their killing requires moist heat at 100–120°C for 10 minutes while vegetative cells can be killed by heating at 60°C for 10 minutes. Marked resistance of the spores is due to:

- the impermeability of their cortex and outer coat,
- their high content of calcium and dipicolinic acid,
- their low content of water, and
- their very low metabolic and enzymatic activity.

Germination

Spores are able to **germinate** when the external conditions become favourable to growth by access to moisture and nutrients particularly trigger nutrients such as a particular amino acid, pyrimidine or sugar in a suitable aqueous environment. Within a short period of time spore loses its heat resistance, refractility, dipicolinic acid and calcium. It then swells and absorbs water, after which the spore coat ruptures, and a new vegetative cell grows out.

Demonstration

- In unstained preparations, the spore is recognized within the parent cell by its greater refractility. In simple stains like Gram it remains unstained and appears as a clear space within the stained cell protoplasm (Fig. 2.10).
- They are slightly acid-fast and may be demonstrated by modified Ziehl-Neelsen staining.

L-FORMS OF BACTERIA

L-forms (after Lister Institute, London) of bacteria are cell wall deficient bacteria derived by variation, usually in the laboratory, from bacteria of normal morphology. They are stable in the sense

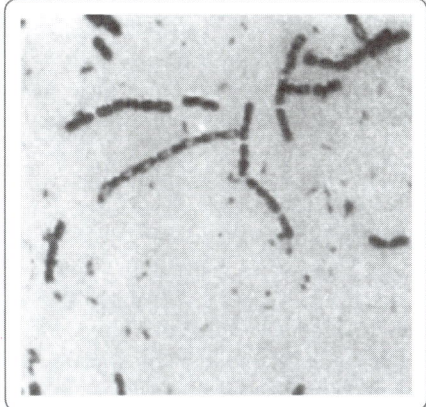

Fig. 2.10: Gram-stained smear of *Bacillus subtilis* showing Gram-positive bacilli in chains with spores which appear as unstained areas within the bacilli (× 1000).

that special conditions of culture, such as presence of penicillin, are not required to prevent their reversion to the parental bacterial forms. They lack regular size and shape. They may be spherical or disc-like and measure 0.1–20 μm in diameter.

Cultural Characteristics

L-forms are difficult to grow and usually require a medium that is solidified with agar as well as having the right osmotic strength. L-forms are produced more readily with penicillin than with lysozyme.

Colonies of L-forms of bacteria on agar medium show a characteristic '**fried-egg**' appearance with a dark thick centre, where many of the organisms embed themselves and grow within the agar, and a lighter periphery consisting of organisms lying on the surface of the agar. In liquid medium they grow in the form of clumps. Some L-forms are capable of reverting to normal bacillary forms upon removal of the inducing stimulus. Other L-forms are, however, stable

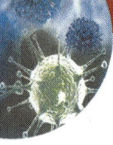

and never revert. Presence of residual peptidoglycan is essential for reversion. It acts as a primer in its own biosynthesis.

CLASSIFICATION OF BACTERIA

The taxonomy of bacteria refers to three basic concepts: classification, nomenclature and identification.

Classification

Classification can be defined as the arrangement of organisms into taxonomic groups (taxa) on the basis of genotypic (genetic) and phenotypic (observable) similarities and differences. It allows the orderly grouping of microorganisms. For bacteriological classification, three main approaches are followed. These include phylogenetic, Adansonian, genetic and intraspecies classification.

Phylogenetic Classification

It is a hierarchical classification. It represents a branching tree-like arrangement, one characteristic being employed for division at each branch or level. This system is called phylogenetic because it denotes an evolutionary arrangement of species. Here some characteristics are given special weightage. For example, Gram staining, spore formation, lactose fermentation, etc. are used to differentiate major groups, whereas less important properties such as nutritional requirements for growth of bacteria, production of certain enzymes by bacteria, etc. are employed to distinguish minor groups such as genera and species.

Formal levels of classification in successive subsets are kingdom, phylum or division, class, order, family, tribe, genus and species. At present, no standard classification of bacteria is universally accepted and applied, although **Bergey's Manual of Systematic Bacteriology** is widely used as authoritative source.

Adansonian Classification

Adansonian classification makes no phylogenetic assumption but merely takes into account all characteristics expressed at the time of study. Hence it is called **phonetic system**. It gives equal weightage to all measurable features, and groups the organisms on the basis of similarities of several characteristics. The availability of computers has extended the scope of phonetic classification by permitting comparison of very large number of properties of several organisms at the same time. This is known as **numerical taxonomy**.

Genetic Classification

This is based on homology of DNA base sequences of the microorganisms. DNA relatedness is determined by studying the nucleotide sequence of DNA by DNA hybridization or recombination methods. The study of messenger RNA and ribosomal RNA also provides useful information on genetic relatedness among bacteria. Genetic classification has been used more with viruses than with bacteria.

Intraspecies Classification

Intraspecies classification is based on biochemical properties (biotypes), antigenic properties (serotypes), susceptibility to bacteriophages (phage types), resistance to various chemicals (resistotypes) or production of bacteriocins (colcin types).

Nomenclature

It refers to the naming of microorganisms. It is governed by the *International Committee on Systematic Bacteriology* and published as *Approved List of Bacterial Names* in the *International Journal of Systematic Bacteriology*. By accepted taxonomic convention, order names have the endings -ales (e.g. the order Eubacteriales), family names have the latinised ending -aceae (e.g. the family Enterobacteriaceae), and tribe names end in -eae (e.g. the tribe Proteae). The order, family and tribe names are capitalized. The genus name is also capitalized followed by species name which is not capitalized. Both the genus or species are either italicized or underlined when appearing in print. Often, the genus name is abbreviated by using the first letter of the genus followed by a period and the full species name, which is never abbreviated, such as *S. pneumoniae*, *S. pyogenes*, *S. agalactiae* and *S. bovis*. The genus name followed by the word species (e.g. *Staphylococcus* species) may be used to refer to the genus as a whole. Species abbreviated sp. (singular) or spp. (plural) is used when the species is not specified. When the bacteria are referred to as a group, their names are neither capitalized nor underlined (e.g. staphylococci).

Identification

Suitable criteria for the purpose of microbial identification include cell shape, Gram reaction and the presence or absence of specialized structures such as spores or flagella. Staining procedures such as Gram stain can provide reliable assessment of the nature of cell surfaces. Some bacteria produce characteristic pigments and others can be differentiated on the basis of their complement of extracellular enzymes (e.g. haemolysins). Tests such as oxidase test can be used to distinguish organisms on the basis of the presence of a respiratory enzyme, cytochrome C.

The traditional method of placing an organism into a particular genus and species is based on the similarity of all members in a number of phenotypic characteristics. This is accomplished by testing each bacterial culture for a variety of metabolic characteristics and comparing the results with those listed in established charts.

In rapid identification systems, a numerical taxonomy (also called computer taxonomy, phenetics, or taxometrics) is used. Numerical classification schemes use a large number (frequently 100 or more) of taxonomically useful characteristics. All these characteristics are assigned numerical value. The computer clusters different strains at selected levels of overall similarity (usually 80% at the species level) on the basis of the frequency with which they share traits.

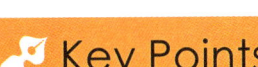 Key Points

- Prokaryotes such as **bacteria are simple cells** with no internal membranes or organelles.
- **Eukaryotes have a nucleus and organelles** such as mitochondria, and complex **internal membranes** (e.g. fungi and human cells).
- **Structures external** to cell wall of bacteria are **flagella, pili** or **fimbriae, capsule** and **slime layer**.
- Flagella are used for movement, pili for adhesion, and capsules protect the bacteria from antibacterial agents such as lytic enzymes and inhibit phagocytosis thus contributing to the virulence of bacteria.
- **Bacterial cytoplasm contains** chromosomal nuclear material, ribosomes, mesosomes and inclusions/storage granules.
- **Sporulation** is a response to starvation in **Bacillus** spp. and **Clostridium** spp.

? ASSESS YOURSELF

LONG AND SHORT ANSWER QUESTIONS

1. Differentiate between prokaryotes and eukaryotes in a tabulated form.
2. Draw a labelled diagram of a bacterial cell.
3. Describe the cell wall of bacteria.
4. Write short notes on:
   - (a) Cytoplasmic membrane
   - (b) Spores

MULTIPLE CHOICE QUESTIONS

1. Which of the following bacteria is cell wall deficient?
   - (a) *Mycoplasma*
   - (b) *Treponema*
   - (c) *Staphylococcus*
   - (d) *Klebsiella*

2. Which of the following bacterial structures is/are involved in attachment to cell surface?
   - (a) Flagella
   - (b) Fimbria
   - (c) Capsule
   - (d) Mesosomes

3. Which of the following are eukaryotes?
   - (a) Fungi
   - (b) Bacteria
   - (c) Chlamydiae
   - (d) Mycoplasmas

4. When determining distances and sizes, the smallest unit of measure is:
   - (a) Centimetre
   - (b) Millimetre
   - (c) Micrometre
   - (d) Nanometre

5. What function does a condenser serve in light microscope?
   - (a) Focuses the light onto our eyes
   - (b) Focuses the light rays on the sample
   - (c) Increases light intensity
   - (d) Reduces glare

6. Fimbriae present on the outer surface of bacteria are used for:
   - (a) Inhibition of phagocytosis
   - (b) Bacterial motility
   - (c) Adherence to surfaces
   - (d) Antibiotic resistance

ANSWERS TO MCQs

1. a   **2.** b   **3.** a   **4.** d   **5.** b   **6.** c

SECTION II • GENERAL CHARACTERISTICS OF MICROBES

3 Chapter

Growth and Nutrition of Bacteria

When an inoculum of bacterial cells is introduced into a suitable nutrient medium and incubated under appropriate conditions, each of the growing organisms becomes progressively larger until, at some critical size, it divides to give rise to two identical daughter cells. Nuclear division precedes cell division. The time required for a bacterium to give rise to two daughter cells is known as generation time. In *Escherichia coli* it is 20 minutes, in tubercle bacilli it is 20 hours and in lepra bacilli it is 20 days.

BATCH CULTURE

When bacteria are grown in liquid medium, multiplication is arrested after a few cell divisions due to depletion of nutrients and/or accumulation of toxic products. This is known as batch culture.

CONTINUOUS CULTURE

By use of special devices like **chemostat** or **turbidostat** in which nutrients are replaced and bacteria are removed continuously it is possible to maintain continuous culture of bacteria for industrial and research purposes.

When pathogenic bacteria multiply in the host tissues the situation is intermediate between batch culture and continuous culture because they get inexhaustible source of nutrients but they have to face host defence mechanisms.

In liquid media, growth of bacteria is diffuse and on solid media they form colonies. Each colony consists of a clone of cells derived from a single parent cell. Bacteria in a culture medium or clinical specimen can be counted by two methods:
- **Total count**
  - This is total number of bacteria present in a specimen irrespective of whether they are living or dead. This is done by counting the bacteria under microscope using counting chamber and by comparing the growth with standard opacity tubes.
- **Viable count**
  - This measures only viable (living) cells which are capable of growing and producing colonies on a suitable medium.

BACTERIAL GROWTH CURVE

When a bacterium is inoculated into a suitable culture medium and incubated, its growth follows a characteristic course. If both total and viable counts are made at different intervals and plotted in relation to time, then a characteristic growth curve is obtained. A typical growth curve contains four major phases (Fig. 3.1):
- **Lag phase**
  - When bacteria are seeded into fresh medium, multiplication usually does not begin immediately. The period between inoculation and beginning of multiplication is known as lag phase. **During this period the organisms adapt themselves to growth in fresh medium and increase in size and metabolic activity. Therefore, lag phase is regarded as a period not of rest but of intense metabolic activity**. The duration of lag phase varies with the species, nature of culture medium, temperature of incubation, etc. It is generally shorter in a nutrient-rich than in a minimal medium.
- **Log or exponential growth phase**
  - During this phase the bacteria are multiplying at their maximum rate and their number increases exponentially or by geometric progression with time. **If logarithm of bacterial count is plotted against time a straight line**

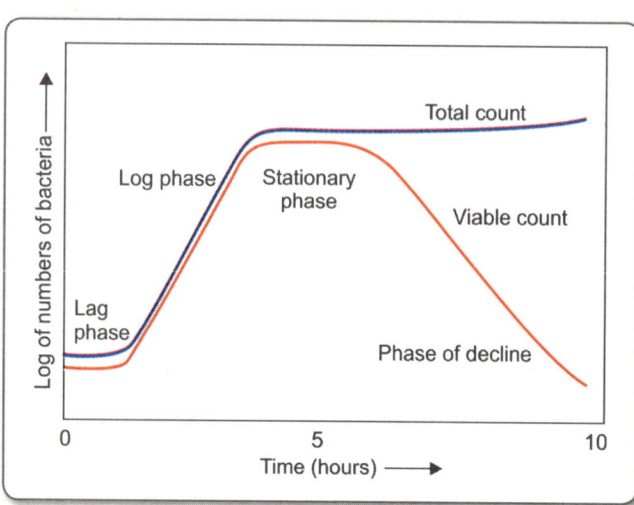

Fig. 3.1: Bacterial growth curves.

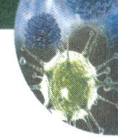

is obtained. **In the log phase, the bacterial cells are small and uniformly stained**. Exponential phase is of limited duration because of:

♦ exhaustion of nutrients,
♦ accumulation of toxic metabolic end products,
♦ rise in cell density,
♦ change in pH, and
♦ decrease in oxygen tension (in case of aerobic organisms).

● **Stationary phase**
  ■ Due to above reasons exponential growth slows down and the bacterial population enters the stationary phase in which the number of viable cells remains constant. There is almost a balance between the bacterial reproduction and bacterial death. **During this phase, bacteria become Gram-variable, show irregular staining and spores start forming in spore forming bacteria**.
● **Phase of decline**
  ■ Stationary phase is followed eventually by the phase of decline because rate of death exceeds the rate of reproduction and the number of viable cells declines. **Finally, after a variable period, all the cells die and culture becomes sterile**.

FACTORS AFFECTING GROWTH OF BACTERIA

Carbon Dioxide

Some organisms such as pneumococci and gonococci grow better in air supplemented with 5–10% CO_2.

Temperature

Each bacterium multiplies best within a restricted temperature range. For most of the pathogenic bacteria optimum temperature for growth is 37°C (our body temperature) with upper and lower temperature limits of 40–50°C and 15–20°C, respectively. The organisms with optimum temperatures of 37°C, less than 20°C and 55–80°C are known as mesophiles, psychrophiles and thermophiles, respectively.

Moisture and Desiccation

Moisture is very essential for the growth of bacteria because 80% of their body weight is made up of water. However, the effect of drying varies in different organisms. For example *Treponema pallidum*, gonococci and human immunodeficiency virus die quickly after drying while tubercle bacilli and staphylococci may survive drying for several weeks. However, bacterial spores can survive for several years, and drying in cold and vacuum (**lyophilization**) is a method for preservation of bacteria and viruses.

pH

Like other living organisms, microorganisms are very susceptible to changes in the acidity or alkalinity of the surrounding medium. Most of the medically important bacteria can grow at neutral or slightly alkaline pH (7.2–7.6). Some bacteria like lactobacilli and cholera vibrio grow at acidic and alkaline pH respectively.

Light and Other Radiations

Darkness provides a favourable condition for growth and viability of bacteria. Ultraviolet rays from direct sunlight or a mercury lamp are bactericidal. Bacteria are also killed by ionizing radiations. Photochromogenic mycobacteria form pigment only on exposure to light.

Osmotic Effect

Because of the mechanical strength of the cell wall, bacteria are more tolerant to osmotic variation, therefore, they can grow in media with widely varying contents of salt, sugar and other solutes. Sudden exposure of bacteria to solutions of high salt concentration may cause **plasmolysis**. This is due to osmotic withdrawal of water leading to shrinkage of protoplast and its retraction from the cell wall. This occurs more readily in Gram-negative than Gram-positive bacteria. On the other hand, sudden transfer of bacteria from concentrated solution to distilled water may cause **plasmoptysis** due to excessive osmotic imbibition of water leading to swelling and bursting of cell.

Mechanical and Sonic Stresses

In spite of the mechanical strength of the cell wall, bacteria can be ruptured and killed by vigorous shaking with glass beads and ultrasonic vibrations.

CULTURE METHODS

The methods of bacterial culture used in the clinical laboratory include streak culture, lawn culture, stroke culture, stab culture, pour-plate culture, shake culture and liquid culture.

Streak Culture

This method is routinely employed for the isolation of bacteria in pure culture from clinical specimens. A platinum or nichrome wire loop of 2–4 mm diameter is used. The loop is first sterilized in the bunsen flame by making it red hot and cooled by touching on uninoculated part of the medium. Then a loopful of the specimen is smeared thoroughly over area *A* (Fig. 3.2), on the surface of a well dried plate, to give a well-inoculum or 'well'. The loop is re-sterilized and drawn from the well in 2 or 3 parallel lines onto the fresh surface of the medium (*B*). This process is repeated as shown (*C*, *D* and *E*), care being taken to sterilized the

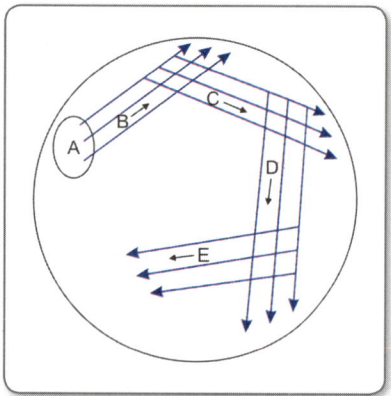

Fig. 3.2: Streak culture.

loop, and cool it on unseeded medium, between each sequence. On incubation, growth may be confluent at the site 'well', but becomes progressively thinner, and well separated colonies are obtained over the final streaks.

Lawn Culture

Lawn cultures are prepared by flooding the surface of the plate with a liquid culture or suspension of bacteria and pipetting off the excess inoculum or by applying a swab soaked in the bacterial culture or suspension. After incubation, lawn culture provides a uniform surface growth. It is useful for antibiotic susceptibility testing by disc diffusion method and bacteriophage typing.

Stroke Culture

Stroke culture is made in tubes containing agar slope or slant. Slopes are seeded by lightly smearing the surface of agar with loop in a zig-zag pattern taking care not to cut the agar. It is used for obtaining pure growth for slide agglutination and other diagnostic tests.

Stab Culture

Stab cultures in solid media (nutrient gelatin or glucose agar) are inoculated by plunging the charged wire into the centre of the medium and withdrawing it in the same line to avoid splitting the medium. These are employed mainly for demonstration of gelatin liquefaction and for the maintenance of stock culture.

Pour-plate Culture

This method is used for counting the number of living bacteria or groups of bacteria in a liquid culture or suspension. Prepare serial 10-fold dilutions of the bacterial suspension over a range (6–9 tubes) ensuring that one dilution will contain between 50 and 500 viable bacteria/ml (number which can be accurately counted). Starting with the greatest dilution, pipette 1 ml amounts of each dilution into each of three 9 cm petri dishes.

Then pour into each dish about 10 ml of clear nutrient agar, melted, and cooled at 45–50°C. Mix well by rapidly moving the plate for about 10 seconds. Allow the agar to set and incubate at 37°C for 48 hours. After incubation, colonies will be seen well distributed throughout the depth of the medium and can be enumerated using colony counters. Count the colonies in three plates containing 50–500 colonies/plate. Multiply the average number/plate by the dilution factor to obtain the viable count/ml in the original suspension.

Shake Culture

It is made by melting nutrient agar in a test tube, cooling it to 45°C and inoculating it while molten from a liquid medium with a drop from a capillary pipette. Withdraw the pipette, replace the cap or plug and discard the pipette into disinfectant. Mix the contents of the tube by rotation between the palms of the hands before the agar solidifies and incubate it at 37°C for 24 hours and look for the growth of the organisms.

Liquid Culture

Liquid cultures in tubes, bottles or flasks may be inoculated by touching with a charged loop or by adding the inoculum with pipettes or syringes. Large inocula can be employed in liquid cultures and hence this method is adopted for blood culture and for sterility tests, where the concentration of bacteria in inocula are expected to be small. Liquid cultures are also preferred when large yields are desired.

CULTURE MEDIA

Numerous culture media have been devised. The original media used by Louis Pasteur were liquids such as urine or meat broth. Liquid media have many disadvantages. Bacteria growing in these media may not exhibit specific characteristics for their identification. With liquid media it is difficult to isolate different types of bacteria from mixed populations. However, liquid media are used for obtaining bacterial growth from blood or water when large volumes have to be used as inoculum, for preparing bulk cultures for antigens and vaccines, and for preparation of inoculum for biochemical reactions and antibiotic susceptibility testing.

In 1881, Robert Koch described means of cultivating bacteria on solid media. First he used as his growth medium pieces of potato, then 2.5–5.0% gelatin to prepare solid media fortifying them with 1% meat extract as an essential ingredient. But gelatin is not satisfactory as it liquefies at 24°C (incubation temperature for most pathogenic bacteria is 37°C) and many proteolytic bacteria liquify gelatin. At the suggestion of Anglina Hesse, the American wife of his assistant, he substituted agar-agar in place of gelatin as solidifying agent for the media.

Agar-agar or '**agar**' for short is prepared from a variety of seaweeds; the product is clarified, dried and supplied as a powder. It does not add to the nutritive properties of medium and is not

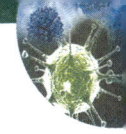

affected by the growth of bacteria. The exact concentration to be used may require some adjustment according to the batch of agar. A concentration of 1–2% usually yields a suitable gel. In preparing agar media, the appropriate amount of agar powder is added to the liquid medium and dissolved by placing the mixture in a steamer at 100°C for 1 hour or longer. Most agars dissolve to give a clear solution but sometimes it is necessary to filter off particulate impurities.

The melting and solidifying points of agar solutions are not the same. At the concentrations normally used, most bacteriological agars melt at about 95°C and solidify only when cooled to about 42°C. Agar can be added to any nutrient liquid medium if the advantages of a solid medium are desired. Most of the culture media are sterilized by autoclaving at 121°C for 15 minutes. Nutrients that are damaged by autoclaving are sterilized separately by filtration, etc. The sterilized agar base is then melted in the steamer and cooled to about 45–50°C followed by addition of heat-labile ingredients, but once these are added the medium must at once be poured into Petri dishes because it cannot be remelted without damaging the heat-sensitive ingredients.

Another important ingredient of common media is **peptone**. It consists of water-soluble products obtained from lean meat or other protein material such as heart muscle, casein, fibrin or soya flour, usually by digestion with the proteolytic enzymes pepsin, trypsin or papain. Its constituents are peptones, proteoses, amino acids, a variety of inorganic salts including phosphates, potassium and magnesium, and certain accessory growth factors such as nicotinic acid and riboflavin. Special brands of peptone such as neopeptone and proteose peptone are available for special use.

Other common ingredients of the culture media include casein hydrolysate, meat extract, yeast extract, malt extract, blood and serum.

While bacteria grow diffusely in liquid media, they produce discrete visible growth on solid media in Petri dishes. If a mixed culture is inoculated in suitable dilution on solid medium, different bacteria form well-separated colonies, which are clones of cells originating from a single bacterial cell. On solid media, bacteria have distinct colony morphology and exhibit many other characteristic features such as pigment production or haemolysis.

Types of Culture Media

Culture media have been classified in many ways:
- Solid, semisolid and liquid.
- Simple (basal), complex, synthetic, defined, semidefined and special media. Special media are further divided into enriched, selective, enrichment, indicator or differential, sugar media and transport media.
- Aerobic media and anaerobic media.

Basal Media

These include peptone water, and nutrient broths which form the basis of most media used in the study of the common pathogenic bacteria.

Meat extract broth is most commonly used nutrient broth. It can be made solid by addition of 1–2% agar. If the concentration of agar is reduced to 0.2–0.5%, it is called **semisolid agar**. If its concentration is raised to 6%, it is called **hard agar**. In semisolid agar the motile organisms show growth in entire medium, and on surface of hard agar swarming of *Proteus* is inhibited.

Enriched Media

These are prepared to meet the nutritional requirements of fastidious organisms by addition of substances such as blood, serum and egg to a basal medium. Important examples of enriched media are blood agar for isolation of *Streptococcus*, chocolate agar for isolation of *Neisseria* and *Haemophilus*, and Loeffler's serum slope for the isolation of *Corynebacterium diphtheriae*.

Selective Media

When a substance is added to a solid medium which inhibits the growth of unwanted bacteria but permits the growth of wanted bacteria in the form of colonies, it is known as selective medium. Important examples of this type of media are MacConkey agar for *E. coli*, deoxycholate citrate agar (DCA) for *Salmonella* and *Shigella*, Wilson and Blair's medium for *Salmonella* and Lowenstein-Jensen medium for *Mycobacterium tuberculosis*.

Enrichment Media

When a substance is added to a liquid medium which inhibits the growth of unwanted bacteria and favours the growth of wanted bacteria it is known as enrichment medium. Important examples of this type of media are tetrathionate broth and selenite F broth for *Salmonella* and *Shigella*, and alkaline peptone water for *Vibrio cholerae*.

Indicator Media or Differential Media

When a substance is added into a medium which would produce a visible change in the medium following the growth of a particular organism, it is designated as indicator or differential medium. For example, MacConkey medium contains lactose and neutral red. Lactose-fermenting organisms after growth on this medium produce acid and in acidic pH neutral red becomes red in colour. Thus, *E. coli* which is lactose fermenter produces red or pink colonies on this medium. Christensen's medium contains urea and phenol red indicator. When urease producing organisms like *Proteus* and *Klebsiella* grow on this medium, urea is split up into ammonia and carbon dioxide. Ammonia makes the medium alkaline and in alkaline pH the medium becomes pink in colour (in alkaline pH phenol red is pink in colour).

Transport Media

When a clinical sample is being transported from the hospital to the laboratory delicate organisms like *N. gonorrhoeae* may not

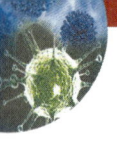

survive or the normal flora (*E. coli*) may overgrow pathogenic flora (*Salmonella, Shigella* and *V. cholerae*). To avoid this, media have been devised to maintain the viability of the pathogen. These media typically contain only buffers and salts. They lack carbon, nitrogen and organic growth factors hence do not facilitate microbial multiplication. Stuart's transport medium and Amies transport medium are examples of transport media.

Storage Media

Bacteria are best preserved and stored by lyophilization. But, for preservation and storage for a few months or so, they can be stab inoculated on semisolid agar or on Dorset egg medium followed by incubation. When growth appears they can be stored in refrigerator.

Defined Synthetic Media

These media are prepared from pure chemical substances, therefore, their exact composition is known. These are used for research purposes.

Sugar Media

For the identification of most of the organisms, sugar fermentation reactions are carried out. Glucose, lactose, sucrose and mannitol are widely used sugars.

For the preparation of sugar media, 1% of the concerned sugar is added to peptone water with a suitable indicator. Durham's tube (a small tube) is kept inverted in the tube containing this medium to detect gas production. For fastidious organisms like *C. diphtheriae* and pneumococci, Hiss's serum sugar media are used.

Anaerobic Media

For the growth of anaerobes, the media used contain reducing substances. These include thioglycollate broth and cooked meat broth.

Aerobic Culture

For cultivation of aerobes the incubation is done in an incubator under normal atmospheric condition. The temperature of incubation for most of the human pathogenic bacteria is 37°C. For cultivation of many fungi incubation of the inoculated media should be carried out at 25–28°C. To prevent drying of the medium when prolonged incubation is necessary, as in the cultivation of the tubercle bacilli, screw-capped bottles should be used instead of test tubes or plates.

Culture in an Atmosphere with added Carbon Dioxide

Some organisms, such as capnophilic streptococci, require extra CO_2 in the air in which they are grown and others, such as the pneumococcus and gonococcus, grow better in air supplemented with 5–10% CO_2. For this CO_2 jars are used. The required amount of air is withdrawn with a vacuum pump and replaced with CO_2 from a cylinder. CO_2 incubators which provide a predetermined and regulated amount of CO_2 in a suitably humid atmosphere are commercially available. Screw caps on containers of liquid media must not be tight and should preferably be replaced by a closure that allows entry of CO_2.

Culture in Microaerophilic Atmosphere

Microorganisms like *Actinomyces israelii* are microaerophilic. This is done by an evacuation replacement method with 5% O_2, 10% CO_2 and 85% N_2.

Anaerobic Culture

A variety of methods are available for the culture of anaerobic organisms in the clinical laboratory. Exclusion of oxygen from the medium is the simplest method, and is effected by growing the organisms within the culture medium such as freshly steamed liquid media, and deep nutrient agar with 0.5% glucose and minimal shaking and solidified rapidly by placing the tube in cold water. Liquid media soon become aerobic unless a reducing agent such as glucose 0.5–1.0%, ascorbic acid 0.1%, cysteine 0.1%, sodium thioglycollate 0.1%, or particles of meat in cooked meat broth are added. Liquid media should be prereduced by holding in a boiling water bath for 10 minutes to drive off dissolved oxygen, then quickly cooled to 37°C just before use.

Cooked meat broth, CMB (original medium known as 'Robertson's bullock-heart medium') has a special place in anaerobic bacteriology; and thioglycollate broth and its modifications are also very useful. CMB is suitable for growing anaerobes in air and also for the preservation of stock cultures of aerobic organisms. The inoculum is introduced deep in the medium in contact with the meat. Meat particles are placed in 30 ml bottles to a depth of about 2.5 cm and covered with about 15 ml broth.

Anaerobes have special nutritional requirements for vitamin K, haemin and yeast extract, and all primary isolation media for anaerobes should contain these three ingredients.

Anaerobic Jars

When an oxygen-free or anaerobic atmosphere is required for obtaining surface growths of anaerobes, anaerobic jars provide the method of choice. The most reliable and widely used anaerobic jar is the McIntosh-Fildes' anaerobic jar. It is a cylindrical vessel made of glass or metal with a metal lid which is held firmly in place by a clamp (Fig. 3.3). The lid has two tubes with taps, one acting as gas inlet and the other as the outlet. On its undersurface it carries a gauze sachet carrying alumina pellets coated with palladium. It acts as a room temperature catalyst for the conversion of hydrogen and oxygen into water. It acts as a catalyst, as long as the sachet is kept dry.

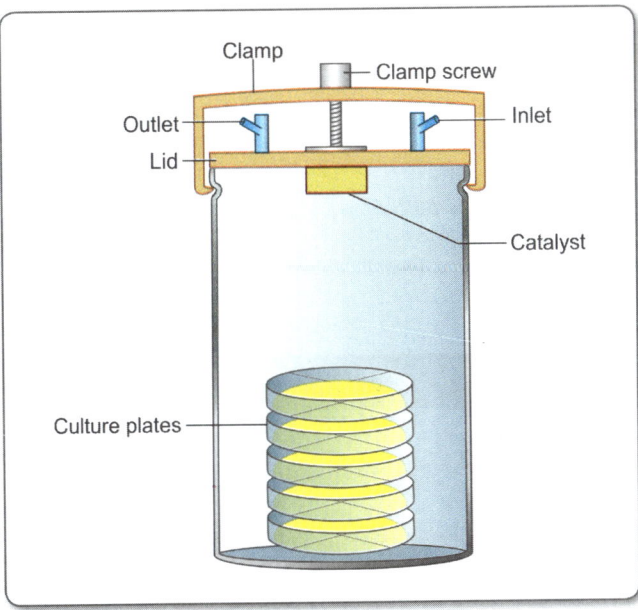

Fig. 3.3: Anaerobic jar.

Inoculated culture plates are placed inside the jar and the lid clamped tight. The outlet tube is connected to a vacuum pump and the air inside is evacuated. The outlet tap is then closed and the inlet tube connected to a hydrogen supply. Hydrogen is drawn in rapidly. As soon as this inrush of gas has ceased the inlet tap is also closed. After about 5 minute inlet tap is again opened. There occurs again an immediate inrush of hydrogen since the catalyst creates a reduced pressure within the jar due to the conversion of hydrogen and leftover oxygen into water. If there is no inrush of hydrogen, it means the catalyst is inactive and must be replaced. The jar is left connected to the hydrogen supply for about 5 minutes, then the inlet tap is closed and the jar is placed in the incubator, catalysis will continue until all the oxygen in the jar has been used up.

The **GasPak** is now the method of choice for preparing anaerobic jar. The GasPak is commercially available as a disposable envelope containing chemicals which generate hydrogen and carbon dioxide on the addition of water. After the inoculated plates are kept in the jar, the GasPak envelope, with water added, is placed inside and the lid screwed tight. Hydrogen and carbon dioxide are liberated and the presence of a cold catalyst in the envelope permits the combination of hydrogen and oxygen to produce an anaerobic environment. The outstanding feature of the GasPak system is the disposable gas generator envelope, which does away with the need for a vacuum pump and cylinders of compressed gas; the operation of the jar is consequently very quick and simple. As the standard GasPak jar is not evacuated before use a relatively large volume of water is formed during catalysis.

An **indicator** should be used for verifying the anaerobic condition in the jar. Methylene blue is generally used for this purpose. When it is placed in an anaerobic environment it is reduced from its coloured oxidized form to a colourless reduced leuco compound.

In addition to, or instead of, using a chemical indicator, some workers include in the jar a plate inoculated with a known strict anaerobe such as *Clostridium tetani* or *Bacteroides fragilis*, and of a strict aerobe, such as *Pseudomonas aeruginosa*. This method is quite reliable if the indicator anaerobe grows and the aerobe does not.

The major disadvantage of any anaerobic jar system is that the plates have to be removed from the jar to be examined. This, of course, exposes the colonies to oxygen, which is especially hazardous to the anaerobes during their first 48 hours of growth. For this reason, a suitable holding system should always be used in conjunction with anaerobic jars, placed in an oxygen-free holding system, removed one by one for rapid microscopic examination of colonies, and then quickly returned to the holding system. Plates never should remain in room air on the open bench.

Anaerobic Chamber

This is an ideal anaerobic incubation system which provides oxygen free environment for inoculating media and incubating cultures. Identification and susceptibility tests can also be performed in anaerobic chambers.

Anaerobic chambers may be fitted with airtight rubber gloves to insert hands and manipulate specimens, plates, tubes or they may be gloveless where airtight rubber sleeves fit tightly against user's bare forearms. All anaerobic chambers contain a catalyst, dessicant, H_2 gas (5–10%), CO_2 gas (5–10%), N_2 gas (80–90%) and an indicator.

Anaerobic Bags or Pouches

These bags are available commercially and one or two inoculated plates are placed into a bag and an oxygen removal system is activated and the bag is sealed and incubated. Plates can be examined for growth without removing the plates from bag, thus without exposing the colonies to oxygen. But as with anaerobic jar, plates must be removed from the bags in order to work with the colonies at the bench. These bags are also useful in transport of biopsy specimen for anaerobic cultures.

INCUBATION

Inoculated plates should be incubated at 37°C for at least 48 hours, and reincubated for another 2–4 days to allow slow-growing organisms (certain species of *Actinomyces*) to form colonies.

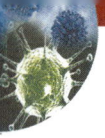

🔖 Key Points

- Bacterial **growth** in laboratory media can be divided into a **lag** phase, **log** phase, **stationary** phase and **decline** phase.
- For *cultivation* and *identification* of bacteria, basal media, enriched media, selective media, enrichment media, differential media, etc. are used.
- Depending upon the expected organisms, the inoculated media are incubated in **aerobic culture, culture in an atmosphere with added carbon dioxide, culture in microaerophilic atmosphere and anaerobic culture**.

❓ Assess Yourself

Long and Short Answer Questions

1. Describe bacterial growth curve.
2. Define generation time of bacteria. Discuss briefly batch culture and continuous culture.
3. What are culture media? Classify and discuss them in brief.
4. Describe bacterial culture methods.
5. What is the influence of temperature on the bacterial growth?
6. Write short notes on:
   (a) Selective media   (b) Enrichment media

Multiple Choice Questions

1. The period between inoculation of bacteria in a culture medium and beginning of multiplication is known as:
   (a) Lag phase   (b) Log phase
   (c) Stationary phase   (d) Decline phase

2. When a substance is added to a liquid medium which inhibits the growth of unwanted bacteria and favours the growth of wanted bacteria, it is known as:
   (a) Selective medium   (b) Enrichment medium
   (c) Enriched medium   (d) Differential medium

3. Which of the following bacteria can grow in alkaline pH?
   (a) Lactobacilli   (b) *Vibrio cholerae*
   (c) *Salmonella*   (d) *Shigella*

4. Which of the following bacteria can grow in acidic pH?
   (a) Lactobacilli   (b) *Vibrio cholerae*
   (c) *Salmonella*   (d) *Shigella*

5. Chocolate agar is an example of which of the following?
   (a) Nonselective media   (b) Selective media
   (c) Differential media   (d) Enriched media

Answers to MCQs

1. a   **2.** b   **3.** b   **4.** a   **5.** d

Chapter 4

Collection of Specimens and Identification of Bacteria

The laboratory diagnosis of an infectious disease begins with the collection of a clinical specimen. Proper collection of an appropriate clinical specimen is the first step in obtaining an accurate laboratory diagnosis of an infectious disease. A poorly collected specimen not only may result in failure to recover important microorganisms, but may also lead to incorrect or even harmful therapy if treatment is directed towards a commensal or contaminant.

GENERAL RULES FOR COLLECTION OF SPECIMEN

- Apply strict aseptic techniques throughout the procedure.
- Wash hands before and after the collection.
- Collect the specimen before the administration of antimicrobial agents.
- Prevent contamination of the specimen with externally present organisms or normal flora of the body.
- Collect the specimen at the appropriate phase of disease.
- Collect the specimen from the actual infection site.
- Collect adequate quantity for the desired tests.
- Collect the specimen aseptically in a sterile and appropriate container.
- Close the container tightly so that its contents do not leak during transportaion.
- Ensure that the outside of the specimen container is clean and uncontaminated.
- Label the container appropriately and complete the requisition form.
- Immediately transport the specimen to the laboratory.

CRITERIA FOR REJECTION OF SPECIMENS

- Missing or inadequate identifications.
- Incomplete forms.
- Leaking container or blood stained containers.
- Specimens collected in an inappropriate container.
- Haemolysed blood sample.
- Insufficient quantity.
- Dried-up specimen.
- Contamination suspected.
- Specimen collected in formalin.
- Inappropriate transport or storage.

Blood for Culture

- Using a pressure cuff, locate a suitable vein in the arm.
- Wearing sterile gloves thoroughly disinfect the venepuncture site as follows:
  - Using spirit (70% ethanol) swab, cleanse an area about 50 mm in diameter. Allow to air-dry.
  - Using 2% tincture of iodine and a circular action, swab the area beginning at the point where the needle will enter the vein. Allow the iodine to dry on skin for at least 1 minute.
- Lift the tape or remove the protective cover from the top of culture bottle. Wipe the top of the bottle using spirit swab.
- Using a sterile syringe and needle withdraw 5 ml of blood from an adult and 1 ml from a young child.
- Insert the needle through a hole in the cap and through rubber or plastic liner of the bottle cap, and dispense 5 ml of blood from an adult and 1 ml from a young child into the culture medium bottles (Fig. 4.1a), respectively. Cap must not be removed for introduction of the blood. In adults large quantity (5 ml) of blood is required since the number of organisms in the blood particularly in mild and recovering cases may be quite small, even as few as one per ml. As blood's natural bactericidal or bacteriostatic action may interfere with the growth of any bacteria present, this effect is annulled by diluting (inoculating) 5 ml of blood in an adult and 1 ml of blood in a young child in 50 ml and 10 ml of the medium (10-fold dilution), respectively. **Organisms causing baceteraemia in young children are usually present in sufficient concentration to be detected in small volume (1 ml) of blood**.
- Using a fresh spirit swab wipe the top of the culture bottle and replace the tape or protective cover. Without delay, mix the blood with the broth. Blood must not be allowed to clot in the culture medium because the bacteria will become trapped in the clot.
- Clearly label the bottle with the name and number of the patient, and the date and time of collection.
- As soon as possible, incubate the inoculated medium.

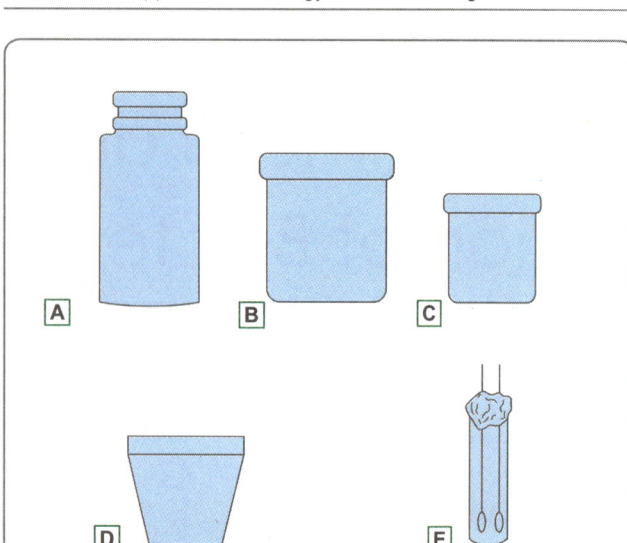

Fig. 4.1: (A) McCartney bottle, (B) Urine/stool container, (C) CSF container, (D) Sputum container, (E) Throat swabs.

- Collect blood during early stages of disease since the number of bacteria is higher in acute and early stages of disease.
- Collect blood during paroxysm of fever since the number of bacteria is higher at high temperature in patients with fever.
- In the absence of antibiotic administration, 99% culture positivity can be seen with three blood cultures.
- Transport the specimen to the laboratory. If not possible keep in incubator or at room temperature. Do not refrigerate.

Anticoagulated Blood Specimen

If anticoagulated blood specimen is required, use suitable anticoagulant, e.g. EDTA for malaria parasites and trypanosomes, and sodium citrate for microfilariae. Mix blood well but gently with anticoagulant. The blood must be examined within one hour of collection to avoid morphological changes in the appearance of parasites.

Blood for Serological Tests

For serological tests collect about 5 ml of blood to ensure there will be enough serum for all the tests that may be required. Immediately transfer the blood from the syringe into a dry stoppered sterile tube or bottle (without anticoagulant) and allow to clot. When the serum has separated, pipette it off into a sterile tube.

Urine

- Mid-stream urine sample is collected after giving proper instructions to the patient.
  - Clean the genitalia properly. (In case of male, retract the prepuce, clean it with sterile normal saline. In case of female, wash perineum and periurethral area with soap and water. Separate apart labia with fingers of one hand).
  - Collect a "clean-catch" mid-stream urine sample in a sterile container (Fig. 4.1b).
- Transport immediately to the laboratory. If a delay of more than 1–2 hours is unavoidable, refrigerate at 4°C.
- In catheterized patients, do not collect urine from collection bag or after opening the closed drainage. Clean the area over the collecting tubes and puncture with the help of a sterile needle and syringe and draw out the sample.
- Suprapubic aspiration under aseptic condition may be done in infants.

Cerebrospinal Fluid (CSF)

Cerebrospinal fluid must be collected by an experienced physician. Rigorous aseptic precautions must be observed to prevent the introduction of infection into the central nervous system. The fluid is usually collected from the arachnoid space.

- Skin between fourth and fifth lumbar vertebrae is decontaminated with spirit and tincture iodine.
- A sterile wide-bore needle is inserted between fourth and fifth lumber vertebrae and the CSF is allowed to drip into a sterile dry container (Fig. 4.1c).
- Only 3–5 ml of fluid should be collected, because the removal of a larger volume may lead to headache.
- Immediately deliver the sample with a request form to the laboratory.
- CSF must be examined without delay and the results of the tests reported to the medical officer as soon as they become available. If delay in processing is inevitable then store it at 37° C. Do not refrigerate.
- The fluid should be handled with special care because a lumber puncture is required to collect the specimen.

Sputum

- Collect the sputum in a wide-mouthed container, which is preferably disposable, made up of transparent thin plastic, unbreakable and leak-proof (Fig. 4.1d).
- Ask the patient to rinse the mouth with plain water and then inhale deeply 2–3 times, cough up deeply and spit in the sputum container by bringing it close to the mouth. If the patient has difficulty in coughing sputum, postural drainage, and appropriate physiotherapy often cause exudate to move in the bronchi and stimulate productive coughing.
- Make sure the sputum sample is of good quality and not just the saliva. A good sputum sample is thick, purulent and sufficient in amount (2–3 ml).
- Sputum sample may be refrigerated up to 3–4 hours.

Throat Swab

- Two swabs should be collected (Fig. 4.1e).
- Depress the tongue with a tongue blade.

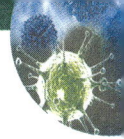

- Swab the inflammed area of the throat, pharynx or tonsils with a sterile swab taking care to collect the pus or piece of membrane.
- Take care not to contaminate the swab with saliva.

Pus and Other Discharge

- Do not apply antiseptic before collection.
- Clean with normal saline.
- In case of discharge, 1–2 ml of sample is collected in a sterile vial.
- If swabs are to be collected then 2 swabs, in a sterile container, should be collected (one for direct microscopic examination and the other for culture).

Bone Marrow

- Decontaminate the skin, overlying the site from where specimen is to be collected, with spirit and tincture iodine.
- Aspirate 1 ml or more of bone marrow by sterile percutaneous aspiration with bone marrow aspiration needle.
- Collect in a sterile screw capped tube.
- Immediately transport to the laboratory.

Stool

- Should be collected in early stage of disease and prior to treatment with antimicrobials.
- Do not collect the specimen from bed pan.
- Should not be contaminated with urine.
- Collect about a spoonful of the specimen, especially that which contains mucus, pus or blood, into a clean, dry, leak proof container (Fig. 4.1b).
- If possible, submit more than one specimen on different days.
- The fresh stool specimen must be processed within 1–2 hours of passage.
- If delay is unavoidable then store it at 2–8°C.

Rectal Swab

- Collect the swab only if stool collection is not possible.
- Insert swab at least 2.5 cm beyond the anal sphincter so that it enters the rectum.
- Rotate it once before withdrawing.
- Transport in Cary-Blair or other transport medium.

IDENTIFICATION OF BACTERIA

Isolation and accurate identification of disease causing microorganism from morbid material and its antibiotic susceptibility is very important. Identification of the isolate is carried out by examination of stained and unstained smears of the morbid material, isolation in pure culture on appropriate culture media, study of macroscopic (colonial characters) and microscopic morphology of the isolate and biochemical characters. Finally, antibiotic susceptibility of the isolate is carried out and specific chemotherapy initiated.

Unstained Wet Film

An unstained wet film or **hanging drop preparation** (*see* Chapter 2) is examined under light microscope for observation of motility, and an unstained wet film may be examined under **dark-ground microscope** for demonstration of motility of spirochaetes. Presence of *Treponema pallidum*, with characteristic spiral shape and motility, in exudate from a chancre is sufficient for presumptive diagnosis of syphilis.

Staining Techniques

A number of staining techniques for the identification of bacteria are available. Of these, Gram stain and Ziehl-Neelsen are most important. A Gram-stained smear shows the Gram reaction, size, shape and grouping pattern of bacteria, absence or presence of spores, their shape, size and intracellular position. Presence of Gram-negative diplococci inside the polymorphs in cerebrospinal fluid (CSF) and urethral discharge gives the provisional diagnosis of meningococcal meningitis and gonorrhoea, respectively. With Ziehl-Neelsen staining, it is possible to identify tubercle bacilli, lepra bacilli and *Nocardia*. They resist decolourization with 20%, 5% and 1% sulphuric acid respectively.

Gram Stain

This staining method is most frequently used in diagnostic bacteriology. The smear is first stained with one of the basic pararosaniline dyes such as crystal violet, methyl violet, or gentian violet which is a mixture of the two preceding dyes. It is then treated with iodine solution which acts as a mordant. Next it is washed with decolourizing agent, e.g. alcohol or acetone and finally stained with a dye of contrasting colour, e.g. dilute carbol fuchsin, safranine, etc. On the basis of their reaction to the Gram stain, bacteria can be divided into two groups, i.e. Gram-positive and Gram-negative. Both Gram-positive and Gram-negative bacteria take up violet colour with pararosaniline dyes. After treatment with decolourizing agent, Gram-positive bacteria retain this dye and violet colour while Gram-negative lose the dye and become colourless. They then take up counterstain and appear red in colour.

Mechanism of Gram Staining

The exact mechanism of Gram reaction is not known. It may, however, be attributed to:
- Gram-positive bacteria have a more acidic protoplasm, which may account for their retaining the basic primary dye more strongly than Gram-negative bacteria.

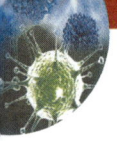

- The violet basic dye and the iodine form a dye-iodine complex inside both Gram-positive and Gram-negative bacteria but during alcohol or acetone wash, cell membranes (outer membrane of cell wall of Gram-negative bacteria and cytoplasmic membrane) of Gram-negative bacteria are dissolved. However, dye-iodine complex is retained in Gram-positive cells by the thick peptidoglycan mesh, whereas it is readily washed out through the very thin peptidoglycan layer remaining in Gram-negative cells after both membranes have been dissolved. Gram-negative bacteria do not retain the stain, but Gram-positive may fail to do so when overdecolourization is done or the smears are made from old cultures. This appears to be due to the fact that such cultures consist largely of dead, dying or degenerated cells, the physical and chemical properties of which are altered.

Method

- Prepare smear from clinical specimen, culture smear of colony or broth culture on a clean glass slide by spreading thinly on the slide.
- Allow it to dry in air and fix it by passing the dried slide, film downwards, three times slowly through the flame.
- Cover the smear with crystal violet (primary stain) for one minute. Other pararosaniline dyes such as methyl violet or gentian violet may also be used as primary stain.
- Pour Gram's iodine over the slide for two minutes.
- Decolourize with alcohol or acetone for 10–30 seconds.
- Counterstain with dilute carbol fuchsin or safranin for 30 seconds.
- Wash thoroughly with water; blot and dry in air.
- Examine under oil-immersion lens.

Ziehl-Neelsen Stain

Next to Gram stain, this is the method most frequently used in diagnostic bacteriology. It is of value in distinguishing a few bacterial species, e.g. tubercle bacilli, non-tuberculous mycobacteria, lepra bacilli and *Nocardia* from all others. Tubercle bacilli, non-tuberculous mycobacteria and lepra bacilli are relatively impermeable to simple stains but when stained with hot concentrated carbol fuchsin, subsequently resist decolourization with 20%, 20% and 5% sulphuric acid, respectively. Decolourized non-acid-fast organisms are counterstained with methylene blue. However, *Nocardia* which resists decolourization with 1% sulphuric acid, can be easily stained with Gram stain and is Gram-positive. Acid-fastness has been attributed to the high content of lipids, fatty acids and higher alcohols found in acid-fast bacteria. Of the lipids, mycolic acid, a high molecular weight hydroxy acid wax containing carboxyl groups, is most important because it is acid-fast even in free state.

Method

- Cover the slide with filtered carbol fuchsin and heat until steam rises. Allow the preparation to stain for 5 minutes, heat being applied at intervals to keep the stain hot. The stain must not be allowed to evaporate and dry on the slide. If necessary, pour more carbol fuchsin to keep the whole slide covered with carbol fuchsin.
- Wash with water.
- The stained smear is decolourized with 20% sulphuric acid and washed with water. This step is repeated till the film is only very faintly pink.
- Wash the slide well with water.
- Counterstain it with 2% methylene blue for 15–20 seconds.
- Wash, blot dry the smear and examine under oil-immersion lens.

Result

Acid-fast bacilli stain bright red, while the tissue cells and other organisms are stained blue.

Negative Capsular Staining

In case of **negative staining**, bacteria (spirochaetes) or fungi (*Cryptococcus*) are mixed with India ink or nigrosin that provide a uniform coloured background against which the unstained organisms can be seen. Bacterial capsules which do not take simple stains can be seen by negative staining.

Staining of Spores

If spore-bearing organisms are stained with ordinary dyes or by Gram stain, the body of the bacillus is deeply coloured, whereas the spore is unstained and appears as a clear area in the organism. However, the spores can be stained by acid-fast stain and malachite green stain.

Acid-fast Stain for Spores

- Prepare smear from clinical specimen, culture smear of colony or broth culture on a clean glass slide by spreading thinly on the slide.
- Allow it to dry in air and fix it by passing the dried slide, film downwards, three times slowly through the flame.
- Stain with Ziehl-Neelsen carbol fuchsin for 3–5 minutes, heating the preparation until steam rises.
- Wash with water.
- Treat with 0.25 or 0.5% sulphuric acid for one to several minutes. This step is repeated till the film is only very thinly pink.
- Wash with water.
- Counterstain with 1% aqueous methylene blue for 3 minutes.
- Wash with water, blot and dry.

The spores tend to retain carbol fuchsin dye after treatment with decolourizing agent, therefore, these appear red in colour.

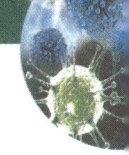

KOH Wet Mount

A 10–20% solution of KOH is useful for detecting fungal elements in skin, hair, nails, and tissue. In this procedure, KOH is mixed in equal proportions with the specimen on a slide and the specimen material is teased with two inoculating needles. A coverslip is placed over it and heated gently. Preparation with KOH clears the tissue and cellular debris from all types of clinical specimens without damaging the fungal cells.

Lactophenol Cotton Blue (LPCB)

- Place a drop of LPCB on a clean glass slide.
- With a bent dissecting needle, remove a small portion of the colony from the agar surface and place it in the drop of LPCB.
- With 2 dissecting needles gently tease apart the mycelial mass of the colony on the slide, cover with coverslip, and observe under the microscope with low-power and high-dry magnifications.

Teasing the colony often disrupts the delicate fruiting structures of the filamentous molds, making it difficult in some instances to observe the characteristic spore arrangements or hyphal attachments necessary for a definitive identification. In such cases, a cellophane tape mount or slide culture may be required.

Differential Identification Characteristics

Accurate identification can be accomplished by isolation of bacteria in pure form followed by study of colonial morphology, examination of stained smear, biochemical reactions, antigenic structure, serotyping, biotyping, bacteriocin typing, phage typing, animal pathogenicity and antibiotic susceptibility determination. Clinical material is inoculated onto a solid medium (nutrient agar, blood agar or MacConkey agar) in such a way so as to ensure isolated discrete colonies.

Enriched, enrichment, selective and differential media, depending upon the organism suspected, are employed. Selective growth conditions, i.e. presence or absence of oxygen and presence of CO_2, etc. are also employed keeping in view the organisms suspected. The culture plates are incubated at optimum temperature. Most of the pathogenic bacteria grow best at 37°C.

Biochemical Reactions

A large number of biochemical tests can be employed for the identification of different bacteria. These include:

Indole Production

Certain bacteria which possess enzyme tryptophanase, degrade amino acid tryptophan to indole, pyruvic acid and ammonia. Indole production is detected by inoculating the test organism into peptone water and incubating it at 37°C for 48–96 hours. Then add 0.5 ml of Kovac's reagent and shake gently. A **red colour** in the alcohol layer indicates a positive reaction. Kovac's reagent consists of:

Paradimethylaminobenzaldehyde	:	10 g
Amyl or isoamyl alcohol	:	150 ml
Conc. hydrochloric acid	:	50 ml

Dissolve aldehyde in alcohol and slowly add the acid and store in refrigerator. Shake gently before use. Indole is extracted from the medium by amyl or isoamyl alcohol and forms red colour ring by forming a red coloured complex with paradimethylaminobenzaldehyde. Negative test will show yellow coloured ring (colour of Kovac's reagent).

Methyl Red (MR) Test

This test detects the production of sufficient acid by fermentation of glucose, so that pH of the medium falls and it is maintained below 4.5. Inoculate the test organism in glucose phosphate broth and incubate at 37°C for 2–5 days. Then add five drops of 0.04% solution of methyl red, mix well and read the result immediately. Positive tests are bright red and negative are yellow. If the test is negative after 2 days repeat it after 5 days.

Voges-Proskauer (VP) Test for Acetoin Production

Many bacteria ferment carbohydrates with the production of acetyl methyl carbinol (acetoin). In the presence of potassium hydroxide and atmospheric oxygen, acetoin is converted to diacetyl, and α-naphthol serves as a catalyst to form a pink complex. This test is usually done in conjunction with the methyl red test. An organism of the family Enterobacteriaceae is usually either methyl-red-positive and Voges-Proskauer-negative or methyl-red-negative and Voges-Proskauer-positive.

Inoculate test organism in glucose phosphate broth and incubate at 37°C for 48 hours. Then add 1 ml potassium hydroxide and 3 ml of 5% solution of α-naphthol in absolute alcohol. A positive reaction is indicated by the development of **pink colour** in 2–5 minutes and crimson in 30 minutes.

Citrate Utilization

This test is used to study the ability of an organism to utilize citrate as sole source of carbon for the growth. Liquid (Koser's) and solid (Simmon's) media containing citrate as sole source of carbon can be used. A part of colony is picked up by a straight wire and inoculated into either of these media. The ability of an organism to utilize citrate as a sole source of carbon is detected by the production of turbidity (due to growth) in liquid medium. Solid medium also contains bromothymol blue as indicator, therefore, on the solid medium the **appearance of growth and blue colour** is positive and original green colour and no growth is negative.

Indole, MR, VP and citrate tests are done in routine for the classification of Gram-negative enteric bacteria. They are commonly referred to as IMViC tests.

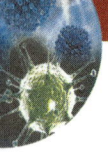

Sugar Fermentation

The ability of an organism to ferment various sugars is tested by inoculation of the test organism in different sugar media containing Andrade's indicator. A small inverted tube (Durham's tube) completely filled with liquid and containing no air bubbles is usually included in each culture tube. Production of acid is indicated by the change of the colour of the medium to red or pink and the gas, if produced, collects in Durham's tube.

Nitrate Reduction

This test detects the production of enzyme nitrate reductase which reduces nitrate to nitrite. All the organisms of the family Enterobacteriaceae are positive for this test. Inoculate test organism in 5 ml medium containing potassium nitrate, peptone and distilled water. Incubate it at 37°C for 96 hours. Then add 0.1 ml test reagent which consists of equal volumes of sulphanilic acid and α-naphthylamine in 5 N acetic acid mixed just before use. A **red colour** developing within a few minutes indicates the presence of nitrite and hence the ability of test organism to reduce nitrate to nitrite.

Urease Test

This test detects the ability of an organism to produce urease enzyme. The test organism is inoculated on the entire slope of Christensen's medium which contains urea and phenol red indicator in addition to other constituents including agar. It is incubated at 37°C and examined after 4 hours and after overnight incubation. Development of **purple-pink colour** indicates production of urease. The latter in the presence of water converts urea into ammonia and carbon dioxide. Ammonia makes the medium alkaline and phenol red indicator changes to purple-pink in colour.

Hydrogen Sulphide Production

Some organisms produce hydrogen sulphide from sulphur-containing amino acids. It may be detected by suspending strips of filter paper impregnated with lead acetate between the cotton plug and the tube. It has variable sensitivity. When cultured in media containing lead acetate or ferric ammonium citrate or ferrous acetate they turn them black or brown. This method is more sensitive than lead acetate strip method.

Potassium Cyanide Test

This tests the ability of an organism to grow in the presence of potassium cyanide. Inoculate buffered peptone water medium, containing 1 in 13,000 concentration of potassium cyanide, with test organism. Incubate at 37°C for 24–48 hours. Development of **turbidity** in the medium indicates the ability of the organism to grow in the presence of potassium cyanide.

Catalase Production

Put a loopful of 10% hydrogen peroxide on colonies of the test organism on nutrient agar. Alternatively, pick up a few colonies of the test organism with platinum loop from nutrient agar plate and dip it in a drop of 10% hydrogen peroxide on a clean glass slide. The production of **gas bubbles** from the culture indicates a positive reaction. A false positive result may be obtained if the growth is picked up from medium containing catalase, e.g. blood agar or if an iron wire loop is used.

Oxidase Test

This test depends on the presence, in bacteria, of certain oxidases that catalyse the oxidation of reduced tetramethyl-p-phenylene-diamine dihydrochloride (oxidase reagent) by molecular oxygen. Put a drop of freshly prepared 1% solution of oxidase reagent on a piece of filter paper. Then rub a few colonies of test organism on it. If it is oxidase positive, it will produce a **deep purple colour** within 10 seconds. Alternatively, pour oxidase reagent over the colonies of the test organism on the culture plate. The colonies of oxidase positive organisms rapidly develop a deep purple colour.

Bacteriocin, Bacteriophage and Serotyping

Each species of an organism contains a number of different strains. These epidemiological markers are useful for intraspecies differentiation of various strains.

Animal Pathogenicity

Various experimental models used in diagnostic microbiology laboratory are mouse, rat, guinea pig, rabbit, nine-banded armadillo and monkey. Various routes of inoculation are intradermal, subcutaneous, intramuscular, intraperitoneal, intracerebral and intravenous. Oral and nasal routes can also be used. The identification of the organism is carried out on the basis of clinical and postmortem findings and cultural characteristics.

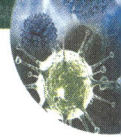

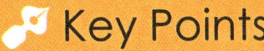 Key Points

- **Microorganisms** may be observed by *hanging drop preparation, dark-ground microscopy, Gram staining, Ziehl-Neelsen staining, negative staining*, etc.
- Bacteria are divided into two major classes according to staining characteristics – *Gram-positive* (violet) and *Gram-negative* (red).
- Cell walls of some bacteria such as the **mycobacteria** contain lipids (mycolic acids); they are relatively impermeable to simple stains but when treated with hot concentrated carbol fuchsin, subsequently resist decolourization by 20% sulphuric acid, these bacteria are called *acid-fast organisms*.
- Identity of the **microorganisms** can be confirmed by various *biochemical reactions*.

? ASSESS YOURSELF

LONG AND SHORT ANSWER QUESTIONS

1. Discuss methods of collection and transportation of specimens.
2. Write short notes on:
   - (a) Gram stain
   - (b) Ziehl-Neelsen stain
   - (c) Indole production
   - (d) Oxidase test

MULTIPLE CHOICE QUESTIONS

1. Which of the following organisms is **not** acid-fast?
   - (a) Tubercle bacilli
   - (b) Lepra bacilli
   - (c) *Nocardia*
   - (d) *Corynebacterium diphtheriae*

2. Which of the following organisms is Gram-negative?
   - (a) *Clostridium*
   - (b) *Bacillus*
   - (c) *Actinomyces*
   - (d) *Bacteroides*

3. Urease test is positive in:
   - (a) *Klebsiella pneumoniae*
   - (b) *Escherichia coli*
   - (c) *Salmonella* Typhi
   - (d) *Shigella flexneri*

4. Oxidase test is negative in:
   - (a) *Neisseria*
   - (b) *Pseudomonas*
   - (c) *Vibrio*
   - (d) *Proteus*

5. Catalase production is negative in:
   - (a) *Staphylococcus*
   - (b) *Streptococcus*
   - (c) *Proteus*
   - (d) *Salmonella*

6. Which of the following is/are reason(s) to reject a specimen for culture?
   - (a) The specimen is preserved in formalin
   - (b) The information on the requisition does not match information on the specimen label
   - (c) A second stool sample is submitted from the same patient on the same day
   - (d) All of the above

ANSWERS TO MCQs

1. d **2.** d **3.** a **4.** d **5.** b **6.** d

NOTES

Infection Control and Safety

Section Summary

Chapter 5

Bacteria in Health and Disease

Skin, alimentary tract and other mucous membranes are continually contaminated by microorganisms from the environment. Based on their relationship they can be divided into saprophytes and parasites.

SAPROPHYTES

Saprophytes are free-living microbes that live on dead or decaying organic matter. They are found in soil and water. They are, generally, incapable of multiplying on living tissues. However, sometimes when host resistance is lowered some saprophytes like *Bacillus subtilis* may cause infection.

PARASITES

Parasites are the microorganisms that can enter and multiply in hosts. They are of two types—**microparasites** which include viruses, bacteria, fungi and protozoa, and **macroparasites** which include helminths.

PATHOGENS

Pathogens are the microorganisms which are capable of producing disease in man and animals. They are of two types—**opportunistic pathogens** and **primary pathogens**.

Opportunistic Pathogens

Opportunistic pathogens rarely cause disease in individuals with intact immunological and anatomical defences. In immunocompromised hosts these bacteria are able to cause disease. Coagulase-negative staphylococci are normally carried on the human skin where they cause no harm. However, introduction of these organisms into anatomical sites in which they are not normally found may lead to infection. Similarly, *Escherichia coli* is normally carried in human intestine. If they enter into urinary tract they lead to urinary tract infection.

Primary Pathogens

Primary pathogens are the organisms which are capable of causing disease in previously healthy individuals with intact immunity.

COMMENSALS

Commensals (organisms of normal flora or normal microbiota) are the microorganisms which live in complete harmony with the host without causing any damage to it.

Table 5.1 enlists the normal flora at various sites of the body.

SOURCES OF INFECTION

Infections may be endogenous, due to the organisms of the normal flora, and exogenous, due to the organisms derived from a source outside the body.

Endogenous Infections

These are also referred to as autoinfections. Organisms of normal flora are usually non-pathogenic but occasionally they may lead to infection:

- *E. coli* and *Enterococcus faecalis*, the normal flora of the intestines, may cause urinary tract infection.
- Viridans streptococci, the normal flora of the mouth, may cause infective endocarditis.

Exogenous Infections

Most of the infections are exogenous in origin. The sources of exogenous infections are as under:

- Human cases and carriers
- Animal cases and carriers
- Insects
- Environment

Human Cases and Carriers

The commonest source of human infection is man himself who may be a patient or a carrier. A **carrier** is a person who harbours the pathogenic microorganisms without suffering from it. There are several types of carriers.

- *Healthy carrier:* One who harbours the pathogen but has never suffered from the disease caused by it.
- *Convalescent carrier:* One who has recovered from the disease but continues to harbour the pathogen on his body.

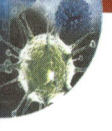

TABLE 5.1: Normal flora at various sites of the body

Site	Organisms
Skin	*Staphylococcus epidermidis, S. aureus, Micrococcus* spp., *Candida* spp. *Clostridium* spp., diphtheroids, α-haemolytic and non-haemolytic streptococci, *Acinetobacter* spp., *Bacteroides* spp., Gram-negative rods (fermenters and non-fermenters), *Moraxella* spp.
Nares and nasopharynx	*S. aureus, S. epidermidis, Corynebacterium* spp., *Peptostreptococcus* spp., *Fusobacterium* spp, *Streptococcus* spp., *Neisseria* spp. including *N. meningitidis, S. pneumoniae, Prevotella* spp., *Haemophilus* spp., yeasts.
Mouth	*S. epidermidis, S. aureus, S. mitis, S. sanguis, S. salivarius, S. mutans, Peptostreptococcus* spp., *Veillonella* spp., *Actinomyces israelii, Bacteroides* spp., *Treponema denticola, T. refringens, Neisseria* spp., lactobacilli, *Candida* spp., *Entamoeba gingivalis, Trichomonas tenax.*
Oropharynx	*S. aureus, S. epidermidis, S. pneumoniae, S. mitis, S. mutans, S. milleri, S. sanguis, S. salivarius, Moraxella catarrhalis, H. parainfluenzae, H. influenzae,* anaerobic streptococci, *Bacteroides* spp., *Prevotella* spp., *Porphyromonas* spp., *Fusobacterium necrophorum, S. pyogenes, N. meningitidis.*
Gastrointestinal tract	*Bacteroides* spp., *Clostridium* spp., Enterobacteriaceae, *Eubacterium* spp., *Fusobacterium* spp., *Enterococcus* spp., *Peptostreptococcus* spp., *Peptococcus* spp., *S. aureus, Lactobacillus* spp., yeasts.
Genitourinary tract	*Lactobacillus* spp., *Bacteroides* spp., *Clostridium* spp., *Peptostreptococcus* spp., *S. aureus, S. epidermidis, Enterococcus* spp., diphtheroids, group B streptococci, Enterobacteriaceae, *Acinetobacter* spp., *Candida albicans.*
Conjunctiva	*Corynebacterium* spp., *S. epidermidis,* nonhaemolytic streptococci, neisseriae.

- *Temporary carrier:* When carrier state lasts for less than six months.
- *Chronic carrier:* When carrier state lasts for years or may be for the life of the patient.
- *Paradoxical carrier:* Who acquires the organisms from another carrier.
- *Contact carrier:* Who acquires the organisms from a patient.

Carriers are very important source of infection. For example, a person acquires organisms from a patient of meningococcal meningitis and becomes a contact carrier. He is then a source of infection for other persons (patient → carrier → patient).

Animal Cases and Carriers

Certain pathogens are capable of causing infection in both man and animals. Therefore, animals may act as a source of infection of such organisms. The infection may be acquired by contact with the animal, animal bite and ingestion of milk or meat. Infection in animals may be asymptomatic and these animals may serve as reservoir for human infections. These are known as **reservoir hosts**. Infectious diseases transmitted from animals to man, either directly or indirectly via a vector, are known as **zoonoses**. For example:
- *Bacterial:* Bovine tuberculosis, bubonic plague, *Salmonella* food poisoning, anthrax.
- *Viral:* Rabies, yellow fever.
- *Fungal :* Microsporum canis, Trichophyton verrucosum.

Vectors

Blood-sucking insects such as mosquitoes, ticks, mites, flies, and lice act as a source of a number of human and animal infections. Insects transmitting pathogens are known as **vectors**. Table 5.2 shows common vectors and diseases transmitted by them.

Environment

This includes soil, water and food. Spores of tetanus and gas gangrene bacilli remain viable in the soil for several decades and serve as a source of infection. The normal habitat of these organisms is the human and animal intestines and they enter the soil through their faeces. Water contaminated with *Shigella, Salmonella, Vibrio cholerae,* poliovirus and hepatitis A and E viruses acts as a source of these infections.

Contaminated food acts as a source of organisms causing food poisoning, gastroenteritis, diarrhoea and dysentery.

MODES OF SPREAD OF INFECTION

Pathogenic organisms can spread from one host to another by a variety of mechanisms. These include:

1. Inhalation

Respiratory infections such as common cold, influenza, measles, mumps, tuberculosis and whooping cough are acquired by inhalation. These organisms are shed into the environment by patients in secretions of nose or throat during sneezing, coughing, talking and other forceful expiratory activities. These activities expel a spray of droplets.

2. Ingestion

Enteric fever, cholera, dysentery, food poisoning, poliomyelitis, hepatitis A and E and most of the parasitic infections are acquired by ingestion. The source of these infections is the faeces of the patients or carriers. The faeces containing pathogens may contaminate food or drink.

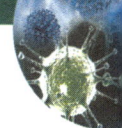

TABLE 5.2: **Vectors and diseases transmitted by them**

Arthropod	Diseases transmitted
1. **Mosquitoes**	
▪ *Anopheles*	Malaria, filariasis
▪ *Cluex*	Filariasis, Japanese encephalitis, West Nile fever
▪ Aedes	Yellow fever, dengue, chikungunya haemorrhagic fever, Rift Valley fever, filariasis
▪ *Mansonia*	Brugain filariasis
2. **Flies**	
▪ Housefly	Typhoid and paratyphoid fever, diarrhoea, dysentery, cholera, gastroenteritis, amoebiasis
▪ Sandfly	Kala-azar, oriental sore, espundia, oroya fever
▪ Tsetse fly	African trypanosomiasis
3. Louse	Epidemic typhus, relapsing fever, trench fever
4. Rat flea	Bubonic plague, endemic typhus, *Hymenolepis diminuta* infection
5. Black fly	Onchocerciasis
6. Reduviid bug	Chagas' disease
7. **Ticks**	
▪ Hard ticks	Spotted fever group, viral encephalitis, Colorado tick typhus, tularaemia, human babesiosis
▪ Soft ticks	Q fever, relapsing fever, Kyasanur Forest disease
8. **Mites**	
▪ Trombiculid mite	Scrub typhus
▪ Gramasid mite	Rickettsial pox
▪ Itch mite	Scabies
9. Body and head lice	Epidemic typhus, relapsing fever
10. Cyclops	Dracunculosis, diphyllobothriasis
11. Cockroaches	Same as in case of housefly

3. Contact

Infection may be acquired by direct or indirect contact with the patient. Sexually transmitted diseases (STD) such as syphilis, gonorrhoea, lymphogranuloma venereum, lymphogranuloma inguinale, trichomoniasis, herpes simplex, hepatitis B and C, and AIDS are acquired by direct contact. The term **contagious disease** is used for the disease acquired by direct contact, and disease acquired by other modes, through inanimate objects, as **infectious disease**.

4. Contamination of Wounds

The infections may be caused by:
- Organisms present in the nose or throat of the patient himself or of nurses or doctors. Pathogenic staphylococci and streptococci derived from respiratory tract are important causes of wound and burn infection.
- Airborne spread of organisms from the infected wounds of other patients.
- Contact with infected hands, clothing or other articles.
- In some instances pathogens may be inoculated directly into the tissues of the host, for example, rabies virus which is present in the saliva of a rabid animal, usually dog, is inoculated directly into the host tissue.

- Spores of *C. tetani* and *C. perfringens* are present in the soil. These get inoculated into the host tissue following severe wounds leading to tetanus and gas gangrene respectively.

5. Blood-sucking Insects

In some diseases, blood-sucking insects play an important role in the spread of infection from one individual to another. Insects normally become infected by biting a human or animal host in whose blood the causative organism is present. After this there is an interval, known as **extrinsic incubation period**, during which the insect is incapable of transmitting the infection. During this period the organisms multiply in the body of the insect. *Ticks which transmit certain rickettsial and arbovirus infections and mites which transmit scrub typhus are unusual in that the infective agent can be transmitted from one generation of the insect to the next through the ovum.*

Arthropods transmit infection in four ways:
- The infective agent gains access to the salivary glands of the insect and the organisms enter into the wound caused by the insect bite along with the saliva, e.g. transmission of malaria by female *Anopheles* mosquito.
- The infective agent multiplies in the intestinal tract of the insect and during feeding it is regurgitated into the wound, e.g. transmission of bubonic plague by rat flea.

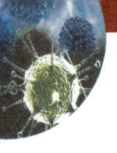

- The agent multiplies in the intestinal tract and is excreted in the faeces. These are deposited by the insect besides the wound when it bites and due to irritation caused by insect bite, are scratched by the victim into the wound, e.g. transmission of rickettsial diseases.
- The infective agent multiplies in the coelomic cavity of the insect and infection is due to contamination of the wound of bite with the coelomic fluid of an insect that has been crushed in its vicinity by the victim, e.g. transmission of louse-borne relapsing fever.

6. Iatrogenic and Laboratory-acquired Infections

If meticulous care in asepsis is not taken, infections like AIDS and hepatitis B, C and D may sometimes be transmitted during therapeutic and investigative procedures. These are known as iatrogenic infections. Laboratory personnel handling infectious material are particularly at risk.

7. Congenital

Some microorganisms like *Toxoplasma*, rubella virus, cytomegalovirus, herpes simplex virus, human immunodeficiency virus, *Treponema pallidum*, malaria parasites, etc. (TORCH complex) can cross the placental barrier and infect the foetus *in utero*. This is known as **vertical transmission**. This may result in abortion, miscarriage or still birth. Live infants may be born with manifestations of the disease.

FACTORS PREDISPOSING TO MICROBIAL PATHOGENICITY

Pathogenicity denotes the ability of a microbial species to cause disease, while the term **virulence** refers to the same property in a strain of the species. Bacterial virulence factors can be defined as the components and products of the bacterial cell which confer on the bacterium the potential to harm the host.

DETERMINANTS OF VIRULENCE

1. Adhesion

Many bacteria possess on their surface colonization factors or adhesins. These usually occur on fimbriae. Through adhesins bacteria attach specifically on the receptors present on the host cells. They are, therefore, responsible for tissue tropism. Adhesion is necessary to avoid innate host defence mechanisms such as peristalsis in the gut and the flushing action of mucus, saliva and urine which remove nonadherent bacteria. Loss of adhesins may render a strain avirulent.

2. Invasion of Tissues

Invasiveness signifies the ability of an organism to penetrate a tissue after it adheres to a cell surface. Some bacteria can invade tissues in the absence of physical injury, e.g. *N. meningitidis* in nasal epithelium and salmonellae in intestinal epithelium. These organisms are endocytosed by epithelial cells, transported across these cells within vacuoles and released into the submucosal space, from which they invade the underlying tissues.

3. Capsules

Cell wall in many bacteria is enclosed by a protective gelatinous covering layer known as capsule. It contributes to the virulence of the bacteria by inhibiting phagocytosis. Virtually all the pathogens associated with meningitis and pneumonia including *H. influenzae*, *N. meningitidis*, and *S. pneumoniae* are capsulated, and non-capsulated variants usually exhibit much reduced virulence. Some bacterial surface antigens such as Vi antigen of *S.* serotype Typhi and K antigen of *E. coli* also help the bacteria to withstand phagocytosis and the lytic activity of complement.

4. Bacterial Toxins

These are substances produced by or present in bacteria, which have a direct toxic action on tissue cells. Two major types of toxin have been described—endotoxins and exotoxins (Table 5.3).

5. Streptococcal M Protein

The M protein present on the surface of *S. pyogenes* binds both fibrinogen and fibrin to the bacterial cell wall thus masking the bacterial receptors from complement.

6. Enzymes

Many species of bacteria produce tissue-degrading enzymes that play important roles in the infection process. Some of these enzymes are lecithinase-C, coagulase, hyaluronidases, streptokinase (fibrinolysin), cytolysins and IgA1 proteases.

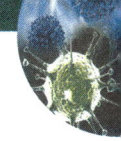

TABLE 5.3: Differences between exotoxins and endotoxins

Exotoxins	Endotoxins
Proteins with high molecular weight ranging from 10,000 to 900,000.	Lipopolysaccharide in nature. Lipid A portion is probably responsible for the toxicity.
Heat-labile. The toxicity is destroyed by heating above 60°C.	Heat-stable. Can withstand heat over 60°C without losing toxicity.
Highly antigenic; stimulate formation of antitoxin which neutralizes toxin.	Weakly antigenic; do not stimulate the formation of antitoxin. Antibodies against only polysaccharide component are raised
Actively secreted by the cells; diffuse into the surrounding medium.	Form integral part of the cell wall; do not diffuse into surrounding medium. These can be obtained only by cell lysis.
Converted into toxoid by formaldehyde.	Cannot be toxoided.
Action often enzymic.	No enzymic action.
Specific pharmacological effect for each exotoxin.	Non-specific action of all endotoxins.
Highly specific for particular tissue, e.g. tetanus toxin for CNS.	Non-specific in action.
Very high potency (one mg of botulinum or tetanus toxin can kill more than one million guinea pigs).	Low potency (one mg of extracted somatic antigen can kill one mouse).
Do not produce fever in the host.	Usually produce fever in the host.
Produced by both Gram-positive bacteria and Gram-negative bacteria	Produced by Gram-negative bacteria only.
Frequently controlled by extrachromosomal genes (e.g. plasmids).	Synthesis directed by chromosomal genes.

Key Points

- **Pathogens** are microorganisms which are capable of producing disease in man.
- **Commensals** (organisms of normal flora) are the microorganisms which live in complete harmony with the host without causing any damage to it.
- Infection may be **endogenous**, due to the organisms of the normal flora, and **exogenous**, due to the organisms derived from a source outside the body.
- **Endotoxins** are the lipopolysaccharide components of cell walls of Gram-negative bacteria and hence, by definition, Gram-positive bacteria do not have endotoxins.
- **Exotoxins** are produced by both Gram-positive and Gram-negative bacteria.

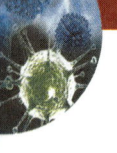

SECTION III • INFECTION CONTROL AND SAFETY

 ## Assess Yourself

LONG ANSWER QUESTIONS

1. What are the various modes of spread of infection? Describe each in brief giving suitable examples.
2. Distinguish between exotoxins and endotoxins in a tabulated form.
3. Define the terms 'pathogenicity' and 'virulence'. Name and discuss various determinants of virulence.

MULTIPLE CHOICE QUESTIONS

1. Tetanus is transmitted by:
   (a) Inoculation
   (b) Inhalation
   (c) Ingestion
   (d) Insect bite

2. Exotoxins **do not** have which of the following characteristics?
   (a) They are produced extracellularly
   (b) They are produced by both Gram-positive and Gram-negative bacteria
   (c) Cannot be converted into toxoids
   (d) They are heat-labile

3. Which of the following infections is acquired from animals?
   (a) Plague
   (b) Diphtheria
   (c) Meningitis
   (d) Poliomyelitis

4. Which of the following infections is **not** spread by the respiratory route?
   (a) Common cold
   (b) Measles
   (c) Mumps
   (d) Hepatitis B

5. Large number of bacteria forming normal flora are found:
   (a) In the mouth
   (b) On the skin
   (c) In the large intestine
   (d) In the nose

6. Infectious agents can enter the body through which of the following routes?
   (a) Inhalation
   (b) Ingestion
   (c) Inoculation
   (d) All of the above

ANSWERS TO MCQs

1. a   **2.** c   **3.** a   **4.** d   **5.** c   **6.** d

Chapter 6

Sterilization and Disinfection, and Biomedical Waste Management

Sterilization and Disinfection

Sterilization is defined as the process by which an article, a surface or a medium is freed of all microorganisms including viruses, bacteria, their spores and fungi, both pathogenic and non-pathogenic.

Disinfection is a process of destruction or removal of organisms capable of giving rise to infection. Disinfectants are capable of killing vegetative bacteria, fungi, viruses and rarely bacterial spores.

Antisepsis is the destruction or inhibition of microorganisms in living tissues thereby limiting or preventing the harmful effects of infection. A disinfectant that is applied to living tissue is referred to as an **antiseptic**.

Various agents used in sterilization and disinfection may be divided into:

- **Physical agents**
  - Sunlight
  - Drying
  - Heat
  - Filtration
  - Radiations
- **Chemical agents**
  - Phenols and cresols
  - Halogens
  - Aldehydes
  - Alcohols
  - Dyes
  - Vapour-phase disinfectants
  - Surface active disinfectants

PHYSICAL AGENTS

Sunlight

Sunlight possesses ultraviolet rays which along with heat rays are responsible for appreciable germicidal activity. These rays, however, cannot penetrate through glass, i.e. window panes. This is one of the natural methods of sterilization of water in tanks, rivers and lakes.

Drying

Water constitutes 80% of the weight of the bacteria and is also essential for the growth of bacteria. Therefore, drying has deleterious effect on many bacteria. However, spores are unaffected by drying.

Heat

Heat is the most reliable, certain and rapid method of sterilization. It can be easily controlled and unlike chemical disinfection, leaves no potentially harmful residue. Unless the material to be sterilized is heat-sensitive, this method should be preferred.

There are two types of heat—dry heat and wet heat.

- **Dry heat:** It is believed to kill microorganisms by causing destructive oxidation of essential cell constituents. Dry heat at 100°C for 60 minutes and 115°C for 60 minutes can kill all vegetative bacteria and fungal spores respectively. Bacterial spores can be killed by dry heat at 160°C for one hour or 180°C for 20 minutes. On the whole dry heat is less efficient sterilization process than moist heat.
- **Moist heat:** It causes denaturation and coagulation of proteins. When steam condenses on cooler surface, it releases its latent heat and raises the temperature of its surface. If spores are present, steam condenses on them and increases their water content leading to hydrolysis and breakdown of bacterial proteins.

Sterilization by Dry Heat

Red Heat

Inoculating wires and *loops*, *points of forceps* and *spatulas* are sterilized by holding them almost vertical in a bunsen burner flame until red hot (Table 6.1).

Flaming

Scalpel blades, *needles*, *mouths of culture tubes* and *bottles*, *glass slides* and *coverslips* are sterilized by passing the article through the Bunsen flame without allowing them to become red hot.

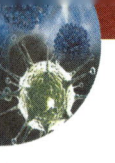

TABLE 6.1: Sterilization by dry heat

Mode of sterilization	Instrument	Temperature and time	Sterilization of	Advantages/disadvantages
Red heat	Bunsen burner	Till red hot	Inoculating wires and loops, points of forceps and spatulas	Sterilization is rapid and thorough
Flaming	Bunsen burner	Waving through the flame	Scalpel blades, needles, mouths of culture tubes and bottles, glass slides and cover slips	1. Surface sterilization is possible 2. Rapid method
Hot air	Hot air oven	160°C for 1 hour or 180°C for 20 minutes	Glassware, metal instruments, sealed materials such as oils, greases, dry powder, etc.	Can be used for loads that cannot be penetrated by steam

Incineration

This is an efficient method for rapidly destroying contaminated materials such as *soiled dressings* and *pathological materials*, etc.

Hot Air Oven

It is a method of choice for sterilization of glassware such as *test tubes, Petri dishes, pipettes* and *flasks, metal instruments* such as *forceps, scissors* and *scalpels,* sealed materials such as *oils, greases* and *dry powder* which are impervious to steam and *swab sticks* packed in test tubes. It is not suitable for materials like fabrics which may be damaged by heat.

Hot air oven is electrically heated and is fitted with a thermostat that maintains the chamber air at a chosen temperature and a fan that distributes hot air in the chamber (Fig. 6.1). It must not be overloaded and spaces must be left for circulation of air through the load. Holding time for sterilization in hot air oven is **one hour at 160°C** or **20 minutes at 180°C**. It is timed as beginning when the thermometer first shows 160°C or 180°C respectively.

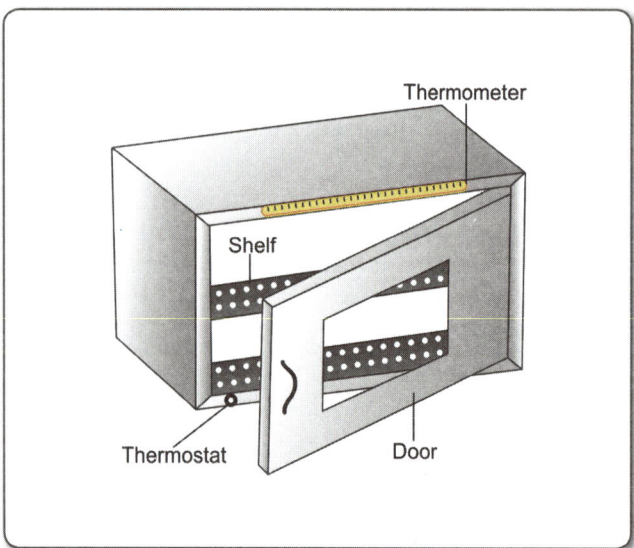

Fig. 6.1: Hot air oven.

Sterilization controls

Two types of controls are available.
- ***Biological control:*** An envelope containing a filter paper strip impregnated with 10^6 spores of *Bacillus subtilis* subsp. *niger* (NCTC 10075 or ATCC 9372) is placed within the load (Table 6.2). After sterilization is over, the strip is removed and inoculated into tryptone soy broth and incubated aerobically at 37°C for five days. No growth of *B. subtilis* subsp. *niger* indicates proper sterilization.
- ***Chemical control:*** A Browne's tube containing red solution is placed within the load. A change of colour of the solution to green indicates proper sterilization.

Sterilization by Moist Heat

Sterilization by moist heat means killing of the microorganisms with hot water or steam. Moist heat is divided into 3 forms (Table 6.3):
- *At temperatures below 100°C.*
- *At a temperature of 100°C.*
  - Boiling water
  - Free steam
- *At temperature above 100°C.*

TABLE 6.2: Biological controls of different sterilization methods

Method of sterilization	Biological control
Hot air oven	*Bacillus subtilis* subsp. *niger*
Autoclave	*Bacillus stearothermophilus*
Ethylene oxide	*Bacillus globigi* (a red-pigmented variant of *Bacillus subtilis*)
Filtration	*Serratia marcescens, Pseudomonas diminuta*
Ionizing radiations	*Bacillus pumilis*

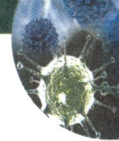

TABLE 6.3: **Sterilization by moist heat**

Mode of sterilization	Instrument	Temperature and time	Sterilization of	Advantages/ disadvantages
Below 100°C	Water bath	56°C for 1 hour	Serum	May be used for disinfection. Most vegetative mesophilic bacteria are killed.
At 100°C	Boiling water bath	100°C for 10–20 min.	Glass, metal and rubber items	Kills all vegetative bacteria and some spores.
Steaming at 100°C	Arnold steamer	100°C for 20 minutes on 3 successive days	Culture media containing sugar and gelatin	Prevents decomposition of media. Spores of bacteria may escape killing.
Steaming above 100°C	Autoclave	121°C for 15–20 minutes	Culture media and other aqueous solutions, dressing material, linen, gloves, etc.	Most reliable method of sterilization.

Moist Heat at Temperatures below 100°C

Heat-labile fluids may be disinfected (not sterilized) by heating at temperatures below 100°C. Such treatment is sufficient to kill mesophilic vegetative bacteria. This includes:

- **Pasteurization** of milk. The temperature employed is either **63°C for 30 minutes** (holder method) or **72°C for 20 seconds** (flash method) followed by rapid cooling to 13°C or lower. By this method non-sporing organisms such as mycobacteria *Brucella* and salmonellae are destroyed. However, *Coxiella burnetii*, causative agent of Q fever, may survive pasteurization by holder method.

  The flash method is preferable for pasteurization of milk because it is less likely to change the flavour and nutrient content, and it is more effective against pathogens such as *C. burnetii*. Although pasteurization inactivates most viruses and vegetative stages of bacteria and fungi, they do not kill spores and thermoresistant species (mostly non-pathogenic lactobacilli, micrococci, and yeasts). Therefore, milk is not sterile after regular pasteurization, which explains why even unopened carton of milk will eventually spoil on prolonged storage. Newer techniques have now been used to produce sterile milk that has storage of 3 months. In this method, the milk is processed **with ultrahigh temperature of 134°C for 1–2 seconds**.

- **Heat-labile fluids** such as serum may be disinfected by heating at 56°C for one hour. If temperature rises above 59°C it will coagulate.

- **Vaccines** prepared from non-sporing bacteria may be inactivated in a water bath at 60°C for one hour.

- **Household utensils and patient's clothing** may be disinfected by washing in water at 70–80°C for several minutes.

- Media such as Lowenstein-Jensen and Loeffler's serum slope are rendered sterile by heating at 80–85°C for half an hour on three successive days in an inspissator.

- Items which cannot withstand heat at 100°C may be disinfected by steam at sub-atmospheric pressure at a temperature of 75°C with formaldehyde vapour. This is known as **low temperature steam-formaldehyde (LTSF) sterilization**.

Moist Heat at a Temperature of 100°C

- **Boiling at 100°C:** Boiling at **100°C for 10–30 minutes** kills all vegetative bacteria and some bacterial spores. Therefore, it is not recommended for sterilization of instruments for surgical procedures.

- **Free steam at 100°C:** Steam at normal atmospheric pressure is at 100°C. But, in addition, it has latent heat which on condensing on the article to be sterilized releases its latent heat. A **Koch** or **Arnold steam sterilizer** consists of a vertical metal cylinder with a removable conical lid having a small opening for the escaping steam. Water is added on the bottom and there is a perforated shelf above water level (Fig. 6.2). On this shelf articles to be sterilized are placed. One single exposure to steam for 90 minutes ensures complete sterilization but for media containing *sugar* and *gelatin*, which may get decomposed on long heating, an exposure of **100°C for 20 minutes on three consecutive days** is employed. This is known as **tyndallization** or **intermittent sterilization**. First exposure to steam kills all vegetative bacteria and any spores present, being in a favourable medium, will germinate and will be killed on the subsequent occasions. Therefore, non nutrient media cannot be sterilized by this method.

Moist Heat at Temperature above 100°C

Steam above 100°C or saturated steam is a more efficient sterilizing agent than hot air because:

- It provides greater lethal action of moist heat.
- It is quicker in heating up the exposed articles.

SECTION III • INFECTION CONTROL AND SAFETY

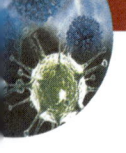

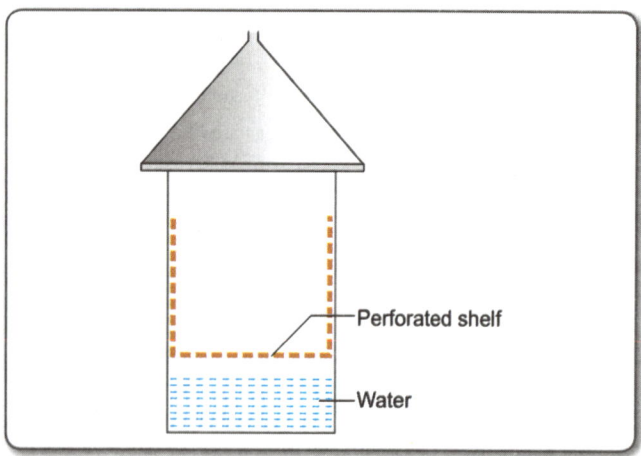

Fig. 6.2: Steam sterilizer.

- It can penetrate easily porous material such as cotton wool stoppers, paper and cloth wrappers, bundles of surgical linen, and hollow apparatus.

When the steam meets the cooler surface of the article, it condenses into a small volume of water and liberates its considerable latent heat to that surface, for example, 1600 ml of steam at 100°C, i.e. at atmospheric pressure condenses into 1 ml of water at 100°C liberating 518 calories of heat. The large contraction in volume brings more steam to the same site and the process continues until the temperature of the article is raised to that of steam. The water of condensation ensures moist conditions for killing of the exposed microorganisms. Pure steam must be used and the presence of air avoided since air hinders penetration by the steam.

Water boils when its pressure equals the pressure of the surrounding atmosphere. When the atmospheric pressure is raised then the boiling temperature is also raised. At normal pressure water boils at 100°C but when it is boiled in a closed vessel at increased pressure the temperature at which it boils and that of the steam it forms rises above 100°C. This principle has been exploited in autoclave and pressure cooker.

Sterilization by **steam under pressure (autoclaving)** is suitable for *culture media* and *aqueous solutions* (since atmosphere of steam prevents evaporation during heating), *dressing material, linen, gloves, etc.* Satisfactory sterilization can be achieved at **15 pounds per square inch** (psi) pressure equivalent to **121°C in 15–20 minutes**. In fact the only practical and dependable method of sterilization is steam under pressure using different types of autoclaves. However, the autoclave is unfit for sterilizing substances that repel moisture (oils, waxes or powders).

All the air must be removed from the autoclave chamber and the articles to be sterilized so that the latter are exposed to pure steam. There are three reasons for this:

- The admixture of air with steam results in lower temperature being achieved.
- Air hinders penetration of steam into the interstices of porous materials, surgical dressings, syringes, etc.

- The air being denser forms a separate and cooler layer in the lower part of the autoclave, so it prevents adequate heating of articles there.

Several types of steam sterilizers are available. The **laboratory autoclave or pressure cooker type autoclave** (Fig. 6.3) consists of a vertical or horizontal cylinder of gun metal or stainless steel in a supporting frame or case. The lid is fastened by screw clamp and rendered air tight by asbestos gasket. Lid bears a pressure gauge and a steam release valve or safety valve. The latter opens and closes when the steam pressure rises or falls the desired level, respectively. On its upper part of the side, the autoclave has a discharge tap for air and steam and an air and steam release knob. Heating is done by electricity. Water is added on the bottom of the autoclave. Above this is a perforated shelf on which articles to be sterilized are placed.

The lid is closed, discharge tap is opened and safety valve is adjusted to the required pressure. As heating continues, the steam and air mixture escapes. To know when all the air inside the autoclave has escaped the discharge tap is connected with one end of a rubber tube and the other end of it is placed in water. When the air bubbles stop coming it indicates that all the air from inside the autoclave has been removed. The discharge tap is now closed. Steam pressure rises inside and when it reaches the desired set level (15 psi) the safety valve opens and excess steam escapes. From this point the **holding time** (15 minutes) is counted.

When the holding time is over, the heating is stopped and autoclave allowed to cool till pressure gauze indicates that inside pressure has reached to the atmospheric pressure. The discharge tap is now opened and air allowed to enter the autoclave. The lid is now opened and the sterilized articles removed. If the tap or lid is opened when the pressure inside is high the liquid media boil violently and may explode. On the other hand, if the articles are not removed for a long time after the normal atmospheric

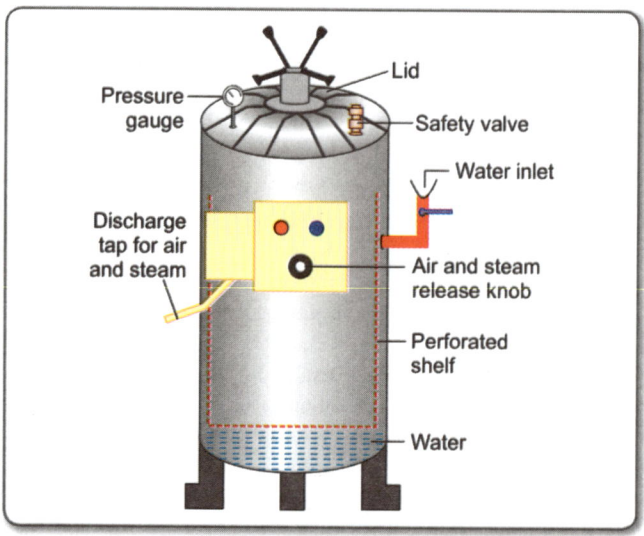

Fig. 6.3: Autoclave.

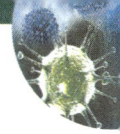

pressure has reached inside the autoclave, an excessive amount of water will be evaporated and lost from the media.

Sterilization controls

Two types of controls are available:

- **Biological control:** An envelope containing a filter paper strip impregnated with 10^6 spores of *Bacillus stearothermophilus* (NCTC 10003 or ATCC 7953) is placed with the load in the coolest and least accessible part of the autoclave chamber (Table 6.2). After sterilization is over the strip is removed and inoculated into tryptone soy broth and incubated aerobically at 56°C for 5 days. No growth of *B. stearothermophilus* indicates proper sterilization. Spores of this organism withstand 121°C for up to 12 minutes and this has made the organism ideal for testing autoclaves.
- **Chemical control:** A Browne's tube containing red solution is placed within the load. A change of colour of the solution red to green indicates proper sterilization.

Filtration

Liquids such as sera and solutions of heat-labile substances such as *sugars* and *urea*, used for preparation of media, can be sterilized by filtration. This method is also useful for:

- sterilization of pharmacological substances,
- *separation of bacteriophages and bacterial toxins from bacteria,* and
- *isolation of organisms which are scanty in fluids.*

The filter disc retains the organisms which can then be cultured.

Limitations

Mycoplasma and viruses, which are very small, cannot be kept back by the bacterial filters, therefore, serum sterilized by filtration cannot be employed for clinical use. *Serratia marcescens* and *Pseudomonas diminuta* have been used to test the efficacy of different filters (Table 6.2). Several types of filters are now available. These include earthenware filters, asbestos (Seitz) filters, sintered glass filters, membrane filters, syringe filters, and air filters.

Radiations

Two types of radiations are used:

- Non-ionizing.
- Ionizing.

Non-ionizing Radiations

- **Ultraviolet (UV) radiations:** Ultraviolet radiations in the range of 250–260 nm wavelength are highly effective. Low pressure mercury vapour lamps emit over 95% of radiations with the wavelength of 253.7 nm. Most vegetative bacteria are susceptible to UV radiations. Spores are highly resistant and susceptibility of viruses is variable. Human immunodeficiency virus is not inactivated by UV radiations. UV radiations induce thymine dimers in DNA and this interferes with DNA replication. They can penetrate only a few mm into liquids and not at all into solids. Therefore, their use is best restricted to disinfection of clean surfaces like *inoculation hoods, laboratories, wards,* and *operation theatres.* Source of UV radiations must be shielded to prevent the radiations falling on eyes and skin because it may damage them.
- **Infrared rays:** Infrared rays bring about sterilization by generation of heat. Articles to be sterilized are placed in a moving conveyor belt and passed through a tunnel that is heated by infrared radiators to a temperature of 180°C. The articles are exposed to that temperature for a period of 7.5 minutes. Articles sterilized include metallic instruments and glassware. It is mainly used in central sterile supply department. Efficiency can be checked by using Browne's tube No. 4 (blue spot).

Ionizing Radiations

These include *X-rays, gamma rays* and *cosmic rays.* These have very high penetrative power and are highly lethal to all cells including bacteria. They damage DNA by various mechanisms. Spores are more resistant than vegetative bacteria. Large commercial plants use gamma radiations for sterilization of prepacked disposable items such as *plastic syringes, transfusion sets, catheters, cannulas, culture plates,* etc. that are unable to withstand heat because there is no appreciable increase in the temperature. Therefore, this method is known as **cold sterilization**. *Bacillus pumilis* has been used to test the efficacy of ionizing radiations (Table 6.2).

CHEMICAL AGENTS

Phenols and Cresols

These are obtained by distillation of coal tar and have a powerful microbicidal action. They cause cell membrane damage thus releasing cell contents and causing cell lysis. They are resistant to inactivation by organic matter and are active against Gram-positive and Gram-negative bacteria, moderately active against mycobacteria and have little activity against spores and viruses. They are used mainly for *discarded cultures, contaminated pipettes and other infected material.* Phenol is bactericidal at a concentration of 1%. At a concentration of 0.5% it is used for preservation of sera and vaccines.

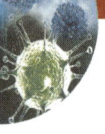

Halogens

Chlorine and iodine are the halogens which are used as disinfectants. They are bactericidal and sporicidal. They are active in very high dilutions and their action is very rapid. In addition to chlorine itself there are three types of chlorine compounds, the hypochlorites, and the inorganic and organic chloramines. The disinfectant action of all the chlorine compounds is due to release of free chlorine. When elemental chlorine or hypochlorites are added to water, the chlorine reacts with water to form hypochlorous acid. It is a strong oxidising agent and effective disinfectant. The activity of chlorine is markedly influenced by the presence of organic matter. Sodium hypochlorite, chloramine and bleaching powder are most widely used for disinfection of HIV infected material. Hypochlorite solution decays rapidly, therefore, it should be prepared daily.

Chlorine has a special place in the *treatment of water supply* and combinations of hypochlorite and detergents are useful for cleansing and disinfection in food and dairy industry. Hypochlorites have a wide spectrum of activity against viruses and very little activity against tubercle bacilli. They are available in liquid or powder form as salts of calcium, lithium and sodium.

Iodine in alcoholic and aqueous solutions is used almost exclusively as a *skin disinfectant* (antiseptic). Like chlorine, it is also inactivated by organic matter. It is also active against tubercle bacilli and a number of viruses. Mixtures of iodine with various surface active agents that act as carriers for iodine are known as **iodophores**, an example of this is **betadine**. It can be used as a *bactericidal antiseptic for intact skin* and for *disinfection of superficial wounds*. It is also active against fungi and *Trichomonas*.

Aldehydes

Two aldehydes (formaldehyde and glutaraldehyde) are currently of considerable importance, although others also possess antimicrobial activity.

- **Formaldehyde:**
  It is an aldehyde generally used as formalin, a 37% aqueous solution of formaldehyde gas. Formaldehyde gas is often used for sterilization of rooms, furniture and a wide variety of articles likely to be damaged by heat, such as clothing, woolen blankets, mattresses, respirators, heat-sensitive instruments, etc. However, its usefulness is limited by its irritability factor and its protential carcinogenicity. Therefore, formaldehyde should not be used as a disinfectant or sterilant on a routine basis.

- **Glutaraldehyde:**
  It is more effective and less irritant than formaldehyde. It possesses high microbicidal activity against bacteria and their spores, mycelial and spore forms of fungi and various types of viruses, including human immunodeficiency viruses and enteroviruses. Two per cent alkaline buffered solution is germicidal in approximately 10 minutes and sporicidal in 3–10 hours. It is used for sterilization of heat-sensitive instruments like *cystoscopes*, *bronchoscopes*, *thermometers*, etc.

Alcohols

Several alcohols possess antimicrobial activity. The antimicrobial activity of alcohols can be attributed to their ability to denature proteins. Alcohol solutions containing 60–70% alcohol are most effective, and higher concentrations are less potent because proteins are not denatured easily in the absence of water. They are active against vegetative bacteria including tubercle bacilli, fungi and lipid-containing viruses but not against spores.

- **Isopropyl alcohol** is preferred over ethyl alcohol as it is a better fat solvent, more bactericidal and less volatile. It is commonly used for *disinfection of clinical thermometers*.
- **Methyl alcohol** is effective against fungal spores.
- **Alcohol based handrubs** are recommended for the decontamination of highly soiled hands in situations where proper hand washing is inconvenient or not possible.

Dyes

Two groups of dyes, the aniline dyes and the acridine dyes have been used extensively as skin and wound antiseptics. Both groups are bacteriostatic in high dilution but have low bactericidal activity. They are much more active against Gram-positive than Gram-negative bacteria.

- **Aniline dyes** include brilliant green, malachite green and crystal violet. Their activity is inhibited by the presence of organic matter like pus. They have no activity against tubercle bacilli, therefore, addition of malachite green to Lowenstein-Jensen medium makes it selective for the isolation of tubercle bacilli. They interfere with the synthesis of the peptidoglycan component of the cell wall.
- **Acridine dyes** include acriflavine, proflavine, euflavine and aminacrine. They are little, if at all, affected by the presence of organic matter. Acridine dyes interfere with the synthesis of nucleic acids and proteins in both bacterial and mammalian cells.

Vapour-phase Disinfectants

Two most important vapour-phase agents are ethylene oxide and formaldehyde.

- **Ethylene oxide:** It is a colourless gas soluble in water. It is highly lethal to all kinds of microbes including spores and tubercle bacilli. It is useful for sterilization of articles liable to be damaged by heat, e.g. *plastic and rubber articles*, *blankets*, *pharmaceutical products* (*crude drugs and powders*) and *complex apparatus* such as *heart-lung machines*. It is highly effective sterilizing agent because it rapidly penetrates packing material, even plastic wraps. It forms explosive mixture when more than 3% is present in air. This hazard can be overcome by using a mixture of 10% ethylene oxide in carbon dioxide. It has an alkylating action on proteins. Inhibition produced by it is irreversible, resulting in enzyme modification and inhibition of enzyme activity. *Bacillus globigi*, a red-pigmented variant of *B. subtilis*, has been used to test ethylene oxide sterilizers (Table 6.2).

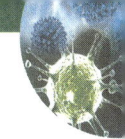

- **Formaldehyde gas:** It is liberated by spraying or heating of formalin, by addition of formalin to potassium permanganate or by volatilization of paraformaldehyde. Its antimicrobial activity depends upon several factors. The atmosphere must have a high relative humidity (more than 60% and preferably 80–90%) and a temperature of at least 18°C.

It is used for fumigation of operation theatres, wards and laboratories. After sealing the windows and other outlets formaldehyde gas is generated by adding 150 g of potassium permanganate to 280 ml of formalin for every 1000 cubic feet of room volume. Rooms are left unopened for 48 hours. Then open the doors and windows to allow vapours to disperse and neutralize any residual formaldehyde with ammonia by exposing 250 ml of SG 880 ammonia per litre of formalin used.

Beta-propiolactone (BPL) is a condensation product of ketone and formaldehyde. It is active against all microorganisms including viruses. In liquid form it is used to sterilize vaccines and sera. It is more efficient than formaldehyde for fumigation purpose. BPL destroys microorganisms more readily than ethylene oxide but does not penetrate materials well and may be carcinogenic. For these reasons, BPL has not been used as extensively as ethylene oxide.

Hydrogen Peroxide Fogging

This is a better method replacing fumigation. It is done by fogging machine using hydrogen peroxide as disinfectant. It has the advantage of short cycle time and is non toxic.

Surface Active Disinfectants

Substances that alter the energy relationships at interfaces leading to reduction of surface or interfacial tension, are known as **surface active agents** or **surfactants**. They possess both hydrophobic (water-repelling) and hydrophilic (water-attracting) groups. On the basis of charge or the absence of ionization of the hydrophilic group, these surfactants are classified into anionic, cationic, non-ionic and amphoteric compounds. **Non-ionic surfactants** do not have antimicrobial activity.

Cationic compounds such as quarternary ammonium compounds are the most important surfactants. They are essentially bacteriostatic and are more active against Gram-positive than Gram-negative bacteria. They are also fungistatic and active against viruses with lipid envelopes (e.g. herpes and influenza) and much less against nonenveloped viruses (e.g. enteroviruses). Commercially available preparations of cationic compounds include cetrimide (cetavalon), benzalkonium chloride and laurodin.

Anionic surfactants such as common soaps usually have strong detergent but weak antimicrobial properties.

Amphoteric agents such as tego compounds possess detergent properties of anionic and antimicrobial activity of cationic compounds.

Table 6.4 gives a list and the recommended concentration of disinfectants commonly used in the hospitals.

TABLE 6.4: List and the recommended concentrations of disinfectants commonly used in the hospitals

Disinfectant	Recommended concentration
Ethanol	70% (700 g/litre)
Methylated spirit	70% (700 g/litre)
Glutaraldehyde	2% activated (available commercially as cidex)
Bleaching powder (calcium hypochlorite)	14 g/litre of water
Sodium hypochlorite	1% solution, 0.1% solution
Hydrogen peroxide	3% solution
Lysol	2.5% solution
Savlon®	2.0%, 5.0%
Dettol®	4.0%
Betadine	2.0%

Biomedical Waste Management

BIOMEDICAL WASTE (BMW)

It is a broader term applied to waste generated in the diagnosis, treatment or immunization of human beings or animals, in research or in the production or testing or biological products. It also includes waste coming out of medical treatment given at home.

Infectious Waste

Medical waste which has the potential to transmit viral, bacterial or parasitic diseases. It includes both human and animal infectious waste and waste generated in laboratories, and veterinary practice. Infectious waste is harzardous in nature.

Hazardous Waste

Waste which has a potential to pose a threat to human health and life. The persons most at risk are the staff of hospitals particularly nurses and waste handlers. In countries such as India, scavengers and ragpickers are at serious risk.

WASTE SEGREGATION

The biomedical waste shall be segregated into containers or bags at the point of generation, since 80% of the waste is non-hazardous and can be disposed of easily into the municipal bin. It is important that hazardous waste component is separated from non-hazardous waste. Mixing of waste will render the entire waste potentially hazardous. Waste should be segregated in bags of different colours to facilitate appropriate treatment and disposal. Table 6.5 shows biomedical waste categories and their segregation, collection, treatment, processing and disposal options.

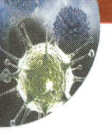

SECTION III • INFECTION CONTROL AND SAFETY

TABLE 6.5: Biomedial waste categories and their segregation, collection, treatment, processing and disposal options

Category	Type of waste	Type of bag or container to be used	Treatment and disposal options
Yellow	(a) **Human anatomical waste**: Human tissues, organs, body parts and foetus below the viability period (as per the Medical Termination of Pregnancy Act 1971, amended from time to time)	Yellow-coloured non-chlorinated plastic bags	Incineration or plasma pyrolysis or deep burial*.
	(b) **Animal anatomical waste**: Experimental animal carcasses, body parts, organs, tissues, including the waste generated from animals used in experiments or testing in veterinary hospitals or colleges or animal houses.		
	(c) **Soiled waste**: Items contaminated with blood, body fluids like dressings, plaster casts, cotton swabs and bags containing residual or discarded blood and blood components.		Incineration or plasma pyrolysis or deep burial*. In the absence of above facilities, autoclaving or microwaving/hydroclaving followed by shredding or multilation or combination of sterilization and shredding. Treated waste to be sent for energy recovery.
	(d) **Expired or discarded medicines:** Pharmaceutical waste like antibiotics, cytotoxic drugs including all items contaminated with cytotoxic drugs along with glass or plastic ampoules vials, etc.	Yellow-coloured non-chlorinated plastic bags of containers	Expired cytotoxic drugs and items contaminated with cytotoxic drugs to be returned to the manufacturer or supplied for incineration at temperature >1200°C or to common biomedical waste treatment facility or hazardous waste treatment, storage and disposal facility for incineration at >1200°C or encapsulation or plasma pyrolysis at >1200°C. All other discarded medicines shall be either sent back to manufacturer or disposed by incineration.
	(e) **Chemical waste:** Chemicals used in production of biologicals and used or discarded disinfectants.	Yellow-coloured containers or non-chlorinated plastic bags	Disposed of by incineration or plasma pyrolysis or encapsulation in hazardous waste treatment, storage and disposal facility.
	(f) **Chemical liquid waste:** Liquid waste generated due to use of chemicals in production of biologicals and used or discarded disinfectants, silver X-ray film developing liquid, discarded formalin, infected secretions, aspirated body fluids, liquid from laboratories and floor washings, cleaning, housekeeping and disinfecting activities, etc.	Separate collection system leading to effluent treatment system	After resource recovery, the chemical liquid waste shall be pre-treated before mixing with other waste water.

Contd...

* Disposal by deep burial is permitted only in rural or remote area where there is no access to common biomedical waste treatment facility. This will be carried out with prior approval from the prescribed authority and as per the standards specified in Schedule III. The deep burial facility shall be located as per the provisions and guidelines issued by Central Pollution Control Board from time to time.

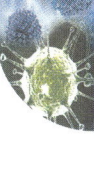

Category	Type of waste	Type of bag or container to be used	Treatment and disposal options
	(g) Discarded linen, mattresses, beddings contaminated with blood or body fluid.	Non-chlorinated yellow plastic bags or suitable packing material	Non-chlorinated chemical disinfection followed by incineration or plasma pyrolysis or for energy recovery. In the absence of above facilities, shredding or mutilation or combination of sterilization and shredding. Treated waste to be sent for energy recovery or incineration or plasma pyrolysis.
	(h) **Microbiology, biotechnology and other clinical laboratory waste:** Blood bags, laboratory cultures, stocks or specimens of microorganisms, live or attenuated vaccines, human and animal cell cultures used in research, industrial laboratories, production of biologicals, residual toxins, dishes and devices used for cultures.	Autoclave-safe plastic bags or containers	Pre-treat to sterilize with non-chlorinated chemicals on-site as per National AIDS Control Organisation or World Health Organisation guidelines thereafter for incineration.
Red	**Contaminated waste (Recyclable):** Wastes generated from disposable items such as tubings, bottles, intravenous tubes and sets, catheters, urine bags, syringes (without needles and fixed needle syringes and vacutainers with their needles cut and gloves.	Red-coloured non-chlorinated plastic bags or containers	Autoclaving or microwaving/hydroclaving followed by shredding or multilation or combination of sterilization and shredding. Treated waste to be sent to registered or authorized recyclers or for energy recovery or plastics to diesel or fuel oil or for road making, whichever is possible. Plastic waste should not be sent to landfill sites.
White (Translucent)	**Waste sharps including metals:** Needles, syringes with fixed needles, needles from needle tip cutter or burner, scalpels, blades, or any other contaminated sharp object that may cause puncture and cuts. This includes both used, discarded and contaminated metal sharps.	Puncture-proof, leak-proof, tamper-proof containers	Autoclaving or dry heat sterilization followed by shredding or mutilation or encapsulation in metal container or cement concrete; combination of shredding-cum-autoclaving; and sent for final disposal to iron foundries (having consent to operate from the State Pollution Control Boards or Pollution Control Committees) or sanitary landfill or designated concrete waste sharp pit.
Blue	(a) **Glassware:** Broken or discarded and contaminated glass including medicine vials and ampoules except those contaminated with cytotoxic wastes.	Cardboard boxes with blue-coloured marking	Disinfection (by soaking the washed glass waste after cleaning the detergent and sodium hypochlorite treatment) or through autoclaving or microwaving or hydroclaving and then sent for recycling.
	(b) **Metallic body implants**	Cardboard boxes with blue-coloured marking	

Note:
1. Microbiological waste and all other clinical laboratory waste shall be pre-treated by sterilization before packing and sending to the common biomedical waste treatment facility.
2. Mutilation or shredding must be to an extent to prevent unauthorized reuse.
3. Autoclaving of medical waste shall be done at a temperature of not less than 121°C and pressure of 15 pounds per square inch for not less than 60 minutes.

SECTION III • INFECTION CONTROL AND SAFETY

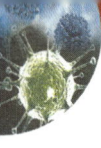

SECTION III • INFECTION CONTROL AND SAFETY

✂ Key Points

- **Sterilization** is a process that *kills* or *removes all* organisms (and their spores) in a material or an object.
- **Disinfection** is a process that *kills* or *removes pathogenic organisms* in a material or an object.
- **Antisepsis** is the application of a chemical agent externally on a *live surface* (skin or mucosa) to destroy organisms or to inhibit their growth (all antiseptics are disinfectants but not vice versa).
- **Sterilization** is usually achieved by *moist heat* (steam under pressure in an autoclave; most popular), *dry heat* (hot air oven) or gaseous chemicals.
- **Biomedical waste** should be *segregated at source*, since 80% of the waste is non-hazardous and can be disposed of easily into the municipal bin; waste should be segregated in bags of different colours to facilitate appropriate treatment and disposal.

? Assess Yourself

Long and Short Answer Questions

1. Define the terms sterilization, disinfection and antisepsis. Name various agents used for sterilization and discuss the role of hot air oven in sterilization.
2. Discuss the role of moist heat in sterilization.
3. Write short notes on:
   - (a) Hot air oven
   - (b) Autoclave
   - (c) Sterilization by filtration
   - (d) Sterilization by radiation

Multiple Choice Questions

1. Destruction or inhibition of microorganisms in living tissues is known as:
   - (a) Sterilization
   - (b) Disinfection
   - (c) Antisepsis
   - (d) None of the above
2. Incineration is an efficient method for:
   - (a) Destroying contaminated materials
   - (b) Sterilizing points of forceps
   - (c) Sterilizing scalpel blades and needles
   - (d) Sterilizing all glass syringes
3. Red heat is used for sterilization of:
   - (a) Inoculating wires and loops
   - (b) All glass syringes
   - (c) Soiled dressings
   - (d) Glass slides
4. Biological control used in an autoclave is the spores of:
   - (a) *Bacillus stearothermophilus*
   - (b) *Clostridium perfringens*
   - (c) *Bacillus cereus*
   - (d) *Clostridium histolyticum*
5. Phenol is bactericidal at a concentration of:
   - (a) 0.1%
   - (b) 0.25%
   - (c) 0.5%
   - (d) 1%
6. The biomedical waste is to be collected in different coloured plastic bags. Which of the following bags contains cadmium and is not to be incinerated because it leads to toxic emissions?
   - (a) Yellow
   - (b) Red
   - (c) Blue
   - (d) Black
7. Which of the following disinfectants have little activity against viruses?
   - (a) Phenols
   - (b) Sodium hypochlorite
   - (c) Iodine
   - (d) Formaldehyde

Answers to MCQs

1. c   **2.** a   **3.** a   **4.** a   **5.** d   **6.** b   **7.** a

Chapter 7

Personal Protective Equipment and Hand Hygiene

Personal protective equipment (PPE) refers to highly specialized clothing or equipment to protect against infection. Healthcare workers (HCW) who work in close proximity of cases who are either carriers or suspected to be carrying infectious agents are recommended to wear PPE for protection against infection. PPE protects the HCW from exposure to blood, body fluids and respiratory secretions of the patient. PPE include:

- Hand gloves
- Surgical mask
- Body gown
- Eye goggles
- Head gear (cover).

Before wearing PPE, there should not be hand accessories, bangles, wrist watch or mobile phone. Hands should be disinfected by washing with soap and running tap water or hand sanitizer. Soap should be applied generously for at least 40 seconds. When applying hand sanitizer, apply liberal quantity, rub vigorously for at least 20 seconds, and make sure no part is left out.

The three layer surgical mask needs to be opened before putting on. Fold should point downwards. Sanitize hands before putting on gloves. Gloves should not come in contact with any of the PPE. If mask becomes damp, it should be replaced immediately with a fresh one. When replacing the gloves, sanitation is must. In routine healthcare three layer surgical mask is good enough. However, when dealing with live virus, suspected patient or performing aerosol generating procedures such as intubation, mechanical ventilation or when collecting samples use N-95 respirator mask.

After attending the patient dispose of PPE in biohazard bag for final disposal as per Biomedical Waste Rules, 2016.

HAND HYGIENE AND PERSONAL PROTECTION

The importance of hand hygiene was, long back, emphasized by Louis Pasteur who said.

'If I had the honour of being surgeon, since I am convinced of the dangerous conditions which can be caused by the germs or microbes which are to be found every where, especially in hospitals, not only would I use only instruments in a perfect state of cleanliness, but also having cleaned my hands with the greatest care I would flame them rapidly'.

Hand washing is the most effective method for prevention of transmission of infection from healthcare worker (HCW) to the patient.

Social hand washing (Fig. 7.1): It is done with plain soap and water. It removes transient organisms by mechanical action. It is indicated before and after handling food, eating food, feeding the patient and after visiting the toilet.

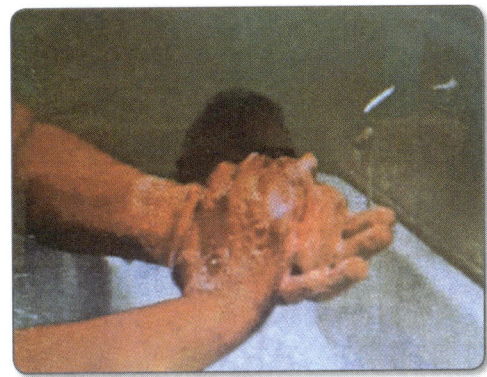

Fig. 7.1: Social hand washing

Hygienic hand washing (Fig. 7.2): Here an antiseptic detergent preparation is used or hands may be disinfected with alocohol-based hand-rub (hand sanitizer).

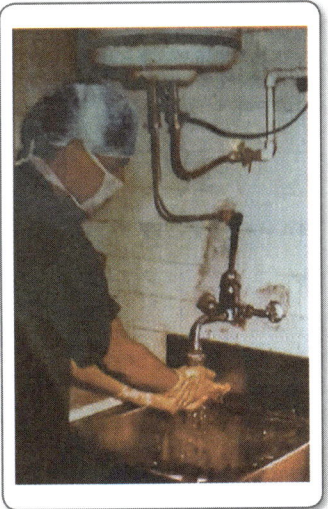

Fig. 7.2: Hygienic hand washing

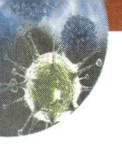

Essentials of Microbiology for BSc Nursing

This is indicated before performing invasive procedure and after contact with blood and body fluids.

Surgical hand washing (Fig. 7.3): Here scrub, the fingers, hands and nails up to elbow.

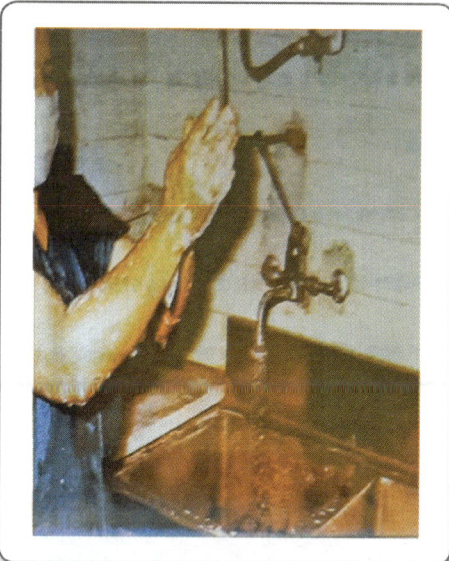

Fig. 7.3: Surgical hand washing

Steps of Effective Hand Washing

Steps of effective hand washing are given in Figure 7.4. For hand washing wash basin with running water should be available. Whenever possible, taps should be operated by wrist or foot pedals. Figure 7.5 shows areas most likely to be missed on hand washing. For drying hand, ideally paper towels should be used. If this is not possible cloth hand towels that are laundered daily should be used.

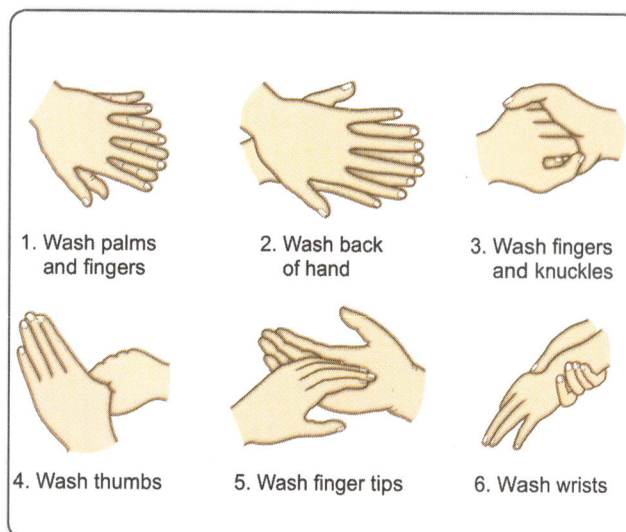

1. Wash palms and fingers
2. Wash back of hand
3. Wash fingers and knuckles
4. Wash thumbs
5. Wash finger tips
6. Wash wrists

Fig. 7.4: Steps of effective hand washing

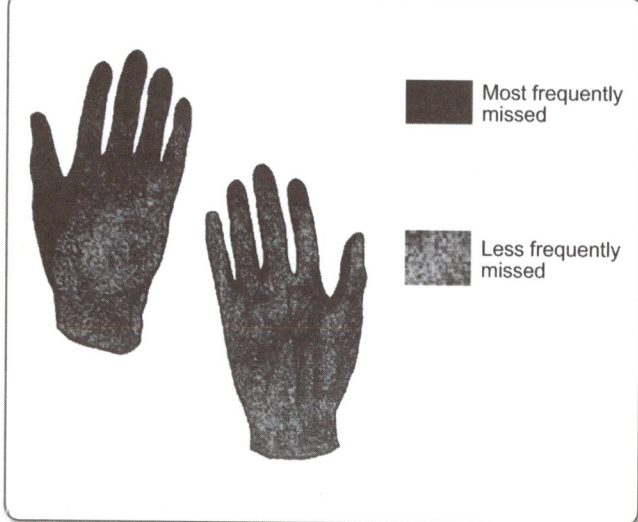

Most frequently missed

Less frequently missed

Fig. 7.5: Areas most likely to be missed on hand washing

Personal Protection

- Cover any cuts, insect bites, open sores or wounds on the hands, or other exposed parts of the body with a water proof adhesive dressing.
- Wear closed shoes and do not walk barefort.
- Do not eat, drink, chew gum or apply cosmetics in the hospital.
- Do not lick gummed labels and do not put pens, pencils, etc. in the mouth, eye or in hair.
- Avoid wearing jewellery particularly pendant necklace and bracelets.
- Wear overall (coverall) over normal clothing.
- When indicated a waterproof apron should also be worn.
- Overall must be worn with buttons. A side closing design is preferable to a front opening because it gives better protection.
- Soiled clothes should be placed in a special bag and prior to laundering, these should be soaked in 1% domestic bleach.
- Protective clothing should always be left in the hospital and never taken home or worn in a room where refreshments are taken.
- Protective gloves should be worn when handling specimens.
- Remove gloves before handling:
  - Door knobs
  - Telephone
  - Pen
  - Performing office work
  - Leaving the hospital.
- Face masks and safety goggles with closed sides should be worn to protect the face and eyes from splashes.
- Safety goggles should fit over spectacles, if worn.
- Get protective inoculation against hepatitis B, tuberculosis, tetanus, etc.

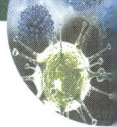

- Never bleed a patient with ungloved hands.
- Do not put blood samples on the laboratory request forms.
- Never separate serum from blood without gloves.
- Do not soil the laboratory slips with blood/body fluids.
- Needles and other sharps should never be passed directly from one person to another. Always use sterile trays and forceps.
- After the blood/clinical sample has been collected the syringe should immediately be submerged in the disinfectant.
- Never recap used needles.
- If by some reason the blood has fallen on floor, the blood spot must be covered with tissue paper/towel and soaked with disinfectant for 30 minutes.
- After 30 minutes the sanitation staff should put on heavy duty gloves and mop the blood spot along with disinfectant.
- Finally, the floor is cleaned with detergent and water in a usual way.

Key Points

- Hand washing is the most effective method for prevention of transmission of infection from healthcare worker to the patient.
- Protective gloves should be worn when handling specimens.
- Face masks and safety goggles with closed sides should be worn to protect the face and eyes from splashes.

? ASSESS YOURSELF

LONG ANSWER QUESTIONS

1. Discuss hand hygiene.
2. Discuss personal protection of healthcare workers.

MULTIPLE CHOICE QUESTION

1. Antiseptic detergent preparation is used in
   - (a) Social hand washing
   - (b) Hygienic hand washing
   - (c) Both above
   - (d) None of the above

ANSWER TO MCQ

1. b

Hospital-acquired Infections

Hospital-acquired infections or nosocomial (nosocomion means hospital) infections represent one of the most common complications of healthcare delivery. A nosocomial infection is defined as infection developing in a patient after admission to the hospital, which was neither present nor in its incubation period when the subject entered the hospital. Such an infection may manifest during the stay in the hospital or sometime after the patient is discharged. To determine whether some infections, such as legionellosis, are hospital-acquired, one must consider the usual incubation periods and determine whether the patient was hospitalized during that time period.

Factors Influencing Nosocomial Infections

A large number of factors contribute towards the development of nosocomial infection. These include the following:

- The hospital environment is heavily laden with a wide variety of pathogens. These may be present in air, dust, antiseptic lotions, water, food or may spread from shedding from the patients.
- Due to injudicious use of antibiotics, the hospital microbial flora is usually multidrug resistant, thus limiting the choice of therapy.
- Hospitalized patients with pre-existing diseases, such as diabetes, immunosuppression and patients with prosthetic implants are more susceptible to nosocomial infection.
- Diagnostic or therapeutic intervention such as insertion of urethral or intravenous catheters may introduce the infection.
- Blood and blood-products used for transfusion and also intravenous fluids, if not properly screened, can transmit many infections.

Source of Infection

The source of the infecting organisms may be exogenous from another patient or a member of the staff or from the inanimate objects in the hospital like medical equipment (endoscopes, cystoscopes, catheters, needles, etc.), bed pans, food, water, hospital air and surfaces contaminated by patients' secretions, excretions, blood and body fluids. It may be endogenous from the patient's own flora which at the time of infection may invade the patient's tissues spontaneously or be introduced into them by surgical operation, instrumental manipulations or nursing procedure.

Nosocomial Infection Sites

Nosocomial infection sites include urinary infection, surgical site infection, nosocomial pneumonia, nosocomial bacteraemia, skin and soft tissue infections, gastroenteritis and endometritis.

Microorganisms causing Nosocomial Infections

The most important microorganisms causing nosocomial infections are given in Table 8.1. Presently, about 60% cases of nosocomial infections are caused by aerobic Gram-negative rods and about 30% by Gram-positive cocci. Remaining 10% are caused by viruses and fungi.

Routes of Transmission of Infection in Hospitals

There are five main routes of spread of infection in hospitals.

1. **Contact spread**

   It is the principal route of transmission of nosocomial infections. It may be by direct contact spread from person to person. *Staphylococcus aureus* and *Streptococcus pyogenes* are two important pathogens spread by hand contact. Certain equipment (endoscope, bronchoscope, cystoscope), if not properly disinfected, may transmit pathogenic organisms, e.g. *Pseudomonas aeruginosa*.

2. **Airborne spread**

   Hospital infection may be acquired by inhalation of droplets, droplet nuclei, dust from bedding and floors, and exudate dispersed from a wound during dressing.

   Aerosols produced by nebulizers, humidifiers and air conditioning apparatus transmit certain pathogens like *Legionella* to the respiratory tract, because these organisms are widespread in water including potable water supplies. Occurrence of legionellae in hospital water supply, and a number of persons with an impaired immune system has led to outbreaks of infection mainly with *Legionella pneumophila*, but also with *L. micdadei*, *L. bozmanii* and *L. longbeachae*. Nosocomial infection occurs in patients rather than in staff who generally have circulating antibodies, which suggest exposure.

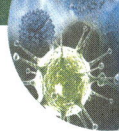

TABLE 8.1: Microorganisms causing nosocomial infections

Hospital infection	Causative agents
Urinary tract infections	*Escherichia coli, Klebsiella, Proteus, Serratia, Pseudomonas, Providencia,* coagulase-negative staphylococci, enterococci and *Candida albicans*
Respiratory infections	*Haemophilus influenzae, Streptococcus pneumoniae, Staphylococcus aureus, Klebsiella, Enterobacter, Serratia, Proteus, Escherichia, Pseudomonas aeruginosa, Acinetobacter, Legionella pneumophila,* respiratory viruses
Wound and skin sepsis	*Staphylococcus aureus, Escherichia coli, Proteus, Bacteroides,* enterococci, coagulase negative staphylococci
Burn infections	*Staphylococcus aureus, Pseudomonas aeruginosa, Acinetobacter, Streptococcus pyogenes*
Gastrointestinal infections	*Salmonella* serotypes, *Shigella sonnei*
Eye infections	*Staphylococcus aureus, Pseudomonas aeruginosa*
Miscellaneous	Hepatitis B virus, human immunodeficiency viruses

3. **Oral route**

Gastrointestinal pathogens may be transmitted by food served to the patients. Hospital food may also be a source of antibiotic-resistant bacteria (*Pseudomonas aeruginosa, Escherichia coli, Klebsiella* spp. and others), which may colonize the gut and later cause infection in susceptible patients.

4. **Parenteral route (inoculation)**

With the use of single-use disposable needles, syringes and other devices and satisfactory procedure for the sterilization of surgical instruments, transmission of infection by parenteral route has been infrequent. However, certain infections may be transmitted by blood transfusion or tissue donation, contaminated blood-products (factor VIII), contaminated infusion fluids and from accidental injury with contaminated sharp instruments (AIDS, hepatitis B and C).

5. **Self-infection**

Self-infection may occur due to transfer into the wounds of staphylococci and streptococci carried by the patient in his nose and over his skin, or of coliform bacilli and anaerobes released from his bowel during surgery.

Prevention

Nosocomial infection can be prevented by:
- The provision of sterile instruments, dressings, surgical gloves, face-masks, theatre clothing and fluids.
- Thorough hand washing after any procedure involving nursing care or close contact with the patient.
- Preoperative disinfection of the patient's skin.
- The use of antiseptics for irrigation of the wound site at operation or for mucosal surfaces such as the bladder after urological surgery and peritoneum during dialysis.
- Rational antibiotic prophylaxis.
- Proper investigation of nosocomial infection and the treatment of the patients and the carriers.

ANTIBIOTIC POLICY

Antibiotic policy constitutes one of the most important aspects of the infection control programme. Often, antibiotics are prescribed when there is no proof of infection. It has been seen that a wrong antibiotic has been chosen, or the timing of the antibiotic used is not in accordance with acceptable standards of practice. It is vital, therefore, that the antibiotic policy is properly framed and formulated. The prerequisites of an antibiotic policy are:
- Data of resistance among commonly encountered pathogens both in the community and in the hospital setting.
- Pattern of resistance to newer antimicrobial agents.
- Recognition of the trends of resistance.

The selection of the antimicrobial agent should be based on the sensitivity reports. Treatment of common infections should conform to standard regimen.

In countries like ours where there is unrestricted sale "over the counter" of antibiotics, uncontrolled misuse of antibiotics is responsible for a general pool of resistant strains in the population. Sale of antibiotics should be restricted to medical prescription only.

Why An Antibiotic Policy?
- To retard the emergence of multiple antibiotic-resistant bacteria.
- To avoid wasteful expenditure of Government/non-Government organization.

Hospital Disinfection Policy

In most hospitals no disinfection policy exists and a number of different disinfectants are used at many different strengths, with particular disinfectant often used for quite unsuitable purposes. The irrational use of disinfectants has both safety and cost implications. The choice of disinfectant for a particular purpose is important because an inappropriate product may be either

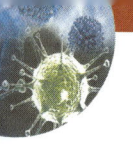

SECTION III ● INFECTION CONTROL AND SAFETY

inherently unsuitable or unnecessarily expensive. The correct-use dilution is important because too low a concentration will be ineffective, and too high a concentration uneconomic and possibly hazardous.

Infection Control Committee

Every hospital should have an infection control committee (ICC) with responsibilities that include the production and implementation of a disinfection policy. List of suggested infection control committee members is given in Table 8.2. Infection control personnel should review microbiology records regularly to identify unusual clusters or a greater-than-usual incidence of certain species or strains of microorganisms. All healthcare facilities must have access to the services of personnel trained and experienced in conducting outbreak investigations. When an outbreak occurs, the infection control team must have adequate resources and authority to ensure a comprehensive and timely investigation and the implementation of appropriate control measures. The ICC should meet regularly, at least once a month and as often as required, to formulate and update policy for the whole hospital matters having implications for infection control and to manage outbreaks of nosocomial infection.

TABLE 8.2: Suggested infection control committee members

Hospital Director/Dean/Principal	Chairman
Microbiologist/Epidemiologist	Infection Control Officer
Chief of medical services	Member
Quality control/assurance officer	Member
Heads of various clinical departments	Members
Head of pharmacy	Member
Head of support services	Member
Chief nurse	Member
Infection control nurses	Members

The functions of ICC include surveillance and control of infection and monitoring of hygiene practices, and the education of all staff in the microbiologically safe performance of procedures. Close working links between the microbiology laboratory and the different clinical specialities and support services (including sterile services, laundry, pharmacy and engineering) are important to establish and maintain the infection control policy, and to ensure that it is rationally based and that the recommended procedures are practicable.

Key Points

- *Hospital-acquired infection may be defined as an infection occurring in a patient in a hospital or other healthcare facility in whom the infection was not present or incubating at the time of admission. This includes infections acquired in the hospital but appearing after discharge, and also occupational infections among staff of the facility.*
- **Factors influencing nosocomial infection** include hospital environment, injudicious use of antibiotics, hospitalized patients with pre-existing diseases such as diabetes, immunosuppression and patients with prosthetic implants, diagnostic or therapeutic intervention and blood and blood products used for transfusion.
- **Routes of transmission of infection** in hospital include contact spread, airborne spread, oral route, parenteral route and self infection.
- *Every hospital should have* **antibiotic policy**, **disinfection policy** *and* **infection control committee**. *The functions of the latter include surveillance and control of infection and monitoring of hygiene practices.*

? ASSESS YOURSELF

LONG AND SHORT ANSWER QUESTIONS

1. Define hospital-acquired infection. Enumerate organisms causing it. What are the factors which influence development of this infection?
2. Write short notes on:
   (a) Routes of transmission of nosocomial infections
   (b) Prevention of nosocomial infections
   (c) Disinfection policy
   (d) Infection control committee
   (e) Antibiotic policy

Contd...

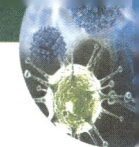

? ASSESS YOURSELF

MULTIPLE CHOICE QUESTIONS

1. Which of the following bacteria can cause urinary tract infections in hospitalized patients?
   - (a) *Escherichia coli*
   - (b) *Klebsiella*
   - (c) *Proteus*
   - (d) All of the above

2. Which of the following bacteria is/are implicated in nosocomial respiratory infections?
   - (a) *Staphylococcus aureus*
   - (b) *Klebsiella*
   - (c) *Enterobacter*
   - (d) All of the above

3. Which of the following bacteria can cause infection of burns in hospital patients?
   - (a) *Pseudomonas aeruginosa*
   - (b) *Acinetobacter*
   - (c) *Staphylococcus aureus*
   - (d) All of the above

4. Hospital-acquired infection can occur by:
   - (a) Contact spread
   - (b) Airborne spread
   - (c) Oral route
   - (d) All of the above

ANSWERS TO MCQS

1. d   **2.** d   **3.** d   **4.** d

NOTES

Pathogenic Organisms-I
Bacteria

Section Summary

Chapter 9

Staphylococcus

Genus *Staphylococcus* contains 40 defined species, 20 of which are known to be associated with colonization and/or infection of man. Of the 20 species found in man, one (*S. aureus*) is coagulase-positive and 19 coagulase-negative. Not all coagulase-negative staphylococci (CoNS) have been isolated from human infections.

STAPHYLOCOCCUS AUREUS

Morphology

They are spherical cocci about 0.8–1.0 µm in diameter. They are arranged characteristically in grape-like clusters. Cluster formation is due to cell division occurring in more than one plane with daughter cells remaining close together. In smear from pus, the cocci appear singly or in pairs, clusters or short chains of three or four cells (Figs 9.1 and 9.2). They are non-motile (non-flagellated), non-sporing and, with the exception of rare strains, non-capsulated. They are Gram-positive but old and phagocytosed organisms may be Gram-negative.

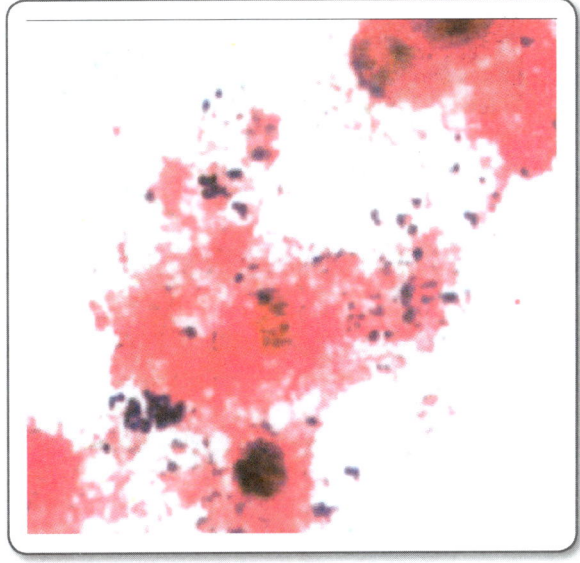

Fig. 9.2: Staphylococci in Gram-stained smear of pus × 1000.

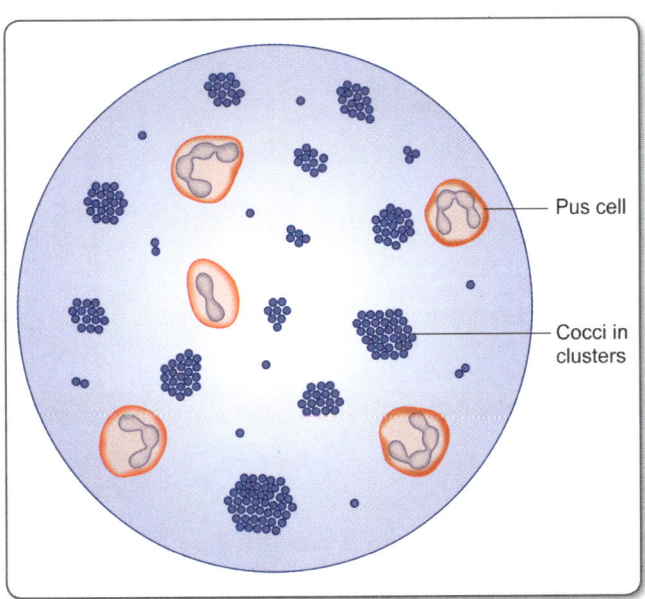

Fig. 9.1: Staphylococci and pus cells.

Pus cell

Cocci in clusters

Cultural Characteristics

They are aerobes and facultative anaerobes. Optimum temperature for growth is 37°C, range being 12–44°C. Optimum pH is 7.5. They can grow well on ordinary media.

- **Nutrient agar:** After overnight incubation at 37°C, colonies are 1–2 mm in diameter with a smooth glistening surface. They are opaque and easily emulsifiable. Most strains produce golden-yellow (*aureus*) pigment, though some strains may form white (non-pigmented) colonies.
- **Blood agar:** Colonies are similar to those on nutrient agar, but may be surrounded by a zone of β-haemolysis (Fig. 9.3), especially when the medium contains sheep, ox, human or rabbit blood.
- **Selective salt media:** Staphylococci can grow in the presence of 10% of sodium chloride, while many other bacteria are inhibited at this concentration. Therefore, 7–10% of sodium chloride may be added to nutrient agar. Salt agar is useful for isolation of staphylococci from food, dust, faeces and pus where mixed bacterial flora are expected. The appearance of colonies on these media is similar to those on nutrient agar.

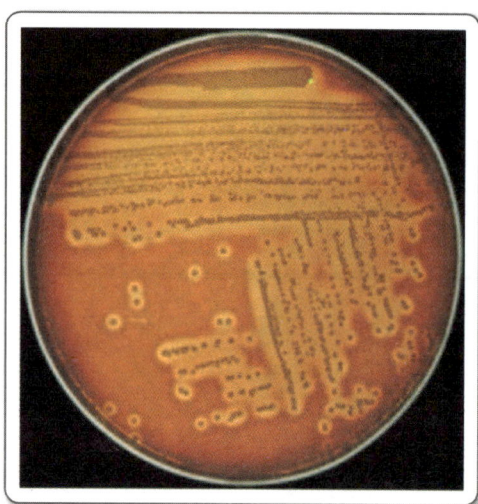

Fig. 9.3: Growth of *Staphylococcus aureus* on blood agar showing β-haemolysis.

Susceptibility to Physical and Chemical Agents

Staphylococci are usually killed by a temperature of 60°C in 30 minutes but some strains are killed by heating at 62°C in 30 minutes. Disinfectants such as chlorhexidine, hexachlorophene and phenol kill staphylococci rapidly. But mercuric chloride is a poor disinfectant for them. They are very sensitive to aniline dyes; thus they are inhibited on blood agar medium containing 1 in 500,000 crystal violet, which permits the growth of streptococci.

Biochemical Reactions

S. aureus is catalase-positive and oxidase-negative. Catalase production by staphylococci may function to inactivate toxic hydrogen peroxide and free radicals formed by myeloperoxidase system within phagocytic cells after ingestion of microorganisms. It ferments glucose, maltose, lactose, sucrose and mannitol with the production of acid but no gas. Of these fermentation reactions, fermentation of mannitol carries diagnostic significance because most strains of *S. aureus* ferment mannitol while most strains of *S. epidermidis* and *S. saprophyticus* are mannitol negative.

Bacteriophage Typing

Phages of *S. aureus* have a narrow host range and lyse only some other strains of the same species. Therefore, for epidemiological studies and tracing the source of infection, strains of *S. aureus* can be distinguished from one another by their patterns of susceptibility to lysis by an internationally recognized set of 23 standard typing phages (Table 9.1). Lysis of a culture by one phage is often associated with lysis by one or more other phages. Staphylococci can seldom be characterized by lysis by a single phage, but many different patterns of lysis are obtained with a set of phages. Differences between these patterns are used to make fine distinction between staphylococcal strains.

TABLE 9.1: Typing set of staphylococcal phages

Lytic group	Designation of phages in lytic group
I	29, 52, 52A, 79, 80
II	3A, 3C, 55, 71
III	6, 42E, 47, 53, 54, 75, 77, 83A, 84, 85
IV	—
V	94, 96
Unclassified	81, 95

The strain to be typed is inoculated on a plate of nutrient agar to produce a lawn culture. Drops of various phages at their routine test dilution (RTD) are applied over marked squares. After overnight incubation at 30°C the culture will be observed to be lysed by some phages but not by others. The phage type of a strain is expressed by designation of the phages that lyse it. Thus, if a strain is lysed only by phages 3C, 55 and 71, it is called phage type 3C/55/71.

Determinants of Pathogenicity or Virulence Factors of *Staphylococcus aureus*

S. aureus possesses a large number of cell-wall associated factors and extracellular toxins and enzymes (Table 9.2 and Fig. 9.4), which contribute to the ability of the organism to overcome the body's defence and to invade, propagate, survive and produce disease in the host.

TABLE 9.2: Determinants of pathogenicity or virulence factors of *Staphylococcus aureus*

I. Cell wall associated
• Capsular polysaccharide
• Teichoic acid
• Peptidoglycan
• Protein A
• Clumping factor
II. Extracellular factors
• Haemolytic toxins
▪ α lysin
▪ β lysin
▪ γ lysin
▪ δ lysin
• Leucocidin
• Epidermolytic toxins
• Enterotoxins
• Toxic shock syndrome toxin
III. Extracellular enzymes
• Coagulase
• Staphylokinase
• Hyaluronidase
• Deoxyribonuclease
• Lipase
• Phospholipases
• Proteases

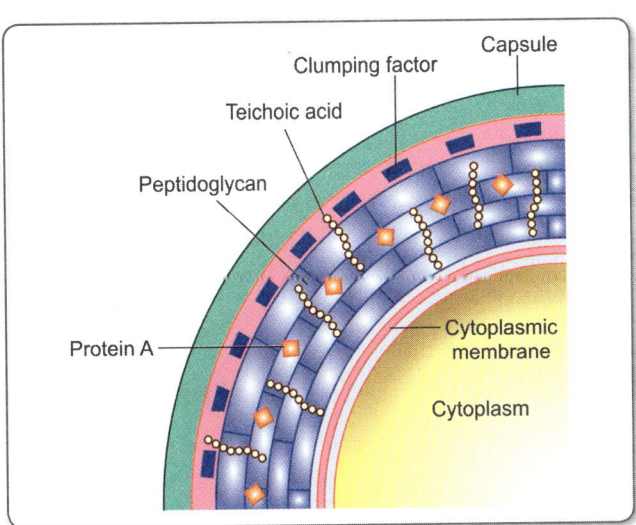

Fig. 9.4: Antigenic structure of *Staphylococcus aureus*.

Cell Wall Associated

- **Capsular polysaccharide**

  A few strains of *S. aureus* are encapsulated and these tend to be more virulent than the non-capsulated strains. The capsule is composed of antigenic polysaccharide. It prevents ingestion of the organism by polymorphonuclear leucocytes. The capsular material may promote the adherence of the organisms to host cells and to prosthetic devices.

- **Teichoic acid**

  It is a major antigenic determinant of all strains of *S. aureus*. It facilitates adhesion of cocci to host cell surface and protects them from complement mediated opsonization.

- **Peptidoglycan**

  It is a polysaccharide polymer which provides rigidity to the cell wall. It stimulates both humoral and cellular immune responses in the host. In addition to their role in providing rigidity and resilience to the staphylococcal cell wall, peptidoglycan and teichoic acid also have several biologic activities that are thought to contribute to virulence.

- **Protein A**

  Protein A is a group-specific antigen found in the cell wall of about 90% strains of *S. aureus* (especially Cowan I strain). It has a molecular weight of 13,000 daltons. It is chemotactic, anticomplementary, antiphagocytic, mitogenic, potentiates natural killer cells, and elicits platelet injury and hypersensitivity reaction.

  Protein A binds IgG molecules, non-specifically, through Fc region leaving specific Fab sites free to combine with specific antigen. When suspension of such sensitized cells is treated with homologous (test) antigen, the antigen combines with free Fab sites of IgG attached to staphylococcal cells. This is known as **coagglutination** (*see* chapter 45).

- **Clumping factor (bound coagulase)**

  It is a surface component that causes the organisms to clump when mixed with plasma. This factor reacts directly with fibrinogen in plasma, causing rapid clumping of the organism. It can be detected by emulsifying a few colonies of the bacteria in a drop of normal saline on a clean glass slide, and mixing it with a drop of rabbit plasma. Prompt clumping of the organisms indicates the presence of clumping factor (bound coagulase). Since this factor is detected by performing the test on a slide, therefore, the test is known as **slide coagulase test**.

Extracellular Toxins

S. aureus produces a variety of extracellular toxins, including haemolysins, leucocidin, epidermolytic toxins, enterotoxins and toxic shock syndrome toxin.

- **Haemolysins**

  Almost every strain of *S. aureus* produces one or more of four haemolytic, membrane-damaging exotoxins known as α, β, γ and δ lysins. They are antigenically distinct and differ from one another in their activity against the red blood cells of different animal species, lethal activity, dermonecrosis and leucocidal activity.

  - α *lysin (α toxin):* Of the four haemolysins produced by *S. aureus*, α lysin is the most important in pathogenicity. In cultures, it is produced only under aerobic conditions and its production is enhanced by a high concentration of carbon dioxide. It is a protein consisting of a single polypeptide chain, with a molecular weight of 28,000–30,000 daltons.

    The α toxin lyses rabbit and sheep erythrocytes. It is leucocidal and when injected intradermally into mice and rabbits it is dermonecrotic and when injected intravenously in these animals it is lethal. It is known to damage smooth muscles, is toxic for human macrophages and platelets and causes degranulation of polymorphonuclear leucocytes through disruption of their lysosomes.

  - β *lysin (β toxin):* β lysin is strongly active on sheep and weakly active on rabbit and human red blood cells. It does not lyse horse red blood cells. It gives rise to '**hot-cold' haemolysis**, the cells that have been exposed to the lysin at 37°C lyse only when cooled to 4°C.

  - γ *lysin (γ toxin):* γ lysin acts on sheep, rabbit and human red blood cells but not on those of horse.

  - δ *lysin (δ toxin):* δ lysin is a polypeptide with a molecular weight of 1600 daltons. It lyses red blood cells of sheep, rabbit, horse and man. It also possesses lethal, dermonecrotic and leucocidal activity.

- **Leucocidin**

  Leucocidin consists of two protein components. On the basis of their migration in carboxymethylcellulose columns they are designated F (fast) and S (slow) components. These components act synergistically to damage polymorphonuclear leucocytes and macrophages and to produce dermonecrosis.

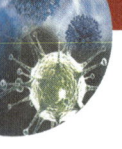

- **Epidermolytic toxins (exfoliative toxins)**

    Many strains of *S. aureus*, mainly belonging to phage group II, produce two types of epidermolytic toxin (types A and B). They are proteins with a molecular weight of 30,000 and 29,500 daltons, respectively. Epidermolytic toxin A is heat-stable and its production is determined by a chromosomal gene. On the other hand, epidermolytic toxin B is heat-labile and plasmid-controlled.

- **Enterotoxins**

    About 40% of all clinical isolates of *S. aureus* produce enterotoxins which are exotoxins that cause food poisoning in man. These have also been implicated in some cases of **pseudomembranous enterocolitis** seen in patients after antibiotic therapy. Enterotoxins are proteins with molecular weights of 26,000–30,000 daltons. These are heat-stable, resisting boiling for 30 minutes. Therefore, once formed enterotoxins might not be destroyed even if food is heated sufficiently to kill all viable staphylococci. These are also not destroyed by gut enzymes. Nine antigenic types (A, B, C_1, C_2, C_3, D, E, H and I) of enterotoxins have been identified. Enterotoxin F is now known as toxic shock syndrome toxin-1. Some strains may form toxin of more than one type.

- **Toxic shock syndrome toxin-1 (TSST-1)**

    TSST-1 is produced by certain strains of *S. aureus*. Most of the strains producing TSST-1 belong to phage group I. TSST-1 is a protein with a molecular weight of 22,000 daltons. It is antigenic and most persons over 30 years of age have circulating antibodies.

> TSST-1 and the enterotoxins are now recognized as super-antigens, i.e. they are potent activators of T lymphocytes resulting in the liberation of cytokines such as tumour necrosis factor, and they bind with high affinity to mononuclear cells. These characteristics partly explain the florid and multisystem nature of the clinical conditions associated with these toxins.

Extracellular Enzymes

- **Coagulase**

    S. aureus produces an extracellular enzyme called coagulase. It activates a coagulase-reacting factor (CRF) normally present in plasma, causing the plasma to clot by the conversion of fibrinogen to fibrin. Clotting does not occur with plasma of certain species like guinea pig which lack CRF. CRF is similar to prothrombin but is probably not identical with it. Coagulase is produced during the logarithmic phase of growth in a variety of media. Eight antigenic types (A–H) have been described. Most human strains produce coagulase A.

All coagulase-producing staphylococci are, by definition, *S. aureus* and as a result, coagulase production is considered the best laboratory evidence for the potential pathogenicity of *Staphylococcus*. However, there is no conclusive proof of the role of coagulase as a virulence factor because coagulase-negative mutants of *S. aureus* are no less virulent than the parent strain. Coagulase may act to coat the bacterial cells with fibrin, rendering them resistant to opsonization and phagocytosis.

Coagulase (tube coagulase) test

0.1 ml of an overnight broth culture or broth suspension from an agar plate culture made up to the same density is mixed with 0.5 ml of a 1 in 10 dilution of human or rabbit plasma. The mixture is incubated in a water bath at 37°C for three to six hours. If positive, the plasma clots and does not flow when the tube is inverted. Continued incubation is not recommended as the clot may be lysed by fibrinolysin produced by some strains. Controls with plasma alone, known coagulase-positive and coagulase-negative cultures must be set up with each batch of tests. Pig plasma which is rich in CRF can also be used. Oxalate, EDTA or heparin are suitable anticoagulants. Citrated plasma should not be used because contaminating Gram-negative bacilli, if present, may utilize the citrate and produce false positive reaction.

For slide coagulase see clumping factor.

- **Staphylokinase (fibrinolysin)**

    Many strains of *S. aureus* that do not produce β lysin may produce staphylokinase. It is a protein with a molecular weight of 13,000–15,000 daltons. It has fibrinolytic activity. It is antigenically and enzymatically distinct from streptokinase produced by *Streptococcus*. Fibrinolysin may breakdown fibrin clots and allow spread of infection to contiguous tissues.

- **Hyaluronidase**

    More than 90% strains of *S. aureus* produce hyaluronidase, but the amount varies widely. It hydrolyses hyaluronic acid present in the intercellular ground substance of connective tissue, thus facilitating the spread of the organisms to adjacent areas.

    Other extracellular enzymes produced by *S. aureus* and their activities are as under:

Extracellular enzyme	Activity
Deoxyribonuclease	Degrades DNA
Lipase	Degrades lipid
Phospholipases	Degrade phospholipids
Proteases	Cause proteolysis

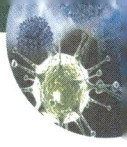

Pathogenicity

About 35–50% of normal adults carry *S. aureus* in the anterior nares. Other sites of colonization include intertriginous skin folds, perineum, axillae, and vagina. Skin carriage rates of 10–20% are found in most areas of the body except the hands, where up to 40% of swabs may yield *S. aureus*. These organisms are acquired from the nose by contact (transients) and their elimination from the nose by antibiotic treatment results in cessation of skin carriage. These can also be removed from the skin by washing.

Staphylococci shed by patients and carriers contaminate fomites such as handkerchiefs, bed linen and blankets, and may persist on them for days or weeks. Staphylococcal disease may follow endogenous or exogenous infection. The mode of transmission may be by contact, direct or through fomites or by airborne droplets.

S. aureus is an opportunistic pathogen in that it causes infection most commonly at sites of lowered host resistance, e.g. damaged skin or mucous membranes or haematomas in the cancellous tissue of a long bone. Those with respiratory tract viral infections, such as influenza and measles, and diabetic patients are also more susceptible to staphylococcal infections.

Staphylococcal diseases may be classified as cutaneous and deep infections, exfoliative diseases, food poisoning and the toxic shock syndrome.

- **Cutaneous infections**
  These include wound and burn infection, pustules (small cutaneous abscesses), furuncles or boils (large cutaneous abscesses), carbuncles, styes, impetigo and pemphigus neonatorum.
- **Deep infections**
  These include osteomyelitis, periostitis, tonsillitis, pharyngitis, sinusitis, bronchopneumonia, empyema, septicaemia, meningitis, endocarditis, breast abscess, renal abscess and abscesses in other organs.
- **Exfoliative diseases**
  These lesions are produced by the strains of *S. aureus* which produce epidermolytic toxins. These toxins separate the outer layer of epidermis from the underlying tissues leading to **blistering disease**. The most dramatic manifestation of these toxins is **staphylococcal scalded skin syndrome (SSSS)** or **Ritter's disease** in which toxin spreads systemically in individuals that lack neutralizing antitoxin. Extensive areas of the skin are involved. Patient develops painful rash which sloughs off and skin surface resembles scalding.

SSSS occurs primarily in newborns and previously healthy young children. In adults, it occurs most commonly among patients with chronic renal failure and those with compromised immune systems. Although the mortality rate is low (0–7%) in cases seen among children, the rate in adults is as high as 50%.

- **Food poisoning**
  Staphylococcal food poisoning (nausea, vomiting and diarrhoea) may follow 2–6 hours after the ingestion of food in which *S. aureus* has multiplied and formed enterotoxin.

The types of food usually responsible are meat, fish, milk and milk products. The duration of acute symptoms is usually less than 24 hours. The illness is rarely fatal.

- **Toxic shock syndrome (TSS)**
  It is a multisystem illness characterized by high fever, headache, confusion, conjunctival reddening, subcutaneous oedema, vomiting, diarrhoea, scarlatiniform rash and fine desquamation of the hands and feet. Severe cases progress to acute renal failure, disseminated intravascular coagulation, peripheral gangrene, profound hypotensive shock and death.

Laboratory Diagnosis

Specimens

Specimens to be collected include pus from suppurative lesions, blood from a patient with pyrexia of unknown origin, mid-stream urine from a patient with urinary tract infection, sputum from a patient with bronchopneumonia and faeces, food remains and vomit from cases of food poisoning. Nasal and perineal swabs may be collected from suspected carriers.

Microscopy

Examine a Gram-stained smear of pus or wound exudate which may show pus cells and Gram-positive cocci in clusters (Fig. 9.2).

Culture

The specimens are cultured on a blood agar plate. Specimens, where staphylococci are expected to be outnumbered by other bacteria (e.g. wound swab and faeces), are inoculated on selective media like salt agar. The inoculated media are incubated at 37°C for 24 hours. Next day, the plates are inspected for golden-yellow or white colonies and are confirmed by slide coagulase test. On blood agar plate, look for haemolysis around the colonies (Fig. 9.3). Other tests which may be carried out include tube coagulase, mannitol fermentation, DNAse and phosphatase production, and gelatin liquefaction. As a guide to treatment, antibiotic sensitivity tests should be done and for epidemiological purposes bacteriophage typing may be done.

Treatment

Since drug resistance is common among staphylococci, therefore, appropriate antibiotic should be chosen by antibiotic sensitivity test. Benzyl penicillin is the most effective antibiotic, if the strain is sensitive. Cloxacillin, oxacillin, flucloxacillin and methicillin are penicillinase-resistant penicillins. In serious infections they may be combined with an aminoglycoside or fusidic acid. First and second-generation cephalosporins are also effective but third-generation cephalosporins should be avoided. Clindamycin is useful in cases of osteomyelitis. Patients allergic to penicillins may be given erythromycin, vancomycin or first-generation cephalosporins. Methicillin-resistant strains are also

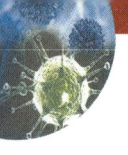

resistant to other penicillins and cephalosporins. However, they may be sensitive to vancomycin, rifampicin, fusidic acid and ciprofloxacin.

COAGULASE-NEGATIVE STAPHYLOCOCCI

Coagulase-negative staphylococci (CoNS) form part of the normal flora of the skin. Some species of CoNS, e.g. *S. epidermidis* and *S. saprophyticus*, can produce human infections. CoNS are morphologically similar to *S. aureus* and the methods for isolation are the same. Their colonies are white (non-pigmented) and they can be distinguished from *S. aureus* by their failure to coagulate plasma and by their lack of clumping factor and DNAse.

Staphylococcus Epidermidis

The role of *S. epidermidis* as an aetiologic agent of disease has become increasingly evident. Infections caused by *S. epidermidis* are predominantly hospital-acquired. Some of the predisposing factors are instrumentation procedures such as catheterization, prosthetic heart valve implantation, and immunosuppressive therapy. Infections caused by this organism include endocarditis of native and prosthetic valves, intravenous catheter infections, CSF shunt infections, peritoneal dialysis, catheter-associated peritonitis, bacteraemia, osteomyelitis, wound infections, vascular graft infections, prosthetic joint infections and mediastinitis.

S. epidermidis is probably the most common cause of hospital-acquired urinary tract infections.

Many strains of *S. epidermidis* can adhere to plastic catheters and prosthetic devices. Adherence of CoNS to plastic prosthetics is, most likely, facilitated by non-specific binding related to electrical charge and/or hydrophobic interactions between the bacterial surface and the surface of plastic devices. Many strains of *S. epidermidis* are capable of producing large amounts of polysaccharide glycocalyx known as slime. It is produced readily when the bacteria are growing on a solid surface such as a plastic catheter allowing the formation of microcolonies. Slime has been thought to play a role in the adherence of staphylococci to surfaces. Slime-producing strains also utilize this adherence factor to inhibit the action of lymphocytes and neutrophils.

Staphylococcus Saprophyticus

S. saprophyticus is a well documented pathogen causing primarily acute urinary tract infection in young healthy sexually active women. In this population *S. saprophyticus* is the most common cause of cystitis after *Escherichia coli*. When present in urine cultures, it may be found in low numbers and yet considered significant. It is found to adhere more effectively to the epithelial cells lining the urogenital tract.

S. saprophyticus can be differentiated from *S. epidermidis* from its novobiocin resistance (Table 9.3).

TABLE 9.3: Differences between three species of *Staphylococcus*

Character	S. aureus	S. epidermidis	S. saprophyticus
Production of			
• Coagulase	+	–	–
• DNase	+	–	–
• Phosphatase	+	– / weak +	–
• Toxin	+	–	–
Anaerobic fermentation of mannitol	+	–	–
Protein A in the cell wall	+	–	–
Novobiocin resistance	–	–	+

Key Points

- **Staphylococci with streptococci** constitute the main group of **medically important Gram-positive cocci**. The former occur in clumps and are catalase-positive and the latter occur in chains and are catalase-negative.
- Staphylococcal infections range from the trivial to the rapidly fatal. They can be very difficult-to-treat, especially those contracted in hospitals, because of remarkable ability of staphylococci to acquire antibiotic resistance determinants.
- *Staphylococcus aureus* is one of the most common causes of **bacterial infections**, and is also an important cause of intoxications such as **food poisoning** and **toxic shock syndrome**.
- *Staphylococcus epidermidis* is an important cause of **prosthetic implant infections**.

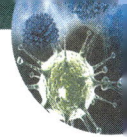

? ASSESS YOURSELF

LONG AND SHORT ANSWER QUESTIONS

1. Name various virulence factors of *Staphylococcus aureus*.
2. Write short notes on:
   (a) Epidermolytic toxins of *Staphylococcus aureus*
   (b) Enterotoxins of *Staphylococcus aureus*
   (c) Toxic shock syndrome
   (d) Coagulase
3. Discuss pathogenicity and laboratory diagnosis of *Staphylococcus aureus*.

MULTIPLE CHOICE QUESTIONS

1. Most strains of *Staphylococcus aureus* show:
   (a) A golden-yellow pigment
   (b) β-haemolysis on sheep blood agar
   (c) Phosphatase production
   (d) All of the above

2. Which of the following bacteria is catalase-positive and oxidase-negative?
   (a) *Staphylococcus*
   (b) *Micrococcus*
   (c) *Neisseria*
   (d) *Pseudomonas*

3. Scalded skin syndrome is due to which toxin of *Staphylococcus aureus*?
   (a) Epidermolytic toxin
   (b) Enterotoxin
   (c) Leucocidin
   (d) Haemolysin

4. Staphylococcal food poisoning usually manifests itself within how much time after ingestion of contaminated food?
   (a) 2–6 hours
   (b) 6–12 hours
   (c) 12–24 hours
   (d) 24–48 hours

5. Which of the following cocci are oxidase-positive?
   (a) Staphylococci
   (b) Streptococci
   (c) Enterococci
   (d) Micrococci

6. Scalded skin syndrome is caused by exotoxin produced by:
   (a) *Staphylococcus aureus*
   (b) *Streptococcus pyogenes*
   (c) *Pseudomonas aeruginosa*
   (d) *Propionibacterium acnes*

ANSWERS TO MCQs

1. d **2.** a **3.** a **4.** a **5.** d **6.** a

10 Chapter

Streptococcus

Streptococci are catalase-negative, Gram-positive, non-sporing, spherical or ovoid cells. Most group A, B, and C strains produce capsules composed of hyaluronic acid. Cell division occurs in one plane, therefore, they are arranged in pairs or chains. With the exception of some species, they are non-motile. Majority of them are aerobes and facultative anaerobes but some are obligate anaerobes. Most of the former grow in air but some require the addition of CO_2 for growth. Streptococci form part of the normal flora of man and animals. They inhabit various sites, notably the upper respiratory tract, and usually live harmlessly as commensals. However, some species, of which *S. pyogenes* is the most important, are highly pathogenic.

CLASSIFICATION

Streptococci are divided into aerobes and facultative anaerobes, and obligate anaerobes. Genus *Peptostreptococcus* is obligate anaerobe. Based upon their haemolytic properties, aerobic and facultative anaerobic streptococci can be classified into three groups:

1. **β-haemolytic streptococci**
   These cause complete lysis of RBCs (2–4 mm wide) resulting in clear area surrounding the colony.
2. **α-haemolytic streptococci**
   These cause partial lysis of RBCs resulting in a greenish discoloration of the area surrounding the colony.
3. **Non-haemolytic streptococci**
   These organisms do not produce any haemolysis or discoloration on blood agar. Earlier these were termed γ-haemolytic streptococci. However, because no lysis of RBCs, occurs, the term γ-haemolytic is confusing.

STREPTOCOCCUS PYOGENES

Morphology

They are Gram-positive, spherical cocci about 0.6–1.0 μm in diameter. They occur in chains of varying lengths. Chain formation is due to the cocci dividing in one plane only and the daughter cells failing to separate completely (Fig. 10.1). In actively spreading lesions within the tissues, diplococcal and individual coccal forms

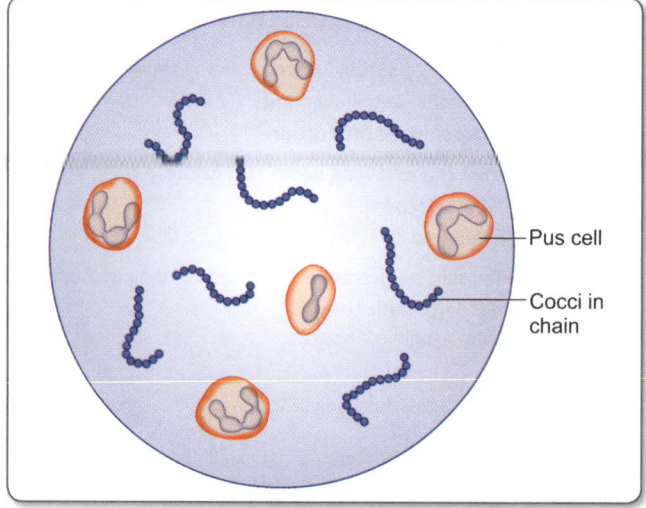

Fig. 10.1: Streptococci in Gram-stained smear of pus.

are common, whereas in purulent exudates from walled-off lesions and in artificial culture media, chain formation is a rule. Chains are longer in liquid than in solid media. They are non-motile, non-sporing and some strains produce a capsule of hyaluronic acid, which may be demonstrable during the first 2–4 hours of growth. Because many strains also produce the enzyme hyaluronidase later during the growth cycle, capsules may not be seen in older cultures. Since hyaluronic acid is a normal component of connective tissue, therefore, anticapsular antibodies are not formed.

Cultural Characteristics

They are aerobes and facultative anaerobes. Temperature range is 22–40°C, optimum temperature being 37°C. They can grow on blood and serum agar.

- After 24 hours incubation, colonies of *S. pyogenes* on blood agar are small (0.5–1 mm in diameter), semitransparent, grey-white with a matt or glossy surface. The colonies are surrounded by a wide zone of β-haemolysis.
- The addition of 0.0002% crystal violet to blood agar inhibits the growth of some bacteria, notably staphylococci, while permitting the growth of streptococci. Crystal violet blood agar is, therefore, a selective medium for isolation of *S. pyogenes*.

Susceptibility to Physical and Chemical Agents

S. pyogenes is a delicate organism. It can be killed by heating at 54°C for 30 minutes. However, if protected from sunlight, it can survive in dust for months. It is also killed by usual strengths of disinfectants, but is more resistant to crystal violet than many other bacteria including *Staphylococcus aureus* hence it is used for preparation of selective media. It is sensitive to benzylpenicillin and a wide range of other antimicrobial agents. It is naturally resistant to aminoglycosides and has acquired resistance to sulphonamides, tetracyclines and less commonly to clindamycin and macrolides. It is sensitive to bacitracin. This property is made use in differentiation of *S. pyogenes* from other haemolytic streptococci.

Biochemical Reactions

It is catalase-negative and, unlike *S. pneumoniae*, insoluble in 10% bile. It ferments several sugars with the production of acid but no gas.

Antigenic structure

Several components of bacterial cell of *S. pyogenes* (Fig. 10.2) are antigenic. These include:

Capsule

The hyaluronic acid of the capsule is non-antigenic, presumably because it is chemically indistinguishable from the hyaluronic acid of ground substance of animal connective tissue. Capsule has only a weak antiphagocytic effect.

Cell Wall

Cell wall is composed of an outer layer of protein, a middle layer of group-specific carbohydrate and an inner layer of peptidoglycan.

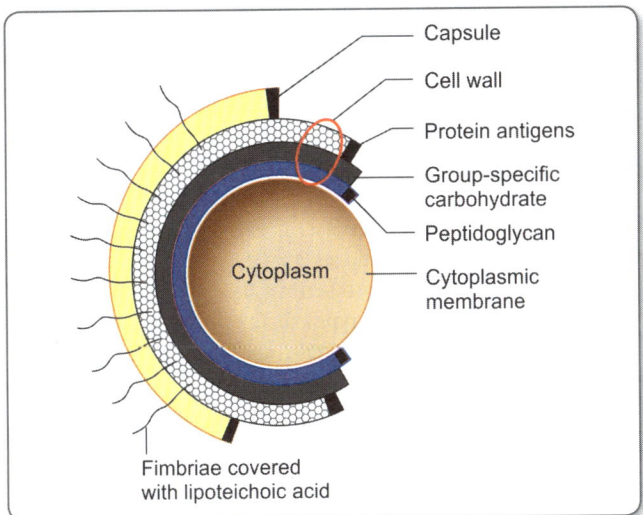

Fig. 10.2: Antigenic structure of *Streptococcus pyogenes*.

- **Peptidoglycan:** Peptidoglycan is responsible for cell wall rigidity. It also has biologic properties such as pyrogenic and thrombolytic activity.
- **Group-specific carbohydrate:** Carbohydrate antigen of haemolytic streptococci can be extracted by a number of methods like Lancefield acid extraction, enzyme (produced by *Streptomyces albus*) extraction and formamide extraction. It gives specific precipitate with sera prepared by injecting killed whole cells into rabbits. On the basis of group-specific carbohydrate antigens contained in the cell wall, haemolytic streptococci have been divided into 20 groups (A to V except I and J). These are known as Lancefield groups. *S. pyogenes* belongs to Lancefield group A. All streptococci except the viridans group have a layer of carbohydrate.
- **Proteins:** *S. pyogenes* produces three surface protein antigens (M, T and R) that are useful in serologic typing.
- **M protein:** It is the most important. It acts as a virulence factor by inhibiting phagocytosis. Specific anti-M antibody develops after infection which enhances phagocytosis. M protein extends through the capsule as fine fimbriae. They are covered with lipoteichoic acid. They enable the organism to attach to epithelial cells. M protein is acid- and heat-stable and trypsin-sensitive. It is antigenic and antisera can be raised against it. On the basis of antigenic differences in the M protein, *S. pyogenes* is divided into more than 120 M types. M protein can be extracted by Lancefield acid extraction method and M typing is performed by capillary tube precipitation tests using type-specific antisera and acid extract.
- **T protein:** It is resistant to pepsin and trypsin but is heat- and acid-stable. It is present in many serotypes of *S. pyogenes*. T typing is done by slide agglutination test using trypsin-treated whole streptococci.
- **R protein:** It is destroyed by pepsin and not by trypsin. Typing systems employing the R surface antigens are not commonly used.

Various structural components of *S. pyogenes* exhibit antigenic **cross reaction with different tissues** of the human body, e.g. capsular hyaluronic acid, cell wall protein, cell wall carbohydrate, cytoplasmic membrane and peptidoglycan cross react with human synovial fluid, myocardium, cardiac valves, vascular intima and skin antigens, respectively (Table 10.1).

TABLE 10.1: Structural components of *Streptococcus pyogenes* which cross react with human tissues

Structural component of *S. pyogenes*	Human tissue with which it cross reacts
Capsular hyaluronic acid	Synovial fluid
Cell wall protein	Myocardium
Cell wall carbohydrate	Cardiac valves
Cytoplasmic membrane	Vascular intima
Peptidoglycan	Skin antigens

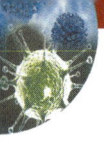

Toxins and Enzymes

S. pyogenes produces several exotoxins and enzymes which contribute to its pathogenicity and identification.

Streptococcal Pyrogenic Exotoxin (Erythrogenic Toxin)

There are three antigenically distinct erythrogenic toxins A, B and C (streptococcal pyrogenic exotoxins; SPE A, SPE B and SPE C). Type A toxin is encoded by bacteriophage gene *speA*, type B toxin by chromosomal gene *speB* and toxin C by bacteriophage gene *speC*. **These exotoxins are superantigens and have been associated with streptococcal toxic shock syndrome and scarlet fever.**

Dick Test

When 0.2 ml of suitably diluted toxin is injected intradermally in the susceptible individual, it causes localized erythematous reaction at least 1 cm in diameter in 12–24 hours. This indicates susceptibility to the toxin and thus to scarlet fever. This test is known as Dick test. This toxin is antigenic. It is neutralized by antibodies found in convalescent sera.

Schultz-Charlton Test

When the patient serum contains demonstrable antitoxin, the Dick test-becomes negative and an injection of homologous antitoxin intradermally in a patient of scarlet fever causes local blanching of the rash. This is known as Schultz-Charlton test.

Haemolysins (Streptolysins)

S. pyogenes produces two types of haemolysins. One of these is oxygen-labile hence designated as streptolysin O (SLO) and the other is oxygen-stable and soluble in serum hence designated as streptolysin S (SLS).

- **Streptolysin O:** It is a heat-labile protein with a molecular weight of 50,000–75,000 daltons. It binds to the cholesterol containing erythrocyte membrane and produces large holes in it, leading to complete lysis. On blood agar, SLO activity is seen only in pour plates and in anaerobic cultures.

  It is strongly antigenic. It induces brisk antibody response, usually within 10–14 days. Antistreptolysin O (ASO) may be demonstrated, *in vitro*, by its capacity to inhibit the haemolytic action of the toxin. It provides a very important tool for determining a recent group A streptococcal infection. Such information is an important aid in the diagnosis of the late complications of streptococcal infections, which usually occur after the organisms have been eliminated from the host.

- **Streptolysin S:** It is a small polypeptide with a molecular weight of less than 20,000 daltons. It is non-antigenic. It is oxygen-stable, so it is responsible for haemolysis around the surface colonies. In addition to causing β-haemolysis, it is able to inhibit chemotaxis and phagocytosis.

Streptokinase

Streptococci of groups A, C and G produce a substance called streptokinase which is actively fibrinolytic for human fibrin (blood clot) and can be recovered in streptococcal culture filtrates. It is an antigenic protein and neutralizing antibodies appear in convalescent sera. It acts on plasminogen, a factor present in normal plasma, which is converted into plasmin, an active proteolytic enzyme that lyses fibrin. It is thought to be at least partially responsible for the rapid spread of streptococcal infection by preventing the formation of a fibrin barrier around the infected site. It is given intravenously for the treatment of early myocardial infarction and other thromboembolic disorders.

Deoxyribonucleases (Streptodornases)

S. pyogenes also elaborates enzymes that degrade DNA. Four immunologically and electrophoretically different types (A, B, C and D) of deoxyribonucleases have been found in streptococcal culture filtrates. Of these, B is most antigenic in man and demonstration of antideoxyribonuclease B is useful in the retrospective diagnosis particularly of skin infections, where ASO titre may be low. One or more of these enzymes are produced by all strains of *S. pyogenes*. These are capable of depolymerizing the highly viscous DNA which accumulates in thick pus as a result of disintegration of polymorphonuclear leucocytes. Thus these enzymes are probably responsible for serous character of streptococcal pus. Mixtures of streptokinase and streptodornase have been used therapeutically for breaking down blood clots, thick pus and fibrinous exudates in closed spaces such as joints or pleural cavity.

Hyaluronidase (Spreading Factor)

It is an enzyme which splits hyaluronic acid binding tissue cells together and also that of streptococcal capsules, consequently strains which produce large amounts of hyaluronidase produce little hyaluronic acid capsule. This enzyme is expected to play a part in the virulence of *S. pyogenes* by facilitating its spread. It is antigenic and antibodies to the enzyme are formed after infection. Hyaluronidase is produced by strains of group A, B, C and G streptococci.

Serum Opacity Factor (SOF)

SOF is an enzyme, lipoproteinase. It exists both as cell-bound and released from it. It produces opacity when applied to agar gel containing horse or swine serum. It is produced by group A streptococci of certain M types. It thus provides a means of classifying group A streptococci into two categories—SOF-producing and non-SOF-producing strains.

Pathogenicity

S. pyogenes causes:
- Suppurative diseases
- Non-suppurative sequelae

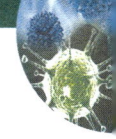

Suppurative Diseases

- **Tonsillitis and pharyngitis:** The main site of streptococcal infection is the throat where purulent tonsillitis is the most typical lesion. This condition characteristically occurs in older children and adults where it may constitute 30–40% of all cases of sore throat. In younger children, the infection is more diffuse (pharyngitis rather than tonsillitis) and less acute in character. The more acute localized lesion of older persons is believed to depend on a previous acquired allergy.

- **Scarlet fever:** Scarlet fever may be caused by any type of group A *Streptococcus* that produces erythrogenic toxin. The disease consists of a combination of a streptococcal sore throat and a generalized erythema, although occasionally the rash can accompany a streptococcal wound infection. The rash consists of widespread erythema with punctate spots. The skin of the face is generally clear.

- **Impetigo:** It is a skin infection that occurs most often in young children, particularly those living in crowded, low socioeconomic conditions. Streptococcal impetigo is characterized by occurrence on the skin of a superficial discrete crusted spot seldom exceeding an inch in diameter, which lasts for 1–2 weeks and heals spontaneously without leaving a scar.

- **Erysipelas:** This is an acute, spreading, intensely erythematous skin lesion with a sharply demarcated but irregular edge and sometimes with superficial vesicles and bullae.

- **Other group A streptococcal infections:** *S. pyogenes* is the most important cause of **puerperal sepsis**. In this condition, the organisms are almost invariably derived from attendant nurses or doctors or from contaminated instruments. It may also cause wound and burn infections.

Non-suppurative Sequelae

There is a considerable evidence that *S. pyogenes* is in some way the cause of acute rheumatic fever (ARF) involving the heart and joints, and acute glomerulonephritis (AGN) involving the kidneys. These conditions differ from suppurative infections in that:

- These conditions appear only between 1–3 weeks after infection with *S. pyogenes*.
- Many cases are not preceded by overt streptococcal infection but in many of these, high titres of antibodies to streptococcal extracellular antigens, particularly to streptolysin O, are frequently demonstrable.
- Streptococci are not directly demonstrable in the lesions in these conditions.

Acute Rheumatic Fever (ARF)

ARF develops in a small percentage (roughly 3%) of individuals, 2–3 weeks after the onset of acute streptococcal pharyngitis caused by any type of group A streptococci. It is characterized by fever, migrating polyarthritis, and carditis, and is frequently associated with subcutaneous nodules. Recovery from ARF occurs without residual injury to the joints, but permanent damage to the heart may occur. The mechanism by which streptococci produce rheumatic fever is still obscure.

There have been reports that a common cross reacting antigen exists in some group A streptococci and the heart. In this case, antibodies synthesized in response to the streptococcal infection could react with antigens in the heart, causing cellular destruction and permanent damage. This theory is supported by the observation that following a streptococcal epidemic, most patients who develop ARF have higher titre of anti-streptococcal antibodies in their sera than do those who escape the disease. Circulating immune complexes have also been found in serum of the patients with ARF.

Acute Glomerulonephritis

AGN is less frequently a consequence of streptococcal infection than is ARF. It is almost always produced by group A streptococci but group C streptococci may also be involved. In contrast to ARF which occurs only after pharyngitis, AGN may be seen after a pharyngeal or cutaneous infection. Most cases of AGN occur 2–3 weeks following skin infection or pharyngitis caused by certain pyodermal (M types 1 and 12) and pharyngeal (M types 49, 53–55 and 59–61) strains of *S. pyogenes*. These strains are known as **nephritogenic strains**.

Poststreptococcal AGN probably develops because some components of glomerular basement membrane are antigenically similar to the cell membranes of nephritogenic β-haemolytic streptococci. Therefore, antibodies which are produced by the host against the latter cross react with the former. Alternatively, streptococcal antigen-antibody complexes may lodge in the glomeruli. In either case, the activation of the C3 and C5 components of complement leads to tissue destruction. This is supported by the detection of C3 as well as γ-globulin and streptococcal antigens in the glomerular lesion.

Laboratory Diagnosis

In acute infections, diagnosis is established by identification of β-haemolytic streptococci that have been isolated from the patient, while in non-suppurative complications, diagnosis is based on the demonstration of rising titre of antibody to one or more streptococcal antigens.

Specimens

Throat and nose swabs from cases of sore throat or from suspected carriers, high vaginal swabs from cases of puerperal sepsis, pus or pus swabs from suppurative infections, and blood from cases of systemic infections are the usual specimens collected.

Gram Staining

The observation of typical Gram-positive cocci arranged in chains on microscopic examination of smear of pus or CSF may indicate the likelihood of the presence of streptococci.

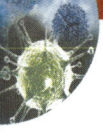

Fluorescent Antibody Technique

The examination of throat swab by the direct fluorescent antibody technique may be used for rapid identification of group A streptococci.

Culture

Inoculate pus or swab on blood agar plate immediately. Incubate it at 37°C for 24 hours and look for β-haemolytic colonies of streptococci. If there is likely to be delay, swab should be sent to the laboratory in Pike's medium (blood agar containing 1 in 1,000,000 crystal violet and 1 in 16,000 sodium azide distributed as for stab cultures in tubes). In case of bacteriological examination of skin lesions, crystal violet blood agar medium is useful selective medium that inhibits many commensal organisms.

Identification

Streptococcal colonies that produce β-haemolysis are subjected to:

- **Lancefield grouping** and in case the isolate belongs to group A, it is further subjected to **M typing**.
- A rapid method for identification of group A streptococci is based on **Maxted's observation** that they are more sensitive to bacitracin than other streptococci. The plate is inoculated with a pure culture of β-haemolytic *Streptococcus*, a 0.04 μg bacitracin disc is placed in the area of inoculation and the plate is incubated at 37°C for 24 hours. The inhibition of growth around the disc is seen with *S. pyogenes* but not with other streptococci. However, this test is not totally reliable as 5–15% of bacitracin-susceptible streptococci recovered from clinical sources may belong to groups other than group A. For example, 6% of group B and 7.5% of group C and G β-haemolytic streptococci are bacitracin-sensitive. About 7.5% of α-haemolytic streptococci are also bacitracin-sensitive.

Serological Tests

In ARF and AGN, a retrospective diagnosis of streptococcal infection may be established by serological tests, preferably with paired sera, to detect a rise in antibody titre to one or more of the extracellular products of *S. pyogenes*.

- **Antistreptolysin O** (ASO) test is used most frequently. ASO titres higher than 200 Todd units/ml are indicative of prior streptococcal infection.
- **Antideoxyribonuclease B** (anti-DNase B) estimation is also commonly employed. Titres higher than 300 or 350 are taken as significant.
- **Streptozyme test**, which is a passive slide haemagglutination test using erythrocytes sensitized with a crude preparation of extracellular antigens of streptococci, is a convenient, sensitive and specific screening test.

Treatment

Penicillin is highly effective in the treatment of all acute infections and penicillin resistance has not yet been observed in *S. pyogenes*. In patients allergic to penicillin, erythromycin or cephalexin may be used. Antimicrobial drugs have no effect on established cases of AGN and ARF.

GROUP B STREPTOCOCCI

Group B streptococci (**S. agalactiae**) are the etiologic agents of bovine mastitis and their association with human disease was recognized in 1930s. In recent years, infections with group B streptococci have been reported with increasing frequency. They are now major streptococcal pathogens in neonates and young children. Infection in the neonate is divided into early-onset-type and late-onset-type.

Early-onset-type

Group B streptococci are present in the vaginal flora of about 25% of all women. Early rupture of the membranes, prolonged labour, prematurity, low birth weight and heavy colonization of mother's vagina by group B streptococci lead to early-onset-type infection. Within first five days of life the neonate develops septicaemia and pneumonia, and in spite of the intensive antibiotic therapy, such infections carry a mortality rate of 50–70%. Meningitis may also develop.

Late-onset-type

This type of infection develops between second to fourth week of life. Baby acquires infection from the hospital personnel during nursing procedures. Baby to baby spread may also occur. The infecting organism is rarely found in the mother's vagina. This type of infection is not as severe as early-onset-type, but has a high incidence of residual effects often of a neurological nature.

Group B streptococci may also cause adult infections, including septicaemia, endocarditis, meningitis and local septic lesions in the female genital tract, the urinary tract, surgical wounds and skin. Occasionally, they may lead to pneumonia, empyema, arthritis and osteomyelitis.

Their ability to hydrolyse hippurate acts as a presumptive identification method. They may be identified by the CAMP reaction (Christie, Atkins and Munch-Peterson), which can be demonstrated as an accentuated zone of haemolysis when *S. agalactiae* is inoculated perpendicular to a streak of *S. aureus* grown on blood agar (Fig. 10.3). Occasional strains are bacitracin-sensitive.

GROUP C STREPTOCOCCI

Group C streptococci comprise four species—*S. equi*, *S. equisimilis*, *S. dysgalactiae* and *S. zooepidemicus*. They produce wide zones of β-haemolysis and can cause sore throat, skin and

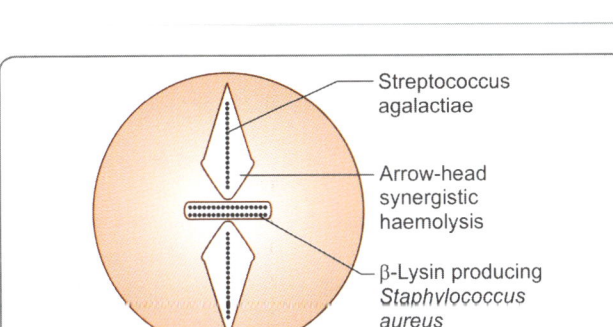

Fig. 10.3: CAMP test.

wound infections, post-partum sepsis, pneumonia, septicaemia, meningitis, endocarditis and AGN.

GROUP G STREPTOCOCCI

These organisms are part of the normal flora of skin, particularly at damp sites, and of gut, pharynx and vagina. These may cause sore throat, pneumonia, septicaemia, endocarditis, and bone, joint, skin and wound infections.

GROUP D STREPTOCOCCI

The Group D streptococci include *S. bovis* and *S. equinus*. Until the mid-1980s, the group D streptococci were divided into the enterococcal and nonenterococcal groups. Those found in the intestinal tract were part of the enterococcal group and have now been placed in a new genus, *Enterococcus*, but nonenterococcal group remains part of the group D streptococci. Both *Enterococcus* and group D streptococci can grow in the presence of 40% bile and also hydrolyse aesculin to aesculetin and glucose.

The species most commonly associated with human disease is *E. faecalis*, but infections caused by *E. faecium, E. durans, E. avium* and other enterococci also occur. Identification of various species of *Enterococcus* is made on biochemical grounds. *E. faecalis* ferments mannitol with gas production. It is VP positive and can grow on blood tellurite agar producing black colonies.

Enterococci may cause urinary tract infection, wound infection, infective endocarditis, biliary tract infection, peritonitis, suppurative abdominal lesions and septicaemia.

VIRIDANS STREPTOCOCCI (ORAL STREPTOCOCCI)

These organisms produce α-haemolysis on 5% sheep blood agar. They are constantly present as commensals in the mouth and oropharynx. At least five species of viridans streptococci have been recognized. These include *S. salivarius, S. sanguis, S. mutans, S. mitior (mitis)* and *S. milleri*. Viridans streptococci, chiefly *S. mutans* and to a lesser extent *S. sanguis*, are involved in the production of **dental caries**. They break down dietary sucrose, producing acid and a tough adhesive dextran. The acid damages dentine and the dextran bind together food debris, epithelial cells, mucus and bacteria to form **dental plaques** which lead to caries.

In persons with predisposing factors, such as valvular disease of heart, viridans streptococci may cause **infective endocarditis** (IE). Tooth extraction and injury of the oral cavity in such persons is dangerous, because from oral cavity they may enter into the blood stream and cause IE. Tooth extraction in such individuals should be done under antibiotic cover. Other organisms which may also cause IE include *E. faecalis* and other enterococci, *S. aureus*, coagulase-negative staphylococci, *Coxiella burnetii* and some fungi.

Diagnosis of IE is established by repeated blood cultures. Viridans streptococci can be recognized by their α-haemolytic colonies on blood agar and their failure to grow on MacConkey medium. When isolated from mouth, throat and respiratory tract, they are regarded as harmless commensals and when isolated from blood or a closed lesion they are likely to be pathogenic. These streptococci are generally susceptible to penicillin, though some strains may be resistant. Therefore, antibiotic sensitivity of these organisms should also be carried out.

STREPTOCOCCUS MG

This belongs to group F streptococci. It has been isolated from the sputum of normal individuals and those suffering from primary atypical pneumonia. These patients frequently have in their sera agglutinins to *Streptococcus* MG.

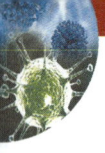

🍂 Key Points

- *Streptococci are Gram-positive, non-motile, catalase-negative cocci.* They are ovoid to spherical in shape and occur in chains (*Streptococcus pyogenes*) or pairs (*Streptococcus pneumoniae*).
- Because of their complex nutritional requirements, **blood-enriched medium** is generally used for their isolation. The diseases caused by this group of organisms are diverse, some of the most prevalent being, for example, acute infections of the throat and skin, caused by group A streptococci (*Streptococcus pyogenes*), genital tract colonization by group B streptococci (*Streptococcus agalactiae*), and endocarditis caused by viridans group of streptococci.
- There is a considerable evidence that *Streptococcus pyogenes* is in some way the cause of **acute rheumatic fever** and **acute glomerulonephritis**.

❓ ASSESS YOURSELF

LONG AND SHORT ANSWER QUESTIONS

1. Discuss the classification of streptococci.
2. Describe the antigenic structure of *Streptococcus pyogenes*, giving suitable diagram.
3. Name various toxins and enzymes produced by *Streptococcus pyogenes* and discuss each of these in brief.
4. Discuss pathogenicity of *Streptococcus pyogenes*.
5. Write short notes on:
   - (a) Streptolysins
   - (b) Streptokinase
   - (c) Streptodornase

MULTIPLE CHOICE QUESTIONS

1. Which type of haemolysis is produced by *Streptococcus pyogenes*?
   - (a) α-haemolysis
   - (b) β-haemolysis
   - (c) γ-haemolysis
   - (d) δ-haemolysis

2. Crystal violet blood agar is a selective medium for:
   - (a) β-haemolytic streptococci
   - (b) *Staphylococcus aureus*
   - (c) *Corynebacterium diphtheriae*
   - (d) *Mycobacterium tuberculosis*

3. Streptolysin O is:
   - (a) Oxygen-labile
   - (b) Heat-labile
   - (c) Antigenic
   - (d) All of the above

4. The most important cause of bacterial sore throat is:
   - (a) *Streptococcus pyogenes*
   - (b) *Staphylococcus aureus*
   - (c) *Haemophilus* spp.
   - (d) *Mycoplasma pneumoniae*

5. CAMP test is useful for identification of:
   - (a) Group A streptococci
   - (b) Group B streptococci
   - (c) Group C streptococci
   - (d) Group D streptococci

6. Which of the following organisms causes scarlet fever?
   - (a) *Staphylococcus aureus*
   - (b) *Streptococcus pyogenes*
   - (c) *Pseudomonas aeruginosa*
   - (d) *Propionibacterium acnes*

ANSWERS TO MCQS

1. b   **2.** a   **3.** d   **4.** a   **5.** b   **6.** b

Chapter 11

Streptococcus pneumoniae (Pneumococcus)

Pneumococcus was first identified in 1881 by Louis Pasteur and Sternberg independently. This organism carries historical importance in that research work with pneumococcal transformations provided the initial proof that **DNA alone is the carrier of genetic information.**

- As a clear halo in India ink preparation.
- By direct special staining techniques.
- It can also be seen and typed by treatment with homologous type-specific antibody which combines with the capsular polysaccharide and renders it refractile – **Quellung reaction**.

MORPHOLOGY

The pneumococcus is a non-motile, non-sporing, Gram-positive coccus. In the material taken from the body, it occurs characteristically in pairs of **flame-shaped** cocci about 1 μm in diameter, the rounded ends of the cocci being adjacent to each other (Figs 11.1 and 11.2). The cell wall of pneumococcus contains an antigen, referred to as C substance, that is similar to the carbohydrate antigens contained in the cell wall of β-haemolytic streptococci. In cultures they usually appear in chains like streptococci. The pneumococcus is capsulated. The capsule encloses each pair and it is best seen in the material taken directly from the exudates and may be lost on repeated cultivation. Pneumococcal capsule can be demonstrated by following methods:

CULTURAL CHARACTERISTICS

Aerobe and facultative anaerobe, may need 5–10% CO_2 for primary isolation. Optimum temperature 37°C (range 25–40°C), pH 7.8 (range 6.5–8.3) and grows only on enriched media.

On **blood agar**, after 18–24 hour incubation at 37°C, virulent strains with abundant capsular polysaccharide produce small (0.5–1 mm in diameter), moist, mucoid, transparent colonies. Poorly encapsulated strains of pneumococci produce small, round, translucent colonies. The colonies are surrounded by a 2–3 mm zone of α-haemolysis. On further incubation, the colonies develop a central depression because of autolysis with raised rim (**draughtsman colony**). Under anaerobic incubation, colonies on blood agar are surrounded by a zone of β-haemolysis due to the liberation of oxygen-labile pneumolysin by pneumococci.

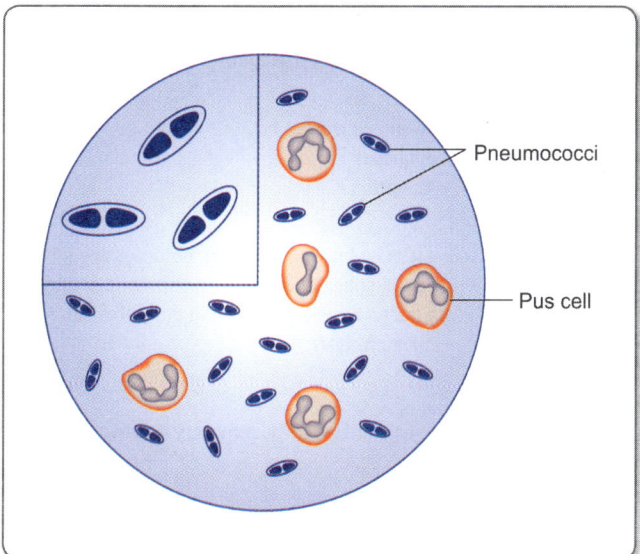

Fig. 11.1: Pneumococci in pus. Inset: enlarged view.

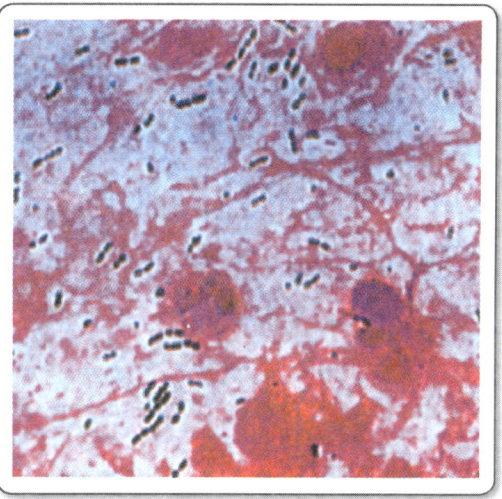

Fig. 11.2: Gram-stained sputum smear showing Gram-positive, encapsulated, extracellular diplococci from a patient of pneumococcal pneumonia (× 1000).

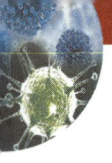

BIOCHEMICAL REACTIONS

Pneumococci ferment glucose, sucrose, lactose and inulin with the production of acid but no gas. Fermentation reactions are tested in Hiss's serum sugar media. **Fermentation of inulin** by pneumococci is a useful test for differentiating them from streptococci which do not ferment it. They are catalase and oxidase negative.

Bile Solubility Test

Pneumococci are bile soluble while viridans and other streptococci are not. Bile salts, (sodium deoxycholate and sodium taurocholate) lyse pneumococci when added to actively growing cultures in an artificial culture medium. Pneumococci produce autolytic enzymes leading to autolysis in older cultures. The addition of bile salts is thought to accelerate this process.

For bile solubility test, inoculate the test organism in 5 ml serum digest broth or infusion broth, incubate it at 37°C for 18 hours. While still warm, add 0.5 ml of 10% sodium deoxycholate solution and reincubate at 37°C. Within 15 minutes initially turbid culture becomes clear and transparent due to the lysis of pneumococci. Alternatively, touch a suspected pneumococcal colony on blood agar plate with a loopful of 2% sodium deoxycholate solution at pH 7. Incubate the plate at 37°C for 30 minutes. The colony disappears, leaving an area of α-haemolysis.

SENSITIVITY TO PHYSICAL AND CHEMICAL AGENTS

Pneumococci are delicate organisms. They can be killed by moist heat at 55°C in 10 minutes and readily by most disinfectants.

They are sensitive to a wide range of antimicrobial drugs including benzylpenicillin, other penicillins, cephalosporins, erythromycin, tetracycline, clindamycin and co-trimoxazole. Some strains resistant to β-lactam antibiotics and erythromycin have been reported.

Optochin Sensitivity Test

Pneumococci are highly sensitive to killing by optochin (ethyl hydrocuprein hydrochloride). Optochin sensitivity test is used for identification of pneumococci and distinguishing them from viridans streptococci, both of which produce α-haemolysis on blood agar. Optochin is a quinine derivative that inhibits the growth of pneumococci but not of viridans streptococci. For testing, a filter paper disc containing 5 μg of optochin is applied to the surface of a blood agar plate streaked with a lawn of pure culture. Plate is incubated at 37°C in air with 5–10% CO_2. Pneumococcus shows a zone of inhibition of 14 mm or more around the 6 mm optochin disc or 16 mm or more if 10 mm disc is used. Viridans streptococci grow right up to the disc. The differences between *S. pneumoniae* and viridans streptococci are given in Table 11.1.

ANTIGENIC STRUCTURE

Capsular Antigen

The most important of pneumococcal antigens is the capsular polysaccharide on the basis of which the pneumococci are divided into more than 90 serologic types named 1, 2, 3, etc. A few more types are awaiting confirmation. As this polysaccharide diffuses into the culture medium or infective exudates and tissues, it is also known as **specific soluble substance** (SSS).

TABLE 11.1: Differences between *Streptococcus pneumoniae* and viridans streptococci

	S. pneumoniae	Viridans streptococci
Morphology		
■ Shape	Flame-shaped cocci	Round or oval cocci
■ Arrangement	In pairs	In chains
■ Capsule	Present	Absent
Cultural characteristics		
■ On blood agar medium	After 24 hour incubation, colonies are round, moist, mucoid, transparent and surrounded by 2–3 mm zone of α-haemolysis. On further incubation, the colonies develop a central depression with raised rim (draughtsman colonies)	After 24 hour incubation, colonies are dome-shaped, opaque and surrounded by a narrow zone (1–2 mm in diameter) of α-haemolysis
■ In liquid medium	Uniform turbidity	Granular turbidity, powdery deposit
Bile solubility	Positive	Negative
Inulin fermentation	Positive	Negative
Optochin sensitivity	Positive	Negative
Intraperitoneal inoculation in mice	Fatal infection, death of mice in 1–3 days	Non-pathogenic

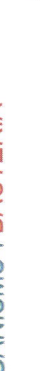

The capsule of the pneumococcus is essential for virulence, its role being to protect the organism from phagocytosis. Only smooth encapsulated (S) strains are pathogenic for man and most laboratory animals. Active or passive immunization against a specific polysaccharide produces a high level of resistance to infection with pneumococci of homologous type. Laboratory strains that have lost the ability to produce a capsule are non-pathogenic.

The typing of individual isolates can be performed by:

- **Quellung reaction** in which the capsules of pneumococci are made more easily visible when acted upon by specific antisera. It is performed by mixing equal quantities of specimen (sputum, pus or sediment of CSF) or light suspension of the test organisms with type-specific pneumococcal antiserum. After waiting for 15–30 minutes, for the reaction to occur, the mixture is examined microscopically using a 100× objective. If Quellung reaction is positive, the capsule of the pneumococci will appear quite prominent as compared with those in the same specimen mixed with saline solution as a control. **The increased prominence of the capsule or swelling is apparently due to an alteration of its refractive index after reacting with the antiserum.** Pooled sera may be tested first and then in turn the individual type-specific antisera until one of them is found to give positive result.
- Agglutination of the cocci with the type-specific antiserum.
- Precipitation of SSS with the specific antiserum.

Somatic Antigen

Pneumococcal cell wall contains a species-specific carbohydrate hapten. It is referred to as pneumococcal C substance. This appears to be analogous to (though antigenically different from) the group-specific C antigens of β-haemolytic streptococci.

Cell Wall Carbohydrate (C-substance)

Pneumococci contain a species-specific somatic carbohydrate antigen which is known as C-substance. C-substance is precipitated by an abnormal protein (β-globulin). It appears in acute phase sera of cases of pneumonia but disappears during convalescence. It also appears in some other pathological conditions. It is known as C-reactive protein because it precipitates with C antigen of pneumococci. It is not an antibody. Its production is stimulated by bacterial infection, inflammation, malignancy and tissue destruction. It disappears when inflammation subsides. It is used as an index of response to treatment in rheumatic fever and certain other conditions. It is tested by:

- capillary precipitation of patient serum with antiserum prepared in rabbits against purified CRP; and
- passive agglutination using latex particles coated with anti-CRP antibody.

PATHOGENICITY

The most important disease caused by *S. pneumoniae* is **pneumonia, either a lobar pneumonia or a bronchopneumonia**. The latter is characteristically a disease of young children and older adults over 50 years, while lobar pneumonia is almost exclusively a disease of the age group 10–50 years. Other pneumococcal lesions are **acute bronchitis, sinusitis, otitis media, mastoiditis, meningitis, endocarditis, suppurative arthritis and peritonitis**. *S. pneumoniae* is the etiologic agent in about half of the children with otitis media. *S. pneumoniae* is a common cause of bacterial meningitis that affects patients of all ages. Pneumococcal meningitis is most often seen in children and the elderly. Pneumococcal meningitis may occur as a complication of otitis media or lobar pneumonia. Sometimes it is a consequence of fracture of skull with tearing of meninges. Bacteraemia may complicate pneumococcal pneumonia in about 15% of patients.

LABORATORY DIAGNOSIS

The diagnosis is carried out by demonstration of pneumococci in sputum (Fig. 11.2), exudate, blood and cerebrospinal fluid (CSF) by Gram staining, culture and by demonstration of pneumococcal antigen by coagglutination (COA), latex agglutination (LA) and counterimmunoelectrophoresis (CIE).

Microscopy

The sputum is homogenized by agitating the specimen for 30 minutes in a mechanical shaker with an equal quantity of distilled water and a small number of glass beads. Gram-stained smears are prepared from homogenized sputum and examined.

Culture

Sputum, after homogenisation, if necessary, is inoculated onto blood agar and heated blood agar media and incubated in air with 5–10% CO_2 for 18–24 hours. If the sputum is unobtainable, as in young children, a serum-coated laryngeal swab is taken and processed. The organisms isolated are identified by their morphological and biochemical characters.

The growth of *S. pneumoniae* may be typed with appropriate antisera. Typing can also be done by Quellung reaction in wet films of sputum, pus or sediment of CSF.

Animal Inoculation

From the specimens where pneumococci are scanty, isolation may be done by intraperitoneal inoculation in mice. Inoculated mice die in one to three days and pneumococci may be demonstrated in the peritoneal exudate and heart blood.

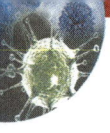

Blood Culture

Since many healthy individuals carry pneumococci in their throats, therefore, demonstration of organisms in sputum or throat culture is not necessarily indicative of pneumococcal disease. Many pneumococcal infections are associated with a bacteraemia or septicaemia. Therefore, if pneumococci are isolated from patient's blood, the diagnosis of a severe pneumococcal infection can be made with certainty. In all cases of suspected acute bacterial pneumonia sample of blood obtained by venipuncture, prior to administration of antimicrobial drugs, should be cultured immediately in beef infusion broth and thioglycollate broth.

Cerebrospinal Fluid

In case of suspected meningitis, a centrifuged deposit of CSF should be examined immediately in a Gram film, cultured on blood agar and heated blood agar, and incubated in air with 5–10% CO_2 for 18–24 hours.

Antigen Detection

In some cases, particularly if antibiotics have been given before collection of the specimen, viable cocci may not be there in the specimen and culture may be negative. In such cases, pneumococcal antigen is often detectable in CSF by COA, LA or CIE. COA test for the detection of antigen gives positive result in larger proportion of specimens than either a Gram film or culture. Moreover, by COA test, result is available within a short time. In addition to CSF, capsular polysaccharide can be demonstrated in blood and urine by CIE.

CHEMOTHERAPY

Treatment with penicillin should be started as soon as pneumococcal pneumonia is suspected. Penicillin-resistant pneumococci do not form penicillinase. The available evidence suggests that the resistance is chromosomally determined and it may be due to the changes in the penicillin-binding proteins in the cell membrane. In case of infection with penicillin-resistant strains or if the patient is penicillin sensitive then any of the cephalosporins, erythromycin, tetracycline, clindamycin, vancomycin, chloramphenicol and sulphonamides may be used.

 Key Points

- Pneumococci are Gram-positive, non-motile cocci occurring in pairs. They are capsulated.
- **Acquisition of DNA** by a bacterium from its environment was first demonstrated in *Streptococcus pneumoniae* by Griffith in 1928.
- Pneumococci cause pneumonia, otitis media and meningitis.

? ASSESS YOURSELF

LONG ANSWER QUESTIONS

1. Discuss the antigenic structure of *Streptococcus pneumoniae*.
2. Describe the pathogenicity of *Streptococcus pneumoniae*.
3. Differentiate between *Streptococcus pneumoniae* and viridans streptococci in a tabulated form.

MULTIPLE CHOICE QUESTIONS

1. Pneumococcal capsule can be demonstrated by:
   - (a) Quellung reaction
   - (b) Negative staining
   - (c) Both of the above
   - (d) None of the above

2. *Streptococcus pneumoniae* can be differentiated from viridans streptococci on the basis of which of the following test/s?
   - (a) Optochin sensitivity test
   - (b) Bile solubility test
   - (c) Inulin fermentation test
   - (d) All of the above

3. Pneumolysin is immunologically related to which of the following haemolysins?
   - (a) *Clostridium tetani* haemolysin
   - (b) *C. perfringens* haemolysin
   - (c) Streptococcal oxygen-labile haemolysin
   - (d) All of the above

4. Pneumococcal antigen in CSF can be detected by:
   - (a) Coagglutination
   - (b) Latex agglutination
   - (c) Counterimmunoelectrophoresis
   - (d) All of the above

ANSWERS TO MCQs

1. c   **2.** d   **3.** d   **4.** d

Neisseria

The genus *Neisseria* has Gram-negative cocci with adjacent sides flattened. *N. gonorrhoeae* and *N. meningitidis* are the primary human pathogens of the genus. *N. gonorrhoeae* is always pathogenic, but *N. meningitidis* may be found as a commensal inhabitant of the upper respiratory tract of carriers.

NEISSERIA MENINGITIDIS (MENINGOCOCCUS)

Morphology

They are Gram-negative cocci, 0.6–1.0 μm in diameter. They usually occur in pairs with adjacent sides flattened or concave and long axes parallel. They are typically seen in large numbers inside polymorphonuclear leucocytes (Fig. 12.1). Fresh isolates of most *N. meningitidis* serogroups are encapsulated. They are non-sporing and non-motile.

Cultural Characteristics

Meningococci have exacting growth requirements and do not grow on ordinary media. Growth occurs on media enriched with

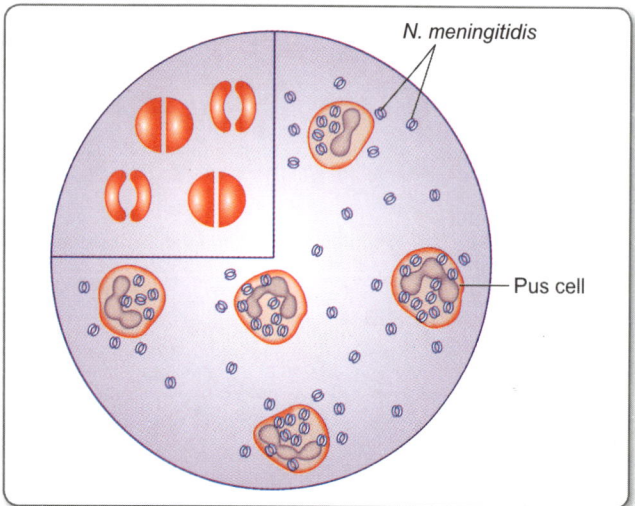

Fig. 12.1: *Neisseria meningitidis* in CSF. Inset: enlarged view showing adjacent sides flattened or concave and long axes parallel.

blood or serum. They are strict aerobes, no growth occurring anaerobically. The growth is facilitated by 5–10% CO_2 and high humidity. The optimum temperature and pH for the growth of meningococci are 35–36°C and 7.0–7.4, respectively.

Colony Morphology

- On **blood agar**, after 24-hour incubation, the colonies of meningococci are small about 1 mm in diameter, round, convex, grey, non-haemolytic and translucent. After 48 hours incubation, colonies are larger with an opaque raised centre and thin transparent margins which may be crenated.
- On **heated blood agar** (chocolate agar), colonies of meningococci are slightly larger than those on ordinary blood agar.

Biochemical Characters

Meningococci are catalase- and oxidase-positive. When 1% solution of oxidase reagent (tetramethyl-*p*-phenylene-diamine dihydrochloride) is poured on culture plate, *Neisseria* colonies quickly turn deep-purple. This **prompt oxidase reaction** helps in the identification of meningococci and gonococci in mixed cultures. This test may also be done by rubbing a few colonies with a glass rod on a strip of filter paper moistened with oxidase reagent. A deep-purple colour develops immediately.

Meningococci utilize glucose and maltose by oxidative method with the production of acid but no gas. They do not attack lactose or sucrose. Indole and hydrogen sulphide are not produced and nitrates are not reduced.

Sensitivity to Physical and Chemical Agents

Meningococci are killed by heating at 55°C in 5 minutes or less. They are highly susceptible to desiccation, death occurring usually within an hour or two. Weak disinfectants such as 1% phenol or 1% mercuric chloride kill them in 1–2 minutes.

Antigenic Structure

N. meningitidis possesses a polysaccharide capsule and on the basis of immunologic specificity of capsular polysaccharide it has been subdivided into 12 serogroups: A, B, C, X, Y, Z, 29E, W-135, H, I, K and L. Most meningococcal infections are caused by strains of groups A, B and C with a small proportion of infections

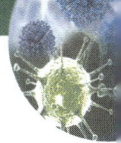

being due to strains of groups Y and W-135. Groups X, Z and 29E are only rarely associated with some form of immune deficiency. Serogroups H, I, K and L have been isolated from carriers and have not been associated with disease.

Pathogenicity

Meningococci are normally carried in nasopharynx of 5–10% of healthy individuals. Like most of the respiratory infections, meningococcal meningitis is disseminated by droplet infection, direct contact and less often by fomites. Infection is spread by patients and convalescents to a limited extent, but the healthy carriers of meningococci are of primary importance. The meningococcal disease can be divided into three stages:

- **First stage**
  The organisms appear in nasopharynx leading to **nasopharyngeal infection**, which is usually asymptomatic but might result in a minor inflammation.
- **Second stage**
  In a small percentage of cases, the meningococci may enter the blood stream from posterior nasopharynx, probably by way of the cervical lymph nodes. This stage is known as **meningococcaemia**. The patient develops fever, malaise and **petechial skin lesions** due to foci of infection in the capillaries. The organisms may also cause lesions in the joints and lungs and, rarely, may cause massive bilateral haemorrhages in the adrenals. This is known as **Waterhouse-Friderichsen syndrome**.
- **Third stage**
  Meningococci infect the meninges causing the major symptoms of severe headache, stiff neck and vomiting accompanied by delirium and confusion. The route of spread of meningococcus from the nasopharynx to the meninges is controversial. The organisms may spread along the perineural sheaths of the olfactory nerves, passing through the cribriform plate may reach the subarachnoid space or it may set up a preliminary sinusitis and reach the brain either via lymphatics or direct extension through the bone. Others believe that the meningococci reach the CNS via blood stream through a preliminary bacteraemia.

Laboratory Diagnosis

Specimens

Specimens may include CSF, blood, aspirate from skin lesions, pus from infected joint, and throat and nasopharyngeal swab. Swab should be transported in Stuart's transport medium. All specimens where meningococcal infection is suspected must be submitted to the laboratory immediately.

Cerebrospinal Fluid

In meningococcal meningitis, CSF is under pressure and is turbid due to a large number of polymorphonuclear leucocytes present in a typical case. For bacteriological examination, the CSF is divided into three portions.

First portion is centrifuged and Gram-stained smears are prepared from the deposit. Meningococci (Gram-negative diplococci) will be seen mainly inside polymorphs, but often extracellularly also. Strains causing meningitis are usually encapsulated and may show a distinct pink halo surrounding the cells. The capsule may also make the cells more resistant to decolourization and they may appear Gram-positive. When present in small numbers, meningococci may be detected by immunofluorescent technique. The supernatant contains meningococcal antigen, which may be demonstrated by precipitation test with polyvalent or monovalent antimeningococcal serum. Counterimmunoelectrophoresis provides a rapid and sensitive method for demonstration of meningococcal antigen.

Second portion of CSF is inoculated on blood agar or chocolate agar and incubated at 35–36°C under 5–10% CO_2. Colonies appear after 18–24 hours which may be identified by morphology and biochemical reactions. The meningococcus isolated may be typed by agglutination with polyvalent or monovalent antimeningococcal serum.

Third portion of CSF is incubated for 18–24 hours, either as such or after adding an equal volume of glucose broth and then subcultured on chocolate agar. This method may sometimes succeed where direct plating fails.

Blood Culture

Blood culture is often positive in meningococcaemia and in early cases of meningitis. Specimen of blood is inoculated into blood culture bottle of trypticase-soy broth. It should be incubated at 35–36°C in 5–10% CO_2 for 4–7 days, with daily subcultures on blood agar. Look for oxidase-positive colonies of Gram-negative diplococci as above.

Serological Diagnosis

This may be attempted in cases of chronic meningococcal septicaemia where no organisms have been isolated. Specific antibodies to capsular polysaccharide may be demonstrated by haemagglutination test.

Treatment

Almost all clinical isolates of *N. meningitidis* are sensitive to penicillin. Penicillin G in high doses, given intravenously or intrathecally, if necessary, is the treatment of choice. In penicillin sensitive individuals, chloramphenicol has been regarded as an alternative to penicillin therapy for meningococcal meningitis but recent studies show that cefotaxime or ceftriaxone are at least as effective and avoid the possibility of blood dyscrasia.

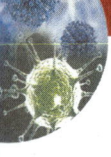
Prophylaxis

Chemoprophylaxis

Outbreaks of disease may be controlled by chemoprophylaxis alone.

- Rifampicin is recommended for chemoprophylaxis in children although it is effective in eradicating meningococcal carriage in only 80–90% of the population treated. After prophylaxis, rifampicin-resistant strains may be found in a small number of patients and may on rare occasions give rise to disease in contacts.
- Ciprofloxacin is widely used as a prophylactic for adolescents and adults as a single oral dose. All household and intimate contacts of a case should be given a chemoprophylaxis as a routine.

Vaccines

Vaccines containing the pure group-specific capsular polysaccharide of meningococci of groups A, C, Y and W-135 are available and are good immunogens.

NEISSERIA GONORRHOEAE (GONOCOCCUS)

Morphology

Morphology and staining characteristics of *N. gonorrhoeae* are similar to those of *N. meningitidis*.

Cultural Characteristics

Gonococci are more difficult to grow than meningococci. They are aerobes, but may grow anaerobically also. Addition of 5–10% CO_2 is essential for primary isolation. Growth occurs best at pH 7.0–7.4 and at a temperature of 35–36°C. They can be isolated on media enriched with blood, either partially lysed by heat (chocolate agar) or completely lysed by saponin.

Heated blood agar may be made selective for the isolation of pathogenic neisseriae by the addition of vancomycin, colistin and nystatin. This selective medium (**Thayer-Martin medium**) is valuable in isolating gonococci from heavily contaminated specimens. Trimethoprim may be added to Thayer-Martin medium to inhibit swarming *Proteus* species that are occasionally present in cervicovaginal and rectal specimens. This chocolate agar medium containing vancomycin, colistin, nystatin and trimethoprim is known as **modified Thayer-Martin medium**.

Colony Morphology

- On **heated blood agar**, after 24 hour incubation, colonies are small about 1 mm in diameter, grey, convex and translucent. After 48 hour incubation, colonies are larger 1.5–2.5 mm in diameter, sometimes with an opaque raised centre and thin transparent margins which may be crenated.
- On **Thayer-Martin medium** growth is slower, although colonies are similar to those on heated blood agar.

Biochemical Reactions

N. gonorrhoeae resembles *N. meningitidis* with the exception that the former can utilize only glucose and the latter glucose and maltose with the production of acid only.

Antigenic Structure

N. gonorrhoeae is antigenically heterogeneous. Surface structures include the following:

- **Pili**
  Pili are nonflagellar surface appendages. These are hair-like structures, several micrometers in length, 7 nm in diameter and are seen on the surface of gonococci of types T1 and T2. These play an important role in attachment of gonococci to the cell. Furthermore, the pili are antiphagocytic. Removal of pili from cells by treatment with trypsin results in their phagocytosis and destruction.
- **Outer membrane proteins**
  Gonococci possess three major outer membrane proteins named proteins I, II and III.
- **Lipooligosaccharide (LOS)**
  It differs in its chemical structure from lipopolysaccharide (LPS) of Gram-negative bacilli. It does not have long O antigenic side chains. Toxicity in gonococcal infections is largely due to the endotoxic effect of LOS.

Sensitivity to Physical and Chemical Agents

N. gonorrhoeae is a very delicate organism. It is readily killed by heat, drying and antiseptics.

Pathogenesis

N. gonorrhoeae causes **gonorrhoea**. It is a sexually transmitted disease that, with few exceptions, is acquired through sexual contact with an infected individual. *N. gonorrhoeae* is exclusively a human pathogen although chimpanzees have been infected by artificial inoculation. It is never found as a commensal although a proportion of those infected, particularly women, may remain asymptomatic. These may develop systemic or ascending infection at a later stage.

Gonococci ordinarily enter the body through the mucous membrane of the genitourinary tract, apparently penetrating between columnar epithelial cells. Stratified squamous epithelium is relatively resistant to infection. After an incubation period of 2–7 days, the organism evokes an acute inflammatory response in the subepithelial tissue giving rise to the purulent urethral or vaginal discharge, dysuria and frequency of micturition. In male,

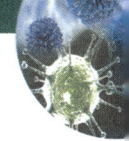

the acute urethritis may extend to the prostate, testes, seminal vesicles, epididymis and sometimes the periurethral tissue. If untreated it is often followed by fibrosis and stricture.

In women, the endocervix is the primary site of infection. The urethra may also become infected. In adult women, the vagina usually escapes because of the acidic pH of the vaginal secretions, but severe vulvovaginitis can occur in prepubertal girls. The primary infection may spread from urethra, vagina and cervix to Bartholin's glands, uterus, fallopian tubes, ovaries and pelvic peritoneum causing a pelvic inflammatory disease resulting in sterility. Bacteraemia may occur in fulminating cases, in both men and women, and is occasionally complicated by endocarditis, acute purulent arthritis or both.

Babies born to infected women may contract serious gonococcal infection of the eye (**ophthalmia neonatorum**) during passage through infected birth canal.

Anorectal infection occurs in both sexes. In men this follows homosexual rectal intercourse. In women, it can follow rectal intercourse, but may also arise as a result of autoinoculation of rectal mucosa with infected vaginal discharge (direct contagious spread). **Gonococcal pharyngitis** may follow orogenital contact in either sex. **Conjunctivitis** may occur usually by autoinoculation with fingers.

Laboratory Diagnosis

Specimens

Specimen swab is collected from urethra, endocervix, anal canal, vagina (in case of paediatric patient), Bartholin's glands, oropharynx and conjunctival swab. These swabs should be either inoculated directly onto growth medium or transported to the laboratory in a transport medium such as Amies medium with charcoal and plated within 6 hours.

Microscopy

Prepare smear by rolling the swab gently over the surface of a glass slide in one direction only. Do not rub swab, it may distort microscopic morphology. Do the Gram staining and see under oil-immersion lens. The observation of characteristic kidney-shaped Gram-negative diplococci lying within polymorphonuclear leucocytes with a few extracellular organisms from a symptomatic male with discharge correlates at a rate of 95% with culture and presumptive evidence of gonococcal infection. If no organisms are visible on Gram staining, report the smear as negative.

Culture

All specimens received in the laboratory for recovery of *Neisseria* species should be held at room temperature and plated as soon as possible. Media should be warmed to room temperature before inoculation, because *Neisseria* species are susceptible to cold. Roll specimen swab firmly in a 'Z' pattern onto selective medium (Thayer-Martin or modified Thayer-Martin) and then cross-streak with a sterile wire loop or needle. In case of specimen from normally sterile sites inoculate nonselective medium (heated blood agar). Incubate the cultures immediately at 35–36°C in 5–10% CO_2.

Observation

Examine plates after 24 hours incubation and test suspected colonies by touching with a cotton bud soaked in oxidase reagent. Oxidase-positive bacteria turn the contact area of the bud purple within 5–15 seconds. If oxidase-positive, prepare a smear from an identical colony and stain it with Gram stain. Gonococci will appear Gram-negative diplococci which can be further confirmed by biochemical reactions. Incubation of primary isolation plate is continued for 48 hours and cultures are re-examined by above procedures before any specimen can be reported negative.

Antibiotic sensitivity of the isolate, especially against penicillin and production of enzyme β-lactamase (penicillinase) should also be carried out for instituting an effective therapy.

Treatment

Large doses of penicillin, 2.4–4.8 million units of aqueous procaine penicillin G intramuscularly, preceded by probenecid 1 gram orally is recommended. Ampicillin 3.5 gram + probenecid 1 gram is an effective oral alternative.

Prophylaxis

Control of gonorrhoea consists of early detection of cases particularly those infected females who have asymptomatic infections. These cases should be treated. Because the incubation period of symptomatic gonorrhoea is short, tracing and treating the recent sexual contacts lessens the spread of the disease. Greater mobility and greater sexual freedom has contributed to the acquisition of gonorrhoea. Use of condom and health education can help in the control of the disease to a great extent.

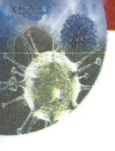

Key Points

- The genus *Neisseria* consists of **Gram-negative cocci**, usually arranged in pairs, and are **oxidase-positive**.
- Two *Neisseria* species are pathogenic for humans – *Neisseria gonorrhoeae* (gonococcus), the causal agent of **gonorrhoea**; and *Neisseria meningitidis* (meningococcus), a frequent cause of **meningitis**.
- Gonococci and meningococci are non-motile and usually occur in **pairs** with adjacent sides flattened or concave and long axes parallel. They are typically seen in large numbers **inside polymorphonuclear leucocytes**. They cannot be differentiated from each other under microscope. However, they can be differentiated in the laboratory by their **sugar utilization patterns**, and by the **sites of their primary infections**.

? ASSESS YOURSELF

LONG ANSWER QUESTIONS

1. Discuss the pathogenicity of *Neisseria meningitidis*.
2. Describe the laboratory diagnosis of meningococcal infections.
3. Describe various culture media for the isolation of *Neisseria gonorrhoeae*.
4. Discuss the pathogenesis of gonorrhoea.
5. Discuss laboratory diagnosis of gonorrhoea.

MULTIPLE CHOICE QUESTIONS

1. How many serogroups of *Neisseria meningitidis* are known?
   - (a) Seven
   - (b) Nine
   - (c) Eleven
   - (d) Twelve
2. Capsule of *Neisseria meningitidis* is made up of:
   - (a) Polysaccharide
   - (b) Polypeptide
   - (c) Hyaluronic acid
   - (d) Polyphosphate

ANSWERS TO MCQs

1. d   2. a

Chapter 13

Corynebacterium diphtheriae

Corynebacteria are pleomorphic, club-shaped, Gram-positive bacilli arranged in V forms or palisades. The most important member of the genus *Corynebacterium* is *C. diphtheriae*. It was first observed and described by Klebs (1883) but was first cultured by Loeffler (1884). Therefore, it is known as the **Klebs-Löeffler bacillus**.

CORYNEBACTERIUM DIPHTHERIAE

Morphology

They are thin, slender, non-sporing, non-capsulated, non-motile, non-acid-fast, Gram-positive bacilli of varying lengths with an average size of 3 × 0.3 μm. They frequently possess club-shaped swellings at one or both ends, a characteristic feature which is responsible for the name of the genus (*coryne* means club). When dividing, the bacilli snap and bend abruptly and appear as angled pairs or parallel rows of 3–4 bacilli (palisades) which resemble Chinese letters (*Chinese letter arrangement or Cuneiform arrangement*) (Figs 13.1 and 13.2).

Although, Gram-positive, *C. diphtheriae* is readily decolourized. Another characteristic of this organism is its granular and uneven staining. When stained with methylene blue or toluidine blue, the granules in the cell stain metachromatically (i.e. granules that stain a colour different from the primary dye colour) bluish-purple. Most cells contain 2 or 3 of these, and they tend to be on the poles. The granules consist of long-chain inorganic polyphosphates. These granules are known as **metachromatic granules** or **volutin granules** or **Babes-Ernst bodies**. In unstained wet preparations, they appear as round refractile bodies within the bacterial cytoplasm.

With Albert stain, the granules stain bluish black and the cytoplasm green (Fig. 13.2). The granules are not seen during active growth, but start to appear towards the end of the logarithmic growth period. The granule formation is best seen on Loeffler's serum slope. It appears that they represent storage depots for materials needed to form high-energy phosphate bonds. Their presence in thin slender bacilli helps to distinguish *C. diphtheriae* from short, thick, plumpy, non-pathogenic diphtheroids which lack them.

Cultural Characteristics

Diphtheria bacillus is an aerobe and facultative anaerobe, has an optimum temperature for growth of 37°C (range 15–40°C). It can grow on ordinary nutrient agar, but its growth is improved by the presence of animal proteins such as serum or blood. Two media are useful for this purpose:

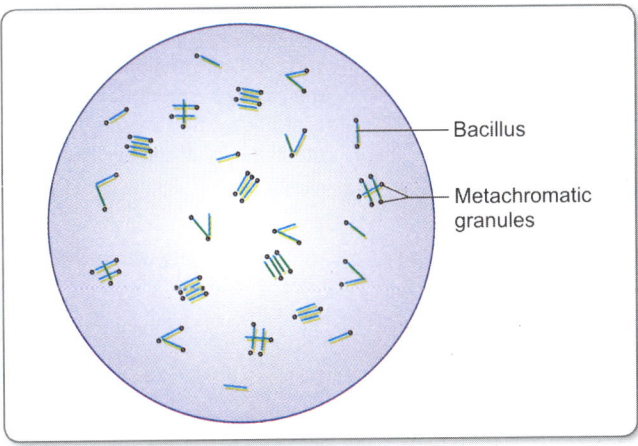

Fig. 13.1: *Corynebacterium diphtheriae* showing metachromatic granules and Chinese letter arrangement.

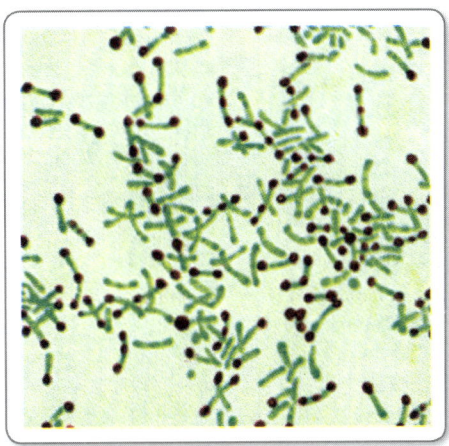

Fig. 13.2: *Corynebacterium diphtheriae* showing metachromatic granules (Albert's stain, × 1000).

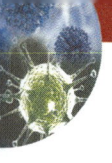

- Loeffler's serum slope.
- Blood tellurite agar (BTA): The addition of 0.03–0.04% potassium tellurite (K_2TeO_3) makes the medium selective for corynebacteria by inhibiting most other pathogenic and commensal bacteria. It may retard the growth even of corynebacteria so that colonies may be very small after 24 hours, therefore, incubation should be continued for 48 hours. On this medium, colonies of *C. diphtheriae* become grey to black because tellurite or tellurous ions are able to diffuse through the cell wall and membrane and are reduced to tellurium metal, which is precipitated inside the cell.

Diphtheria bacilli grow rapidly on Loeffler's serum slope, and colonies can be seen in 6–8 hours, long before other bacteria grow. The colonies are at first small, white, opaque discs, but on continued incubation increase in size and may acquire a yellow tint.

On the basis of colonial morphology on BTA, diphtheria bacilli can be divided into three biotypes—mitis, intermedius and gravis (Table 13.1). These names were originally proposed to relate to the clinical severity of the disease produced by the three biotypes. Mitis, intermedius and gravis biotypes produce disease of mild, intermediate and severe variety respectively. However, this association is not constant. In general, biotype mitis is predominant in endemic areas, while intermedius and gravis tend to be epidemic.

Biochemical Reactions

C. diphtheriae ferments glucose, maltose and on rare occasions sucrose with the production of acid without gas. It does not ferment lactose, mannitol and trehalose. For biochemical differentiation of three biotypes of *C. diphtheriae*, starch and glycogen are used. Gravis strains ferment both but intermedius and mitis strains ferment neither (Table 13.1).

The fermentation tests are usually done by culture for 24 hours at 37°C in Hiss's serum sugar media. Calf or rabbit serum should be used in the medium, because some batches of ox and sheep sera contain a saccharolytic enzyme that gives rise to false positive results.

Susceptibility to Physical and Chemical Agents

C. diphtheriae is readily killed by moist heat at 58°C in 10 minutes, and by the commonly used disinfectants. It is, however, relatively resistant to drying and may remain alive for weeks in dust and on fomites when dry and protected from sunlight.

Toxin Production

Toxigenic strains of *C. diphtheriae* produce a potent exotoxin which is an iron-free, crystalline, heat-labile protein. Its molecular weight is 61,150 daltons and is made up of two parts—A and B with molecular weights of 21,150 and 40,000 daltons respectively. Fragment B is required for transport of fragment A into the cell where it inhibits polypeptide chain elongation at the ribosome. Inhibition of protein synthesis is probably responsible for both the necrotic and neurotoxic effects of the toxin. When the toxin is treated with formalin it is converted into toxoid.

TABLE 13.1: Differentiation of three biotypes of *Corynebacterium diphtheriae*

Character	Gravis	Intermedius	Mitis
Morphology	Uniformly stained short rods. Some degree of pleomorphism with irregularly barred tear-drop forms. Few or no granules	Long, irregularly barred cigar-shaped rods, highly pleomorphic. Poor granulation	Long, curved, pleomorphic, wispy rods with terminal swellings. Prominent granulation
Colony characters on blood tellurite agar after 18–24 hours incubation	Dull greyish black, opaque colonies, 1.5–2.5 mm in diameter. In 2–3 days, 3–5 mm in diameter flat colony with raised dark centre, radially striated periphery and crenated edge – 'daisy-head' colony	Small (0.5–0.75 mm in diameter), grey colony with a darker centre and a shining surface – 'frog's egg' colony. There is little change in size after 48 hours incubation	Grey, opaque colonies, 1.5–2.0 mm in diameter with regular margins and glossy smooth surface. On further incubation the colony becomes flat with central elevation and regular margins – 'poached egg' colony
Haemolysis of sheep, rabbit and horse blood	Weakly haemolytic	Non-haemolytic	β-haemolytic
Growth in broth	Surface pellicle, granular deposit and little or no turbidity	Uniform turbidity with fine granular deposit	Uniform turbidity with pellicle later
Fermentation of starch and glycogen	+	–	–
Phage types	14	3	4
Serotypes	13	4	40
Toxigenic strains	Almost 100%	95–99%	80–85%
Predominant strains in	Epidemic areas	Epidemic areas	Endemic areas

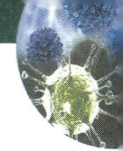

Almost all strains of gravis, 95–99% of intermedius and 80–85% of mitis produce this toxin. However, toxin produced by different biotypes is antigenically similar. The classic Park-Williams strain (PW8) of *C. diphtheriae* isolated in 1896, is still used as a source of toxin for preparation of diphtheria toxoid (vaccine).

Lysogeny and toxin production

Only those strains of *C. diphtheriae* which are lysogenic for β phage or related temperate phages, that contain the structural gene (*tox* gene), produce diphtheria toxin. Non-toxigenic strains may be rendered toxigenic by infecting them with β phage. This is known as **lysogenic** or **phage conversion**. The toxigenicity remains only as long as the bacillus is lysogenic. When the bacillus is cured of its phage, as by growing it in the presence of antiphage serum, it loses the toxigenicity.

Iron concentration and toxin production

Diphtheria toxin is produced most actively, *in vitro*, when iron concentration is decreased, although other factors such as osmotic pressure, amino acid concentrations and pH also have a role. Optimum iron concentration for toxin production is 0.1 mg per litre of the medium. Toxin production stops at 0.5 mg per litre of the medium. Reason for this is not known. The repressor of the *tox* gene appears to be an iron containing protein. When sufficient iron is present suppressor is formed which inhibits toxin production.

Pathogenicity

C. diphtheriae **causes natural infection only in man**. Infection spreads directly from person-to-person via nasopharyngeal secretions. Spread is facilitated by intimate contact. Most clinical infections are probably contracted from carriers rather than symptomatic patients. Nasal carriers are particularly dangerous because they shed large number of bacilli which may survive for many weeks in dust and on dry fomites. Children are susceptible after the age of 3–6 months when passive immunity derived from maternal antibodies has disappeared. Incidence is highest among young children, but outbreaks also occur among teenagers and young adults.

Incubation period is 3–4 days, however, it may be as short as 1 day. When toxigenic diphtheria bacilli become lodged in the throat of a susceptible individual, they first multiply rapidly on epithelial cells and produce an exotoxin (diphtheria toxin) that causes local tissue necrosis. The organisms then multiply in cell debris, produce more toxin leading to enlargement of the lesion. The combination of cell necrosis and an exudative inflammatory response of tissue leads to an accumulation of necrotic cellular material, erythrocytes, fibrin and bacteria,

which forms a characteristic **diphtheritic pseudomembrane** (in Latin *diphtheria* means pseudomembrane) varying in colour from white to grey to yellow. Since epithelial cells of the mucosa are incorporated in the pseudomembrane, therefore, attempts to remove it produce bleeding.

Diphtheritic pseudomembrane usually appears first on tonsils or posterior pharyngeal wall. The infection may then spread either upwards into nasal passages or downwards into the larynx and trachea.

Diphtheria bacilli do not, as a rule, penetrate deeply in the underlying tissues, or the blood, but they produce a powerful exotoxin. Toxin is absorbed into the blood stream from the site of infection and causes toxaemia and various systemic complications. The toxin has a **special affinity for certain tissues, notably heart muscles, nerve endings and adrenal glands**. Death often results from cardiac failure, but necrotic and often haemorrhagic lesions are usually seen in many organs at necropsy, and in laryngeal diphtheria death is due to suffocation caused by mechanical obstruction.

Laboratory Diagnosis

Because early administration of antitoxin is of paramount importance, specific treatment should be instituted immediately on suspicion of diphtheria, without waiting for laboratory confirmation. The disease runs a quick course and any delay may be fatal. Laboratory confirmation of diphtheria is necessary for the initiation of control measures and for epidemiological purposes. Diagnosis of diphtheria is based on isolating *C. diphtheriae* from the infected area and demonstrating its toxin-producing ability.

Specimens

Two swabs are taken from the local lesion which is usually in the throat but may also be in the nose, larynx, ear, conjunctiva, vagina and skin or from the nose and throat of contacts or suspected carriers. No antiseptics, in the form of gargles, etc., must have been applied within 12 hours. The swabs should be rubbed over the affected area and pseudomembrane, if formed, should be scraped with swab stick or where there is no definitely localized lesion the swabs should be rubbed over the mucous membrane of posterior pharyngeal wall and tonsils.

Microscopy and Culture

One swab should be inoculated on Loeffler's serum slope, blood tellurite agar and a plate of ordinary blood agar, the last for differentiating streptococcal or staphylococcal pharyngitis, which may simulate diphtheria. All these media are incubated at 37°C. Loeffler's serum slope is examined after 12–18 hours. If an early result is urgently required then culture may be examined after 6–12 hours, but if it is negative the examination must be repeated after 18–24 hours. The resultant growth on Loeffler's serums slope is mixed by emulsifying it with a wire loop in the condensation fluid and from this smears are made and stained

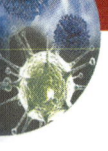

by Gram and Albert methods. Blood tellurite agar is examined after 24 hours, and after 48 hours if no growth is obtained after 24 hours. The growth is identified by colonial morphology, Gram staining, Albert staining and biochemical reactions (Table 13.1).

With the **second swab, two smears** are prepared and stained by Gram and Albert methods, but only in a small proportion of cases can positive results be obtained in this way and cultures should always be made as a routine procedure, irrespective of direct examination. Smear from Loeffler's serum slope may be the first indication of the presence of diphtheria bacillus.

Toxigenicity or Virulence Tests of C. diphtheriae

The identification of an isolate as *C. diphtheriae* does not mean that the patient has diphtheria. Diagnosis of diphtheria depends on showing that the isolate produces diphtheria toxin. This can be done by either *in vivo* or *in vitro* testing. *In vivo* testing is rarely done because the *in vitro* method is reliable, less expensive, and free from the need to use animal.

- *In vivo*
  - Subcutaneous test
  - Intradermal test
- *In vitro*
  - Elek's gel precipitation test

Subcutaneous Test

Emulsify the growth from an overnight culture on Loeffler's serum slope in 2–4 ml broth and inject 0.8 ml of the emulsion subcutaneously into two guinea pigs, one of which has been protected with intramuscular injection of 500 units of diphtheria antitoxin 18–24 hours previously. If the strain is virulent, the unprotected animal will die within four days.

Perform autopsy on any of the animals dying within this period. If the isolate is toxigenic then the unprotected animal shows:

- Gelatinous haemorrhagic oedema at the site of inoculation.
- Blood-stained pleural and peritoneal exudate.
- Haemorrhagic inflammation of adrenal glands.

If neither animal dies, the culture is non-toxigenic. If both animals die, the culture is virulent or toxigenic, but not *C. diphtheriae*. This method is usually not employed because the animal is sacrificed.

Intradermal Test

Inoculate one colony of suspected *C. diphtheriae* isolate from BTA on a moist Loeffler's serum slope. Incubate at 37°C for 24 hours. Prepare a dense suspension of culture on this medium in 3 ml broth and inject 0.1 ml of this intradermally into the shaved side of a guinea pig or rabbit. After four hours, the animal is injected intraperitoneally with 500 units of antitoxin. Thirty minutes later a second sample of the test suspension is injected intradermally on the opposite side.

Non-specific inflammatory reaction may occur at both sites within 24–48 hours, but if toxigenic bacilli are present, only the site injected before the antitoxin was administered will progress to form a characteristic necrotic lesion in 48–72 hours. With this test first injection acts as test and second as control and about five strains (10 injections) can be tested on each animal. Moreover, the animal does not die. Therefore, intradermal test is better than subcutaneous test.

Elek's Gel Precipitation Test

This is a gel precipitation test. Pipette 10 ml of nutrient agar that has been cooled to 55°C in a water bath and 2 ml sterile calf serum in a Petri dish and rotate 20 times to mix. Before the medium solidifies, place a 1 cm × 8 cm filter paper strip that has been soaked in the diphtheria antitoxin 500–1,000 units/ml across the middle of the plate on the surface of the agar. Allow the medium to solidify and then place the plate in the incubator with the lid ajar to allow the surface moisture to evaporate.

Inoculate the plate within 2 hours after drying by streaking a heavy inoculum of the culture to be tested across the plate at right angles to the antitoxin strip. Parallel to this streak, at a distance of about 15 mm from it, streak a known toxigenic strain of *C. diphtheriae* on one side of the test strain and streak a non-toxigenic strain on the other side. Incubate the plate at 37°C and examine after 24 and 48 hours. Look for **white lines of precipitation** a few mm from the paper strip, that extend out from the line of bacterial growth, forming an angle of about 45°.

These white precipitin lines form where the toxin from pathogenic strains of *C. diphtheriae* combines with the antitoxin in optimum concentration from the paper strip, thus identifying the strains of *C. diphtheriae* that produce the toxin. At 24 hours, the line is best seen with the help of a hand lens, at 48 hours it is more obvious. Look for continuity between the line from unknown culture and that from the known toxigenic culture (Fig. 13.3). This test is very convenient and economical.

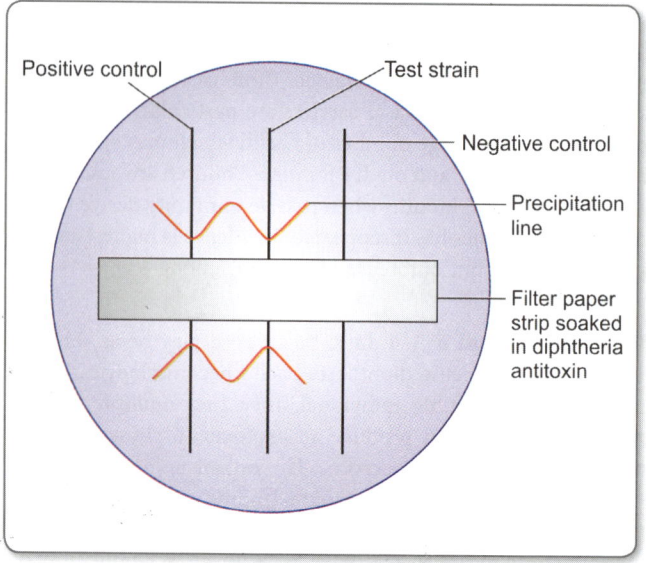

Fig. 13.3: Elek's test.

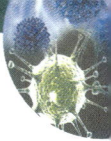

Prophylaxis

Active Immunization

This can be carried out by single and combined vaccines:

Single preparations: These include toxin-antitoxin mixture, formol toxoid, alum-precipitated toxoid, purified toxoid and aluminium phosphate precipitate.

Combined preparations. These consist of diphtheria toxoid in combination with tetanus toxoid (DT) only or tetanus toxoid and killed suspension of pertussis bacilli (DPT or triple vaccine). The component antigens of DPT can be given separately also, but giving them together not only minimizes the number of injections, but also improves immune response because the pertussis vaccine acts as an adjuvant for the toxoids. A quadruple preparation incorporating, in addition, inactivated polio vaccine, has also been used.

DPT and oral polio vaccines are given at the age of 6 weeks, 10 weeks, 14 weeks and 16–24 months followed by DT at the age of 5–6 years.

Passive Immunization

This is an emergency measure, to be employed when susceptible (non-immunized) individuals are exposed to infection. It consists of subcutaneous administration of 500–1,000 units of antitoxin or anti-diphtheritic serum (ADS). Contacts immunized within the previous 5 years should receive a booster dose of toxoid.

Combined Immunization

Since protection conferred by passive immunization is of short duration, therefore, ADS should be administered on one arm and first dose of diphtheria toxoid on the other arm, to be continued by the full course of active immunization.

Treatment

Treatment of diphtheria consists of antitoxic and antibiotic therapy. The antitoxin should be administered promptly, as soon as clinical diagnosis is made to neutralize the toxin being produced, because antitoxin is ineffective if given after the toxin is bound to cell receptor sites. Therefore, for antitoxic therapy, one should not wait for bacteriological confirmation of the diagnosis. The dosage recommended is 20,000 units intramuscularly for moderate cases and 50,000–100,000 units for serious cases, half the dose being given intravenously.

C. diphtheriae is sensitive to penicillin, erythromycin, rifampicin and many other antibiotics, but the antibiotics do not neutralize circulating toxin and, therefore, are of value only when used concurrently with antitoxin. By killing diphtheria bacilli they prevent further toxin production. Diphtheria cases are generally treated with penicillin or erythromycin in addition to antitoxin. Penicillin-sensitive individuals can be given erythromycin. Erythromycin is more active than penicillin in the treatment of carriers.

DIPHTHEROIDS

Corynebacteria resembling *C. diphtheriae*, occur as normal commensals in the throat, skin and other areas. These may be mistaken for diphtheria bacilli and are known as diphtheroids. They stain more uniformly than diphtheria bacilli, are arranged in V forms or palisades rather than Chinese letter arrangement and possess few or no metachromatic granules. They can be differentiated from *C. diphtheriae* on the basis of biochemical characters and toxigenicity tests. The common diphtheroids are *C. pseudodiphtheriticum* and *C. xerosis*.

🔖 Key Points

- *Corynebacterium diphtheriae* (diphtheria bacilli) are thin, slender, Gram-positive bacilli occurring in angled pairs resembling letters V or L, or parallel rows of 3–4 bacilli which resemble **Chinese letters**.
- **Toxigenic** strains of *Corynebacterium diphtheriae* are responsible for **diphtheria**, the sometimes fatal upper respiratory tract infection of childhood.
- The **diphtheria toxin is toxoidable**, and is a **component of the triple (DPT) vaccine**.

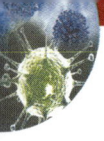

 ASSESS YOURSELF

LONG AND SHORT ANSWER QUESTIONS

1. Name various organisms causing sore throat and discuss in detail laboratory diagnosis of diphtheria.
2. Discuss morphology, biochemical characters, cultural characteristics, toxin production and pathogenesis of diphtheria.
3. Write short notes on:
   (a) Diphtheria toxin
   (b) Prophylaxis of diphtheria

MULTIPLE CHOICE QUESTIONS

1. What is the colour of colonies of *C. diphtheriae* on blood tellurite agar medium?
   (a) White
   (b) Grey to black
   (c) Cream
   (d) Yellow

2. Earliest growth of diphtheria bacilli can be detected on:
   (a) Blood agar
   (b) Blood tellurite agar
   (c) Loeffler's serum slope
   (d) Nutrient agar

3. Which of the following properties is/are shown by diphtheria toxin?
   (a) It is a heat-labile protein
   (b) It inhibits protein synthesis
   (c) It is produced by *Corynebacterium diphtheriae* strains lysogenic for β phage
   (d) All of the above

4. Diphtheria toxin has a special affinity for which of the following tissue/s?
   (a) Heart muscles
   (b) Nerve endings
   (c) Adrenal glands
   (d) All of the above

5. *Corynebacterium diphtheriaeae* is known as:
   (a) Friedlander's bacillus
   (b) Klebs-Loeffler's bacillus
   (c) Koch-Weeks bacillus
   (d) Whitmore's bacillus

6. In order to cause disease, *Corynebacterium diphtheriae* must:
   (a) Be infected with a lysogenic toxin-producing bacteriophage
   (b) Produce a haemolysin
   (c) Invade the blood stream
   (d) Destroy platelets

ANSWERS TO MCQs

1. b   **2.** c   **3.** d   **4.** d   **5.** b   **6.** a

Chapter 14

Bacillus anthracis

MORPHOLOGY

They are large, Gram-positive, catalase-positive, non-acid-fast, non-flagellate, non-motile, spore-forming bacilli, $4-8 \times 1-1.5$ μm in size. In smears from infected tissues these are found singly, in pairs and in short chains, the entire chain being surrounded by a **capsule** (Fig. 14.1A). It is polypeptide in nature. It is not formed under ordinary conditions of culture but only on media containing serum or bicarbonate in the presence of excess CO_2.

Spores are formed in culture or in the soil, but never in the animal body during life. The spores are oval, refractile, central in position and of the same diameter as the bacilli so that they do not cause bulging of the vegetative cell. In cultures, the bacilli are arranged end-to-end in long chains. The ends of the bacilli are truncated and somewhat swollen so that a chain of bacilli presents a **"bamboo-stick" appearance** (Fig. 14.1B).

CULTURAL CHARACTERISTICS

Anthrax bacilli are aerobes and facultative anaerobes. The optimum temperature for growth is 37°C but growth occurs over a wide temperature range of 12–45°C. Optimum pH for growth is 7–7.4. They can grow on ordinary media.

- On **nutrient agar**, the organisms produce large, raised, opaque, greyish-white colonies, 2–3 mm in diameter with an irregular, fringe-like edge. Under low power of the microscope, the edge of the colony is found to be composed of long, interlacing chains of bacilli, resembling curled hair-lock. This gives them the **'medusa head' appearance**. Virulent capsulated strains form rough colonies, while avirulent strains form smooth colonies.
- A selective medium (**PLET medium**) consisting of heart infusion agar with polymyxin, lysozyme, ethylenediaminetetraacetic acid (EDTA) and thallous acetate has been devised to isolate *B. anthracis* from mixtures containing other spore-bearing bacilli.
- In a **gelatin stab** culture, there is growth down the stab line with lateral spikes that are longest near the surface, giving **'inverted fir tree' appearance** with slow liquefaction commencing from the top.

BIOCHEMICAL CHARACTERS

B. anthracis ferments glucose, sucrose, maltose and dextrin with the production of acid but no gas. Nitrate is reduced to nitrite, catalase is produced and VP test is positive.

SUSCEPTIBILITY TO PHYSICAL AND CHEMICAL AGENTS

Because of its ability to produce spores, *B. anthracis* is extremely resistant to adverse physical and chemical environment. In the dry state or in soil, the spores remain viable for many years and serve as a source of infection for long periods of time.

PATHOGENICITY

B. anthracis causes **anthrax**. It is a **zoonosis**—a disease of animals transmissible to man. It is primarily a disease of cattle and sheep and less often of horses and swines, but experimentally most mammals are susceptible. Bacilli are shed in large numbers from all orifices of the infected animal during the terminal stages of the disease. The organisms sporulate in the soil and remain a source of infection for a number of decades.

Man acquires infection through small cuts or abrasions in the skin, by inhalation of spores and rarely by ingestion of infected meat. Depending on the mode of infection, anthrax presents in one of the three forms – cutaneous, pulmonary and intestinal.

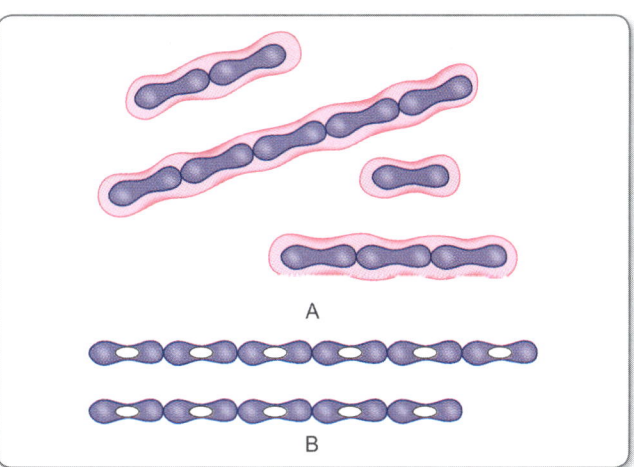

Fig. 14.1: *Bacillus anthracis.*

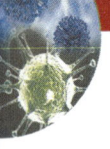

SECTION IV • PATHOGENIC ORGANISMS-I BACTERIA

Cutaneous Anthrax

About 95% of human cases of anthrax are cutaneous infections. It is common in farmers and veterinary surgeons handling infected animals, dock workers, factory workers and persons who handle carcasses, hides and animal hair. The lesion starts as a small, pruritic, painless papule 1–5 days after contact with infected material. The papule then develops into vesicle containing haemorrhagic fluid. Eventually, the vesicle breaks down and is replaced by a **black eschar**, from which it derives its name. Anthrax in Greek means coal. Black eschar is later surrounded by a ring of vesicles containing serous fluid and an area of oedema and induration which may become extensive. This has been called a **malignant pustule**. If the lesion is not treated, the organisms may invade the regional lymph nodes and blood stream causing death.

Pulmonary Anthrax

It is also known as **woolsorter's disease** because it used to be common in workers in wool factories, due to inhalation of spores from infected wool. It may also involve workers who handle animal hides which contain spores. This is a haemorrhagic pneumonia with a high fatality rate.

Intestinal Anthrax

It is extremely rare and occurs in primitive communities who eat improperly cooked carcasses of animals dying of anthrax. Patient develops haemorrhagic diarrhoea after a day or so and dies rapidly from septicaemia.

LABORATORY DIAGNOSIS

Specimens

B. anthracis can be demonstrated in the material from a malignant pustule, sometimes in sputum from pulmonary anthrax, in gastric aspirates, faeces or food in intestinal anthrax and in the blood in the septicaemic stage of all forms of the disease. In case of malignant pustule, necessary specimens include fluid aspirated from the vesicles surrounding black eschar or material beneath the edge of the black eschar. In early cases, fluid may be obtained by scraping the lesion with a needle.

Microscopy

Prepare smears of each specimen and stain with Gram's method. Examine the stained smears under oil-immersion lens for characteristic Gram-positive anthrax bacilli.

When blood films containing anthrax bacilli are stained with **polychrome methylene blue** for a few seconds and examined under microscope, **an amorphous purplish material** is noticed around the bacilli. This represents the capsular material and is characteristic of anthrax bacillus. This is known as **McFadyean's reaction** and is employed for the presumptive diagnosis of anthrax.

Culture

Culture the exudate on nutrient agar, blood agar, PLET medium and nutrient broth. Incubate at 37°C for 24 hours. Examine plates for the medusa-head colonies characteristic of *B. anthracis*. Prepare a smear, stain it by Gram's method and look for tangled chains of large Gram-positive bacilli some of which have central, oval, non-bulging spores. In nutrient broth, look for a pellicle and a deposit.

Animal Inoculation

Anthrax bacilli can often be isolated from contaminated tissue by applying them over shaven skin of a guinea pig. The animal dies in 48–72 hours. Autopsy reveals gelatinous, haemorrhagic oedema at the site of inoculation, petechial haemorrhages in the peritoneum and an enlarged dark red spleen. Make smears from heart blood and spleen, stain by Gram's and McFadyean's methods, and look for typical anthrax bacilli.

Serology

If the sample received is putrid so that viable bacilli are unlikely, diagnosis may be established by **Ascoli's thermoprecipitin test**. The tissue is ground up in saline, boiled for 5 minutes, filtered and layered over antianthrax serum in a narrow tube. If tissue contains anthrax antigen, a ring of precipitation will appear at the junction of the two liquids within 5 minutes at room temperature. Serological diagnosis by ELISA may be of value retrospectively.

PROPHYLAXIS

Animals with known or suspected anthrax should be handled with care and their carcasses should be incinerated or buried deep in quicklime to prevent soil contamination. Animal products like wool, horse hair and hides from areas where epidemic anthrax is present should be gas sterilized.

Alum precipitated toxoid prepared from the protective antigen has been used in persons occupationally exposed to anthrax infection. It is safe and effective. It is given in 3 doses intramuscularly at intervals of 6 weeks and 6 months. A booster dose may be given after one year.

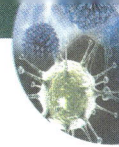

Key Points

- The entire chain of *Bacillus anthracis* is surrounded by a capsule which is **polypeptide** in nature.
- The ends of the bacilli are truncated and somewhat swollen so that a chain of bacilli presents a **"bamboo-stick"** appearance.
- *B. anthracis* does not form spores in animal body during life.
- **Anthrax** in man presents in one of the three forms – *cutaneous, pulmonary and intestinal*.

? ASSESS YOURSELF

LONG AND SHORT ANSWER QUESTIONS

1. Discuss the pathogenesis of anthrax.
2. Discuss laboratory diagnosis of anthrax.
3. Write short notes on:
   - (a) Malignant pustule
   - (b) Prophylaxis of anthrax

MULTIPLE CHOICE QUESTIONS

1. Koch's postulates were satisfied for the first time with:
   - (a) *Bacillus anthracis*
   - (b) *Clostridium tetani*
   - (c) *Corynebacterium diphtheriae*
   - (d) *Salmonella* Typhi

2. 'Medusa head' appearance of the colonies is characteristic of:
   - (a) *Proteus mirabilis*
   - (b) *Clostridium tetani*
   - (c) *Bacillus anthracis*
   - (d) *Pseudomonas aeruginosa*

3. Malignant pustule is characteristic of:
   - (a) cutaneous anthrax
   - (b) pulmonary anthrax
   - (c) intestinal anthrax
   - (d) All of the above

4. An organism that can cause cutaneous infection and can be transmitted by spores is:
   - (a) *Staphylococcus aureus*
   - (b) *Streptococcus pyogenes*
   - (c) *Yersinia pestis*
   - (d) *Bacillus anthracis*

ANSWERS TO MCQs

1. a **2.** c **3.** a **4.** d

15 Chapter

Clostridium (Gas Gangrene, Food-Poisoning and Tetanus)

Anaerobic, Gram-positive, spore-bearing bacilli belong to the genus *Clostridium*. Natural habitat of the clostridia is soil, water, intestinal tract of animals and man, and decomposing plant and animal matter. A few species are opportunistic pathogens and can produce diseases like **gas gangrene** (*C. perfringens*), **tetanus** (*C. tetani*), **botulism** (*C. botulinum*), **food poisoning** (*C. perfringens*) and **pseudomembranous colitis** (*C. difficile*).

CLOSTRIDIUM PERFRINGENS (CLOSTRIDIUM WELCHII)

Morphology

They are large, Gram-positive, spore-bearing bacilli, measuring $4–6 \times 1$ μm with parallel sides and truncated or slightly rounded ends. They occur singly, in pairs or in small bundles. They are non-motile and form capsules in animal body. Spores are oval, subterminal or central and non-bulging (Fig. 15.1A). They are formed under natural conditions, e.g. in the bowel. They are only rarely seen in direct smears from wounds or cultures but can be demonstrated on growth in special media such as Ellner's medium.

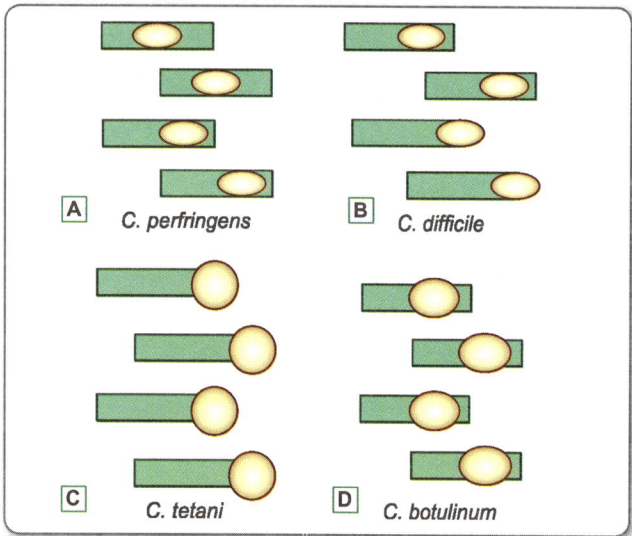

Fig. 15.1: Types of spores in different *Clostridium* species.

Cultural Characteristics

It is an anaerobe, but can grow under microaerophilic conditions. Optimum temperature for growth is 37°C. It grows best on media containing carbohydrate such as **glucose blood agar** and forms two main types of colonies. One is round, 2–4 mm in diameter, smooth, regular, convex, amorphous, greyish-yellow and slightly opaque. Other is umbonate with an opaque brownish centre and a lighter, translucent, radially striated periphery with a crenated edge.

On **horse blood agar**, colonies are usually surrounded by a zone of β-haemolysis and commonly also by an outer wider zone of incomplete haemolysis owing to the action of θ and α toxins respectively (**double zone haemolysis**).

Biochemical Reactions

It is actively saccharolytic and ferments glucose, maltose, sucrose, lactose and starch with the production of acid and gas.

In **litmus milk medium**, it ferments lactose and produces acid and gas. The acid clots the milk and the gas breaks up the clot resulting in **stormy clot reaction**. Production of acid is also indicated by change in the colour of the litmus from blue to red. The culture has sour butyric acid odour. It is indole negative, MR positive, VP negative and H_2S positive.

Gelatin is liquefied but coagulated serum is usually not liquefied. In cooked meat broth (CMB), meat turns pink and is not digested.

Resistance to Physical and Chemical Agents

Vegetative cells of *C. perfringens* are very sensitive to heat and disinfectants. However, spores generally resist routinely used antiseptics and disinfectants except formaldehyde and glutaraldehyde. Spores are usually destroyed within 5 minutes by boiling but those of food poisoning strains of type A and certain type C strains resist boiling for 1–3 hours. Autoclaving at 121°C for 15 minutes is lethal.

Toxins

C. perfringens produces four major lethal, eight minor lethal or non-lethal toxins, and enterotoxin. Major lethal toxins include

TABLE 15.1: Typing of *Clostridium perfringens*

Type	Toxin produced			
	α	β	ε	τ
A	+	−	−	−
B	+	+	+	−
C	+	+	−	−
D	+	−	+	−
E	+	−	−	+

α (alpha), β (beta), ε (epsilon) and ι (iota) and minor lethal toxins include γ (gamma), δ (delta), κ (kappa), λ (lambda), μ (mu), η (eta), θ (theta) and ν (nu).

On the basis of four major toxins, *C. perfringens* can be divided into five types, A to E (Table 15.1). Typing is done by neutralization tests with specific antitoxins by intracutaneous injection in guinea pigs or intravenous injection in mice. Strains of *C. perfringens* type A that produce enterotoxin are associated with a mild form of food poisoning. Typical food poisoning strains (type A2) are non-haemolytic or feebly haemolytic on horse blood agar and have markedly heat-resistant spores but classical (type A1) strains are β-haemolytic and have relatively heat-sensitive spores.

Alpha Toxin

It is produced by all types of *C. perfringens* but most abundantly by type A strains. It is the most important toxin and is responsible for the profound toxaemia of gas gangrene. It is Ca^{++} or Mg^{++} dependent phospholipase (lecithinase-C). In the presence of free Ca^{++} or Mg^{++}, it produces opalescence in serum or egg yolk containing media by splitting phospholipid complexes. This reaction can be inhibited by specific antitoxin. This is the basis of Nagler's reaction.

Nagler's reaction

A culture plate containing 6% agar, 5% peptic digest of sheep blood and 20% human serum or 5% egg yolk is prepared. The plate is dried. On one half of the plate, 2–3 drops of *C. perfringens* antitoxin are spread and allowed to dry. The plate is then inoculated with the test organisms or the exudate under study and incubated anaerobically at 37°C for 18 hours. On the section containing no antitoxin, *C. perfringens* colonies show surrounding zone of opalescence, i.e. Nagler's reaction whereas colonies of the remainder half of the plate show no change (Fig. 15.2).

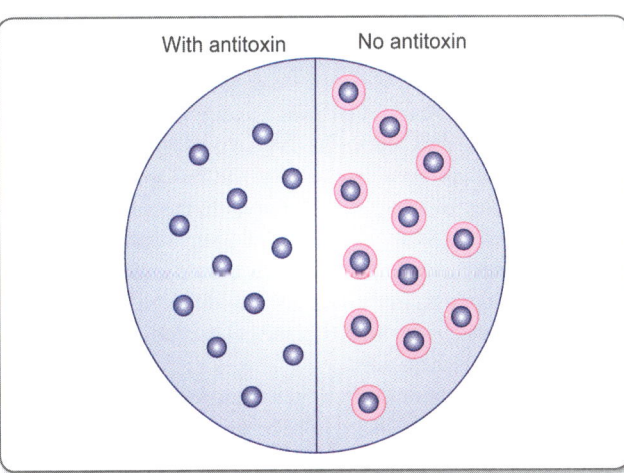

Fig. 15.2: Nagler's reaction.

Other Major and Minor Toxins

- *Beta toxin* is not haemolytic, it is lethal to mice, and when given intradermally in guinea pigs and rabbits it produces necrotic lesions.
- *Epsilon* and *iota toxins* are lethal and necrotizing, and non-haemolytic.
- *Gamma* and *eta toxins* are minor lethal toxins. They are neither necrotizing nor haemolytic.
- *Delta toxin* is lethal and actively haemolytic for the red cells of sheep, goat, pig and cattle.
- *Theta toxin* is oxygen-labile haemolysin antigenically related to streptolysin O. It is moderately lethal.
- *Lambda toxin* is non-lethal, non-necrotizing proteinase and gelatinase.
- *Kappa*, *mu* and *nu toxins* are collagenase, hyaluronidase and deoxyribonuclease respectively.

Enterotoxin

C. perfringens type A strains produce a potent enterotoxin. It is a heat-labile, non-diffusible protein with a polypeptide chain and a molecular weight of 34,000–35,000 daltons. It is formed in the intestine at the time of sporulation.

Pathogenesis

C. perfringens may lead to following infections:

Wound Infection

C. perfringens occurs normally in the soil, particularly that of manured and cultivated land, and animal and human excreta. The infection usually results from contamination of a wound with these. Wound may get contaminated with patient's own faeces during surgery or after accident. Clostridia may also be present on the normal skin, especially on the perineum and thigh. These may also cause infection.

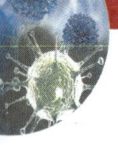
The presence of devitalized or dead tissue due to crushing of tissues and the severing of arteries in accidental and war injuries, blood clots, extravasated fluid, foreign bodies (bullets, shell fragments and bits of clothing) and coincident infection with aerobic organisms reduce the oxygen tension in the infected tissue. This leads to germination of clostridial spores followed by multiplication of vegetative forms with the production of exotoxins and enzymes into the surrounding environment causing more tissue destruction and resulting in a rapid and fulminating spread of the organism in the necrotic environment. In addition, carbohydrates may be fermented, resulting in production of large quantities of gas in the tissues.

The pressure resulting from gas formation may cause still more restriction of the blood supply to adjoining tissue and hence more necrosis. Hyaluronidase produced by *C. perfringens* breaks down intercellular cement substance and promotes the spread of the infection along tissue planes. Collagenase and proteinase produced by this organism break down tissues and virtually liquefy muscles. In the absence of surgical and antitoxic treatment, severe toxaemia and death frequently ensue. Three types of clostridial wound infections are recognized:

- **Wound contamination:** Here one or more clostridia are present in the traumatized tissue without evidence of infection. Up to 80–90% isolates of *C. perfringens* from hospitalized patients represent simple saprophytic wound contamination.
- **Clostridial cellulitis:** In this condition, infection is confined to local fascial planes in the absence of significant toxaemia. The infecting clostridia are of low invasive power and poor toxigenicity. There is a seropurulent discharge from the wound with an offensive odour and prognosis is good.
- **Clostridial myonecrosis or gas gangrene:** In this condition, there is invasion of healthy muscle tissue and striking systemic intoxication.

The **incubation period** of gas gangrene is 2–3 days. The disease develops with increasing pain, tenderness and oedema of the affected part along with systemic signs of toxaemia. There is a thin watery discharge from the wound, which later becomes profuse and serosanguinous. Accumulation of gas (predominantly hydrogen which is less soluble than carbon dioxide) makes the tissue crepitant.

Food Poisoning

Enterotoxin producing strains of *C. perfringens* are associated with a mild form of food poisoning. It is third most common etiologic agent of food poisoning after *Salmonella* serotypes and *S. aureus*. Both heat-resistant (A2) and heat-sensitive (A1) strains of *C. perfringens* are capable of causing food poisoning. The incriminated food is usually meat that has been cooked hours in advance and then cooled slowly, or even allowed to stand at room temperature for several hours before being served. Before cooking, the meat may get contaminated with heat-resistant spores from the animal's intestine at the abattoir or from soil and

dust during transit to shops and then from shops to houses and catering establishments.

Heat-resistant spores may survive the whole cooking procedure and during cooling period they germinate in the anaerobic environment produced by the cooked meat and multiply. If spores of heat-sensitive strains contaminate uncooked meat, they are not likely to cause food poisoning because they usually do not survive cooking. However, if dust containing heat-sensitive spores contaminates cooked meat, the spores germinate in the meat and multiply during the period of storage before serving.

Virtually 100% of healthy population carries classical β-haemolytic *C. perfringens* in their gut, and 2–30% carry heat-resistant *C. perfringens*. After ingestion of large numbers of vegetative cells in food, multiplication occurs in the intestine for a brief period followed by sporulation and the production of an **enterotoxin**. Patient develops abdominal cramps and diarrhoea with foamy and foul smelling stools 8–12 hours after ingestion of the contaminated food. It usually subsides within 24 hours. There is little vomiting or fever. No specific treatment is indicated.

Necrotizing jejunitis (Enteritis necroticans)

It is a severe and often fatal disease caused by *C. perfringens* type C. In addition, *C. perfringens* may also cause necrotizing colitis, gangrenous appendicitis, biliary tract infection, brain abscess and meningitis, panophthalmitis, thoracic infections, and urogenital infections.

Laboratory Diagnosis

The diagnosis of gas gangrene must primarily be made upon clinical grounds and initiation of treatment should not await full laboratory report. The function of laboratory is only to provide confirmation of clinical diagnosis.

Specimens

- Edges of affected muscles,
- Necrotic tissue, and
- Exudate from the depth of the lesion, where infection seems to be most pronounced, to be collected with a capillary pipette.

Microscopic Examination

Gram smears are prepared. If gas gangrene exists, smear shows typical Gram-positive bacilli often with other bacteria. Thick, stubby, Gram-positive rods suggest *C. perfringens*.

Culture

Specimens are inoculated on fresh blood agar, heated blood agar and cooked meat broth (CMB). Growth in CMB is subcultured on blood agar medium after 24–48 hours incubation at 37°C anaerobically for 48–72 hours. A plate of human serum or egg

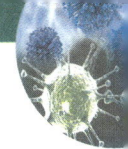

yolk agar with *C. perfringens* antitoxin spread on one-half of the plate is used for Nagler's reaction. The bacterial isolate is identified by morphology, cultural characteristics and biochemical reactions.

Prophylaxis and Treatment of Gas Gangrene

- **Toilet of the wound**
  The most important preventive measure against clostridial myonecrosis is early and adequate wound debridement and irrigation of the wound to remove blood clots, necrotic tissue and foreign material. This ensures elimination of the bulk of the contaminating organisms. Wound is not sutured but is left open after thorough cleansing and loosely packed. Hyperbaric oxygen chamber, in which an infected area is placed in a chamber containing pure oxygen under pressure, has been used with some success to stop the growth of the anaerobes.

- **Chemotherapy**
  Surgical toilet is combined with topical and parenteral antimicrobial therapy in high doses. This should be directed against clostridial element and likely coexistence of aerobic organisms. Therefore, penicillin, metronidazole and an aminoglycoside may be given in combination. Clindamycin or a broad-spectrum β-lactam antibiotic such as cefotaxime or imipenem may also be given.

- **Antitoxic therapy**
  A polyvalent antiserum containing 10,000 units each of *C. perfringens* and *C. novyi* antitoxins and 5,000 units of *C. septicum* antitoxin has been used in the prophylaxis and treatment of gas gangrene. Its efficacy has never been established and intensive antimicrobial therapy has now replaced antitoxic therapy.

CLOSTRIDIUM DIFFICILE

It is a Gram-positive bacillus, 4–8 × 0.5–1 μm in size with oval, subterminal or terminal, non-bulging spores (Fig. 15.1B). It is motile by peritrichate flagella. It is an obligate anaerobe and grows well on blood agar at 37°C. On this medium, after 24 hours incubation, colonies are glossy, greyish, low convex, circular with irregular edges.

Pathogenesis

C. difficile is ubiquitous in nature, and has been isolated from soil, water, intestinal contents of various animals, vagina and urethra of humans and faeces of 40–50% of neonates and only 3% of healthy adults. It has, however, been implicated as a causative agent in **antibiotic-associated diarrhoea** (AAD), **antibiotic-associated colitis** (AAC) and life-threatening **pseudomembranous colitis** (PMC). These conditions have been associated with a number of antimicrobial agents particularly clindamycin and ampicillin.

Use of these antibiotics leads to killing of antibiotic-sensitive organisms and overgrowth of *C. difficile* in the intestine leading to these conditions. Most of the cases of PMC are caused by *C. difficile* but infrequently it may also be caused by *S. aureus* and *C. perfringens*.

C. difficile produces disease by the elaboration of two distinct exotoxins:
- **Toxin A:** It is an enterotoxin that is primarily responsible for diarrhoea.
- **Toxin B:** It is a potent cytotoxin capable of producing cytopathogenic effects in several tissue culture cell lines.

Laboratory Diagnosis

Laboratory diagnosis can be accomplished by demonstrating the toxin in the faeces of the patients by its characteristic effect on HEp2 and human diploid cell cultures or by ELISA. *C. difficile* can also be grown from the faeces of the patient.

Treatment

Discontinue the antibiotic that is presumed to have precipitated the disease, and suppress growth and toxin production of *C. difficile* by giving vancomycin or metronidazole.

CLOSTRIDIUM TETANI

Morphology

C. tetani is a slender, Gram-positive bacillus, 4–8 × 0.5 μm with rounded ends. It tends to be pleomorphic and filamentous. It is non-capsulated and motile by peritrichate flagella. However, type VI strains which do not possess flagella, are non-motile. Young cultures of the organisms usually stain Gram-positive but in older cultures and in smears made from the wounds, they are Gram-variable and even frank Gram-negative. The spores are spherical, terminal and twice the diameter of vegetative cells giving them typical **drumstick appearance** (Fig. 15.1C). The spores do not take up the Gram stain and appear as colourless round structures.

Cultural Characteristics

C. tetani is an obligate anaerobe. The optimum temperature and pH for its growth are 37°C and 7.4 respectively. It can grow well on ordinary media, but its growth is improved by the addition of blood or serum.
- **Colonies on solid media** are irregularly round, 2–5 mm in diameter with fine branching projections. Isolated colonies of *C. tetani* may not be obtained because of the tendency of the organism to swarm over the surface of the medium. However, non-motile variants may produce isolated colonies.
- **On horse blood agar**, the colonies of *C. tetani* are surrounded by a zone of α-haemolysis, which subsequently develops into

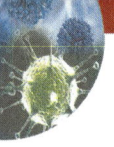

β-haemolysis owing to the production of an oxygen-labile haemolysin known as tetanolysin.

- **On egg-yolk agar**, it does not produce opalescence or pearly layer.
- It grows well **in CMB**. The meat is not digested but shows slight blackening on prolonged incubation.

Biochemical Reactions

C. tetani has slight proteolytic and no saccharolytic activity. Gelatin is slowly liquefied. Coagulated serum is rendered more transparent and softened but not liquefied.

Sensitivity to Physical and Chemical Agents

Spores of some strains of *C. tetani* are killed by boiling for 10–15 minutes, but some resist boiling for up to 3 hours and dry heat at 160°C for 1 hour. They can, however, be killed by autoclaving at 121°C for 15 minutes.

Antigenic Structure

Flagellar (H), somatic (O) and spore antigens have been demonstrated in *C. tetani*. Spore antigens are different from H and O antigens. On the basis of agglutination and complement fixation tests, the strains of the organism have been divided into 10 (I–X) types of which types I and III are the commonest. This typing is on the basis of their H antigens. Type VI consists of non-flagellate strains. All the strains carry same O antigen. This permits identification of the organism by use of fluorescein-labelled antisera. Toxins formed by all types are pharmacologically and antigenically identical and are neutralized by antitoxin prepared against any one type. However, within the same type some strains may be toxigenic and others non-toxigenic.

Tetanus Toxins

C. tetani produces an oxygen-labile haemolysin (tetanolysin) but all the symptoms in tetanus are attributable to a potent neurotoxin (tetanospasmin). Different strains vary from completely non-toxigenic to very highly toxigenic.

Pathogenesis

The spores of *C. tetani* are ubiquitous. They occur in the gastrointestinal tracts of man and animals. They are also present in the soil especially in manured soil. Tetanus develops following the contamination of wound with *C. tetani* spores. The source of infection may be soil, dirty clothing or faeces. Germination of spores is dependent upon the reduced oxygen tension occurring in devitalized tissue.

Infection strictly remains localized in the wound and the disease is due to the effect of a potent diffusible exotoxin (tetanospasmin). Conditions that favour the germination of spores and the multiplication of the organisms in the tissues are similar to those of *C. perfringens*. However, tetanus may also develop following superficial abrasion, septic abortion, thorn prick, and cleansing of auditory meatus with a small stick.

Tetanus neonatorum follows infection of umbilical wound of newborn infants. Postoperative tetanus may be due to imperfectly sterilized catgut, intestinal contents during abdominal surgery and air of the operation theatre containing spore-bearing dust.

C. tetani remains localized at the site of initial infection and produces tetanus toxin. It is absorbed from the site of its production and ascends to the central nervous system via motor nerves. However, some toxin may be delivered from the site of infection via the blood to all nerves in the body and the subsequent transmission to the central nervous system depends upon uptake through neuromuscular nerve endings and intra-axonal transport. Therefore, the first symptoms in human tetanus appear in head and neck because of the shorter length of the cranial nerves.

Tetanospasmin resembles strychnine in its effect. It appears to act by interfering with the normal inhibition of motor impulses exercised by the upper motor neuron over the lower. This results in sustained muscle spasm and characteristic signs of spasm of jaw muscles (**lock jaw, trismus**) and facial muscles (**risus sardonicus**), and arching of the body (**opisthotonicus**).

The incubation period of tetanus varies from 2 days to several weeks but commonly it is 6–12 days. Tetanus is a serious disease with a high mortality rate of 80–90% without proper treatment and even with proper treatment it is 15–50%. Tetanus neonatorum and uterine tetanus have very high fatality rates (70–100%). In rural India, it is fourth commonest cause of death.

Laboratory Diagnosis

The diagnosis is usually based on clinical findings alone because the isolation of the organism can occur in the absence of the disease, and it is also possible to have tetanus and never isolate the organism.

Microscopy

Collect pus or necrotic material from the wound, prepare a smear and stain it by Gram's method. Examine under microscope for typical 'drumstick' bacilli. But only a minority of specimens will show these. Direct immunofluorescence microscopy can also be employed for the demonstration of *C. tetani*.

Culture

Diagnosis by culture is more dependable. Pus or wound scrapings or excised bits of tissue from the necrotic depths of wound should be plated on one half of a blood agar plate and 3 bottles of CMB. Blood agar plate is incubated anaerobically at 37°C. *C. tetani* produces swarming growth which may be detected on opposite half of the plate after 1–2 days. Of the 3 inoculated CMB bottles, one should be incubated unheated, second is heated in a water bath at 80°C for 5 minutes and third for 20 minutes. The purpose

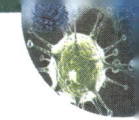

of heating for different periods is to kill non-sporing bacilli, while leaving tetanus spores undamaged, which vary widely in heat-resistance. The heated bottles are also incubated anaerobically at 37°C.

Subcultures from all these bottles are made on half of a blood agar plate daily for 4 days. The plates are incubated anaerobically at 37°C and examined for the swarming edge of *C. tetani*. Incorporation of polymyxin B, to which clostridia are resistant, makes the medium selective.

In vitro Toxigenicity Test

A blood agar plate containing 4% agar, to minimize swarming, is divided into 2 halves. One half is smeared with tetanus antitoxin. Both halves are then inoculated with growth assumed to be *C. tetani* and incubated anaerobically for 2 days. Colonies haemolytic on the untreated half, but not on the antitoxin half, are of *C. tetani*.

The toxigenicity of the organisms is confirmed by demonstrating the production of tetanospasmin. Two mice, one unprotected and other protected, by giving 1,000 units of tetanus antitoxin intraperitoneally 1 hour before the test, are challenged with an intramuscular injection in the hind leg of 0.1 ml of a 48 hour CMB culture supernate of the isolate. The protected mouse remains well. Signs of ascending tetanus develop in the unprotected animal after several hours, they begin in the inoculated leg and extend to the tail, then the other hind limb is affected and then generalized signs appear. The animal dies within 2 days.

Prophylaxis

It is of 3 types:

Surgical Prophylaxis

This includes prompt and adequate wound debridement, removal of foreign material, necrotic tissue and blood clots. This ensures elimination of the bulk of the contaminating organisms and an anaerobic environment for the growth of *C. tetani* is not provided. Clean superficial wounds that receive prompt attention may not require specific protection against tetanus.

Antibiotic Prophylaxis

This includes prompt administration of antibiotics to destroy or inhibit *C. tetani* and pyogenic bacteria in the wound, so that the production of the toxin can be prevented. A long-acting penicillin or one tablet of erythromycin 500 mg twice daily for 5 days may be given preferably before the wound toilet. However, antibiotics have no effect on the toxin, therefore, antibiotic prophylaxis does not replace immunoprophylaxis.

Immunoprophylaxis

It includes 3 types of immunization.

Active Immunization

All persons should be actively immunized against tetanus in infancy and their immunity maintained by booster doses. DPT and oral polio vaccines are given at the age of 6 weeks, 10 weeks, 14 weeks and 16–24 months followed by DT vaccine at the age of 5–6 years. Thereafter, booster doses of TT are given at the age of 10 and 16 years. Subsequently, immunity to tetanus can be maintained by booster doses of toxoid every 10 years.

If the individual has not been immunized in infancy, then immunization should be carried out with 3 spaced intramuscular injections. The intervals recommended are 6–8 weeks between the first and second injections and 4–6 months between the second and third, and booster doses every 10 years.

Passive Immunization

Tetanus antitoxin often called antitetanus serum (ATS) can be obtained by immunizing horses with TT. This serum is of value if given immediately after wounding. The usual prophylactic dose is 1,500 international units given intramuscularly or subcutaneously as soon as possible after injury. The injection may be repeated at a weekly interval till the danger of tetanus persists. Larger initial dose of 3,000–10,000 international units may be given when the wound is severe.

Disadvantages of ATS:
- *Immune elimination:* The half life of ATS in man is about 7 days, and in persons who have had prior injections of horse serum (antigenic for man) it is eliminated much quicker by combination with pre-existing antibodies to horse serum developed in response to earlier injections of ATS.
- *Hypersensitivity reactions:* Administration of ATS may lead to hypersensitivity reactions like fatal anaphylaxis and serum sickness. It is, therefore, mandatory to test for hyper-sensitivity before administration of ATS. The intradermal test for hypersensitivity is unreliable. A dose of 0.05 ml of ATS is given subcutaneously and patient is observed for at least half an hour for general reactions. Since even this may lead to anaphylaxis in some individuals, therefore, a syringe loaded with adrenaline (1/1,000) should invariably be kept ready.

Human tetanus immunoglobulin (HTIG) has replaced ATS for tetanus prophylaxis in many countries, because it has considerable advantage of a longer half life (3–5 weeks) and freedom from risks of hypersensitivity reactions. This is prepared by immunization of human volunteers who are free from hepatitis B, C and D, and human immunodeficiency viruses. Since HTIG is not antigenic for man, therefore, immune elimination is not seen with HTIG. The prophylactic dose of HTIG is 250–500 units by intramuscular injection.

Combined Immunization

It consists of administering to a non-immune person ATS or HTIG at one site, along with the first dose of TT at another site, followed by second and third doses of TT at appropriate intervals.

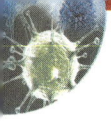

CLOSTRIDIUM BOTULINUM

Morphology

C. botulinum is a straight or slightly curved Gram-positive bacillus with rounded ends. It measures about 5 × 1 µm (range 3.4–8.6 × 0.5–1.3 µm) in size. It is non-capsulated and motile by peritrichate flagella. It produces heat-resistant spores that are oval, subterminal and bulging (Fig. 15.1D).

Cultural Characteristics

It is an obligate anaerobe. Optimum temperature for growth is 35°C, but some strains can grow and produce toxin at 1–5°C. It can grow well on routine culture media. Surface colonies are large, irregular, smooth, semitransparent with fimbriate border. On horse blood agar, all strains except those of type G are β-haemolytic. All types except G produce opalescence and a pearly effect on egg-yolk agar (EYA).

Biochemical Reactions

It ferments glucose, fructose and maltose. Type A, B and F are proteolytic; they liquefy gelatin and coagulated serum and digest meat in cooked meat broth, blacken it and produce a foul smell. They produce hydrogen sulphide. All types are indole-negative and calase-negative.

Susceptibility to Physical and Chemical Agents

Spores of *C. botulinum* are highly resistant, surviving boiling for several hours and some strains can even survive autoclaving at 121°C for 10 minutes.

Antigenic Types

On the basis of the type of toxin produced, *C. botulinum* has been divided into 8 serologically distinct types, A, B, C_1, C_2, D, E, F and G. The toxins produced by different types are antigenically distinct but pharmacologically similar. Types A, B and E are the principal causes of human illness.

Properties of Botulinum Toxin

Botulinum toxin is probably the most toxic substance known to mankind. It is a small protein with 19 amino acids and a molecular weight of about 150,000 daltons. Minimum lethal dose, of this toxin, for a mouse is 0.03 ng and that for humans may be 1 µg. It acts slowly taking several hours to kill. It is a neurotoxin which apparently acts by inhibiting the release of acetylcholine from the motor nerve endings of the parasympathetic system. The toxin is relatively stable being inactivated at 80°C for 30–40 minutes and at 100°C for 10 minutes. It resists digestion in the intestine and is absorbed through intestinal mucosa in an active form. It can be toxoided. It is a good antigen and is specifically neutralized by the antitoxin.

Pathogenicity

C. botulinum is widely distributed in soil and decaying vegetation, thus, many foods, both vegetables and meats, may become contaminated with these organisms. It is non-invasive and its pathogenicity is entirely due to the toxin produced by it. The disease caused by this organism is known as botulism. It is of 3 types:

1. **Food-borne botulism**

   It is due to the ingestion of preformed toxin. The causative organism, *C. botulinum*, multiplies in the food before it is consumed, and produces a powerful soluble toxin. The source of botulism is usually preserved food such as meat and meat products, fish, and vegetables. Food responsible for botulism is usually abnormal in appearance and odour. Bulging of this and the presence of gas bubbles on opening suggest contamination with *C. botulinum*. However, at times food may look normal.

   Symptoms usually begin 18–36 hours after ingestion of food and may include nausea, vomiting, thirst, constipation, double vision, difficulty in swallowing, speaking and breathing. This may be followed by muscular weakness, blurred vision, and death as a result of respiratory failure. Case fatality varies from 25–70%.

2. **Wound botulism**

   C. botulinum has occasionally been isolated from wound in man. Toxin is produced at the site of infection and is absorbed. The symptoms are those of food-borne botulism except those of gastrointestinal system. Symptoms appear 4–14 days after injury, in persons with *C. botulinum* infection.

3. **Infant botulism**

   This entity was recognized in 1976. Affected infants have ranged from 3 weeks to 9 months in age and both sexes have been affected equally. Older children and adults are not susceptible. The infants ingest spores, but not preformed toxin, from soil, household dust, honey, etc. About 10% of honey samples have been shown to contain type A and B spores of *C. botulinum*. Within the intestine, *C. botulinum* multiplies and elaborates toxin. After a period of normal development, the infant develops constipation, listlessness, difficulty in sucking and swallowing, weak or altered cry, muscle weakness, ptosis, and loss of head control. Eventually the baby appears 'floppy' (**floppy child syndrome**) and develops respiratory insufficiency or respiratory arrest. Patient excretes toxin and spores in the faeces. Management consists of supportive care and assisted feeding.

Laboratory Diagnosis

Diagnosis may be made by demonstration of the bacillus or the toxin in suspected residual food or in faeces.

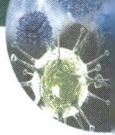

Demonstration of toxin

Botulinum toxin may be demonstrated in the food or faeces. The food is macerated in sterile saline, and the filtrate inoculated into mice or guinea pigs intraperitoneally. The test animal develops dyspnoea, flaccid paralysis and dies within 24 hours. Control animals protected by polyvalent antitoxin remain healthy. Toxin may also be demonstrated in patient serum.

Demonstration of the Organism

Gram-positive sporing bacilli may be demonstrable in smears made from the residual food. For the isolation of *C. botulinum*, the specimen is inoculated on EYA, blood agar and three bottles of CMB. Hold one of these three bottles in a water bath at 80°C for 10 minutes and another for 20 minutes and third is unheated. This procedure selects heat-resistant spores and also allows heat-sensitive spores to grow in unheated CMB. The culture media are incubated anaerobically at 30°C for 3–5 days. Cultures in CMB are screened at intervals for toxin production in mice and presence of the organisms may be detected by fluorescent antibody test. Absence of toxin production up to 5 days usually rules out botulism. Subculture toxin-positive CMB culture onto EYA and blood agar. Incubate anaerobically at 30°C for 48 hours. The growth on EYA and blood agar (direct as well as subculture) is identified by Gram staining, fluorescent antibody procedure, colonial morphology and biochemical characters.

Treatment

The toxin still remaining in the stomach should be removed by lavage with 2–5% bicarbonate solution because toxin is labile in alkaline pH. Saline enemas may be given to remove toxin from the colon. Polyvalent antitoxin against common types, i.e. A, B and E or monovalent when the type of intoxication is known should be given as soon as possible. The antitoxin cannot reverse the effect of toxin already affecting the nerves but will neutralize unfixed toxin. Intensive nursing care and the use of mechanical respirator, when necessary, is of great importance.

Prophylaxis

Since botulism follows consumption of inadequately canned or preserved food, it can be prevented by proper canning and preservation of food. The food that exhibits the signs of spoilage (inflated cans, gas bubbles on opening and abnormal odour) should not be consumed. When an outbreak occurs, a prophylactic dose of polyvalent antitoxin should be given intramuscularly to all those who have consumed that food. Those who may be exposed to the hazards of intoxication in the laboratory or of deliberate intoxication, as in biological warfare, may be protected by injecting three doses of mixed toxoid at two month intervals.

Key Points

- Clostridia are *anaerobic, spore-bearing, Gram-positive bacilli*. They are anaerobic because they *cannot utilize molecular oxygen* (aerobic metabolism) for production of energy.
- Clostridia are also, in varying degrees, *damaged by free oxygen*, which limits the condition under which these organisms can colonize the human body or cause disease. These organisms synthesize some of the *most potent exotoxins* known. For example, the toxins of specific clostridial species cause *botulism, tetanus, gas gangrene* and *pseudomembranous colitis*.
- **Tetanus** causes **sustained muscle spasm** and the characteristic signs of spasm of jaw muscles (lockjaw, *trismus*) and facial muscles (*risus sardonicus*), and arching of the body (*opisthotonicus*).
- Tetanus toxin (*tetanospasmin*) can be *attenuated to form a toxoid*. The latter is *a component of the DPT* (diphtheria-pertussis-tetanus) *vaccine*.

? Assess Yourself

Long and Short Answer Questions

1. Discuss the pathogenicity of *Clostridium perfringens*.
2. Define gas gangrene and discuss its bacteriology and pathogenesis.
3. Write short notes on:
   - (a) Nagler's reaction
   - (b) Alpha toxin
   - (c) Tetanospasmin
   - (d) Pathogenesis and prophylaxis of tetanus
   - (e) Pathogenicity and prevention of *Clostridium botulinum*
   - (f) *Clostridium difficile*

Contd...

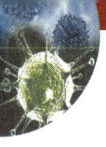

? ASSESS YOURSELF

MULTIPLE CHOICE QUESTIONS

1. Which of the following types of *Clostridium perfringens* produces alpha toxin most abundantly?
   - (a) Type A
   - (b) Type B
   - (c) Type C
   - (d) Type D
2. Contamination of umbilical cord at birth may lead to infection by:
   - (a) *Clostridium perfringens*
   - (b) *C. tetani*
   - (c) *C. botulinum*
   - (d) *C. histolyticum*
3. Which of the following exotoxins resembles strychnine in its effect?
   - (a) Botulinum toxin
   - (b) Tetanus toxin
   - (c) Diphtheria toxin
   - (d) None of the above
4. Nagler's reaction is mediated by:
   - (a) Coagulase
   - (b) Hyaluronidase
   - (c) Deoxyribonuclease
   - (d) Phospholipase

ANSWERS TO MCQs

1. a   2. b   3. b   4. d

Chapter 16

Non-sporing Anaerobes

Nonsporing anaerobes constitute an important cause of human and animal infections. Many of these bacteria form commensal flora of man and animals in mouth and oropharynx, gastrointestinal tract and genitourinary tract. Some of these nonsporing anaerobes act as opportunistic pathogens when body resistance is lowered. They are particularly likely to set up infections in situations in which there is damaged and necrotic tissue. Anaerobic infections of the head, neck and respiratory tract are often associated with organisms found in the mouth, whilst infection in the abdominal and pelvic regions are more commonly associated with gut bacteria.

On the basis of morphology and staining characters, nonsporing anaerobes have been classified as under:

I. **Cocci**
  - Gram-positive
    - *Peptococcus*
    - *Peptostreptococcus*
  - Gram-negative
    Veillonella
II. **Bacilli**
  - Gram-positive
    - *Lactobacillus*
    - *Bifidobacterium*
    - *Propionibacterium*
    - *Actinomyces*
    - *Mobiluncus*
    - *Eubacterium*
  - Gram-negative
    - *Bacteroides*
    - *Fusobacterium*
    - *Leptotrichia*
    - *Porphyromonas*
    - *Prevotella*
III. **Spirochaetes**
  - *Treponema*
  - *Borrelia*

PEPTOCOCCUS

This genus has one species: *P. niger*. They are Gram-positive, non-sporing, anaerobic cocci with G+C content of DNA 50 mol %. They measure 0.4–1.2 μm in diameter and occur singly or in pairs or in clumps. They produce **black colonies on blood agar** after prolonged incubation and produce H_2S. They do not produce catalase and indole and do not reduce nitrate to nitrite.

They occur as normal flora of skin, gastrointestinal tract and genitourinary tract. However, they may cause pyogenic infections of wounds, puerperal sepsis and urinary tract infection.

PEPTOSTREPTOCOCCUS

This genus has 9 species—*P. anaerobius*, *P. asaccharolyticus*, *P. prevotii*, *P. magnus*, *P. indolicus*, *P. micros*, *P. productus*, *P. heliotrinreducens* and *P. tetradius* (formerly *Gafficia anaerobia*). They are Gram-positive cocci occurring in pairs, chains or irregular masses. They are **obligate anaerobes**, measure 0.5–2 μm in diameter, non-haemolytic, catalase-variable, indole production and nitrate reduction variable. Some strains ferment carbohydrates but others are asaccharolytic.

They occur as normal flora of skin, mouth, gastrointestinal tract and genitourinary tract and are the commonest anaerobic organisms recovered from human infections like pleuropulmonary disease, chronic otitis media, brain abscess, puerperal sepsis and urinary tract infections.

P. anaerobius and *P. magnus* are the commonest anaerobic Gram-positive cocci isolated from wound infections. *P. anaerobius* is the anaerobic coccus most commonly associated with puerperal infection.

VEILLONELLA

These are Gram-negative cocci occurring in pairs, short chains and clumps. They are obligate anaerobes, oxidase-negative, catalase-negative, non-motile and measure 0.3–2.5 μm in diameter. They are present as normal flora of the mouth, gastrointestinal and genital tracts. Colonies on blood agar, after 24 hours incubation are small, round, convex, shiny, opaque, light grey and non-haemolytic. In the broth culture, abundant gas is produced. *V. parvula* is isolated from clinical specimens, but little is known of its role in the production of infection.

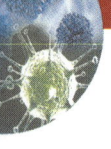

LACTOBACILLUS

These are straight or curved rods that, like corynebacteria, frequently show bipolar bodies due to the presence of **metachromatic granules**. They are Gram-positive and non-sporing. Most strains are non-motile, while a few strains are motile by peritrichous flagella. The bacilli are of varying length and thickness with parallel sides. On an average they measure 1.5×1 µm in size and tend to occur singly or in chains. Occasionally, they may show filamentous forms.

Lactobacilli are normally present in mouth (*L. casei, L. fermentum, L. acidophilus* and *L. brevis*), gut (*L. acidophilus, L. fermentum* and *L. salivarius*) and in vagina (*L. acidophilus, L. fermentum, L. casei* and *L. cellobiosus*). In the mouth, they have been incriminated in the pathogenesis of **dental caries**. The mineral components of enamel and dentine are believed to be dissolved by the acid formed by the fermentation of sucrose and other dietary carbohydrates by lactobacilli. In the intestine, they synthesize vitamins such as biotin, vitamin B_{12} and vitamin K which may be absorbed by the host.

In the adult vagina, lactobacilli ferment glycogen which is deposited in the vaginal epithelial cells and form lactic acid, which accounts for the highly acidic pH of the vagina. This protects adult vagina from infection with gonococci. In prepubertal and postmenopausal vagina, lactobacilli are scanty. Lactobacilli occurring in vagina are collectively known as **Doderlein's bacilli**.

Lactobacilli are also found in plant materials such as silage and in food stuffs and agricultural products, particularly milk, cheese and fermented milk products and in fermented beverages such as wine and cider. In some of these products the multiplication of lactobacilli brings about desirable changes, in others it causes spoilage.

Lactobacilli grow best under microaerophilic conditions in the presence of 5% CO_2 and at pH 6. Better growth is obtained in media enriched with glucose or blood. Colonies on agar media are usually small, 1–3 mm in diameter, with entire margins. Some species form rough colonies. Selective media include Hadley's tomato juice agar (pH 5) and glucose yeast extract acetic acid agar of Rogosa et al., 1951.

BIFIDOBACTERIUM

They are non-motile, non-sporing and pleomorphic Gram-positive rods showing true and false branching. The name is derived from the frequent bifid Y-shaped cells. Most species are obligate anaerobes, but a few species, isolated from animals and bees, can grow in the presence of 90% air and 10% CO_2. Various bifidobacteria occur as normal flora in the mouth, gastrointestinal and genitourinary tracts. *B. bifidum* is common in the faeces of breast-fed and bottle-fed infants and in the faeces of adults and of animals. Bifidobacteria are non-pathogenic to man or laboratory animals.

PROPIONIBACTERIUM

Propionibacteria are pleomorphic, Gram-positive, coryneform rods, non-acid-fast, non-motile and are often arranged in short chains or clumps. They are commonly found on the skin, conjunctiva, external ear, and in the oropharynx and female genital tract. They are aerotolerant, and growth may occasionally be obtained aerobically. Two most commonly isolated species are *Propionibacterium acnes* and *P. propionicum*. *P. acnes* is responsible for two types of infections – (1) **acne vulgaris** in teenagers and young adults, and (2) **opportunistic infections** in patients with prosthetic devices (e.g. artificial heart valves or joints) or intravascular lines (e.g. catheters, cerebrospinal fluid shunts).

MOBILUNCUS

Mobiluncus is the generic name given by Spiegel and Roberts (1984) to a group of curved, motile Gram-variable, anaerobic, non-sporing rods isolated from human vagina in cases of bacterial vaginosis. This genus was tentatively placed in family Bacteroidaceae by them, but its taxonomic position is uncertain. Recent studies suggest that genus *Mobiluncus* belongs to the order Actinomycetales and is closely related to the genus *Actinomyces*. This genus has two species—*M. curtisii* and *M. mulieris*.

Morphology

Both species are highly curved rods and occur singly or in pairs. *M. curtisii* is short, 1.7×0.5 µm and Gram-variable while *M. mulieris* is long, 2.9×0.5 µm and Gram-negative. Both species are motile by means of multiple subpolar flagella.

Cultural Characteristics

They are essentially anaerobes but can grow in an atmosphere of 5% O_2 and 95% N_2. They are fastidious and grow slowly at 33–37°C producing round, entire, low convex, smooth, translucent, colourless colonies, 2–3 mm in diameter, after anaerobic incubation on blood agar medium for five days. Addition of 10 µg/ml each of colistin and nalidixic acid to blood agar makes it selective for isolation of these organisms.

Biochemical Reactions

They are oxidase- and catalase-negative. Small amounts of acetic acid and major amounts of succinic acid are produced in glycogen-containing media. Differentiating biochemical characters of both the species are given in Table 16.1.

Pathogenicity

In association with *Bacteroides* species and *Gardnerella vaginalis*, *M. curtisii* and *M. mulieris* have been blamed to cause **bacterial**

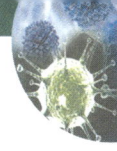

TABLE 16.1: Differentiating characters of species of *Mobiluncus*

Character	M. curtisii	M. mulieris
Mean size of the bacterial cell	1.7 × 0.5 μm	2.9 × 0.5 μm
Gram staining reaction	Variable	Negative
Arginine hydrolysis	+	–
Hippurate hydrolysis	+	–
ONPG	+	–
Nitrate reduction	+	–

vaginosis. Of these, *Bacteroides* species constitute a major component. There is a foul-smelling but non-purulent vaginal discharge with a raised pH (>4.5).

Laboratory Diagnosis

Microscopic examination of fresh unstained smears of vaginal discharge show epithelial cells coated with bacteria (**'clue cells'**). *M. curtisii* and *M. mulieris* may be isolated from vaginal discharge by inoculation on blood agar and blood agar with colistin and nalidixic acid and identified as above.

Treatment

Mobiluncus species are susceptible to benzylpenicillin, clindamycin, erythromycin and gentamicin. For the treatment of infection by *Mobiluncus* species, penicillins are appropriate drugs. *M. mulieris* is more susceptible than *M. curtisii* to metronidazole.

EUBACTERIUM

Members of the genus *Eubacterium* are obligate anaerobic Gram-positive bacilli. They occur as normal flora of mouth and intestine. Some species (*E. brachy, E. timidum* and *E. nodatum*) are commonly seen in periodontitis. *E. lentum* is commonly isolated from non-oral clinical specimens.

BACTEROIDACEAE

Gram-negative, anaerobic, non-sporing and non-motile bacilli, ranging from short Gram-negative rods to filamentous and fusiform shapes, belong to family Bacteroidaceae. This family possesses five genera—*Bacteroides, Fusobacterium, Leptotrichia, Porphyromonas* and *Prevotella*. These anaerobes occur as commensals in the mouth, gastrointestinal and female genital tracts and are now recognized as **opportunistic pathogens** that may produce disease when the host resistance is lowered such as trauma, tissue necrosis, impaired circulation, administration

of antibiotics, corticosteroids and cytotoxic agents, diabetes, malnutrition and malignancy.

The infections due to anaerobes are usually polymicrobial, more than one anaerobe being involved along with aerobic organisms. In anaerobic infections, the resultant pus is usually putrid (foul-smelling) and cellulitis is a frequent finding.

Bacteroides

Bacteroides occur as commensals in the mouth, gastrointestinal and female genital tracts. This genus comprises the most common anaerobes isolated from clinical specimens. They are non-sporing, non-motile, Gram-negative bacilli. They are very pleomorphic, appearing as slender rods, branching forms or coccobacilli. They occur singly, in pairs or in short chains. They grow readily in media such as brain heart infusion agar in an anaerobic atmosphere containing 10% CO_2. They possess capsular polysaccharide which appears to be virulence factor. The capsule confers resistance to phagocytosis and intracellular killing.

They cause peritonitis following bowel injury, pelvic inflammatory disease, abdominal and brain abscesses, and empyema. Pus is often foul smelling. *B. fragilis* is the most frequent of the non-sporing anaerobes isolated from clinical specimens. *B. melaninogenicus* forms black-pigmented or brown colonies on blood-containing media. The pigment is an intracellular or cell-associated derivative of haemoglobulin (haemin). It has been isolated from lung or liver abscesses, mastoiditis, and lesions of intestine, mouth and gums.

Fusobacterium

Fusobacteria are Gram-negative, **strict anaerobic rods** of varied size and morphology. Some species of *Fusobacterium* produce long slender Gram-negative rods that are wide at the centre and taper towards the ends (fusiform), but others produce coccobacilli to very long and filamentous cells. They are usually non-motile and growth is often improved by 5–10% CO_2. They can be isolated on blood agar plates containing neomycin and vancomycin. After 48 hours incubation at 37°C, the colonies are striate or granular with irregular or crenated edge and a raised centre.

F. nucleatum is the most studied species. It may cause infections of head and neck region including dental and periodontal infections and cerebral abscess. *F. necrophorum* is an important animal pathogen. It may, however, sometimes cause infections in man similar to those caused by *F. nucleatum*.

Leptotrichia

This genus contains only one species, *L. buccalis* which is synonymous with *Fusobacterium fusiforme*. They are anaerobic, non-sporing, non-motile, long, straight or slightly curved Gram-negative bacilli with considerable width and tapering ends. They measure 5–15 × 1–1.5 μm in size. They can be grown on blood agar at 37°C under anaerobic conditions with 5–10% CO_2.

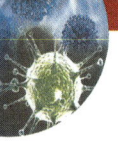

After 48 hours incubation, colonies are 2–3 mm in diameter, irregular and often striate. Many strains become aerotolerant after several subcultures.

L. buccalis is a normal flora of mouth and gastrointestinal tract. However, in association with *Borrelia vincentii* it is believed to cause **acute ulcerative gingivitis** or **Vincent's angina**. It is seen in patients with malnutrition, debility and poor oral hygiene. It is characterized by pain, haemorrhage, foul odour, destruction of interdental papillae, inflammation of the gums and formation of a pseudomembrane. *L. buccalis* and *B. vincentii* are present in the exudate and pseudomembrane, and diagnosis is made by direct microscopy.

Porphyromonas

Porphyromonas spp. are part of normal oral flora. *P. gingivalis* causes periodontal disease and *P. endodontalis* causes dental root infections.

Prevotella

Prevotella contains *P. melaninogenica*, *P. buccalis*, *P. denticola* and other species. *P. melaninogenica* produces black or brown colonies on anaerobic blood agar. The colour is not due to the melanin pigment but is due to hemin derivative. It causes lung or liver abscess, mastoiditis, intestinal lesions and lesions of mouth and gums. Cultures of *P. melaninogenica* and dressings from wounds infected with the bacillus produce a characteristic red fluorescence when exposed to ultraviolet light.

Laboratory Diagnosis

As anaerobic bacteria form part of the normal flora of the skin and mucous surfaces, their isolation from clinical specimens has to be interpreted cautiously. The mere presence of an anaerobe does not prove its causal role.

Specimen Collection and Transport

Specimens should be collected in such a manner as to avoid normal resident flora. For example, the sputum is unsatisfactory for culture from a suspected case of lung abscess. In general, material for anaerobic culture is best obtained by tissue biopsy or by aspiration using a needle and syringe. Swabs are unsatisfactory specimens, but when they are to be used, they should be sent in Stuart's transport medium. Ideally, specimens should be placed in an anaerobic transport device that consists of a tube or vial containing an anaerobic gas mixture substituted for air, which protects the organisms from oxygen exposure and drying during transport to the laboratory. Specimens should be delivered within 20 minutes for culture.

Direct Microscopy

Examination of a Gram-stained smear shows numerous pus cells and a variety of organisms. In case of *P. melaninogenica* infection, examination of the specimen under ultraviolet light may show the bright red fluorescence.

Culture

Freshly prepared blood agar with neomycin, yeast extract, hemin and vitamin K is inoculated and incubated at 37°C in an anaerobic jar, with 10% CO_2. Anaerobiasis can also be maintained by GasPak system. Plates are examined after 24–48 hours. Some anaerobes, such as fusobacteria, require longer period of incubation. Parallel aerobic cultures should also be set up because in most anaerobic infections aerobic bacteria are also involved. Other anaerobic media, such as cooked meat broth and thioglycollate broth, may also be used for isolation of anaerobes.

Definitive identification of the anaerobes depends on colony morphology and various biochemical tests. Gas liquid chromatography is also useful to identify anaerobes in the specimens.

 Key Points

- Many non-sporing anaerobes form **commensal flora** of man and animals in **mouth and oropharynx.**
- Lactobacilli have been incriminated in the pathogenesis of **dental caries**.
- Fusobacteria inhabit **oral cavity, colon and female genital tract**.
- *Fusobacterium nucleatum* causes **dental** and **periodontal disease,** and cerebral abscess.

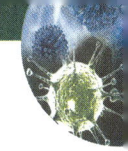

? ASSESS YOURSELF

LONG AND SHORT ANSWER QUESTIONS

1. Discuss the classification of non-sporing anaerobes.
2. Write short notes on:
   (a) Anaerobic cocci
   (b) *Bacteroides*

MULTIPLE CHOICE QUESTIONS

1. Which of the following bacteria are predominant flora of the human gut?
   (a) *Escherichia coli*
   (b) *Clostridium perfringens*
   (c) *Bacteroides*
   (d) *Actinomyces*

2. Which of the following bacteria are Gram-negative cocci?
   (a) *Peptococcus*
   (b) *Peptostreptococcus*
   (c) *Sporosarcina*
   (d) *Veillonella*

3. Lactobacilli constitute the normal flora of:
   (a) Adult vagina
   (b) Prepubertal vagina
   (c) Post-menopausal vagina
   (d) None of the above

4. Which of the following genera is/are included in the family Bacteriodaceae?
   (a) *Bacteroides*
   (b) *Fusobacterium*
   (c) *Leptotrichia*
   (d) All of the above

ANSWERS TO MCQs

1. b   **2.** d   **3.** a   **4.** d

Mycobacterium (Tuberculosis and Leprosy)

Important mycobacteria causing human disease are *Mycobacterium tuberculosis*, *M. bovis*, *M. leprae* and non-tuberculous mycobacteria.

MYCOBACTERIUM TUBERCULOSIS

Morphology

Tubercle bacilli are slender, straight or slightly curved rods with rounded ends. They measure 1–4 × 0.2–0.8 μm (average 3 × 0.3 μm) in size. In sputum and other clinical specimens they may occur singly or in small clumps. True branching is occasionally seen in old cultures and in smears from caseous lymph nodes. They are non-motile, non-sporing, non-capsulated and acid-fast.

The Ziehl-Neelsen acid-fast stain is useful in staining organisms from cultures or from clinical material. With this stain, the tubercle bacilli stain bright red, while the tissue cells and other organisms are stained blue (Fig. 17.1).

Organisms in tissue and sputum smears often stain irregularly and have a beaded or barred appearance, presumably because of their vacuoles and polyphosphate content. Tubercle bacilli may also be stained with auramine O and smears examined by fluorescence microscopy under low magnification. Tubercle bacilli appear yellow luminous rods in a dark-field.

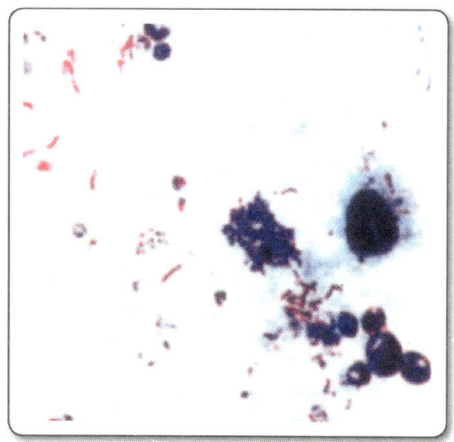

Fig. 17.1: Sputum smear showing acid-fast bacilli (Ziehl-Neelsen staining, × 1000).

When they have been detected under low power, the morphology of the bacilli is confirmed by observation with an oil-immersion objective. Tubercle bacilli are Gram-positive but it is difficult to stain them with the Gram stain. This is because of the failure of the dye to penetrate the cell wall.

Cultural Characteristics

M. tuberculosis is an obligate aerobe. Optimum temperature for growth is 37°C (range 30–40°C) and optimum pH is 7.0 (range 6.0–7.6). Tubercle bacilli can grow on a wide range of enriched culture media but **Lowenstein-Jensen (LJ) medium** is most widely used. This medium consists of whole egg, asparagine, some mineral salts, malachite green and glycerol or sodium pyruvate, and solidified by heating (inspissation). **Malachite green inhibits the growth of organisms other than mycobacteria and provides a colour contrast against which colonies of mycobacteria can be easily seen**. The addition of glycerol improves the growth of *M. tuberculosis*, while it is without any effect or even inhibitory to *M. bovis*. Sodium pyruvate improves the growth of both *M. tuberculosis* and *M. bovis*.

The average generation time of tubercle bacilli is about 14–15 hours, prolonged incubation is, therefore, necessary. *M. tuberculosis* grows well on LJ medium (**eugonic growth**). It produces visible growth on LJ glycerol medium, incubated at 37°C, in 2–8 weeks, although on primary isolation from clinical material, colonies may take up to 12 weeks to appear. They grow as '**rough, tough and buff**' colonies – rough due to dry, irregular growth; tough due to difficulty in lifting the colony from the surface; and buff due to the pale yellow colour. They are tenacious and not easily emulsified. On the other hand, *M. bovis* grows poorly on LJ glycerol medium (**dysgonic growth**) forming small, moist, smooth, flat and white colonies which easily break up when touched.

Sensitivity to Physical and Chemical Agents

Tubercle bacilli are highly resistant to drying. When exposed to direct sunlight, organisms from culture are killed in 2 hours, but bacilli contained in sputum require an exposure of 20–30 hours. In dried sputum, protected from sunlight, they survive for as long as 6 months. The tubercle bacillus is generally more resistant to chemical disinfection than other non-spore-formers, especially when present in sputum.

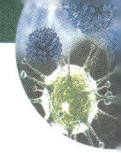

Pathogenesis

Humans become infected with *M. tuberculosis* most frequently by inhaling infective droplets coughed or sneezed into air by a patient with tuberculosis. Bovine tuberculosis is spread from animal-to-animal, and sometimes to human attendants, in moist cough spray. About 1% of infected cows develop lesions in the udder and bacilli are excreted in the milk which can then infect people who drink it raw. Thus, primary human tuberculosis due to *M. bovis* usually involves cervical or mesenteric lymph nodes. Human tuberculosis is divisible into primary and post-primary (secondary) forms.

Primary Tuberculosis

This begins with inhalation of the mycobacteria and ends with a T cell-mediated immune response that induces hypersensitivity to the organisms and controls 95% of infections. Inhaled tubercle bacilli are engulfed by alveolar macrophages in which they replicate to form the initial lesion or **Ghon focus**. It consists of a parenchymal subpleural lesion, often just above or just below the interlobar fissure between the upper and the lower lobes.

Some bacilli are transported by macrophages to the hilar lymph nodes. The Ghon focus together with the enlarged hilar lymph nodes forms the **primary complex**. In addition, the bacilli may be seeded by further lymphatic and haematogenous dissemination in many organs and tissues, including other parts of the lung. In case of *M. bovis* which enters the mouth, as in milk-borne bovine tuberculosis, the primary complexes involve the tonsil and cervical lymph nodes or the intestine, often the ileocaecal region, and the mesenteric lymph nodes.

Post-primary (Secondary) Tuberculosis

It is caused by reactivation of the primary lesion (endogenous), or by exogenous reinfection. Reactivation tuberculosis is particularly likely to occur in immunocompromised individuals including the elderly, transplant recipients and those who are infected with human immunodeficiency virus (HIV). Granulomas of secondary tuberculosis most often occur in the apex of the lungs but may be widely disseminated in the lungs, kidneys, meninges, bones and other organs. The same process of granuloma formation occurs but the necrotic element of the reaction causes tissue destruction and the formation of large areas of caseation termed **tuberculomas**.

Proteases liberated by activated macrophages cause softening and liquefaction of the caseous material. Two special features of secondary tuberculosis are the presence of caseous necrosis and of cavities, which may rupture into blood vessels, spreading myco-bacteria throughout the body, and break into airways, releasing infectious mycobacteria in aerosols and sputum (**open tuberculosis**).

Immunity and Hypersensitivity

Two immunologic responses, antituberculous immunity and tuberculin hypersensitivity, develop simultaneously in naturally infected host. Both these are mediated by T-cells sensitized to bacterial antigen. Humoral immunity appears to be of no relevance in tuberculosis and antibodies do not influence the course of disease. In the non-immune host, the bacilli are able to multiply inside phagocytes and lyse the host cells, while in immune host CD4+ helper T cells and CD8+ suppressor T cells are produced. The former secrete interferon-gamma which activates macrophages to kill intracellular mycobacteria and the latter kill the macrophages that are infected with mycobacteria.

Koch's Phenomenon

The tuberculin reactivity was first demonstrated in guinea pigs by Robert Koch (1890, 1891). The experiment that led to the demonstration of this reactivity is known as **Koch's phenomenon**. When a healthy guinea pig is inoculated subcutaneously with a pure culture of tubercle bacilli, the puncture site heals quickly and there is no immediate visible reaction. But after 10–14 days a hard nodule appears which soon breaks down to form an ulcer that persists till the animal dies of progressive tuberculosis. The regional lymph nodes are enlarged and caseous.

But something totally different develops when a guinea pig already ill with tuberculosis is inoculated. It is best to use animals that have been successfully inoculated 4–6 weeks previously. An indurated lesion appears at the site of second inoculation in a day or two which undergoes necrosis in another day to form a shallow ulcer that heals rapidly without involvement of the regional lymph nodes or other tissues. Koch's phenomenon is a combination of hypersensitivity and immunity.

Tuberculin Test

Principle

Delayed, type IV or cell-mediated hypersensitivity.

Method

- **Mantoux test:** 0.1 ml of purified protein derivative (PPD) containing 5 Tu is injected intradermally into the skin of the volar aspect of the forearm. Those suspected of having tuberculosis, and therefore likely to react strongly, may first be tested with 1 Tu. The site of inoculation is palpated 72 hours later. The development of an area of palpable, firm induration 10 mm or more in diameter is recorded as positive, and those between 5 and 9 mm in diameter as doubtful. The extent of the accompanying erythema is irrelevant and should be ignored. If the reaction is completely negative, the test may be repeated by giving an injection of 100 Tu.
- **Heaf test:** This test is done with a multiple puncture apparatus with 6 needles that prick 1–2 mm deep into the skin. A drop of undiluted PPD is spread on the area of skin selected for inoculation. The multiple puncture apparatus is pressed against this area of skin and needles are released. The test is read after 72 hours. Erythema and induration around at least 4 of the punctures is regarded as positive.

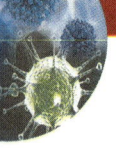

The equipment must be adequately sterilized between each use to prevent transmission of hepatitis and AIDS.

Uses of Tuberculin Test

- To diagnose active infection in infants and young children.
- To measure prevalence of infection in a community.
- To select susceptibles for BCG vaccination.
- Indication of successful BCG vaccination.

False negative (tuberculin anergy)

- Early tuberculosis.
- Advanced tuberculosis.
- Miliary tuberculosis.
- In patients with measles and other exanthematous reactions.
- Occasionally, after chemotherapy and removal of lung lesion.
- Advanced age.
- Immunosuppressive therapy and defective CMI.
- Lymphoreticular malignancy.
- Sarcoidosis.
- Severe malnutrition.

False Positive

False positive reactions may be seen in patients with infection by related mycobacteria (non-tuberculous mycobacteria). These are usually low grade reactions and can be differentiated by testing with tuberculin prepared from these mycobacteria.

Laboratory Diagnosis

Bacteriological diagnosis can be established by demonstration of tubercle bacilli in clinical specimens by microscopy and cultural techniques.

Collection of Specimen

The specimen most commonly collected is sputum which consists of pus and mucus secretions coughed up from the lung.

- Patient is instructed to cough up the sputum into a clean wide-mouthed container. Disposable waxed cardboard containers are ideal. A morning specimen may be collected. If sputum is scanty, a 24 hour specimen may be collected.
- If no sputum is produced, **laryngeal swab or bronchial washings** are examined.
- In children, stomach washings may be examined as they tend to swallow sputum.
- Depending upon the site of involvement, **cerebrospinal fluid, pleural fluid, urine and aspirated fluid from bone and joint** are centrifuged and the deposits are examined.

- **Tissue biopsies** are homogenized and examined by microscopy and culture.
- In pulmonary and renal tuberculosis, three consecutive specimens of **sputum and urine** should be examined respectively.

Direct Microscopy

Pour the sputum in a petri dish and examine. For preparation of smear, select **blood-tinged part** of the sputum, if it is not there then **purulent part** should be selected. The smear is stained by Ziehl-Neelsen technique and examined under oil-immersion lens. Acid-fast bacilli stain bright red against a blue background (Fig. 17.1).

Concentration of Specimens

Mycobacteria in a specimen can be decontaminated and concentrated into a small volume without inactivation. Such concentrate can be used for microscopy, culture and animal inoculation. Several methods are in use:

- *Petroff's method:* It is a simple and widely used technique. Equal volumes of sputum and 4% sodium hydroxide are mixed and incubated at 37°C with frequent shaking till it gets liquefied and becomes clear. On the average, it takes 20–30 minutes. It is then centrifuged at 3,000 rpm for 30 minutes. The supernatant fluid is pipetted off and the deposit is neutralized by adding 8% hydrochloric acid in the presence of a drop of phenol red indicator.
- *Other methods:* Instead of alkali, homogenization can be carried out by treatment with dilute acids (5% oxalic acid, 3% hydrochloric acid or 6% sulphuric acid) or mucolytic agents such as N-acetyl-L-cysteine with sodium hydroxide and pancreatin.

Culture

It is very sensitive for detection of tubercle bacilli. It may be positive with as few as 10–100 bacilli per ml of sputum and it is necessary for antimicrobial drug sensitivity testing. **Concentrate of sputum** is inoculated on two slopes of LJ medium. In case of **laryngeal swab**, add enough 5% oxalic acid to the tube to cover the swab and leave it at room temperature for 30 minutes to kill non-acid-fast contaminants. Squeeze the swab against the side of the tube to remove excess fluid and rub it over the surface of two slopes of LJ medium.

The inoculated media are incubated at 37°C. The cultures are examined weekly for 12 weeks. Growth of most strains of *M. tuberculosis* may appear in 2–8 weeks. But cultures should not be discarded as negative until they have been observed for 12 weeks. Longer incubation is necessary for strains originating from patients treated with antitubercular agents. However, by **radiometric method** the growth may be detected in about a week by using ^{14}C-labelled substrates and measuring ^{14}CO$_2$ evolved due to bacterial metabolism. The sensitivity of radiometric method is slightly more than that of traditional culture method.

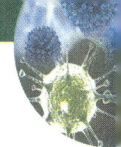

Genexpert System—Xpert MTB/Rif Test

This is a fully automated nucleic acid amplification test (NAAT). This is a rapid test which identifies both the presence of *M. tuberculosis* and resistance to rifampicin.

Nucleic Acid Technology

Polymerase chain reaction (PCR) is a rapid method in diagnosis of tuberculosis. It is based on DNA amplification and has been used to detect *M. tuberculosis* directly in clinical sample.

Prophylaxis

Protection from tuberculosis may be afforded by public health measures, BCG vaccination and by chemoprophylaxis. General measures such as adequate nutrition, good housing and health education are important.

BCG Vaccine

It is a live attenuated vaccine introduced by Calmette and Guerin (1921). This is a strain of *M. bovis* attenuated by repeated subcultures, every 3 weeks, for 230 subcultures on slices of potato soaked in autoclaved bile containing glycerol (5%) over a period of 13 years (1908–1921).

BCG vaccine is available in liquid form and freeze-dried (lyophilized) form. The latter is commonly used. The lyophilized vaccine supplied by BCG vaccine laboratory, Chennai, is reconstituted with sterile physiological saline to make a final concentration of 0.1 mg (moist weight) in 0.1 ml of the vaccine. Once reconstituted, vaccine should be utilized within 3–6 hours. Following injection of 0.1 ml of vaccine intradermally, the organisms grow to a limited extent in the tissues. Immunizing capability of the vaccine depends on this. Dead vaccine or tuberculin is not effective. BCG vaccine should be administered soon after birth failing which it may be given at any time during the first year of life.

A **small nodule** develops at the site of inoculation 2–3 weeks after injection. It increases slowly in size and by about 5 weeks it attains a diameter of 4–8 mm. It then subsides or breaks into a **shallow ulcer** which heals by scarring. Such individuals become **tuberculin-positive** after 4–6 weeks.

Complications of BCG vaccination

- *Local:* (a) abscess, (b) indolent ulcer, (c) keloid, (d) tuberculids (small satellite BCG tubercles developing in the neighbourhood of the site of vaccination).
- *Regional:* Lymphadenitis.
- *Systemic:* (a) Fever, (b) erythema nodosum, (c) otitis media.

Contraindications of BCG

BCG vaccination is contraindicated in patients of tuberculosis, AIDS, measles, pertussis and eczema, and patients on steroids and tuberculin positive individuals.

Chemotherapy

The antituberculous drugs include rifampicin, isoniazid, pyrazinamide, streptomycin, ethambutol and thiacetazone. The first 4 of these are bactericidal and the others are bacteriostatic. Other less often used drugs include ethionamide, cycloserine, capreomycin, kanamycin and *p*-aminosalicylic acid. Tubercle bacilli resistant to a number of antitubercular drugs (**multidrug-resistant tuberculosis**, MDR TB) is a growing problem. Another serious condition **extensively drug resistant tuberculosis (XDR-TB)** has emerged recently.

MYCOBACTERIUM LEPRAE

Morphology

Lepra bacilli are straight or slightly curved slender bacilli about the same size as tubercle bacilli (average size: 3 × 0.3 μm). They have pointed, rounded or club-shaped ends. They are non-motile and non-sporing. They are Gram-positive and stain more readily than *M. tuberculosis*. With Ziehl-Neelsen stain, they are less acid-fast than tubercle bacilli, so 5% sulphuric acid is employed for decolourization after staining with carbol fuchsin.

The bacilli are seen singly and in groups, intracellularly and lying free outside the cell. Inside the cells they are usually present in parallel bundles of 50 or more organisms bound together by a lipid-like substance, the **glia**. These masses of bacteria are known as **globi** which are seen inside the histiocytes which have a foamy appearance. These are known as **lepra cells** (Fig. 17.2).

Live bacilli in the smear appear solid and uniformly stained, while dead or dying forms appear fragmented, beaded and granular. The percentage of uniformly stained bacilli in the tissues is known as **morphological index** (MI). This provides a method for assessing the progress of patients on chemotherapy and is more meaningful than the old criterion, the bacteriological index (BI). Poorly stained bacilli are probably dead. A continuing fall in the MI is encouraging, and a fall succeeded by a rise indicates

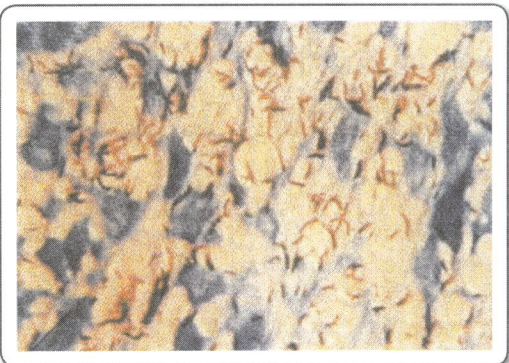

Fig. 17.2: Lepromatous leprosy showing acid-fast bacilli in histiocytes (Ziehl-Neelsen staining, × 1000).

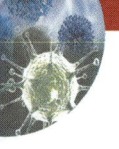
TABLE 17.1: Bacteriological index (Ridley's scale)

Bacteriological index	Number of acid-fast bacilli
6+	More than 1000 per oil–immersion field
5+	100–1000 per oil–immersion field
4+	10–100 per oil–immersion field
3+	1–10 per oil–immersion field
2+	1–10 per 10 oil–immersion fields
1+	1–10 per 100 oil–immersion fields

development of drug resistance in the bacteria. **Bacteriological index** of a smear is the total number of acid-fast bacilli in an oil immersion field. It can be expressed from 1+ to 6+ by Ridley's scale (Table 17.1).

Cultivation

A large number of attempts at cultivation of *M. leprae*, in artificial culture media and in tissue culture, have been made and success has been claimed from time to time, but none has been confirmed so far.

There have been many attempts to transmit leprosy to various experimental animals. But the first breakthrough was achieved by Shepard (1960) when he reported a limited localized multiplication of *M. leprae* in the **foot-pad of mouse** in 1–6 months.

Nine-banded armadillo (*Dasypus novemcinctus*) is highly susceptible to leprosy. This is presumably due to low body temperature. When inoculated with *M. leprae*, about 40% armadillos develop generalized infection with extensive multiplication of *M. leprae*. Involvement of skin, nerves, lymph nodes, larynx and eye is similar to that of man. In addition, in armadillo, it involves lungs, oesophagus, meninges and cerebral cortex. In armadillo, *M. leprae* survives for about 400 days.

Pathogenesis

Leprosy is an exclusively human disease and the only source of infection is the patient. The exact mode of infection is not clear. Very large number of bacilli are shed in nasal secretions (over 10^8 organisms per ml) and in discharges from superficial lesions of the cases of lepromatous leprosy. Organisms may be acquired by a susceptible person by way of skin to skin contact or through respiratory tract. Once worldwide in distribution, leprosy is now confined mainly, but not exclusively, to the underdeveloped areas of tropics and southern hemisphere.

M. leprae causes **chronic granulomatous lesions** closely resembling those of tuberculosis with epithelioid cells and giant cells but **without caseation**. The organisms in the lesion are predominantly intracellular and like tubercle bacilli can proliferate in macrophages. The organism has predilection for skin, nerves

and nasal mucosa though it is capable of affecting any tissue or organ.

- In **cutaneous form** of the disease, large, firm nodules are distributed widely and on the face they create a characteristic **leonine appearance**.
- In the **neural form**, segments of peripheral nerves are involved leading to localized patches of anaesthesia. The loss of sensations in fingers and toes increases the frequency of minor trauma, leading to secondary infection and mutilating injuries. Both forms may be present in the same patient.

SPECTRUM OF LEPROSY

On the basis of clinical, histopathologic and immunologic findings, Ridley and Joplings (1966) introduced a scale for classifying the spectrum of leprosy into 5 groups with hyper-reactive tuberculoid (TT) leprosy at one pole and anergic lepromatous (LL) leprosy at the other.

- **Tuberculoid type:** It is seen in patients with high degree of resistance where cell-mediated immunity is intact. The skin lesions are few and consist of nonelevated hypo- or hyperpigmented macular anaesthetic patches involving the face, trunk and limbs. There are very few acid-fast bacilli (AFB) so that they are generally not seen microscopically (**paucibacillary disease**), and numerous epithelioid cells, giant cells and lymphocytes as in tuberculosis. The local nerves are involved in the early stage and gradually the infection extends into the bigger nerve trunks which are thickened, hard and tender. This leads to deformities of hand and feet. In tuberculoid leprosy, lepromin test is positive due to intact CMI. Antimycobacterial and autoantibodies are rarely produced.
- **Lepromatous type:** It is the generalized form of the disease and is found in individuals where the host resistance is low. Patient develops numerous nodular skin lesions (lepromata) on face, ear lobes, hands, feet and less commonly trunk. Skin lesions contain many macrophages, often seen as large foamy cells packed with AFB. In advanced cases, there may be 10^9 *M. leprae*/g of skin (**multibacillary disease**). Cooler parts of the body, such as ear lobes, are particularly infiltrated by bacilli. Blood stream may be invaded, with resulting foci in the liver, spleen, adrenals, testicles and bone marrow and excretion of the organisms in milk. In addition, there is heavy infection of upper respiratory tract, particularly the nasal mucosa, from which the organisms are shed.

There is slow and symmetric thickening of nerves and anaesthesia. Nodular skin lesions ulcerate due to repeated trauma as a result of loss of sensation. The ulcerated nodules become secondarily infected that leads to distortion and mutilation of extremities. **Lepromatous leprosy is more infectious than other types and has a poor prognosis.** Because of deficient CMI, lepromin test is negative. Humoral antibodies against mycobacterial antigens are produced in high concentrations which play no protective role. **Autoantibodies are also produced.**

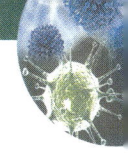

TABLE 17.2: Characteristics of 5 forms of leprosy

	TT	BT	BB	BL	LL
AFB in the skin	−	+/−	+	+++	++++
AFB in nasal secretions	−	−	−	+	++++
Granuloma formation	++++	+++	+	−	−
Lepromin reaction	++++	+	+/−	−	−
Antibodies to *M. leprae*	+/−	+/−	+	+++	++++

Borderline or Dimorphous Type

Many patients occupy an intermediate position on the spectrum and are classified as borderline tuberculoid (BT), mid-borderline (BB) and borderline lepromatous (BL). The characteristics of these five forms are shown in Table 17.2.

Lepromin Test

This reaction was first described by Mitsuda in Japan in 1919.

Lepromins

The lepromins used as antigen in lepromin test may be of human origin (lepromin-H) or of armadillo origin (lepromin-A).

Procedure

The test is carried out by the intradermal injection of 0.1 ml of lepromin. The response to this is biphasic:
- **Early or Fernandez reaction:** It is characterized by an acute localized area of inflammation with congestion and oedema, more than 10 mm in diameter, appearing usually in 24–48 hours and tending to disappear in 3–4 days. Histologically, it consists of serous exudate with lymphocytic infiltration.
- **Late or Mitsuda reaction:** It appears 1–2 weeks after the injection in the form of a nodule that may undergo central necrosis and ulceration. It takes several weeks to heal.

Uses of Lepromin Reaction

- To classify the lesions of leprosy patients. The reaction is positive in tuberculoid and negative in lepromatous leprosy patients.
- To assess the prognosis and response to treatment. A positive reaction indicates a good prognosis and a negative one a bad prognosis. Conversion to lepromin positivity during treatment is the evidence of improvement.
- To assess the resistance of an individual to leprosy.
- For recruitment of persons to work in leprosy homes. Only lepromin-positive persons are recommended to be appointed.
- To verify the identity of candidate *M. leprae*. Cultivable AFB, claimed to be *M. leprae*, should give matching results when tested in parallel with standard lepromin.

Laboratory Diagnosis

As a routine, smears are made from affected parts of the skin and nasal mucous membrane. Material for smear is, however, sometimes taken from lymph nodes and affected nerves.
- **In lepromatous cases**, bacilli are always found in large numbers and about equally frequently in skin and nose.
- **In tuberculoid cases**, as a rule, the bacilli are very few and found with great difficulty, or not at all. The characteristic histologic response in biopsy material is helpful in such cases and is essential for accurate classification of the disease within the disease spectrum.

Skin Smears

The selection of site for taking smear is of great importance. Places where leprous lesions are most prominent, such as nodules, thick patches and areas of infiltration, should be selected. In case of patches, smears should be made from the thickened margins. In a patient with only diffuse infiltration, about 5–6 different areas of the skin should be sampled, including the skin over the ear lobes, buttocks, forehead, chin and cheeks. The specimen is obtained by **slit and scrape method**.

Nasal Scrapings

Smears from the nose are made by scraping a little material from the nasal septum, particularly from inferior turbinate bones, with a small-bladed knife.

When smears dry, these are fixed by passing the slide twice or thrice over a flame with the surface carrying the smears uppermost. The smears are then stained by the Ziehl-Neelsen technique using 5%, instead of 20%, sulphuric acid for decolourization. Bacteriological and morphological indices (as already discussed) are also determined.

Skin and Nerve Biopsy

Skin biopsy is collected from active edge of the patches, and nerve biopsy from thickened nerve for histological confirmation of tuberculoid leprosy when acid-fast bacilli cannot be demonstrated in direct smear. Skin biopsy is useful in the diagnosis and accurate classification of leprosy lesion but nerve biopsy is not required if a skin lesion is present.

Animal Inoculation

- Injection of ground tissue from lepromatous nodules and nasal scraping from leprosy patient into the **footpad of mouse** produces typical granuloma at the site of inoculation in 1–6 months.
- **Nine-banded armadillo** is highly susceptible to leprosy. Such an animal, when inoculated with ground tissue from lepromatous nodules and nasal scrapings from leprosy patient, develops generalized infection with extensive

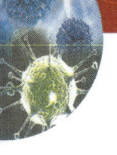

multiplication of bacilli and the lesions produced resemble lepromatous leprosy.

The lesions which develop in the mouse and armadillo can be identified by histological examination and Ziehl-Neelsen staining.

Lepromin Test or Mitsuda Reaction

It is not a diagnostic test but is a guide to the resistance of the patient to *M. leprae* infection.

Serological Test

Serodiagnosis of leprosy may be carried out by detection of antiphenolic glycolipid 1 antibodies by latex agglutination, *M. leprae* particle agglutination and ELISA test.

Polymerase Chain Reaction (PCR)

PCR can be used for the diagnosis at an early stage, before appearance of clinical symptoms. It is effective even in the diagnosis of paucibacillary leprosy, as **the detection limit of PCR is as low as one bacillus**. The PCR assay can be performed on biopsy specimens, skin scrapings and nasal secretions.

Treatment

Dapsone (4,4′-diaminodiphenyl sulphone, DDS) monotherapy was the standard treatment for all types of leprosy for a number of years. However, there is evidence that *M. leprae* is acquiring dapsone resistance. In view of this, multiple drug therapy is now recommended for the treatment of leprosy. Patients with paucibacillary lesions (TT, BT) are given rifampicin 600 mg once a month and dapsone 100 mg daily for six months. For multibacillary lesions (BB, BL, LL), patient is administered rifampicin 600 mg once a month, dapsone 100 mg daily and clofazimine 50 mg daily for 2 years.

🔖 Key Points

- Mycobacteria are **acid-fast beaded bacilli** and resist decolorization with dilute mineral acids. Hence, a special stain, the **Ziehl-Neelsen stain**, is used to visualize them.
- The above property is due to the high lipid content (40–60%) of the cell wall (**mycolic acid**), which is also an effective defence mechanism resisting phagocytosis.
- *Mycobacterium tuberculosis* grows slowly (up to **8–12 weeks**) on Lowenstein-Jensen medium as **'rough, tough and buff'** colonies.
- *Mycobacterium leprae* is **less acid-fast** than tubercle bacilli, so 5% sulphuric acid is employed for decolourization after staining with carbol fuchsin.
- *M. leprae* invades both sensory and motor nerves and **destroys nerve fibres**.
- Leprosy may be classified into **five groups** with hyper-reactive tuberculoid (TT) leprosy at one pole and anergic lepromatous (LL) leprosy at the other.
- Prevalence of leprosy is **highest in India**.

❓ Assess Yourself

Long and Short Answer Questions

1. Discuss pathogenesis and laboratory diagnosis of tuberculosis.
2. Write short notes on:
   - (a) Tuberculin test
   - (b) BCG vaccine
   - (c) Lowenstein-Jensen medium
   - (d) Pathogenesis of leprosy
   - (e) Laboratory diagnosis of leprosy
   - (f) Lepromin test

Contd...

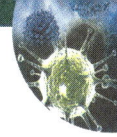

? ASSESS YOURSELF

MULTIPLE CHOICE QUESTIONS

1. Which of the following bacteria cause/s tuberculosis in man?
   (a) *Mycobacterium tuberculosis*   (b) *M. bovis*
   (c) *M. africanum*   (d) All of the above

2. Eugonic growth on Lowenstein-Jensen medium is produced by:
   (a) *Mycobacterium tuberculosis*   (b) *M. bovis*
   (c) Both of the above   (d) None of the above

3. BCG vaccine is a:
   (a) Live attenuated preparation   (b) Killed preparation
   (c) Toxoid preparation   (d) Recombinant preparation

4. Mitsuda reaction in lepromin test appears after:
   (a) 24–48 hours   (b) 3 days
   (c) 5 days   (d) 1–2 weeks

5. Fernandez reaction in lepromin test appears in:
   (a) 1–2 days   (b) 3 days
   (c) 2 weeks   (d) 3–4 weeks

ANSWERS TO MCQs

1. d   **2.** a   **3.** a   **4.** d   **5.** a

Spirochaetes

The spirochaetes have **Gram-negative-type** cell wall composed of an outer membrane, a peptidoglycan layer and a cytoplasmic membrane. They are thin helical, motile, and flexible bacteria, twisted spirally along the long axis, giving these bacteria the name spirochaetes (*spira* meaning coiled and *chaite* meaning hair). They possess a varying number of fine fibrils which are attached subterminally at each pole of the cell and extend towards the opposite pole between outer membrane and peptidoglycan layer. Because of their similarity to other bacterial flagella they are known as **endoflagella**. The number of endoflagella per cell end is a morphologic characteristic of each species, in *Treponema* pathogenic for humans, the number is 3 but occasionally 4, in most *Borrelia* it is 15–20, and in *Leptospira* it is one. The spiral shape and serpentine motility of the spirochaetes depend upon the integrity of these endoflagella.

TREPONEMA PALLIDUM

Morphology

It is a thin, delicate, long, motile, flexible organism which is twisted spirally round its long axis. It is 6–14 μm long. Its width is 0.13 μm in dried state, but is about 0.2 μm in the wet living state, which is just great enough for resolution with the light microscope. It has 6–12 coils which are remarkably evenly disposed at 1 μm intervals and the amplitude of spirals is 1–1.5 μm. They have tapering ends. It is actively motile exhibiting flexion and extension, translatory and corkscrew-like motility. As the spirochaete moves across the dark-field of the microscope, it often displays **a characteristic tendency to bend at right angles near its midpoint**. These secondary curves appear and disappear but its primary spirals remain unchanged.

Because of its weak refractility and slender thickness, about the limit of resolution by the light microscope, it is best seen in wet living preparation with the **dark-ground microscope**. In dried preparations, it needs to be thickened by **silver impregnation methods (Fontana's method is useful for staining films, and Levaditi's for tissue sections)**. It cannot be stained by simple aniline dyes or by Gram's method. By prolonged Giemsa staining it stains pale pink. By immunofluorescence method, treponemes can be detected in tissues and body fluids.

Ultrastructurally, *T. pallidum* possesses usually three but occasionally four endoflagella attached subterminally at each end of the cell and extend towards the opposite pole between outer membrane layer and peptidoglycan layer of the cell wall.

Cultivation

Pathogenic treponemes cannot be cultivated in artificial media and are maintained by subculture in susceptible animals. **Nichol's strain** of *T. pallidum* has been maintained, in rabbit testis, for several decades by serial testicular passage since it was isolated in 1913 from CSF of a patient with neurosyphilis.

Cultivable treponemes such as *T. phagedenis* (**Reiter treponeme**) and *T. refringens* are non-pathogenic. They can be grown under strict anaerobic conditions in Smith-Noguchi medium or in digest broth enriched with serum.

Sensitivity to Physical and Chemical Agents

T. pallidum is a very delicate organism, therefore, syphilis is ordinarily acquired by sexual intercourse. It is readily inactivated by heating at 41.5°C for 1 hour.

Antigenic Structure

The antigenic structure of *T. pallidum* is poorly understood. Infection with these treponemes leads to the production of three types of antibodies. On the basis of these antibodies, the treponemal antigens may be divided into specific and non-specific antigens.

Specific Antigens

- **Group-specific antigen:** It is a protein antigen present in *T. pallidum* as well as in non-pathogenic treponemes, such as Reiter treponeme. Antibody to this antigen appears in serum of syphilitic patients. The antigen used in tests to detect group-specific antibodies is derived from the Reiter treponeme.
- **Species-specific treponemal antigen:** It appears to be polysaccharide in nature. *T. pallidum* is used as antigen for detection of species-specific antibody.

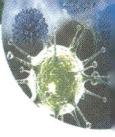

Non-specific Antigen

A non-specific antibody (reagin) appears in blood of syphilitic patients that reacts with a lipid hapten extracted from beef heart. The hapten is known as **cardiolipin**.

Pathogenesis

T. pallidum is a **strict parasite** and its life outside the animal body is short. Most cases of syphilis are **contracted during sexual intercourse**. The treponemes are present in the superficial genital lesions and pass from one partner to the other through **intact mucous membranes or through minor skin abrasions**. The disease may also be transmitted congenitally, by close contact with mucous membrane lesions as in **kissing** and through blood transfusions. Medical personnel are occasionally infected by an **accidental finger prick** with an infected needle.

In venereal syphilis, the treponemes penetrate mucosal surfaces or abraded skin and multiply at the site of entry and after an incubation period of about a month (range 10–90 days), the clinical disease sets in. The clinical manifestations fall into four stages—primary, secondary, latent and tertiary.

Primary Syphilis

The primary lesion of syphilis is the **chancre** which is painless, relatively avascular, circumscribed, indurated, 1–2 cm in diameter. It ulcerates in the centre. It is known as hard chancre to distinguish it from non-indurated lesion (soft sore) caused by *Haemophilus ducreyi*.

Most frequently chancre appears on the external genitalia—prepuce, corona of the penis (Fig. 18.1), labia and vaginal wall. It may also occur on the cervix, perianal area, anal canal or on the tongue and other oral mucous membrane. In some cases it may be on lips, cheeks and nipples (when it is acquired through kissing).

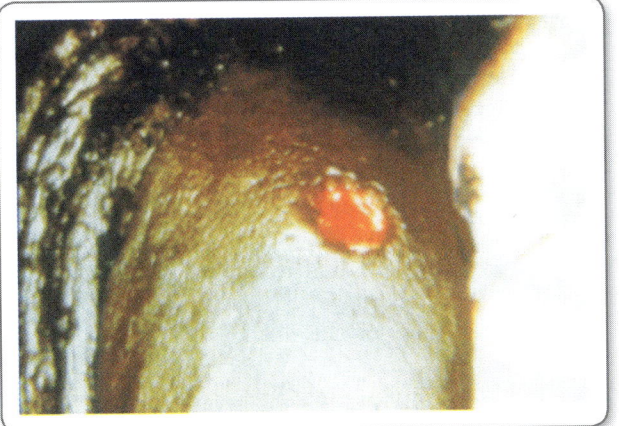

Fig. 18.1: Chancre caused by *Treponema pallidum* on the penis.

Secondary Syphilis

This sets in 2–6 months after the primary lesion heals during which period the patient is asymptomatic. The secondary lesions are due to widespread multiplication of the treponemes and their dissemination through the blood. Patient develops marked constitutional symptoms, **diffuse erythematous cutaneous lesions**, particularly on the trunk and extremities, mucous patches in the oropharynx and **condylomata** at mucocutaneous junctions. There may also be enlargement of the lymph nodes. *Lesions of secondary syphilis undergo spontaneous healing in 4–5 years.*

Latent Syphilis

After the secondary lesions disappear, the disease becomes latent and can be detected only by serological tests. In many cases, this is followed by natural cure but in others, after several years, manifestations of tertiary syphilis appear.

Tertiary Syphilis

Decades after the primary infection, patient may develop late or tertiary syphilis. It is a slowly progressive, destructive inflammatory disease that may affect any organ. It may lead to relatively benign ulcerating lesions of the skin, mucous membranes or bones, or **gummata** of the internal organs. More serious are lesions of heart and aorta that may lead to the formation of **aneurysms**, or of the central nervous system, of which **tabes dorsalis** and **general paralysis of the insane** are the most common. The lesions of tertiary syphilis contain very few organisms and the remarkable severity of the lesions is attributed to an intense cellular immune response to the organisms and their products.

Laboratory Diagnosis (Flowchart 18.1)

The clinical diagnosis of syphilis is confirmed in the laboratory by:

Demonstration of Treponemes in the Exudate

- **Dark-ground microscopy:** To avoid the risk of acquiring infection, it is important to wear gloves and exercise great care in handling the lesions. The surface of the lesion is cleansed carefully with a gauze swab soaked in warm normal saline and the margins are gently scrapped so that superficial epithelium is abraded. Gentle pressure is applied to the base of the lesion until serum exudes from its surface. If it is blood stained, it should be wiped away and process repeated until a clear fluid is obtained. The material is collected directly on a coverslip which is then placed on a glass slide and examined under dark-ground microscope.

   T. pallidum is recognized by its slender structure, regularity of its spirals and slightly pointed ends. Other spirochaetes are usually thicker and have rounded ends. It is motile with a to and fro drilling motion and occasional flexion of the body.

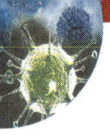

Flowchart 18.1: Laboratory diagnosis of syphilis

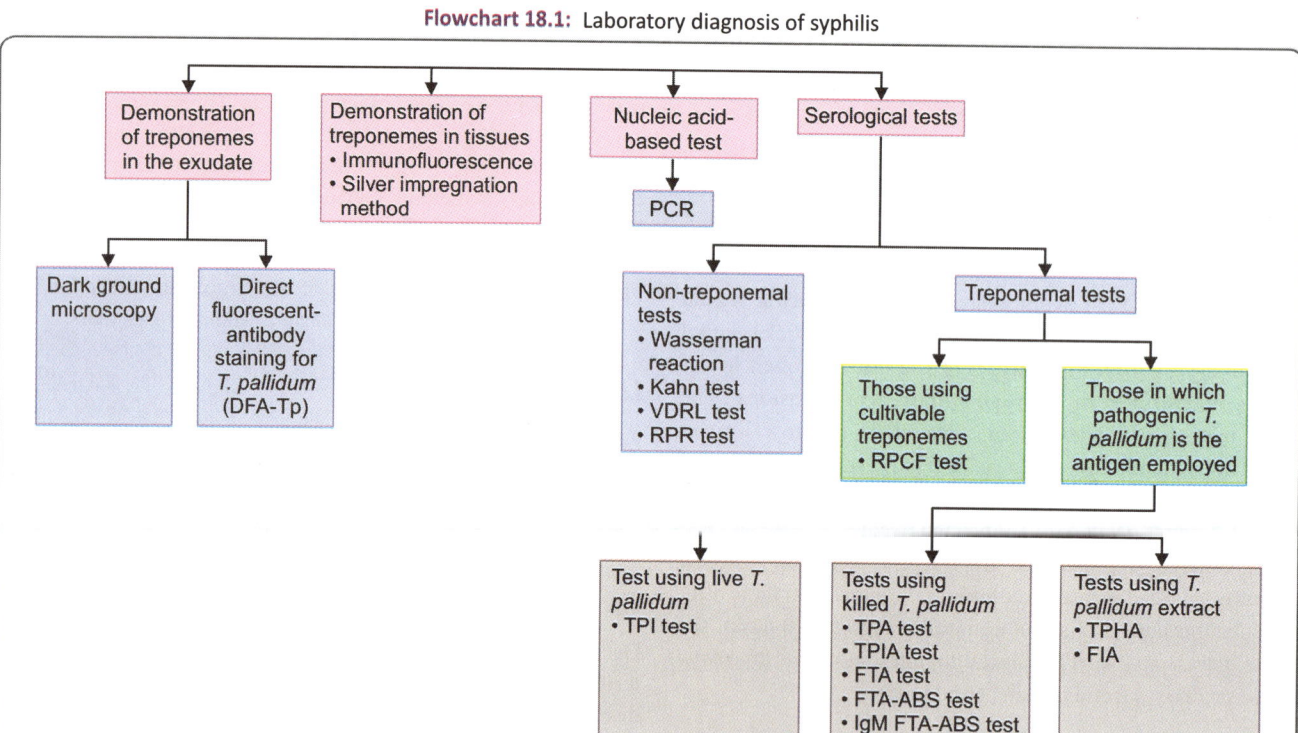

- **Direct fluorescent-antibody staining for T. pallidum (DFA-Tp):** A more definite approach to diagnosis is provided by DFA-Tp. It has the advantage that a smear of the material to be tested is made on a glass slide, fixed in acetone and sent to the laboratory. The smear is then stained with fluorescein-labelled pathogen-specific monoclonal antibody. The treponemes appear distinct, sharply outlined and have an apple-green fluorescence.

Demonstration of Treponemes in Tissues

Treponemes in the tissues can be demonstrated by immuno-fluorescence or silver staining.

Nucleic Acid-based Test

Nucleic acid amplification test (polymerase chain reaction) has been developed for detecting *T. pallidum* in genital lesion, infant blood, and cerebrospinal fluid.

Serological Diagnosis of Syphilis

Non-treponemal Tests

Non-treponemal tests that can be employed are Wassermann, Kahn, Venereal Diseases Research Laboratory (VDRL) and the rapid plasma reagin (RPR) tests. The antigen used in these tests is an alcoholic extract of beef heart tissue (cardiolipin) to which lecithin and cholesterol are added.

- **VDRL test:** VDRL is the most widely used simple and rapid test which requires only a small quantity of serum. It is performed as a slide test in which inactivated patient serum is mixed with a freshly prepared suspension of cardiolipin-lecithin-cholesterol antigen on a glass slide. The mixture is rotated, usually mechanically, for 4 minutes after which the flocculation (aggregation of antigen-antibody complexes in suspension) can be detected under a low power objective of a microscope.

- **RPR test:** In rapid plasma reagin test, VDRL antigen is adsorbed on finely divided carbon particles. This test is performed by mixing one drop of patient serum or plasma (50 μl) with a drop of this modified antigen (20 μl), on a disposable plastic card (12.5 × 7 cm in size with 10 clearly defined test areas) using a disposable stick. The card is then rocked gently to and fro for 8 minutes and observed under strong source of light. In a positive test, the flocculation of carbon particles (black aggregates) is visible with naked eye. Black aggregates may be deposited at the periphery of the liquid. In a negative test, there is a complete absence of black aggregates with a uniform greyish background. Any specimen giving a positive reaction should then be tested quantitatively using doubling dilutions of serum (1 : 2, 1 : 4, 1 : 8, 1 : 16, 1 : 32, etc.).

   Antibodies against cardiolipin may be detected in the absence of *T. pallidum* infection and give what is known as **biological false positive (BFP) reaction**. In such cases,

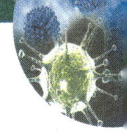

specific treponemal tests are negative and there is no history of present or past treponemal infection. These reactions are of two types:

- **Acute or transient BFP reaction** which may develop shortly after an acute febrile infectious disease and will disappear within a few weeks or months after the illness has subsided.
- **Chronic BFP reactions** persist longer than 6 months. These may occur in a wide variety of infectious and noninfectious conditions associated with tissue damage. These include autoimmune diseases particularly systemic lupus erythematosus, leprosy particularly lepromatous leprosy, malaria, relapsing fever, infectious mononucleosis, hepatitis and tropical eosinophilia.

Treponemal Tests

- **Those using cultivable treponemes**
  The antigen used to detect group-specific antibody is derived from *T. phagedenis* (Reiter treponeme). It is protein in nature, most probably derived from endoflagella and the test is known as **Reiter protein complement fixation (RPCF) test**.
- **Those in which pathogenic T. pallidum is the antigen employed:** A number of specific tests are now available for the definite diagnosis of syphilis. All these tests require live or killed or extracts of *T. pallidum* (Nichol's strain) grown in rabbit testes.
  - **Test using live T. pallidum:**
    - **Treponema pallidum immobilization (TPI) test**
      This test determines the ability of patient serum to immobilize motile virulent *T. pallidum*. The test serum is incubated anaerobically with a suspension of the treponemes and complement. If antibodies are present, the treponemes will be found to be immobilized, when examined under dark-ground microscope. The test is considered reactive if more than 50% of the treponemes are immobilized, and non-reactive if less than 20% are immobilized. The test is doubtful if 20–50% treponemes are immobilized.
  - **Tests using killed T. pallidum:**
    - **Treponema pallidum agglutination (TPA) test**
      In this test, a suspension of *T. pallidum*, inactivated by formalin, is mixed with test serum and incubated. The mixture is then examined under dark-ground microscope. In the presence of antibody, treponemes are found to be agglutinated.
    - **Treponema pallidum immune adherence (TPIA) test**
      Suspension of inactivated treponemes is mixed with test serum, complement and fresh heparinised whole blood from a normal individual, and incubated. In the presence of antibodies, the treponemes will be found to adhere to the erythrocytes. In the absence of antibody, immune adherence does not take place.
- **Fluorescent treponemal antibody (FTA) test**
  It is an indirect immunofluorescence test. Smears of *T. pallidum* are prepared on slides and fixed with acetone. These slides can be stored in the deep freezer for several months. The patient serum is added on the smear and incubated for the antibody to react with the treponemes. The excess serum is then washed off and the antibodies that bind to the fixed organisms are detected by treating the smear with fluorescein-labelled antihuman immunoglobulin. After incubation and washing off the unfixed conjugate, slide is examined under fluorescence microscope. In a positive test, treponemes fluoresce.

  Originally, patient serum was used in a dilution of 1 in 5. At this dilution, the test has high sensitivity and poor specificity. Therefore, the dilution of the serum was raised to 1 in 200. In this test, called **FTA-200**, the specificity was improved but sensitivity was decreased. Therefore, this test was further modified to **fluorescent treponemal antibody absorption (FTA-ABS) test**. Here the patient serum is first absorbed with an extract of non-pathogenic *T. phagedenis* (Reiter treponemes) to remove group-reactive antibody. FTA-ABS test has high specificity and sensitivity.

  Another modification of this test, the **IgM FTA-ABS test, can detect IgM antibodies in congenital syphilis** thus distinguishing it from seropositivity due to passively transferred maternal antibodies which are IgG in nature. In addition, in the former repeated tests will show an increase in titre, whereas in the latter titre will fall.
  - **Tests using T. pallidum extract**
    - **Treponema pallidum haemagglutination test (TPHA)**
      In this test, *T. pallidum* antigen is adsorbed onto the surface of red blood cells. When these red blood cells are mixed with patient serum, specific antibody, if present, causes haemagglutination. As in FTA-ABS test patient serum is pre-absorbed with an extract of Reiter treponemes to remove group-reactive antibody.
    - **Enzyme immunoassay (EIA)**
      Ultrasonicate of *T. pallidum* antigen is coated on tubes or ferrous metal beads as a solid-phase carrier for antigen. Antibody in the patient serum is detected by enzyme immunoassay. Sensitivity and specificity of this test has been reported to be 90% and 98% respectively.

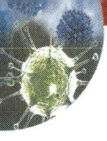
SECTION IV • PATHOGENIC ORGANISMS-I BACTERIA

Prophylaxis

At present, there is no effective vaccine against syphilis. An infected individual may serve as a source of infection for 3–5 years during early syphilis. As transmission of the infection is by direct contact, it is possible to protect against syphilis by avoidance of sexual contact with an infected individual. The contacts are examined and given treatment. Other forms of prevention include:

- The use of **mechanical barriers** such as condoms in which prevention of direct contact between infected mucous membranes is achieved.
- The use of **antibiotic (penicillin) prophylaxis**. It, however, carries the danger that it may suppress the primary lesion without eliminating the infection.

LEPTOSPIRA INTERROGANS

Morphology

L. interrogans are spiral bacteria, 5–15 μm long and 0.1 μm in diameter. They are actively motile and possess tightly coiled spirals and hooked ends. Because of their narrow diameter, leptospires are best observed by dark-ground, phase-contrast and electron microscopy. Leptospires rotate rapidly along their long axes and also glide across the field with either end foremost. They occasionally form secondary coils and then straighten again. They stain poorly with aniline dyes but can be demonstrated by fluorescent antibody technique and silver impregnation techniques of Levaditi and Fontana.

Cultural Characteristics

L. interrogans are obligate aerobes. Optimum pH and temperature for their growth are 7.2 and 28–32°C respectively. They do not grow at 13°C and for primary isolation from infected tissues, incubation at 37°C may be advantageous. *L. interrogans* can be grown in artificial media supplemented with sterile rabbit serum or bovine serum albumin with Tween 80. A semisolid medium prepared by adding 0.2–0.5% agar to liquid medium may be used for isolation of *L. interrogans* from animal tissues. Leptospires may be grown on the chorioallantoic membrane of chick embryo. They may be demonstrated in the blood of allantoic vessels 4–5 days after inoculation.

Pathogenesis

L. interrogans causes leptospirosis. It is primarily a parasite of vertebrates other than humans, such as rodents, dogs, pigs and cattle. Leptospires localize in the kidneys, colonizing the convoluted tubules and are continuously shed in the urine of some infected animals, thereby contaminating the environment.

Man acquires infection mainly through contact with water, soil or vegetation contaminated with animal urine. The pathogenic leptospires enter the body through cuts or abrasions of the skin. They may also enter through the mucous membranes of the nose, mouth or eyes. The organisms enter the blood and invade various tissues and organs, particularly the kidney, liver, meninges and conjunctiva.

After an incubation period of 1–2 weeks, the patient develops muscular pain, headache, vomiting, photophobia, fever and chills. Jaundice occurs in about 10–20% of cases by second or third day. Purpuric haemorrhages sometimes occur on the skin and mucosa. Albuminuria is a constant feature. Leptospires can be seen in the blood during acute phase of the disease, but can seldom be demonstrated after 8–10 days. However, they persist in internal organs, particularly in the kidneys so that they may be demonstrated in the urine in the later stages of the disease. *L. interrogans* serovar *icterohaemorrhagiae* produces a more severe illness. It is known as **Weil's disease** (infectious jaundice).

Laboratory Diagnosis

The diagnosis of leptospirosis may be established by: (I) demonstration of leptospires, and (II) serological diagnosis.

Demonstration of Leptospires

Leptospires may be demonstrated in (1) the blood and (2) the urine.

- **Demonstration of leptospires in the blood**
  - Leptospires can be demonstrated in the blood, by dark-ground microscopy, especially after differential centrifugation of blood. As leptospires disappear from blood after 8 days, therefore, blood examination is useful only in the early stages of the disease.
  - Inoculate a number of bijou bottles containing 3 ml of modified Korthof's medium with varying amounts of blood ranging from 1–4 drops. Incubate at 28–32°C and examine by dark-ground microscopy every 3 days up to 6 weeks before discarding it as negative. The blood from the patient is also inoculated intraperitoneally into young guinea pigs, followed some days later by culture of the animal blood obtained by cardiac puncture.
- **Demonstration of leptospires in the urine**
  Leptospires may be present in the urine in the second week of the disease and intermittently thereafter for 4–6 weeks. Centrifuged deposit of fresh urine may be examined by dark-ground microscopy and by culture on Fletcher's semi-solid medium containing neomycin sulphate.

Serological Diagnosis

Antibodies appear in the serum towards the end of the first week of the disease, they continue to rise for several weeks and then begin to decline. Serological tests fall into two categories:

- **Genus-specific tests:** These tests detect leptospiral infection without indicating the exact infecting serovar. These tests

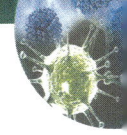

include complement fixation test, sensitized erythrocyte lysis and haemagglutination test, and enzyme-linked immunosorbent assay (ELISA) which is capable of detecting IgM and IgG leptospiral antibodies.

- **Serogroup and serovar-specific tests:** These tests identify the infecting serovar by demonstrating specific antibodies. Macroscopic and microscopic agglutination tests have been widely used. In the macroscopic agglutination test, commercially available, formalin-killed suspensions of a number of reference strains (concentrated by centrifugation so that results can be read with naked eye) are tested for macroscopic agglutination with serial dilutions of the test serum. The microscopic agglutination test uses formalinized or live suspensions of well grown cultures and the results are read by low-power dark-ground microscopy.

BORRELIA

Borreliae are large, motile, refractile spirochaetes with 3–10 irregular, wide and open coils. Two important human diseases associated with borreliae are relapsing fever, caused by *Borrelia recurrentis* and several other *Borrelia* species, and Lyme disease caused by *B. burgdorferi*.

Relapsing Fever

It is characterized by the occurrence of one or more relapses after the subsidence of primary febrile paroxysm. It occurs worldwide as epidemic or louse-borne relapsing fever, and endemic or tick-borne relapsing fever. The former is caused by *B. recurrentis* and the latter by several *Borrelia* species, including, *B. duttoni*, *B. hermsii*, *B. parkeri* and *B. turicatae*.

Morphology

Various *Borrelia* species causing **relapsing fever** are morphologically indistinguishable, but exhibit some antigenic differences. They are 3–20 μm long and 0.2–0.5 μm wide. They possess 15–20 endoflagella per cell end and 3–10 loose, uneven spiral coils. Spirals are coarser and more irregular than those of the treponemes or leptospires and can usually be seen with light microscopy in preparations stained with aniline dyes such as Wright or Giemsa stains. The spirochaetes may be demonstrated in the peripheral blood by direct stain. In fresh blood the organisms are actively motile, they move in forward and backward waves and in a corkscrew-like motion.

Cultural Characteristics

Borrelia are microaerophilic. Optimum temperature for growth is 28–30°C. These may be grown in fluid media containing blood, serum or tissue, on chorioallantoic membrane of chick embryo and in peritoneal cavity of mouse or rat.

Pathogenesis

Relapsing fever is transmitted by infected vectors—body louse (*Pediculus corporis*) in case of *B. recurrentis*, and tick (*Ornithodoros*) in case of *B. duttoni* and others. After an infected blood meal, spirochaetes may be demonstrated in the stomach of the louse for 24 hours. Thereafter, they grow in the haemolymph of the louse but do not invade tissues. They are not found in the salivary glands, the gut or the genital organs. As a result, the excrement of the louse is non-infectious and the bacterium is not transferred transovarially to the progeny. However, once the louse is infected, it remains so for the rest of its life (usually about 3 weeks).

The disease is transmitted to man not by the bite of the louse, but by contamination of the wounds made by the bite itself or by scratching, with body fluids of the louse which is crushed by scratching releasing spirochaetes. The latter then enter into the tissues through damaged or intact skin or mucous membranes.

Spirochaetes causing tick-borne relapsing fever invade all the tissues of the tick, including the salivary glands, genitalia and excretory system. Infection is transmitted to man through the bite of the ticks or through their excrements. **Transovarial transmission** to the tick progeny maintains the spirochaete in the tick population.

In both forms of relapsing fever, after an incubation period of 2–14 days, the disease sets in abruptly with high fever (up to 40°C), rigors, headache, myalgia, arthralgia, photophobia and sometimes nausea and vomiting. The spleen and liver are enlarged and tender. Some patients develop jaundice, bronchitis and skin rash. During acute phase, there may be up to 10^5 spirochaetes per ml of blood. The primary illness subsides in 3–9 days. After an afebrile period of 11–15 days, during which borreliae are not demonstrable in blood, a relapse follows which is less severe and shorter than the primary attack. The borreliae reappear in blood during the relapse of fever. The disease ultimately subsides after 3–4 relapses. In general, tick-borne relapsing fever has shorter febrile and afebrile periods than louse-borne infection.

Laboratory Diagnosis

Wet Preparation

Blood is collected during pyrexial period and a drop of it is examined as a wet film under the dark-ground or phase-contrast microscope. Borreliae can be detected by their active movements.

Staining

Thick or thin blood smears may be stained with Giemsa and Leishman stain and examined for *Borrelia*.

Animal Inoculation

If direct microscopy is negative, 1–2 ml of fresh whole blood or of clot ground up in saline, is injected intraperitoneally into

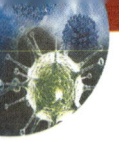

a newborn mouse or rat. The borreliae multiply in the animal and appear in large numbers in peripheral blood within two days and remain for 5–6 days if the animal does not die. Smears are prepared from the tail vein and examined.

Prevention and Treatment

Since the organisms are transmitted only by vectors, therefore, tick and louse control, and maintenance of good personal hygiene are effective measures for the control of relapsing fever. Tetracycline, chloramphenicol, penicillin and erythromycin have been used successfully for the treatment of relapsing fever.

BORRELIA BURGDORFERI

It was first identified in 1975 in Lyme, Connecticut, USA.

Morphology

It measures 4–30 μm in length and 0.2 μm in diameter. It is flexible, helical and Gram-negative.

Culture

It is a microaerophilic spirochaete. It can be grown on BSK medium which contains N-acetyl glucosamine, yeast extract, amino acids, vitamins, nucleotides and serum. Optimum temperature for growth is 34–37°C.

Pathogenesis

B. burgdorferi causes **Lyme disease**. It is widespread in the USA, where it is most common vector-borne infection. It has been reported from other parts of the world also. Wild and domestic animals, including mice and other rodents, deer, sheep, cattle, horses and dogs are the natural hosts of *B. burgdorferi*. It is transmitted to man by ixodid ticks that become infected whilst feeding on infected animals. The organisms grow in the midgut of the tick and transmission to man occurs by regurgitation of the gut contents during the blood meal.

Patient develops a small red macule or papule at the site of bite. Three to 22 days later, redness spreads centrifugally surrounded by an induration about 2 cm wide. It is known as **erythema chronicum migrans (ECM)**. The centre of the lesion may become vesicular or necrotic. Commonly affected sites are the thigh, groin and axilla. The organism also spreads to a variety of other organs. In about one-half of the patients, multiple skin lesions develop several days after the appearance of the initial lesion. ECM is frequently accompanied with headache, fever, stiff neck, malaise and lymphadenopathy. Weeks to months later, some patients develop meningoencephalitis, myocarditis or migratory musculoskeletal pain and intermittent arthritis.

Laboratory Diagnosis

The diagnosis of Lyme disease is made mainly on clinical grounds. The presence of an ECM lesion at the site of vector bite, which was followed by an expanding bright red rash would be suggestive of a positive diagnosis. However, a definitive diagnosis can be made by the isolation and identification of *B. burgdorferi* from skin lesions or blood of the infected patient. However, the culture is too slow and gives too low a yield of positive results for routine use. Microscopic detection of borreliae by dark-ground microscopy, phase-contrast microscopy, silver staining and immunofluorescence methods also lacks sensitivity. DNA probes have been developed for a gene encoding a specific outer membrane protein, however, their efficiency in detecting this in tissue samples is yet to be established.

For the **serological diagnosis**, ELISA, indirect immuno-fluorescence and haemagglutination tests are commonly used. However, these tests lack specificity and may give positive results in cases of relapsing fever, syphilis, yaws, pinta, leptospiral infections and collagen disorders. Lyme disease patients may give a positive FTA-ABS test, though the VDRL test is negative.

Treatment

Doxycycline, amoxicillin and cefuroxime are useful for the treatment of Lyme disease. Jarisch-Herxheimer reactions occur in 15% of patients following antibiotics therapy.

Key Points

- **Spirochaetes are long, slender**, coiled and highly **motile** bacteria that do not take up the Gram stain.
- **Spirochaetes** comprise three genera – *Treponema*, *Borrelia* and *Leptospira*.
- *Treponema pallidum*, the agent of **syphilis**, cannot be cultivated *in vitro* and is uniformly sensitive to **penicillin**.
- Syphilis can be diagnosed by demonstration of treponemes, treponemal antigens and by serological tests.
- Two important human diseases associated with borreliae are **relapsing fever** caused by *Borrelia recurrentis* and several other *Borrelia* spp., and **Lyme disease** caused by *B. burgdorferi*.
- *Leptospira interrogans* serovar *icterohaemorrhagiae* causes **Weil's disease**.

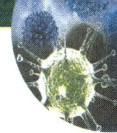

? ASSESS YOURSELF

LONG AND SHORT ANSWER QUESTIONS

1. Discuss laboratory diagnosis of syphilis.
2. Discuss pathogenesis of syphilis.
3. Write short notes on:
   - (a) VDRL test
   - (b) Non-treponemal tests for serodiagnosis of syphilis
   - (c) Treponemal tests for serodiagnosis of syphilis
   - (d) Lyme disease

MULTIPLE CHOICE QUESTIONS

1. Which of the following genus/genera belongs to family Spirochaetaceae?
   - (a) *Spirochaeta*
   - (b) *Treponema*
   - (c) *Borrelia*
   - (d) All of the above

2. Three or occasionally four endoflagella are present at each pole in:
   - (a) *Treponema*
   - (b) *Borrelia*
   - (c) *Leptospira*
   - (d) *Vibrio cholerae*

3. Spirochaetes exhibit:
   - (a) Flexion and extension motility
   - (b) Corkscrew-like rotatory movement
   - (c) Translatory motion
   - (d) All of the above

4. Group-specific antigen of *Treponema* is chemically a:
   - (a) Protein
   - (b) Polysaccharide
   - (c) Lipid
   - (d) Nucleic acid

5. Appearance of a hard chancre is characteristic of:
   - (a) Primary syphilis
   - (b) Secondary syphilis
   - (c) Latent syphilis
   - (d) Tertiary syphilis

6. Lyme disease is caused by:
   - (a) *Borrelia recurrentis*
   - (b) *B. duttoni*
   - (c) *B. burgdorferi*
   - (d) *B. hermsii*

ANSWERS TO MCQS

1. d   **2.** a   **3.** d   **4.** a   **5.** a   **6.** c

Enterobacteriaceae: *Escherichia, Klebsiella* and Other Genera

Organisms of the family Enterobacteriaceae are Gram-negative, capsulated or non-capsulated, non-acid-fast, non-sporing bacilli that are either motile by means of peritrichous flagella or non-motile. They are oxidase-negative, catalase-positive. They are aerobes and facultative anaerobes, grow readily on ordinary media including MacConkey agar and ferment glucose in peptone water with the production of either acid or acid and gas.

ESCHERICHIA COLI

Morphology

It is a Gram-negative, non-capsulated bacillus measuring 1–3 × 0.4–0.7 μm in size. Most (about 80%) strains are motile by peritrichous flagella. The fimbriae are present on 80% of the strains. A few strains, especially those from extra-intestinal infections, possess polysaccharide capsule.

Cultural Characteristics

It is an aerobe and a facultative anaerobe. Optimum temperature for its growth is 37°C (range 10–45°C). It can grow on ordinary media like **nutrient agar** forming large (2–3 mm in diameter), circular, low convex, colourless, opaque or partially translucent colonies after 18 hours incubation at 37°C. Since most strains ferment lactose rapidly the colonies on **MacConkey agar** medium are red or pink in colour. On **blood agar**, colonies of some strains of *E. coli* (especially those isolated from pathologic conditions) are surrounded by a complete zone of haemolysis.

Biochemical Reactions

E. coli is indole and methyl red reaction positive and it is negative for Voges-Proskauer reaction and citrate utilization. It ferments glucose, mannitol, maltose, lactose, and many other sugars with the production of acid and gas. Typical strains do not ferment sucrose. Some strains of *E. coli* are late lactose or non-lactose-fermenters. Indole production and fermentation of sugars takes place both at 37°C and 44°C.

Antigenic Structure

E. coli possesses 4 types of antigens.

- H (flagellar) antigens,
- O (somatic) antigens,
- K (capsular) antigens, and
- F (fimbrial) antigens.

H Antigens

So far **75 H antigens** have been recognized. These are thermolabile. All of them are usually monophasic, but rare diphasic strains have been reported.

O Antigens

These are heat-stable, lipopolysaccharide antigens of cell wall. One hundred and seventy three different O antigens have been described which are designated 1, 2, 3, 4, etc.

K Antigens

The term K antigen (K for kappa, in German *kappa* means capsule) refers to the acidic polysaccharide capsular antigens. One hundred and three K antigens of *E. coli* are known.

F Antigens

These are thermolabile proteins and heating the organisms at 100°C detaches their fimbriae. *E. coli* possesses common fimbriae which are chromosomally determined and sex pili, which are determined by conjugative plasmids and appear to be organelles of conjugation.

A number of filamentous protein structures resembling fimbriae have been described in *E. coli*. These cause mannose-resistant haemagglutination. They probably play a significant role in the pathogenesis of diarrhoeal disease and in urinary tract infection. These include K88, K99 and colonization factor antigens (CFAs).

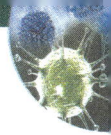

Toxins

Some strains of *E. coli* produce enterotoxins, haemolysin and Verocytotoxin.

Enterotoxins

Enterotoxigenic strains of *E. coli* (ETEC) produce one or both of two different toxins, a heat-labile toxin (LT) and a heat-stable toxin (ST).

Heat-labile Toxin

It is a heat-labile protein which is destroyed by heating at 65°C for 30 minutes. It is composed of one enzymatically active polypeptide A (active) subunit and five identical B (binding) subunits. The B subunits of LT bind to the Gm$_1$ ganglioside at the brush border of epithelial cells of the small intestine. This binding facilitates the entry of subunit A into the cell, which then activates **adenylate cyclase**. This results in conversion of adenosine triphosphate (ATP) to cyclic adenosine monophosphate (cAMP). The accumulation of cAMP in the intestinal mucosa initiates the hypersecretion of electrolytes and fluids into the lumen, resulting in a watery diarrhoea.

Various strains of *E. coli* produce two types of LT toxin: LT-I and LT-II. LT-I is structurally and antigenically related to enterotoxin produced by *Vibrio cholerae* (CT). Anti-CT can neutralize LT-I. LT-II is biologically similar to LT-I, but it is not neutralized by either anti-LT-I or anti-CT. LT can be assayed by ligated rabbit ileal loop (read at 18 hours), adult rabbit skin (vascular permeability factor), steroid production in Y1 mouse adrenal cell culture, morphological changes in Chinese hamster ovary cells, agar gel diffusion, reversed passive latex agglutination, enzyme-linked immunosorbent assay, solid phase radioimmunoassay and DNA probes (Table 19.1).

Heat-stable Toxin

In contrast to LT, ST is a low molecular weight polypeptide and poorly immunogenic. Two major classes of *E. coli* ST are known. They are known as ST-I and ST-II. ST-I is not destroyed by heating at 100°C for 30 minutes. It activates **guanylate cyclase** causing the increased production of cyclic guanosine monophosphate (cGMP) and subsequent hypersecretion. ST-I has no effect on the concentration of cAMP. It can be assayed by injecting the toxin intragastrically into a 1–4 days old suckling mouse and measuring intestinal fluid accumulation (ratio of intestinal/remaining body weight) after 4 hours. It can also be assayed by ligated rabbit ileal loop (read at 6 hours).

ST-II is produced by some strains of *E. coli*. It stimulates fluid accumulation in ligated intestinal loops of piglets ranging in age from a few days to 9 weeks but not in infant mouse test. Unlike ST-I, ST-II is insoluble in methanol. The mechanism of action of ST-II is not known but it appears not to act via cAMP or cGMP.

TABLE 19.1: Differences between heat-labile (LT) and heat-stable (ST) enterotoxins of *Escherichia coli*

Test	LT	ST
In vivo tests		
• Ligated rabbit ileal loop		
Read at 6 hours	±	+
Read at 18 hours	+	−
• Adult rabbit skin (vascular permeability factor)	+	−
• Intragastric into 1–4 day old suckling mouse after 4 hours	−	+
In vitro tests		
• Steroid production in Y1 mouse adrenal cell culture	+	−
• Elongation of Chinese hamster ovary cells	+	−
• Agar gel diffusion	+	−
• Reversed passive latex agglutination	+	−
• Enzyme-linked immunosorbent assay	+	+*
• Solid phase radioimmunoassay	+	−
• DNA probes	+	+

* With monoclonal antibodies

The enterotoxin alone is not sufficient to cause diarrhoea. It must also be able to adhere to the mucosal surface of the epithelial cells of the small intestine. In humans, it is mediated by colonization factors.

Verocytotoxin

E. coli O157: H7 produces two cytotoxins—verocytotoxin 1 (VT1) and verocytotoxin 2 (VT2). VT1 is a phage encoded cytotoxin identical to the Shiga toxin (Stx) produced by *S. dysenteriae* type 1. This verocytotoxin is cytotoxic to Vero cells (African green monkey kidney cells), hence the term verocytotoxin. It also reacts with and is neutralized by the antibody against Shiga toxin. In contrast with VT1, VT2 is not neutralized by the antibody to Shiga toxin and is immunologically different from but biologically similar to VT1. These verocytotoxins have also been called Shiga-like toxins but are more recently referred to as Shiga toxin 1 (Stx 1) and Shiga toxin 2 (Stx 2). *E. coli* strains that produce these toxins are known as Shiga toxigenic *E. coli* (STEC) or verotoxigenic *E. coli* (VTEC).

Haemolysin

Many strains of *E. coli* produce a haemolysin which can bring about lysis of RBCs of some species. A larger proportion of strains of *E. coli* recovered from extra-intestinal lesions of man are haemolytic than are those isolated from human faeces.

Pathogenesis

E. coli forms a part of normal intestinal flora of man and animals. It can cause four main types of clinical syndrome:

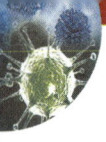

- Urinary tract infection,
- Diarrhoea and dysentery,
- Pyogenic infections, and
- Septicaemia.

Urinary Tract Infection

E. coli is the commonest organism causing urinary tract infection (UTI).

It occurs more often in females than in males. This is due to short urethra, pregnancy, infrequent voiding and sexual intercourse which may lead to **'honey-moon' cystitis**. Shorter and wider female urethra appears to be less effective in preventing access of the bacteria to the bladder. The high incidence of UTI in pregnant women can be attributed to impairment of urine flow due to pressure on the urinary tract and due to hormonal changes.

Relative infrequency of UTI in men may be due to longer male urethra and the bactericidal activity of the prostatic fluid. Other causes of urinary stagnation that may predispose to UTI include enlarged prostate, urinary calculi, congenital malformations and neurological disorders. Catheterization and cystoscopy may introduce endogenous or exogenous bacteria into the bladder leading to infection.

Diarrhoea and Dysentery

E. coli causing diarrhoeal diseases are divisible into six groups. They produce diarrhoea with different pathogenic mechanisms.

Enteropathogenic E. coli (EPEC)

They cause infantile enteritis, especially in tropical countries. The pathogenic mechanism is not clear, however, the inflammatory reactions and epithelial degenerative changes that are observed in tissue sections may be secondary to adhesive properties of the bacteria. Common serogroups of EPEC are O26, O55, O86, O111, O114, O119, O125, O126, O127, O128 and O142.

Enterotoxigenic E. coli (ETEC)

These strains produce LT or ST or both. They are associated with diarrhoea in infants and adults in tropical and subtropical climates, especially in developing countries, where it is one of the major causes of infantile bacterial diarrhoea. In the United States and other developed countries, ETEC diarrhoea is the most common cause of diarrhoeal disease referred to as **traveller's diarrhoea**. The diarrhoeal illness is acquired by travellers from developed countries when they visit developing countries.

ETEC infection is commonly acquired by consuming contaminated food or water. In addition, they possess colonization factors that are specific for the host animal species. These enable the organisms to adhere to the epithelium of the small intestine. Surface attachment of the bacterial cells to the intestinal epithelial cells is a prerequisite to toxin production. Common serogroups of ETEC are: O6, O8, O15, O25, O27, O63, O78, O115, O148, O153, O159 and O167.

Enteroinvasive E. coli (EIEC)

These strains are capable of penetrating the intestinal epithelial cells and producing an illness identical to that caused by *Shigella* in patients of all ages. This strain can be suspected when observing blood, mucus and neutrophils in faecal smears. Common serogroups of EIEC are: O28, O112, O124, O136, O143, O144, O152 and O164.

Verotoxigenic E. coli (VTEC)

In 1982, one particular serovar of *E. coli* (O157: H7) was identified as the causative agent involved in two outbreaks of a distinctive **bloody diarrhoeal syndrome**. Soon after it was recognized that some strains of other *E. coli* serovars may exhibit a similar virulence potential. The ability to cause haemorrhagic colitis has led some workers to refer to these strains as **enterohaemorrhagic E. coli or EHEC**.

These strains cause **haemorrhagic colitis (HC)** and **haemolytic uraemic syndrome (HUS)**. In HC, patient develops blood-stained diarrhoea, usually without fever. It may often be preceded by abdominal pain and watery diarrhoea. HUS is characterized by acute renal failure, microangiopathic haemolytic anaemia and thrombocytopenia. It occurs in all age groups but is most common in infants and young children. It is a major cause of renal failure in childhood.

Enteroaggregative E. coli

Enteroaggregative *E. coli* (EAEC) cause acute and chronic diarrhoea in developing countries by adhering to the mucosal surface of the intestine. These strains are found to adhere to HEp-2 cells, packed in an aggregative pattern on the cells and in between the cells. These organisms produce symptoms such as watery diarrhoea, vomiting, dehydration and occasionally abdominal pain. These symptoms persist for more than 2 weeks.

Diffusely Adherent E. coli (DAEC)

These strains adhere to epithelial cells in a diffuse pattern and carry a gene encoding surface fimbria designated F1845. Majority of the patients infected with DAEC develop watery diarrhoea without blood or faecal leucocytes.

Pyogenic Infections

E. coli may cause wound infection, peritonitis, biliary tract infection, and meningitis. *E. coli* is a common cause of meningitis in the newborn, but is much less so in older patients.

Septicaemia

E. coli is a very common cause of septicaemia in many hospitals. It leads to fever, hypotension and disseminated intravascular coagulation (endotoxic shock) with high mortality. This condition usually develops in debilitated patients.

Laboratory Diagnosis

Urinary Tract Infection

Collection of Specimen

Normal urine is sterile, but during voiding may become contaminated with genital commensals. Therefore, **clean-voided midstream sample** of urine is employed for culture. The normal flora of anterior urethra must be adequately flushed out by passing some urine before the specimen is obtained.

- **In case of male**, retract the prepuce, clean it with sterile normal saline and collect midstream specimen.
- **In case of female**, anogenital toilet is more important. Remove underclothing completely, sit comfortably on the seat and swing one leg to the side as far off as possible. Wash perineum and periurethral area with soap and water. Then clean with nonirritant antiseptic such as chlorhexidine. Separate apart labia with fingers of one hand and collect midstream urine.
- **In newborn infants and young children**, urine may be aspirated from the bladder into a syringe with a needle introduced aseptically through the abdominal wall just above the pubis.
- **In catheterized patient** collect urine with sterile needle and syringe through the catheter port, after cleaning with alcohol.

Urine is an excellent culture medium, therefore, contaminating bacteria, from the anterior urethra, can readily multiply to reach significant numbers. Therefore, the urine must be processed immediately. If a delay of more than 1–2 hours is unavoidable, the specimen should be stored in a refrigerator at 4°C.

Microscopy

Microscopic examination of urine is done to detect the presence of increased number of polymorphs (pyuria) which is an indication of UTI. The deposit of the centrifuged urine can be examined under microscope to find out the presence of pus cells, red blood cells and bacteria in it. Presence of more than 3 pus cells per high power field is suggestive of infection. Red blood cells indicate damage to urinary tract hence increased susceptibility to infection.

Culture

Measured quantity of urine (0.001 ml or 1/1000 ml) with the help of standardized loop (internal diameter 3.26 mm) of nichrome or platinum wire of SWG 28 is inoculated on blood agar and MacConkey media and incubated overnight at 37°C. The number of colonies is counted and multiplied by 1000 to get the bacterial count per ml. For example, growth of 100 colonies indicates the presence of 10^5 bacteria/ml of urine (100×1000). On the basis of this result, it can be reported whether the patient has significant bacteriuria or not. The identification of the isolate is carried out by culture characteristics and biochemical reactions.

Diarrhoea and Dysentery

Faeces or rectal swab is inoculated on MacConkey agar. For detection of EPEC, *E. coli* colonies are emulsified in saline on a slide and tested by agglutination with polyvalent and monovalent O antisera against enteropathogenic serogroups. As more than one serogroup may be present in faecal cultures, it is essential to test at least 10 isolated colonies by agglutination.

EIEC can be detected by **Sereny test** in which the organism is instilled into the conjunctival sac of guinea pig. The animal is examined after 72 hours for the production of **keratoconjunctivitis**. Simpler tests using HeLa cells or HEp-2 cells have also been described. Monolayers of these cells are exposed to suspension of test organisms. Extracellular organisms are removed after an appropriate infection period by washing with a solution containing gentamicin and lysozyme. After a further period of intracellular growth, cells are examined microscopically for the presence of intracellular organisms. Methods of detection of ETEC and VTEC have been discussed above.

Pyogenic Infections

For the diagnosis of pyogenic infections caused by *E. coli* pus, wound swab, CSF, etc. are inoculated on MacConkey agar and blood agar followed by incubation at 37°C for 24 hours. The isolate is identified by its morphological and biochemical characters.

Septicaemia

Diagnosis of septicaemia caused by *E. coli* depends on the isolation of the organism by blood culture. Five to 10 ml of blood is inoculated into 50–100 ml glucose broth. It is incubated at 37°C for up to 7 days. After overnight incubation, subculture is made on MacConkey agar and blood agar, and processed as above. If no growth is obtained from first subculture, then subcultures should be repeated daily up to 7 days.

EDWARDSIELLA

Genus *Edwardsiella* is separated from *Escherichia* by its ability to produce hydrogen sulphide in triple sugar iron agar. *E. tarda* is the only recognized human pathogen and the term tarda refers to slow or weak fermentation of sugars by the organism. It is a motile, non-capsulated, Gram-negative bacillus and ferments only glucose and maltose with the production of acid and some gas. It is indole and MR positive, and VP and citrate negative. It produces H_2S and is negative for urease test, gelatin liquefaction, growth in the presence of KCN and malonate utilization (Table 19.2).

E. tarda mainly inhabits the intestinal tract of cold-blooded animals and their environment, particularly fresh water. It is pathogenic for eels, catfish and other animals. It is an occasional pathogen of man causing wound infection. It has rarely been

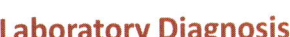

SECTION IV • PATHOGENIC ORGANISMS-I BACTERIA

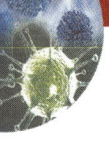

found in the faeces of healthy people. A higher isolation rate of *E. tarda* has been found in patients with diarrhoea, however, its role in the causation of diarrhoea has yet to be established.

CITROBACTER

Members of the genus *Citrobacter* are motile, indole positive or negative, MR positive, VP negative, citrate positive, urease weak positive and may or may not ferment lactose but they nearly always produce β-galactosidase (ONPG positive). Lactose fermentation may be rapid or late. They do not decarboxylate lysine but most strains decarboxylate ornithine.

Genus *Citrobacter* has three species—*C. freundii*, *C. koseri* (*C. diversus*) and *C. amalonaticus* (Table 19.2). They can grow well on ordinary media like nutrient agar producing smooth convex colonies 2–4 mm in diameter. They are not pigmented. Rough or mucoid forms sometimes occur. On MacConkey and DCA media, they form pale colonies and share somatic antigens with salmonellae. Therefore, when encountered in cultures of faeces they may be mistaken for salmonellae. However, they can be distinguished by their negative lysine decarboxylase and positive KCN reactions. Some strains possess a K antigen closely related to Vi antigen of *S.* serotype Typhi and *S.* serotype Paratyphi C.

Citrobacter is a normal inhabitant of human intestine and may cause urinary tract, gall bladder and middle ear infections. *C. koseri* may occasionally cause neonatal meningitis.

KLEBSIELLA

Members of the genus *Klebsiella* are Gram-negative, non-sporing, non-motile capsulated bacilli, 1–2 µm long and 0.5–0.8 µm wide with parallel or bulging sides and slightly pointed or rounded

TABLE 19.2: Differentiation of three species of the genus *Citrobacter*

Biochemical test	C. freundii	C. koseri	C. amalo-naticus
Indole production	−	+	+
H$_2$S production	+	−	−
Growth in KCN medium	+	−	+
Ornithine decarboxylase	v	+	+
Acid from:			
• Malonate	−	+	−
• Adonitol	−	+	−
• Salicin	−	+	+

v, variable.

ends. They occur either in end-to-end pairs (diplobacilli, like pneumococci) or are arranged singly.

Freshly isolated strains possess a well defined polysaccharide capsule. It is produced in greater amounts in media rich in carbohydrates. It can be demonstrated by India ink preparation, Quellung reaction and even by Gram staining. In the Gram-stained smear, capsule appears as an empty halo around the bacterium. Some extracellular polysaccharide is also secreted from the bacteria as loose soluble slime, accumulation of which gives mucoid appearance to the colonies.

Genus *Klebsiella* has 2 species *K. pneumoniae* and *K. oxytoca*. *K. pneumoniae* is further subdivided into *K. pneumoniae* subspecies *pneumoniae*, *K. pneumoniae* subspecies *ozaenae* and *K. pneumoniae* subspecies *rhinoscleromatis*.

Cultural Characteristics

Klebsiellae grow well on ordinary media in a temperature range of 12–43°C with optimum growth at 37°C. On MacConkey agar, the colonies typically appear large, mucoid and red. However, some strains are not mucoid.

Biochemical Reactions

Biochemical reactions of different subspecies of *K. pneumoniae* and *K. oxytoca* are given in Table 19.3.

Antigenic Structure

Somatic (O) Antigen

Klebsiellae possess five O antigens (O1–O5).

Capsular (K) Antigen

On the basis of capsular (K) antigens, the klebsiellae have been differentiated into 80 (1–80) serotypes, which is usually done by the microscopic demonstration of capsule swelling in wet films with capsular antiserum. Capsular type 2 is immunologically similar to type 2 pneumococcus. Human respiratory tract infection is mostly caused by capsular types 1–6.

Methods of Typing

Klebsiellae can be typed by serotyping. Other typing methods such as phage typing, biotyping, bacteriocin (klebocin or pneumocin) typing and resistotyping have also been tried. Bacteriocin (klebocin) production in *Klebsiella* has been found to be determined by conjugative (transmissible) plasmids (Arora and Chugh, 1982).

Pathogenicity

Klebsiellae are widely distributed in nature and in the gastrointestinal tracts of humans and animals. They are found in

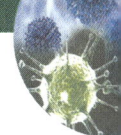

TABLE 19.3: Differentiation of species and subspecies of Klebsiella

Property	pneumoniae	ozaenae	rhinoscleromatis	K. oxytoca
Indole	–	–	–	+
MR	+	+	+	v
VP	–	–	–	v
Citrate	+	v	–	+
Urease	+	–	–	+
Gelatin liquefaction	–	–	–	v
Lactose (acid)	+	+	–	+
ONPG	+	+	–	+
Lysine decarboxylase	+	v	–	+
Ornithine decarboxylase	–	–	–	–
Growth in KCN medium	+	+	+	+

v, variable.

the oropharynx of 1–6% of normal healthy individuals, however, a prevalence as high as 20% may be seen in hospitalized patients. This colonization may prove to be the source of lung infections such as severe bronchopneumonia, sometimes with chronic destructive lesions, pleuritis and multiple abscess formation in the lungs (**Friedlander's pneumonia**). Many of these patients may develop septicaemia with high mortality.

Klebsiellae, in general, are more frequently involved in healthcare-associated (nosocomial) urinary tract infections, wound and burn infections and as secondary invaders in other respiratory infections. In fact, they are the most frequently encountered Gram-negative pathogens causing nosocomial infections of the lower respiratory tract and are second only to *E. coli* as a cause of primary bacteraemia by Gram-negative organisms. They may also cause meningitis and diarrhoea. The latter may be due to the production of heat-labile and heat-stable enterotoxins by these organisms (Arora et al., 1983).

K. pneumoniae subsp. *ozaenae* has been associated with atrophic rhinitis, a condition known as **ozaena**, and purulent infection of nasal mucous membrane. *K. pneumoniae* subsp. *rhinoscleromatis* causes a granulomatous disease called **rhino-scleroma**. It is a chronic upper respiratory tract disease. The lesions occur in the nose, larynx, throat and to a lesser extent, in the trachea and consist of granulomatous infiltrations of the submucosa.

Laboratory Diagnosis

Laboratory diagnosis is made by culturing appropriate specimens on MacConkey agar and blood agar media. The isolate is identified by colony morphology, Gram staining, motility and biochemical reactions. For the purpose of treatment antimicrobial susceptibility testing is done.

Treatment

Virtually all clinical isolates of *Klebsiella* contain R plasmids and are usually resistant to ampicillin, amoxycillin and other penicillins, but combination of these drugs with β-lactamase inhibitors such as clavulanic acid are generally effective. Klebsiellae are normally susceptible to cephalosporins, especially β-lactamase stable derivatives such as cefuroxime and cefotaxime, and to fluoroquinolones. They are often sensitive to gentamicin and other aminoglycosides, but transferable enzymatic resistance to aminoglycosides and other antimicrobial agents has become common in strains found in some hospitals. Resistance to chloramphenicol and tetracycline varies from strain to strain. *Klebsiella* infection of the urinary tract often responds to trimethoprim, nitrofurantoin, co-amoxiclav or oral cephalosporins.

ENTEROBACTER

Enterobacter belongs to the tribe Klebsielleae but can be differentiated from *Klebsiella* because it is motile and ornithine positive. *Enterobacter* is less often and less heavily capsulated than *Klebsiella*. Therefore, the colonies of *Enterobacter* are less mucoid. Genus *Enterobacter* has 12 species of which *E. aerogenes* and *E. cloacae* are most commonly encountered in clinical specimens. Some strains of *E. cloacae* are non-motile.

Pathogenicity

E. aerogenes and *E. cloacae* are widely distributed in water, sewage, soil and on vegetables. They are occasionally found in faeces and the respiratory tract of man. They are also associated with a variety of opportunistic infections involving the urinary

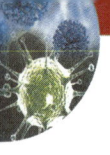

tract, respiratory tract and cutaneous wounds. They may occasionally cause meningitis and septicaemia. In recent years, infection of hospital patients with *E. aerogenes* and *E. cloacae* has been reported more frequently, but *Enterobacter* species are a much less important cause of hospital infection than *Klebsiella* species. Aminoglycosides are often effective in the treatment of *E. aerogenes* and *E. cloacae* infections.

HAFNIA

Genus *Hafnia* has only one species, *H. alvei*. It is usually motile. Its biochemical characteristics are similar to those of *Enterobacter* species except that it does not produce acid from lactose. Biochemical reactions are evident best at 22°C. At 37°C, they may be negative or irregular. *H. alvei* can be distinguished from *Serratia* species because it does not produce lipase or deoxyribonuclease. It is found in human and animal faeces, sewage, soil and water. It has been recovered from wounds, abscesses, sputum, urine, blood and other sites. However, its role in infection is difficult to discern because it is often associated with other bacterial species. It is, therefore, believed that *H. alvei* is at the most an opportunistic pathogen.

SERRATIA

These are small (0.7–1.5 × 0.7 μm), motile, Gram-negative coccobacilli. Several species of *Serratia* have been described. *S. marcescens* is the most important member of this genus.

After 24–48 hours incubation, colonies of *S. marcescens*, on nutrient agar, are usually homogeneous and then may develop a convex, pigmented (red) and relatively opaque centre, and colourless, transparent periphery with crenated edge. The red pigment, prodigiosin, is insoluble in water and does not diffuse away from the colonies. Therefore, the colonies are red or pink. The pigment is soluble in absolute alcohol, ether, chloroform, acetone, benzol and carbon disulphide. Many strains grow best at 30–37°C but pigmentation may be poor at such temperatures whereas at lower temperatures, e.g. 15–20°C, growth is poorer and pigment formation is abundant. The pigment is formed only in cultures grown aerobically and non-pigmented variant strains may originate by mutation in laboratory cultures. *Serratia* species are ONPG positive but fail to ferment lactose, therefore, unless pigment is produced, they form pale colonies on MacConkey agar.

Pathogenicity

Serratia is a saprophyte found in water, soil and food. However, it can lead to serious nosocomial infections particularly in the newborn, the debilitated or the patient receiving immunosuppressive drugs. These include infections of wound, urinary and respiratory tracts, meningitis, endocarditis, septicaemia and endotoxic shock.

Serratia is commonly resistant to cephalosporins. Resistance to ampicillin and gentamicin varies from strain to strain. In hospital strains, multiple drug resistance is common.

Key Points

- Organisms of family Enterobacteriaceae are **Gram-negative, aerobes** and **facultative anaerobes** that ferment glucose and usually **live in the intestinal tract**.
- *Escherichia coli is the predominant facultative inhabitant of human intestinal tract.*
- *Diarrhoea-producing Escherichia coli can be divided into enteropathogenic (**EPEC**), enteroinvasive (**EIEC**), enterotoxigenic (**ETEC**), verocytotoxigenic (**VTEC**), enteroaggregative (**EAEC**) and diffusely adherent E. coli (**DAEC**) types.*
- **Enterotoxin produced by *E. coli*** is of two types – heat-labile toxin (**LT**) and heat stable toxin (**ST**).
- *Klebsiella pneumoniae* may cause **severe destructive pneumonia** and **nosocomial urinary tract infection**.

ASSESS YOURSELF

LONG AND SHORT ANSWER QUESTIONS

1. Write short notes on:
   - (a) Enterotoxins of *Escherichia coli*
   - (b) *Enterobacter*
   - (c) *Serratia*
   - (d) Pathogenicity of *Klebsiella*
2. Discuss the pathogenicity of *Escherichia coli*.
3. Discuss the laboratory diagnosis of various infections caused by *Escherichia coli*.

MULTIPLE CHOICE QUESTIONS

1. Which of the following bacteria does not belong to the family Enterobacteriaceae?
   - (a) *Shigella*
   - (b) *Salmonella*
   - (c) *Yersinia*
   - (d) *Acinetobacter*
2. Which of the following bacteria is not known as coliform bacilli?
   - (a) *Escherichia*
   - (b) *Klebsiella*
   - (c) *Enterobacter*
   - (d) *Salmonella*
3. Heat-labile enterotoxin of *Escherichia coli* activates:
   - (a) Adenylate cyclase
   - (b) Guanylate cyclase
   - (c) Both of the above
   - (d) None of the above
4. Traveller's diarrhoea is caused by:
   - (a) Enteropathogenic *Escherichia coli*
   - (b) Enterotoxigenic *E. coli*
   - (c) Enteroinvasive *E. coli*
   - (d) Verocytotoxigenic *E. coli*
5. Haemolytic uraemic syndrome is caused by:
   - (a) Enteropathogenic *Escherichia coli*
   - (b) Enterotoxigenic *E. coli*
   - (c) Enteroaggregative *E. coli*
   - (d) Verocytotoxigenic *E. coli*
6. Which of the following produces indole?
   - (a) *Salmonella* serotype Typhi
   - (b) *K. oxytoca*
   - (c) *K. pneumoniae* subspecies *pneumoniae*
   - (d) *K. pneumoniae* subspecies *rhinoscleromatis*
7. On the basis of capsular antigens, klebsiellae have been differentiated into:
   - (a) 20 serotypes
   - (b) 40 serotypes
   - (c) 80 serotypes
   - (d) 100 serotypes

ANSWERS TO MCQs

1. d   **2.** d   **3.** a   **4.** b   **5.** d   **6.** b   **7.** c

20 Chapter

Proteus, Morganella and Providencia

Tribe Proteeae, in the family Enterobacteriaceae, comprises three genera—*Proteus*, *Morganella* and *Providencia*.

PROTEUS

Genus *Proteus* has four species—*P. mirabilis, P. vulgaris, P. myxofaciens* and *P. penneri*.

Morphology

They are Gram-negative coccobacilli, 1–3 μm long and 0.6 μm wide. In young cultures, most of them are long (up to 80 μm) curved and filamentous. They may be arranged singly, in pairs or in short chains. They are actively motile by peritrichous flagella. However, non-flagellate and non-motile variants are also encountered.

Cultural Characteristics

They can grow on ordinary media like nutrient agar and culture emits characteristic putrefactive (fishy or seminal) odour. *P. mirabilis* and *P. vulgaris* possess the **ability to swarm** (spread) on solid media. A group of cells at the edge of a developing microcolony migrate to an uninoculated area of the medium. Swarming growth on a plate may eventually appear either as a uniform film of growth extending over the whole plate (**continuous swarming**) or as a series of concentric circles of growth around the point of inoculation (**discontinuous swarming**). Swarming of *Proteus* appears to be due to vigorous motility of the organism although the exact cause is not yet established. Swarming can be inhibited by:

- Increasing the concentration of agar in the medium from 1–2% to 6%
- Incorporating chloral hydrate (1 in 500), sodium azide (1 in 500) or boric acid (1 in 100) in the medium.

Swarming does not occur on MacConkey agar on which smooth, colourless colonies are formed. Non-motile variants do not swarm.

Dienes phenomenon

When two identical strains of *Proteus* are inoculated at different points of the same culture plate, without any swarming inhibiting substance, the resulting swarms of growth coalesce without signs of demarcation. When, however, two different strains of *Proteus* species are inoculated, the spreading films of growth fail to coalesce and remain separated by a narrow but easily visible furrow. This is known as Dienes phenomenon. **It has been used to determine the identity or non-identity of various strains of *Proteus*.**

Biochemical Reactions

All species of *Proteus* produce acid from glucose. Lactose is not fermented. Other biochemical characters of four species of *Proteus* are given in Table 20.1.

Antigenic Structure

Motile strains of *Proteus* possess O (somatic) and H (flagellar) antigens. Weil and Felix (1916) observed that flagellated strains growing on agar formed a thin surface film resembling the mist produced by breathing on glass and named this variety the 'Hauch' form (from Hauch meaning film of breath). Non-flagellated variants grew as colonies without the surface film and were called 'Ohne Hauch' (maening without film of breath). These names came to be abbreviated as the H and O forms. Subsequently, H and O were used to refer to the flagellar and somatic antigens of other bacilli as well.

O antigen has got alkali-labile and alkali-stable fractions. The alkali-stable fraction of O antigen (polysaccharide) of non-motile *Proteus* strains OX19, OX2 and OXK is shared by some rickettsiae. This is the basis of **Weil-Felix reaction** for the diagnosis of some rickettsial diseases. OX19, OX2, and OXK are the strains of *P. vulgaris* serotype O1 and serotype O2, and *P. mirabilis* serotype O3, respectively.

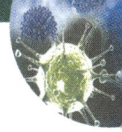

TABLE 20.1: Differentiation of four species of *Proteus* and *Morganella morganii*

Property	Proteus				M. morganii
	mirabilis	*vulgaris*	*penneri*	*myxofaciens*	
Motility	+	+	+	+	+
Swarming on solid nutrient media	+	+	–	–	–
Indole	–	+	–	–	+
Methyl red	+	+	v	+	+
Voges-Proskauer	v	–	–	+	–
Citrate	v	v	–	v	–
Phenylalanine deaminase test	+	+	+	+	+
Urease	+	+	+	+	+
H$_2$S	+	+	–	+	–
Gelatin liquefaction	+	+	v	+	–
Lipase production	+	+	v	+	–
Ornithine decarboxylation	+	–	–	–	+
Gas from glucose	+	+	v	+	+
Acid from:					
• Mannose	–	–	–	–	+
• Maltose	–	+	+	+	–
• Xylose	+	+	+	–	–
• Trehalose	+	v	v	+	–

v, variable.

Typing Methods

The available typing systems for various species of *Proteus* and *Providencia* are serotyping, phage typing, Dienes typing and bacteriocin (proticin) typing. Of these methods, proticin typing method appears to be promising. Al-Jumali (1975) claimed 100% typability with his method of proticin sensitivity typing using 12 standard proticin producing strains. However, using the same set of producer strains the author (Arora et al., 1988) obtained 85% typability.

Pathogenicity

The genus *Proteus* is found in soil, water and faecally contaminated materials. *P. mirabilis* is the most important species (70–90%) recovered from humans, particularly as a causative agent of urinary tract and wound infections. After *Escherichia coli*, *P. mirabilis* is the most frequently associated bacterium with urinary tract infection (UTI). It commonly involves young boys and elderly people of both sexes often with diabetes or structural abnormalities of the urinary tract. In the hospital patients, it may lead to UTI following various forms of urological instrumentation. *P. vulgaris* is more commonly recovered from infected sites in immunosuppressed hosts, particularly those receiving prolonged regimens of antibiotics.

UTI caused by *Proteus* tends to be more serious than that caused by *E. coli* and other coliforms, because these organisms are usually confined to the bladder whereas *Proteus* has a predilection for the upper urinary tract. It produces urease which liberates ammonia from urea. Ammonia inactivates complement, damages renal epithelium and makes the urine alkaline. The alkaline conditions lead to the precipitation of phosphates and the formation of calculi in the urinary tract. It may also lead to hyperammonaemic encephalopathy and coma. Occasionally, *Proteus* may cause wound infection, bed sores, osteomyelitis and in neonates it may cause infection of the umbilical stump which often leads to bacteraemia and meningitis. *P. penneri* and *P. myxofaciens* are rarely encountered in clinical laboratory.

MORGANELLA

This genus has only one species—*M. morganii*. It is motile, but does not swarm on solid nutrient media. Biochemical reactions of this organism are shown in Table 20.1.

M. morganii is frequently found in human faeces and sometimes in the faeces of other animals and reptiles. It has also been isolated from diarrhoeic stools in the absence of other known bacterial enteropathogens. However, its role in the causation of enteritis has not as yet been established. It may also cause nosocomial urinary tract infection, pneumonia and wound infection. Occasionally, it is isolated from blood.

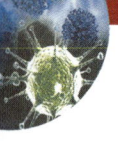

PROVIDENCIA

Genus *Providencia* has three species—*P. rettgeri*, *P. alcalifaciens* and *P. stuartii*. All the three species of *Providencia* are motile but do not swarm on solid nutrient media. The colonies emit 'fruity' smell. All the species of *Providencia* deaminate phenylalanine, but only *P. rettgeri* consistently hydrolyses urea. Biochemical properties of all the species of *Providencia* are given in Table 20.2.

P. stuartii may occasionally cause hospital-associated urinary tract infection, particularly in patients undergoing long-term catheterization and in those with urinary tract abnormalities. It may also cause infection of burns and pneumonia. In elderly and immunodeficient patients, it may lead to septicaemia. All species may be recovered from faeces, however, only *P. alcalifaciens* may be associated with diarrhoea. *P. rettgeri* has been associated with hospital-associated infections of urinary tract, wounds, burns and of blood.

Laboratory Diagnosis

Laboratory diagnosis of the infections caused by species of *Proteus*, *Morganella* and *Providencia* can be carried out by culture of the specimen on MacConkey agar or DCA. The isolate is identified by its morphological and biochemical tests and agglutination reactions.

Treatment

Members of the tribe Proteeae are resistant to polymyxin B and colistin. Urinary tract infection produced by *P. mirabilis* usually responds to ampicillin and trimethoprim but nitrofurantoin is not effective. Strains of *P. mirabilis* that do not form β-lactamases are sensitive to benzyl penicillin, ampicillin, carbenicillin and cephalosporins. However, β-lactamase-producing strains are resistant to the first three antibiotics and may remain sensitive to cephalosporins. *P. vulgaris* and *P. penneri* strains are resistant to benzyl penicillin, ampicillin and many cephalosporins but are sensitive to some of the newer cephalosporins such as cefotaxime and cefuroxime. Most strains of *Proteus* are susceptible to aminoglycosides but they may acquire plasmids coding for resistance to aminoglycosides, trimethoprim and other antibiotics to which they are normally sensitive. Therefore, treatment should be guided by antibiotic susceptibility testing *in vitro*.

TABLE 20.2: Differentiation of three species of *Providencia*

Property	Providencia		
	rettgeri	*alcalifaciens*	*stuartii*
Motility	+	+	+
Swarming on solid nutrient media	–	–	–
Indole	+	+	+
Methyl red	+	+	+
Voges-Proskauer	–	–	–
Citrate	+	+	+
Phenylalanine deaminase test	+	+	+
Urease	+	–	v
Ornithine decarboxylation	–	–	–
H$_2$S	–	–	–
Gelatin liquefaction	–	–	–
Lipase production	–	–	–
Gas from glucose	–	+	–
Acid from:			
• Glucose	+	+	+
• Mannose	+	+	+
• Inositol	+	–	+
• Adonitol	+	+	v
• Trehalose	–	–	+

v, variable.

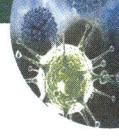

Key Points

- **Phenylalanine deaminase test** distinguishes tribe Proteeae from all other members of the Enterobacteriaceae.
- After *Escherichia coli*, *P. mirabilis* is the most frequently associated bacterium with **urinary tract infection** (UTI).
- UTI caused by *Proteus* tends to be more serious than that caused by *E. coli* and other coliforms.

? ASSESS YOURSELF

SHORT ANSWER QUESTION

Write short notes on:

(a) Dienes phenomenon

(b) Antigenic structure of *Proteus*

(c) Genus *Morganella*

(d) Genus *Providencia*

(e) Pathogenicity of *Proteus*

MULTIPLE CHOICE QUESTIONS

1. Which of the following bacteria is **not** included in the tribe Proteeae?

   (a) *Proteus*

   (b) *Morganella*

   (c) *Providencia*

   (d) *Edwardsiella*

2. Which of the following species is **not** included in the genus *Proteus*?

   (a) *Mirabilis*

   (b) *Vulgaris*

   (c) *Penneri*

   (d) *Morganii*

3. Phenylalanine deaminase test is positive in:

   (a) *Proteus*

   (b) *Morganella*

   (c) *Providencia*

   (d) All of the above

4. Dienes phenomenon is used to determine the identity or non-identity of strains of:

   (a) *Proteus*

   (b) *Salmonella*

   (c) *Shigella*

   (d) *Klebsiella*

ANSWERS TO MCQs

1. d   **2.** d   **3.** d   **4.** a

Shigella

The genus *Shigella* has four species. They cause bacillary dysentery in man.

MORPHOLOGY

Shigellae are non-motile, non-flagellate, non-sporing, non-capsulate, Gram-negative bacilli measuring 2–4 × 0.6 μm.

CULTURAL CHARACTERISTICS

They are aerobes and facultative anaerobes, growing within a temperature range of 10–40°C, with an optimum temperature of 37°C and pH of 7.4. They can grow on ordinary media.

- On **nutrient agar** or **blood agar**, colonies are 2–3 mm in diameter, circular, convex, smooth, greyish or colourless and translucent. Colonies of *S. sonnei* are slightly larger and more opaque than those of other shigellae.
- On **MacConkey agar**, colonies are colourless due to the absence of lactose fermentation. However, colonies of *S. sonnei*, a late lactose-fermenter, become pink when incubation is prolonged beyond 24 hours.
- Colonies of *Shigella* on **deoxycholate citrate agar** (DCA), a selective medium for isolation of shigellae from faeces, are smaller (1–1.5 mm in diameter) and do not form a black centre. On prolonged incubation, colonies of *S. sonnei* form pink papillae due to late lactose fermentation.
- **Xylose lysine deoxycholate (XLD) agar** is a better selective medium than DCA because it is less inhibitory to *S. dysenteriae* and *S. flexneri* than DCA. On this medium, colonies of *Shigella* are red and unlike those of most salmonellae, without black centres.
- *Salmonella-Shigella* **(SS) agar** is a highly selective medium for the isolation of *Salmonella* and *Shigella*. The high bile salt concentration and sodium citrate, in this medium, inhibit all Gram-positive bacteria, coliforms and many other Gram-negative organisms. Colonies of *Shigella* on this medium are colourless with no blackening, while those of *Salmonella* are colourless with black centres.

Enrichment Media

Enrichment media or broths are helpful in the recovery of *Shigella* and *Salmonella*, whose number in the faeces may be as low as 200/gram while that of *E. coli* and other enteric bacilli (normal flora) may be as high as 10^9/gram. Inhibitory chemical substances in the enrichment media maintain the normal flora in a prolonged lag phase, while *Shigella* and *Salmonella* species are far less inhibited, enter into a log phase of growth and are more readily recovered from faecal samples. However, after several hours, the enrichment media no longer suppress the growth of normal flora that will ultimately overgrow the culture.

- **Selenite F broth:** Sodium selenite in this enrichment medium inhibits coliform bacilli while permitting salmonellae and many shigellae to grow. Therefore, it is recommended for the isolation of these organisms from faeces.
- **Gram-negative (GN) broth:** Most strains of *Shigella* and *Salmonella* grow well in this medium. Therefore, it is useful for isolation of these organisms.

SUSCEPTIBILITY TO PHYSICAL AND CHEMICAL AGENTS

Shigellae are killed by moist heat at 56°C in one hour and by 1% phenol in 15 minutes. In stools that are allowed to become acid through growth of coliforms or other bacteria they tend to die within a few hours, but can survive for several days in faeces kept non-acid in buffered glycerol solution or preserved at 4°C. When dried on linen and kept in dark at room temperature, they survive for 5–46 days. **S. sonnei is more resistant to adverse environmental conditions as compared to other species.**

CLASSIFICATION

On the basis of biochemical reactions and antigenic structure, shigellae are classified into four groups (A, B, C and D) or species: *S. dysenteriae*, *S. flexneri*, *S. boydii* and *S. sonnei* (Table 21.1). Shigellae are methyl red positive and negative for Voges-Proskauer reaction, citrate and malonate utilization, lysine decarboxylation, urease and H_2S production, gelatin liquefaction, phenylalanine deamination and are unable to grow in the presence of KCN. All the shigellae produce acid from glucose and with the exception of *S. dysenteriae*, from mannitol. *S. dysenteriae* serotype 1, *S. flexneri* serotype 6 and *S. sonnei* are always indole negative. Strains of other serotypes differ in their reactions.

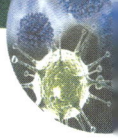

TABLE 21.1: Differentiation of *Shigella* species

Species	Acid produced in fermentation of					Indole	Lysine decarbo-xylase	Ornithine decarbo-xylase	Number of serotypes
	Lactose	**Sucrose**	**Mannitol**	**Dulcitol**	**Xylose**				
S. dysenteriae	–	–	–	–	–	v	–	–	15
S. flexneri	–	–	+	–	–	v	–	–	6 + 2 variants
S. boydii	–	–	+	v	v	v	–	–	19
S. sonnei	–*	–*	+	–	v	–	–	+	2 phases; 26 colicin types

* negative at 24 hours, late positive at 2–8 days; v, variable.

S. sonnei **is a late-lactose fermenter**, and colonies growing on MacConkey or DCA medium for more than 24 hours develop pink colour. Other three species are non-lactose-fermenters. Only *S. sonnei* forms ornithine decarboxylase.

ANTIGENIC STRUCTURE

All *Shigella* species possess O antigens, and certain strains may possess K antigens. *Shigella* K antigens, when present, interfere with the detection of the O antigen during serologic grouping. The K antigen is heat-labile and may be removed by boiling the organism in a cell suspension. On the basis of somatic (O) antigens, shigellae can be subdivided into serotypes. This is carried out by agglutination tests with absorbed specific antisera.

Group A (*S. dysenteriae*)

It is subdivided into 15 serotypes of which serotypes 1 and 2 are also known as Shiga's bacillus (*S. shigae*) and Schmitz's bacillus (*S. schmitzi*), respectively. Each serotype is characterized by a different type antigen.

Group B (*S. flexneri*)

Among shigellae, this group is the most complex antigenically. Based on type-specific (I–VI) and group-specific (1–8) antigens, they have been classified into 6 serotypes (1–6) and several subtypes (1a, 1b, 2a, 2b, 3a, 3b, 3c, 4a, 4b, 5a, 5b). In addition, 2 antigenic variants called X and Y are recognized which lack the type-specific antigen (Table 21.2). Serotype 6 is always indole negative and can be subdivided into three biotypes: Boyd 88, Manchester and Newcastle (Table 21.3).

Group C (*S. boydii*)

Dysentery bacilli of this group resemble those of *S. flexneri* biochemically but not antigenically.

Group D (*S. sonnei*)

It is antigenically homogeneous. It may, however, undergo an antigenic variation that affects the somatic antigens and has been

TABLE 21.2: Antigens of various serotypes of *Shigella flexneri*

Serotype	Subserotype antigen	Type-specific antigens	Group-specific antigens
1	1a	I	1, 2, 4
	1b	I	1, 2, 4, 6
2	2a	II	1, 3, 4
	2b	II	1, 7, 8
3	3a	III	1, 6, 7, 8
	3b	III	1, 3, 4, 6, 7, 8
	3c	III	1, 6
4	4a	IV	1, 3, 4
	4b	IV	1, 3, 4, 6
5	5a	V	1, 3, 4
	5b	V	1, 7, 8
6		VI	1, 2, 4
X variant		–	1, 7, 8
Y variant		–	1, 3, 4

TABLE 21.3: Biotypes of *Shigella flexneri* serotype 6

Biotype	Indole	Fermentation of	
		Glucose	**Mannitol**
Boyd 88	–	⊥	⊥
Manchester	–	+	+
Newcastle	–	⊥ or +	–

⊥, acid only; +, acid and gas.

referred to as phase or form variation. These 2 phases or forms of the culture are known as phase S or form I and phase R or form II. The former gives rise to smooth colonies while the colonies of the latter are larger, flatter and irregular. Cultures often contain a mixture of both forms, but the colonies of one form can be selected by addition of antiserum of the other form to the culture medium because form II variant is antigenically different from

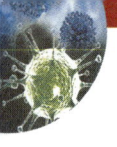

form I variant. By using 33 indicator strains, Horak (1980) could divide *S. sonnei* into 26 colicin types. The ability to produce a particular colicin is a fairly stable character, therefore, the results of colicin typing are of value for epidemiological purposes.

TOXIN FORMATION

Endotoxin

All shigellae release an endotoxin after autolysis. It is thermostable lipopolysaccharide of the cell wall. It has irritating action on the intestinal wall which causes diarrhoea and subsequent ulcers.

Exotoxin

S. dysenteriae serotype 1, in addition to endotoxin, produces a powerful exotoxin. It is a heat labile protein and acts as enterotoxin and neurotoxin. As enterotoxin, it acts on the intestinal mucosa causing transudation of fluid in the lumen and as neurotoxin, it damages endothelial cells of small blood vessels of the central nervous system which results in neurological complications like polyneuritis, coma and meningism.

Verocytotoxin

S. dysenteriae serotype 1 produces a potent toxin (shiga toxin) very similar to VT1 expressed by strains of verocytotoxigenic *E. coli* (VTEC).

PATHOGENICITY

Members of the genus *Shigella* produce a serious illness known as **bacillary dysentery**. It is an acute diarrhoeal disease characterized in the more severe infection by the presence of blood and mucus in the stools. Humans appear to be the only natural hosts for shigellae and they become infected by ingestion of contaminated food or water. **The only source of infection is man – cases or carriers. The infecting dose is small between 10–100 organisms**, and the bacteria seem relatively unaffected by gastric acid or bile.

A patient or a carrier after contaminating his hands while cleansing himself at toilet, touches and contaminates objects like toilet seat, toilet chain, door handles, wash-basin taps, hand towels, etc. and these objects when used by other person may lead to infection. Infection may also spread via flies, fingers, food and faeces. Flies contaminate food mainly by carrying infective material on their feet (mechanical carriage) rather than in their intestines. Faeces of the patient or a carrier may also contaminate water supply.

After reaching the large intestine, the shigellae multiply in the gut lumen. Many bacteria adhere to the epithelial cells of the gut mucosa and induce these cells to ingest them. They then multiply within the epithelial cells and spread laterally into adjacent cells and deep into the lamina propria. Inflammatory reaction

develops with capillary thrombosis, leading to necrosis of patches of epithelium, which slough off, leaving behind **superficial ulcers**. The cellular response is mainly by polymorphonuclear leucocytes which can be seen on microscopic examination of stool, together with red cells and sloughed epithelium.

The ulcers of the bacillary dysentery are much shallower than amoebic ulcers. The **intervening mucosa is inflamed and oedematous**. Thus, there is diffuse involvement, unlike the amoebic dysentery in which the mucosa in between the ulcerative lesions is healthy. Dysentery bacilli rarely invade other tissues and bacteraemia has been reported in only 2–4% of cases of bacillary dysentery particularly in malnourished children and in AIDS cases.

The incubation period is usually between 2–3 days, but may be as short as 12 hours. In the typical case there is diarrhoea, often bloody, and tenesmus. The severity of disease varies widely. A considerable proportion of patients suffer from a simple diarrhoea, but in most of them there is usually some constitutional disturbance. In severe infections, toxaemia is profound and bacterial endotoxin can often be detected in the blood by means of the *Limulus* test.

The severity of the clinical illness is to some extent associated with the particular species involved. Infection with *S. dysenteriae* is usually associated with a severe illness in which there is a sudden onset of abdominal pain, tenesmus, pyrexia (due to absorption of exotoxins from gut), prostration and sometimes convulsions. The stools loose their usual faecal character, are small and frequent, and are composed mainly of **fresh blood, pus and mucus**. Exotoxin produced by *S. dysenteriae* serotype 1 appears to be much less important in pathogenesis than the ability of the pathogens to adhere, penetrate and multiply. Invasive and non-toxigenic mutants can still cause dysentery, while toxigenic and non-invasive cannot do so.

Complications are most often seen in patients with *S. dysenteriae* serotype 1 infection. These include arthritis, toxic neuritis, conjunctivitis, parotitis, intussusception and haemolytic uraemic syndrome (HUS). HUS is characterized by haemolytic anaemia, thrombocytopenia and acute renal failure. It can be caused by many pathogens particularly *E. coli* O157. It is associated with complement activation and disseminated intravascular coagulation.

On the other extreme, the disease caused by *S. sonnei* is of mild type and may be associated with a few loose stools with vague abdominal discomfort. The illness caused by *S. flexneri* and *S. boydii* is more severe than that caused by *S. sonnei* and sometimes may be as severe as that caused by *S. dysenteriae*.

Epidemiology

Bacillary dysentery has a global distribution. It is commoner in countries with a warm than a temperate climate and in poor than in affluent countries. It is mostly associated with the overcrowding and bad hygienic conditions encountered in times of war and other disasters, and in jails and mental institutions.

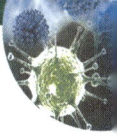

The most prevalent species of *Shigella* in the United States is *S. sonnei* which can survive for many days on lavatory seats, particularly in conditions of low temperature and high humidity. It is transmitted by faecal-oral route and majority of the patients are pre-school age children, particularly those in day-care centres. In India, *S. flexneri* has always been the predominant species (50–85%) followed by *S. dysenteriae* (8–25%), *S. sonnei* (2–24%) and *S. boydii* (0–8%).

LABORATORY DIAGNOSIS

Specimens

The laboratory diagnosis of bacillary dysentery can be made by the isolation of *Shigella* from faeces. It should be inoculated without delay. If this is impossible, the mucus or faeces should be transported in a buffered 30% glycerol saline solution, which prevents the dysentery bacilli from being destroyed by the acid produced during the growth of other organisms. A direct swab may be taken from the ulcer by sigmoidoscopic examination. Rectal swabs which do not allow adequate macroscopic and microscopic examination of faeces should be avoided.

Direct Microscopy

Microscopic examination of the faeces or mucus shows numerous erythrocytes and polymorphonuclear leucocytes and a few macrophages. The latter must be carefully differentiated from vegetative forms of *Entamoeba histolytica* which have relatively smaller nuclei with a central karyosome.

Culture

The mucus or faeces are inoculated on MacConkey agar and DCA. SS agar and XLD medium can also be used. After overnight incubation at 37°C, the plates are inspected for pale (non-lactose-fermenting) colonies on MacConkey agar and DCA, and red and colourless colonies with no blackening on XLD and SS agar, respectively. These are tested for motility and biochemical reactions.

Slide Agglutination

The colonies that give the characteristic biochemical reactions should be identified further by serological investigation with species-specific sera and then with type-specific sera unless the strain is *S. sonnei*.

Enrichment Media Inoculation

Along with the inoculation of plating media, selenite F broth and GN broth (enrichment media) may also be inoculated. Subcultures are made on plating media after 8–12 hours and 4–6 hours respectively and processed as above.

TREATMENT

Most of the cases of bacillary dysentery especially those due to *S. sonnei*, are mild and self-limiting and do not require antibiotic therapy. Replacement of fluids and electrolytes by oral rehydration salt solution is all that is required. Intravenous replacement of fluids and electrolytes plus antibiotic therapy is necessary in the very young, the aged or debilitated and in severe cases of shigellosis. Ampicillin, co-trimoxazole, tetracycline, the quinolone antibiotics such as nalidixic acid and ciprofloxacin are appropriate choices.

 Key Points

- Members of the genus *Shigella* produce a serious illness known as **bacillary dysentery**.
- The **infective dose of shigellae** is small (10–100 organisms), and the bacteria seem relatively unaffected by gastric acid or bile.
- Shigellae produce **superficial ulcers** in the large intestine, the intervening mucosa is inflamed and oedematous.

SECTION IV • PATHOGENIC ORGANISMS-I BACTERIA

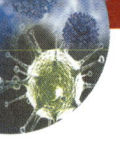

? ASSESS YOURSELF

LONG ANSWER QUESTIONS

1. Discuss various culture media employed for the isolation of *Shigella*.
2. Discuss the antigenic structure and toxins of *Shigella*.
3. Discuss pathogenicity of *Shigella*.
4. Discuss laboratory diagnosis of shigellosis.

MULTIPLE CHOICE QUESTIONS

1. Selective medium/media for the isolation of *Shigella* is/are:
   (a) Xylose lysine deoxycholate agar
   (b) *Salmonella-Shigella* agar
   (c) Hektoen enteric agar
   (d) All of the above

2. Which of the following bacteria is/are always indole-negative?
   (a) *Shigella dysenteriae* serotype 1
   (b) *S. flexneri* serotype 6
   (c) *S. sonnei*
   (d) All of the above

3. Which of the following bacteria is negative for fermentation of mannitol?
   (a) *Shigella dysenteriae*
   (b) *S. flexneri*
   (c) *S. boydii*
   (d) *S. sonnei*

4. Which of the following complications can be associated with *Shigella dysenteriae* serotype 1 infection?
   (a) Arthritis
   (b) Toxic neuritis
   (c) Haemolytic uraemic syndrome
   (d) All of the above

ANSWERS TO MCQs

1. d   **2.** d   **3.** a   **4.** d

Chapter 22

Salmonella

The genus *Salmonella* is the most complex, with more than 2,500 serotypes currently, described in Kauffman-White scheme. According to this scheme, each named serotype was regarded as a separate *Salmonella* species and the convention was adopted that each new serotype should be given the name of the place where it was first isolated.

It is now generally accepted that all salmonellae belong to two species. *S. enterica* and *S. bongori*. There are six subspecies of *S. enterica*, the most important of which is *S. enterica* subsp. *enterica* (subspecies I) which includes the typhoid and paratyphoid bacilli and most other serotypes responsible for causing disease in mammals. Salmonellae are named as, for example, *S. enterica* subsp. *enterica* serotype Enteritidis. For convenience it is usual to abbreviate this to *S.* serotype Enteritidis, or just Enteritidis for use in clinical situations. Serotype names are capitalized and not in italics.

MORPHOLOGY

These are Gram-negative, non-sporing, non-acid-fast, non-capsulated bacilli measuring $2–4 \times 0.6$ μm. Most strains are motile by means of peritrichous flagella except *S.* serotype Gallinarum and *S.* serotype Pullorum which are non-motile. Non-motile mutants of other serotypes may sometimes be found.

CULTURAL CHARACTERISTICS

Salmonellae are aerobes and facultative anaerobes, growing within a temperature range of 15–45°C (optimum temperature 37°C). They can grow on ordinary media.

- On **nutrient agar** or **blood agar**, colonies are 2–3 mm in diameter, greyish-white, circular, moist, convex and translucent.
- On **MacConkey agar**, after overnight incubation at 37°C, the colonies are 1–3 mm in diameter and pale yellow or colourless due to the absence of lactose fermentation.
- The colonies of *Salmonella* on **deoxycholate citrate agar (DCA)**, a selective medium for isolation of shigellae and salmonellae from faeces, are similar to or slightly smaller in size than those on MacConkey agar. After 48 hours incubation, the colonies may develop a black centre.

- On **Wilson and Blair's brilliant-green bismuth sulphite agar** medium, *S.* serotype Typhi and *S.* serotype Paratyphi B form small (about 1 mm in diameter) black colonies.
- For the appearance of colonies of *Salmonella* on **xylose lysine deoxycholate (XLD) agar**, and **Salmonella-Shigella (SS) agar**, see cultural characteristics of *Shigella*.

Enrichment Media

Selenite F and tetrathionate broth are commonly employed as enrichment media.

BIOCHEMICAL REACTIONS

Salmonellae are indole negative, methyl red reaction positive, Voges-Proskauer negative and citrate positive (except *S.* serotype Typhi and *S.* serotype Paratyphi A which are citrate negative). Most salmonellae give a positive reaction for H_2S in triple sugar iron agar, but exceptions include strains of *S.* serotype Paratyphi A and *S.* serotype Choleraesuis. They fail to hydrolyse urea and deaminate phenylalanine. They are gelatin liquefaction and malonate utilization negative and are unable to grow in the presence of KCN.

Salmonellae ferment glucose, mannitol, maltose and sorbitol with the production of acid and gas. *S.* serotype Typhi, *S.* serotype Gallinarum and rare anaerogenic variants in other serotypes, e.g. *S.* serotype Typhimurium form acid only. Salmonellae do not ferment lactose, sucrose, salicin and adonitol. They decarboxylate lysine, ornithine and arginine but not glutamic acid. However, *S.* serotype Typhi and *S.* serotype Paratyphi A do not decarboxylate ornithine and lysine, respectively.

SENSITIVITY TO PHYSICAL AND CHEMICAL AGENTS

Salmonellae are readily killed by moist heat at 55°C for one hour and at 60°C for 15 minutes. They are also killed by pasteurization, boiling and chlorination of water. In polluted water, they can survive for weeks and in ice for months.

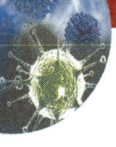

ANTIGENIC STRUCTURE

Salmonellae possess three main types of antigens on the basis of which they are serologically typed. These are:

- Flagellar (H) antigens
- Somatic (O) antigens
- Surface (Vi) antigens.

In addition, several strains carry fimbriae. Fimbrial (F) antigens are not important in identification, but may cause confusion due to their nonspecific nature and widespread sharing amongst enterobacteria.

PATHOGENESIS

S. serotype Typhi, *S.* serotype Paratyphi A, B and C are **primarily human pathogens**. On the other hand, many serotypes such as *S.* serotype Typhimurium have a wide host range affecting animals, birds and man.

Man acquires infection by ingestion of contaminated water or food. Water becomes polluted by the introduction of faeces from any human or animal excreting salmonellae. Infection by food usually results either from ingestion of contaminated meat or by way of the hands of the carrier. Poultry and eggs also comprise an important source of salmonellae for humans because a large percentage of chickens are routinely infected with salmonellae. Therefore, man can acquire these organisms through direct contact with uncooked chicken or by ingestion of undercooked chicken. Organisms may also be present on outer shell and in the yolk, therefore, consuming anything containing raw eggs can result in *Salmonella* infection. Slaughterhouse workers are exposed to salmonellosis, as an occupational hazard, primarily from poultry and pigs. **The infective dose of most serotypes including *S.* serotype Typhi, varies from 10^6–10^9 organisms**.

Salmonellae cause the following clinical syndromes in man:

- Enteric fever.
- Septicaemia with or without local suppurative lesions.
- Gastroenteritis or food poisoning.

Enteric Fever

Enteric fever is most usually caused by *S.* serotype Typhi (**typhoid fever**) or *S.* serotype Paratyphi A, B and C (**paratyphoid fever**). On reaching the gut, the bacilli attach themselves to the microvilli of the ileal mucosa by means of adhesins on the bacterial surface, which adhere specifically to mannose-containing receptors on the epithelium. They then penetrate lamina propria and submucosa, where they are phagocytosed by neutrophils and macrophages. They resist intracellular killing and multiply within these cells. These cells enter the mesenteric lymph nodes, where after a period of multiplication, the bacilli invade the blood stream via thoracic duct and a transient bacteraemia (**primary bacteraemia**) follows.

During this period the bacilli are seeded in the liver, gall bladder, spleen, bone marrow, lymph nodes, lungs and kidneys,

where further multiplication takes place. After multiplication in these organs, bacilli pass into the blood, causing a **second and heavier bacteraemia**, heralding the onset of clinical illness.

The organisms multiply abundantly in the gall bladder and are discharged continuously into the intestine where Peyer's patches and other gut lymphoid tissues of ileum become involved. These become inflamed, undergo necrosis and slough off, leaving behind characteristic **typhoid ulcers**. Perforation and haemorrhage are occasional associated accidents.

Incubation period is usually 8–15 days, but can be as short as 5 days or as long as 50 days. The clinical course may vary from a mild undifferentiated pyrexia to a rapidly fatal fulminating disease. The onset is usually gradual with headache, malaise, anorexia, a coated tongue and abdominal discomfort with either constipation or diarrhoea. In the untreated case the temperature shows a step-ladder rise over the first week of illness, remains high for 7–10 days and then falls by lysis during third or fourth week.

Physical signs include a relative bradycardia for the height of the fever, hepatomegaly, splenomegaly and often a rash of **rose spots**. These are 2–4 mm in diameter, slightly raised discrete irregular macules. They are most often found on the front of the chest during the second or third week and fade on pressure. They are seldom noticeable in dark-skinned patients.

The most important complications are intestinal perforation, haemorrhage and circulatory collapse. Other complications include cholecystitis, arthritis, periosteitis, nephritis, haemolytic anaemia, venous thromboses, peripheral neuritis and rarely osteomyelitis. In about 5–10% cases, relapse occurs during convalescence. Mortality in untreated patients is 20%. **The development of cell-mediated immunity is probably the main means by which the infection is overcome**.

LABORATORY DIAGNOSIS

Laboratory diagnosis of enteric fever can be made by:

- Isolation and identification of the causative agent from a specimen of the patient blood, faeces, urine, bone marrow, rose spots, etc.
- Demonstration of circulating antigen.
- Demonstration of antibodies in the patient serum.

Since the onset of symptoms is associated with bacteraemia, blood culture is positive in about 90% of cases in the first week of fever. The frequency with which causative agent can be isolated from the blood falls thereafter so that blood culture is positive in about 75% of cases in the second week, 60% in the third week and 25% after till the fever disappears.

Salmonellae are shed in the faeces throughout the course of the disease and even in convalescence, with varying frequency. During the first week of illness, organisms can be isolated from the faeces in about half the cases and they are most easily isolated between third to fifth week of illness. However, isolation from the faeces is of less certain significance, since salmonellae may be

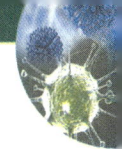

present in the faeces of carriers. Salmonellae are shed in the urine irregularly and infrequently. Urine cultures are generally positive only in the second and third weeks in about 25% of cases.

Testing of patient serum for *Salmonella* antibodies (Widal test) can afford only indirect evidence of infection, and its interpretation may be rendered difficult by past exposure to infection, previous immunization with TAB vaccine or early antibiotic treatment. Therefore, the significance of the result of the Widal test is often doubtful.

Blood Culture

With all aseptic precautions, 5–10 ml of blood is collected by venipuncture and inoculated into a culture bottle containing 50–100 ml of 0.5% bile broth. As far as possible, sample of blood should be collected before starting treatment. Large quantity (5–10 ml) of blood is required, since the number of organisms in the blood, particularly in mild and recovering cases, may be quite small, even as few as one/ml. As the blood's natural bactericidal or bacteriostatic action may interfere with the growth of any bacteria present, this effect is annulled by diluting (inoculating) 5–10 ml of blood in 50–100 ml of the medium (10-fold dilution). The antibacterial effect may be further prevented by the addition of liquoid (sodium polyanethol sulphonate). **Organisms causing bacteraemia in young children are usually present in sufficient concentration, therefore, small volume (1 ml) of blood is inoculated into 10 ml of the medium (10-fold dilution).**

Blood culture bottle is incubated at 37°C for up to 7 days. After overnight incubation, subculture is made on to MacConkey agar, and blood agar (for organisms other than *Salmonella*) media. These plates are incubated at 37°C for 24 hours and the isolate is identified by its morphological and biochemical characters and slide agglutination test. If salmonellae are not obtained from first subculture from bile broth, then subcultures should be repeated every other day up to 7 days. If no growth is obtained after 7 days, then the culture is declared as negative.

For slide agglutination test, a loopful of growth from nutrient agar plate or slope is emulsified in two separate drops of saline on a clean slide. One emulsion acts as a control to show that the strain is not autoagglutinable. If the isolate is anaerogenic (i.e. *S.* serotype Typhi is suspected) then a loopful of factor 9 (typhoid O) antiserum is added to one drop of bacterial emulsion on the slide. The slide is rocked gently. Prompt agglutination indicates that the isolate belongs to *Salmonella* O serogroup D. Its identity as *S.* serotype Typhi is established by agglutination with the flagellar antiserum (anti-d serum). Sometimes, fresh isolates of *S.* serotype Typhi are in the V form and do not agglutinate with O antiserum. Such strains may be tested for agglutination with anti-Vi serum or the growth is scraped off in a small amount of saline, boiled for one hour and tested for agglutination with O antiserum. If the isolate is nontyphoid *Salmonella*, it is tested for agglutination with O and H antisera for serogroups A, B, C, etc.

Clot Culture

With strict aseptic precautions, 5 ml blood is withdrawn from the patient into a sterile test tube and allowed to clot. The separated serum is removed and used for the Widal test. The clot is broken up with a sterile glass rod and added to a bottle of bile broth containing streptokinase (100 units/ml). Streptokinase causes rapid clot lysis with release of bacteria trapped in the clot. Clot culture with streptokinase yields a higher rate of isolation than whole blood culture as the bactericidal action of the serum is obviated. Another advantage is that a sample of serum also becomes available for Widal test.

Faeces Culture

A spoonful of faeces should be collected in a sterile container. Rectal swab is not satisfactory. If there is likely to be a delay of some hours before specimen of faeces for culture reaches the laboratory, the faeces can be placed in a container with 5 ml of buffered glycerol saline transport medium. Faecal samples are plated directly on MacConkey agar, DCA, and Wilson and Blair's brilliant-green bismuth sulphite agar media. The last is highly selective and should be plated heavily.

On MacConkey and DCA media salmonellae appear as pale yellow or colourless colonies after 18–24 hours incubation at 37°C. On Wilson and Blair's brilliant-green bismuth sulphite agar, *S.* serotype Typhi forms black colonies, with a metallic sheen after 24–48 hours incubation at 37°C.

For enrichment, one tube each of selenite F and tetrathionate broth are also inoculated. These are also incubated at 37°C for 8–12 hours with subsequent subculture on MacConkey and DCA media.

Other Materials for Culture

Salmonellae may be isolated from several other sources. These include urine, bone marrow, bile obtained by duodenal aspiration, rose spots, pus from suppurative lesions, CSF and sputum. Bone marrow and bile culture are positive in most cases. The latter may be employed for detection of carriers.

Demonstration of Circulating Antigen

In the early phase of the disease, typhoid bacillus antigens are consistently present in the blood and urine of the patient. *Staphylococcus aureus* containing protein A (Cowan 1 strain) is stabilized with formaldehyde and then coated with *S.* serotype Typhi antibody. When a 1% suspension of such sensitized staphylococcal cells is mixed with patient serum on a slide, typhoid antigen present in the serum combines specifically with the antibody attached to staphylococcal cells producing visible agglutination within 2 minutes. This test is known as **coagglutination**. The test is rapid, sensitive and specific, but is not positive after the first week of illness.

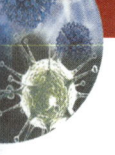

Demonstration of Antibodies in the Patient Serum

- **Widal test**

  It is an **agglutination test** which detects the presence of agglutinins in patient serum against H and O suspensions of the enteric bacteria likely to be encountered, e.g. *S.* serotype Typhi and *S.* serotype Paratyphi A in India. Two types of tubes are used for the test:
- Dreyer's tube (narrow tube with conical bottom) for H agglutination.
- Felix tube (short round bottomed tube) for O agglutination.

Equal volumes (0.4 ml) of serial dilutions of the patient serum (1 : 20 to 1 : 640), and H antigens of *S.* serotype Typhi (TH) and *S.* serotype Paratyphi A (AH), and O antigen of *S.* Typhi (TO), are mixed in Dreyer's and Felix tubes, respectively and incubated in a water bath at 37°C for 4 hours and read after overnight refrigeration at 4°C. O antigen of *S.* serotype Paratyphi A (AO) may not be employed as it cross reacts with TO. Control tubes containing the antigen and normal saline are set to check for autoagglutination. H agglutination leads to the formation of loose and cotton-woolly clumps, while O agglutination appears as a disc-like granular deposit at the bottom of the tube. Control (Felix) tube shows a compact deposit. **The highest dilution of the serum showing agglutination indicates the titre of the antibody**.

Interpretation of Widal Test

- Agglutinins usually appear by seventh to tenth day of the illness in enteric fever, so that a negative result at an early stage is inconclusive. The titre then increases steadily till the third or fourth week, after which it declines gradually.
- Demonstration of rising titre, e.g. four-fold or greater rise, between tests made in the first and third weeks is highly significant. However, if the first sample is taken late in the disease, a rise may not be demonstrable. Instead a fall in titre may be seen in some cases.
- Though it is generally stated that titres of 1: 100 or more for O agglutinins and 1: 200 or more for H agglutinins are significant, the results in a single test by no means prove the presence of enteric fever nor negative results its absence.
- For determining the serotype of infecting organism, H agglutinin is more reliable than O agglutinin because the different serotypes have some O antigens in common. Moreover, O antigens are also widely distributed among other enterobacteria.
- Persons who had past enteric infection or who have been vaccinated may develop anamnestic response during an unrelated fever like malaria, influenza, etc. The anamnestic response shows only a transient rise, while in enteric fever the rise is sustained.
- Test suspensions of bacteria may contain nonspecific antigens such as fimbrial antigens which may produce false positive results.

Best methods of control of enteric fever are:
- Proper sewage disposal.
- Safe water supply.
- Handling of food hygienically.
- Periodic examination of food handlers to ascertain that they are not carriers.

Vaccines against Typhoid Fever

Parenteral Vaccines

- *Killed whole cell vaccine:* Heat killed, phenol preserved, whole cell vaccines containing a mixture of cultures of *S.* serotype Typhi, 1,000 million and *S.* serotype Paratyphi A and B, 750 million each per ml have been used for many years in countries with a high endemic level of typhoid fever. The vaccine is injected in 2 doses of 0.5 ml each at an interval of 4–6 weeks followed by a booster dose every 3 years.
- *Vaccine of purified Vi antigen:* This vaccine contains purified Vi antigen which is injected intramuscularly in a dose of 25 µg.

Oral Vaccine

Oral administration of live avirulent mutant strain of *S.* serotype Typhi (Ty 21a), which is a stable mutant lacking the enzyme UDP-galactose-4-epimerase, has given encouraging results in Egypt. On ingestion, it initiates infection but 'self destructs' after four or five cell divisions, therefore, it cannot induce any illness. Three doses of the vaccine are given on alternate days to children. This oral vaccine is available in enteric coated capsules or in liquid form. It is safe and confers 65–96% protection for 3–5 years.

Typhoid fever responds slowly to ampicillin, amoxycillin, co-trimoxazole or trimethoprim alone. Among newer quinolones, norfloxacin and ciprofloxacin are most widely used antimicrobial agents. They act by inhibiting bacterial enzyme DNA gyrase which is responsible for division, coiling and supercoiling of bacterial DNA during multiplication.

Of the third generation cephalosporins, ceftriaxone, cefotaxime and cefoperazone are effective therapeutic alternative in MDRST infected cases. The results are particularly encouraging with ceftriaxone with overall cure rate of 90%.

Certain salmonellae, *S.* serotype *Choleraesuis* in particular, cause septicaemia. It is characterized by suppurative lesions such as osteomyelitis, deep abscesses, endocarditis, pneumonia and meningitis. Infection occurs by oral route and the incubation period is short. Salmonellae can be isolated from blood or exudate from focal lesions but rarely from faeces.

SALMONELLA GASTROENTERITIS

Salmonella gastroenteritis or food poisoning is generally a **zoonotic disease**. It is caused by ingestion of food like meat, egg, milk and sweets contaminated by certain serotypes of *Salmonella*

which are primarily animal pathogens. In most parts of the world, *S.* serotype Typhimurium is the commonest (30–40%) serotype. Other common serotypes include *S.* serotype Enteritidis, *S.* serotype Newport, *S.* serotypes Dublin, *S.* serotypes Heidelberg and *S.* serotypes Indiana.

The incubation period is 12–24 hours and the illness is characterised by fever, vomiting, abdominal pain and diarrhoea. It may vary in severity from the passage of one or two loose stools to an acute cholera-like disease. It usually subsides in 2–7 days.

🍃 Key Points

- The genus *Salmonella* is the most complex, with **more than 2,500 serotypes** currently described in Kauffmann-White scheme.
- Major types of salmonellosis (diseases caused by *Salmonella*) are **enteric fever**, **gastroenteritis** and **septicaemia**.
- Enteric fever is caused by *S.* serotype Typhi (**typhoid fever**) or *S.* serotype Paratyphi A, B and C (**paratyphoid fever**).
- Laboratory diagnosis of enteric fever can be made by isolation and identification of causative agent from blood, faeces, urine, bone marrow, bile, etc., and by demonstration of circulating antigen and antibodies in the patient serum.

❓ Assess Yourself

LONG AND SHORT ANSWER QUESTIONS

1. Discuss in detail the laboratory diagnosis of enteric fever.
2. Write short notes on:
   - (a) Widal test
   - (b) *Salmonella* septicaemia
   - (c) Culture media for *Salmonella*

MULTIPLE CHOICE QUESTIONS

1. Which of the following media is selective for *Salmonella*?
   - (a) Wilson and Blair's brilliant-green bismuth sulphite agar medium
   - (b) Bile salt agar
   - (c) Thiosulphate citrate bile salt agar
   - (d) Lowenstein-Jensen medium
2. Which of the following media **does not** serve as enrichment medium/media for *Salmonella*?
   - (a) Tetrathionate broth
   - (b) Brilliant green tetrathionate broth
   - (c) Selenite-F broth
   - (d) Alkaline peptone water
3. Most important complication/s of enteric fever is/are:
   - (a) intestinal perforation
   - (b) haemorrhage
   - (c) circulatory collapse
   - (d) All of the above
4. Which of the following media is/are used for blood culture in cases of enteric fever?
   - (a) Bile broth
   - (b) Tetrathionate broth
   - (c) Selenite-F broth
   - (d) Alkaline peptone water
5. In enteric fever, *Salmonella* may be isolated from:
   - (a) urine
   - (b) faeces
   - (c) blood
   - (d) All of the above

Contd...

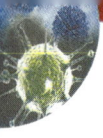

? ASSESS YOURSELF

6. For determining the serotype of infecting organism, detection of which agglutinins is more important in Widal test?
   - (a) O
   - (b) H
   - (c) Fimbrial
   - (d) M

7. In the first week, typhoid is diagnosed by:
   - (a) stool culture
   - (b) urine culture
   - (c) blood culture
   - (d) Widal test

ANSWERS TO MCQS

1. a   **2.** d   **3.** d   **4.** a   **5.** d   **6.** b   **7.** c

Chapter 23

Yersinia

Yersinia pestis, the causative agent of plague, was first isolated independently and almost simultaneously by Yersin (1894) and Kitasato (1894) from patients suffering from plague. It was classified in genus *Pasteurella* and was named as *P. pestis*. In 1944, genus *Yersinia* was created and this was named as *Y. pestis*.

YERSINIA PESTIS

Morphology

They are Gram-negative coccobacilli or rods with rounded ends and straight or convex sides, 1–3 × 0.5–0.8 µm, occurring singly or in pairs or, when in fluid culture, in chains. They are non-sporing, non-acid-fast and non-motile. In exudates from lesions and in cultures grown at 37°C, rather than at the optimum temperature of 27°C, *Y. pestis* exhibits typical capsule. In smears from the tissues stained with methylene blue, the bacilli show characteristic bipolar staining in which the ends of the bacilli stain darker than the central part (Fig. 23.1). In culture, the bipolar staining is less obvious.

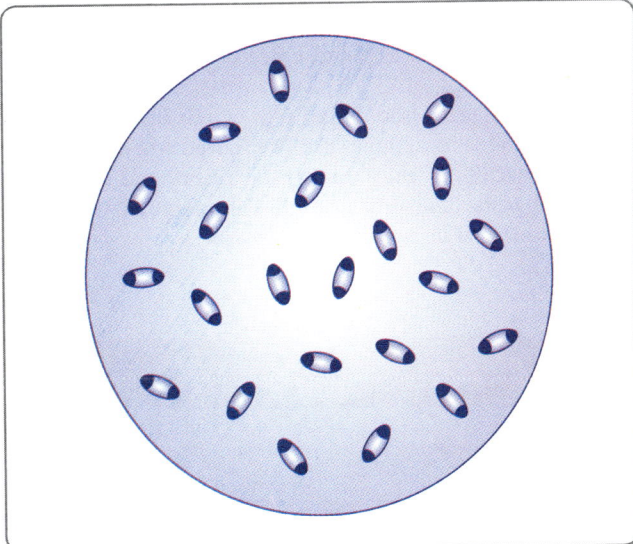

Fig. 23.1: Bipolar staining of *Yersinia pestis*.

Cultural Characteristics

Plague bacilli are aerobes and facultative anaerobes. Optimum (and range) pH and temperature for the growth of these organisms are 7.2 (5.0–9.6) and 27°C (14–37°C), respectively.

- On **nutrient agar** medium, after overnight incubation, *Y. pestis* forms transparent, minute, pin-point colonies.
- On **blood agar**, colonies are dark brown due to absorption of the haemin pigment.
- On **MacConkey agar** colourless colonies are formed.

In **broth**, it produces little turbidity but results in a granular deposit at the bottom and the sides of the tube. On prolonged incubation, a surface pellicle may appear. If a drop of sterile oil is allowed to float on the surface of an inoculated broth and provided the flask is not shaken, a characteristic growth appears which hangs down into the broth from the oil drop resembling stalactites (**stalactite growth**).

Biochemical Reactions

Y. pestis is catalase-positive, indole negative, methyl red reaction positive, and Voges-Proskauer and citrate negative. It is nitrate reduction positive, and urease and gelatin liquefaction negative. It ferments glucose, mannitol and maltose with the production of acid but no gas. Lactose and sucrose are not fermented.

Susceptibility to Physical and Chemical Agents

Y. pestis is easily destroyed by heat at 55°C and 0.5% phenol within 15 minutes. Exposure to sunlight for 3–4 hours is also lethal. It remains viable for long periods in cold and moist environments. It can survive for many months in the soil of rodent burrows.

Pathogenesis

Y. pestis is a natural pathogen of rodents. It causes **zoonotic disease** called **plague**. Infection is transmitted from one animal to another by the bite of rat flea.

Infection in Man

When a rat flea, commonly *Xenopsylla cheopis*, bites a diseased rat, it sucks about 0.5 ml of blood per feed which contains about

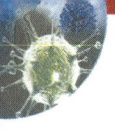

5,000 to 50,000 bacilli. These are sufficient to infect flea. In the flea, the bacilli multiply in the stomach and block the lumen of proventriculus. In *X. cheopis* it takes about 3 weeks (**extrinsic incubation period**). When such a flea bites another rodent blood cannot pass through. The hungry flea bites ferociously and bacteria are regurgitated into the site of bite, transmitting the infection.

When the diseased rat dies, the flea leaves the carcass and in the absence of another rat may bite man causing bubonic plague. Infection in man may also be transmitted by contamination of the wound of bite with the faeces of infected fleas. In man plague occurs in three forms—bubonic, septicaemic and pneumonic.

Bubonic Plague

After an incubation period of 2–5 days, the lymph nodes draining the site of entry of bacillus become infected. As the plague bacillus usually enters through the bite of infected flea on the legs, the inguinal lymph nodes are involved, hence the name bubonic plague (bubo means enlarged gland in groin). The glands become enlarged and suppurate. Patient develops fever, chills, nausea and malaise. Pain may precede and accompany the bubo. The spread of disease is not stopped by the lymph nodes and hence bacteraemia occurs.

Septicaemic Plague

The presence of bacteria in the blood denotes septicaemic plague. Massive involvement of blood vessels occurs resulting in haemorrhages in the skin and mucosa. This manifestation is responsible for the disease being given the name **'black death'**.

Pneumonic Plague

Bacterial emboli may become trapped in the lungs causing pneumonic plague. It gives an added dimension to the disease since it can be transmitted from man-to-man by droplet infection (airborne route). Pneumonic plague may also occur in epidemic form. Patient develops fever, 40°C or more, and cough with expectoration. The sputum at first is mucoid and blood-tinged later. It is loaded with *Y. pestis*. Patient complains of severe chest pain, difficult and rapid breathing. Towards the end, patient develops cyanosis and circulatory failure. Those who develop pneumonic plague die within 2–3 days if not treated vigorously.

Death rate from bubonic plague is 50–75%, from pneumonic plague almost 100% and with treatment it is 5–30%.

Laboratory Diagnosis

The diagnosis of plague can be confirmed by demonstrating *Y. pestis* in stained films from bubos in bubonic plague or in sputum in pneumonic plague. In septicaemic plague, the bacilli may be demonstrated in blood cultures or from spleen on postmortem.

Bubonic Plague

- Puncture the bubo with a hypodermic syringe and draw the exudate for examination.
- Prepare the films of the exudate and stain by Gram staining and methylene blue. Characteristic Gram-negative coccobacilli and bacilli showing bipolar staining with methylene blue are suggestive of plague bacilli.
- Culture the exudate on blood agar plate, incubate at 27°C. Pick up single colony and subculture to obtain a pure growth. Carry out biochemical tests to confirm the diagnosis.
- Inoculate guinea pigs or white rats subcutaneously with exudate from bubo or with 24 hours broth culture. Infected animals die in 2–5 days. Postmortem reveals marked local inflammatory condition at the site of inoculation, with necrosis and oedema. Regional lymph nodes are enlarged and congested and may show greyish-white patches in the tissue. Prepare films from local lesions, lymph nodes, spleen and heart blood. Stain films with Gram and methylene blue stains and examine under microscope for characteristic *Y. pestis*.

Pneumonic Plague

- Prepare films from sputum and stain by Gram and methylene blue stains. Examine stained films microscopically for characteristic Gram-negative and bipolar stained coccobacilli respectively.
- Inoculate on blood agar and proceed further as in case of bubonic plague.
- Inoculate sputum into guinea pigs or rats by applying the sputum to the nasal mucosa or to a shaved area of skin. The plague bacilli can enter through microabrasions caused by shaving while other organisms in sputum cannot. Carry out postmortem as in case of bubonic plague.

Key Points

- *Yersinia pestis* is a natural pathogen of rodents causing *zoonotic disease* called **plague**.
- In man plague occurs in 3 forms – *bubonic*, *septicaemic* and *pneumonic*.
- In smears from tissues stained with methylene blue, *Y. pestis* shows characteristic **bipolar staining** in which the ends of the bacilli stain darker than the central part.

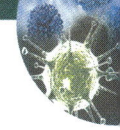

? ASSESS YOURSELF

LONG AND SHORT ANSWER QUESTIONS

1. Discuss pathogenesis of plague.
2. Write short notes on:
   - (a) Bubonic plague
   - (b) Pneumonic plague
   - (c) Septicaemic plague

MULTIPLE CHOICE QUESTIONS

1. In *Yersinia pestis*, capsule is best demonstrated in cultures grown at:
   - (a) 22°C
   - (b) 27°C
   - (c) 37°C
   - (d) 42°C
2. Which of the following agents can cause plague?
   - (a) *Yersinia pestis*
   - (b) *Y. pseudotuberculosis*
   - (c) *Y. enterocolitica*
   - (d) *Pasteurella multocida*
3. Plague is transmitted by:
   - (a) Sandflies
   - (b) Rat fleas
   - (c) Mites
   - (d) Ticks
4. The name 'black death' is given to which of the following diseases?
   - (a) Tuberculosis
   - (b) Black water fever
   - (c) Plague
   - (d) AIDS
5. Bubonic plague can be diagnosed in the laboratory by:
   - (a) Demonstration of Gram-negative coccobacilli
   - (b) Culture on blood agar
   - (c) Inoculation in guinea pigs
   - (d) All of the above

ANSWERS TO MCQs

1. c   **2.** a   **3.** b   **4.** c   **5.** d

Vibrio cholerae

VIBRIO CHOLERAE

Morphology

These are short, curved or comma-shaped rods with rounded or pointed ends and 1.5–2.5 × 0.5–0.8 μm in size. S forms or spirals may be seen due to two or more cells lying end-to-end (Fig. 24.1). They show vigorous **darting motility** which is mediated by a single polar flagellum. They are Gram-negative, non-sporing, non-capsulated and non-acid-fast.

Cultural Characteristics

V. cholerae is aerobe and facultative anaerobe. It grows within a temperature range of 16–40°C (optimum temperature 37°C). Growth occurs freely between pH 7.4 and 9.6 (optimum pH 8.2).

- On **nutrient agar**, after overnight incubation at 37°C, the colonies are glistening translucent discs, 1–2 mm in diameter with bluish or greenish tinge in transmitted light.
- On **MacConkey agar**, they are smaller than those on nutrient agar and are colourless, but become reddish on prolonged incubation due to the late fermentation of lactose.
- On **blood agar**, classical biotype does not produce haemolysis although some strains produce greenish discolouration

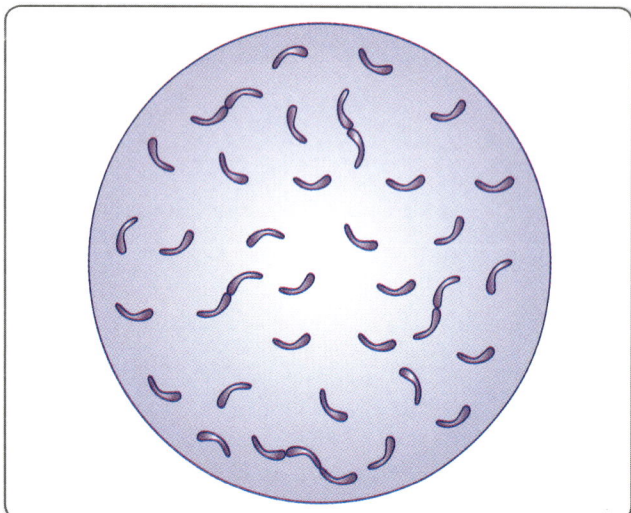

Fig. 24.1: *Vibrio cholerae.*

around individual colonies which later becomes clear due to haemodigestion. However, colonies of El Tor biotype are haemolytic.

Special Media

A number of special culture media have been employed for the cultivation of *V. cholerae*. They may be classified as under:

Transport (Holding) Media

- **Venkatraman-Ramakrishnan (VR) medium:** It is prepared by dissolving 20 g crude sea salt and 5 g prepared in 1 litre of distilled water and pH is adjusted to 8.6–8.8. It is dispensed in screw-capped bottles in 10–15 ml amounts. About 1–3 g of stool is added to each bottle. *V. cholerae* does not multiply in this medium but remains viable for several weeks. Moreover, it prevents overgrowth by other organisms.
- **Cary-Blair medium:** This medium is a buffered solution of disodium hydrogen phosphate, sodium thioglycollate, sodium chloride and calcium chloride at pH 8.4.
- If a transport medium is not available, a 5 × 1.5 cm strip of **thick blotting paper** can be soaked in the faecal matter, then placed in a sealed plastic bag, and sent to the laboratory.

Enrichment Media

- **Alkaline peptone water (APW):** This medium contains 1% each of peptone and sodium chloride at pH 8.6. It is particularly useful when low concentrations of organisms, in the specimen, are anticipated (e.g. in convalescent stage of the disease). High pH of the medium suppresses the growth of many commensal intestinal bacteria while permitting uninhibited growth of *V. cholerae*. Subcultures on plating media should be done within 3–6 hours because other organisms can begin to overgrow after prolonged incubation. APW is also an excellent transport medium. About 1–3 g of the stool or a rectal swab should be placed into 10 ml of APW in a screw-capped tube and transported to the laboratory.
- **Monsur's taurocholate tellurite peptone water:** Place about 1–3 g stool or a rectal swab in this medium and transport to the laboratory. Subculture a loopful onto a selective plating

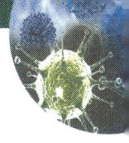

medium within 6–8 hours at ambient temperature. Also incubate it overnight at 37°C and subculture again on a plating medium next day.

Plating Media

These include:

- **Alkaline bile salt agar (BSA) pH 8.2:** This is modified nutrient agar medium containing 0.5% sodium taurocholate (bile salt). The colonies on BSA are similar to those on nutrient agar medium.
- **Monsur's gelatin taurocholate trypticase tellurite agar (GTTA) medium:** This medium is useful for the isolation of cholera and other vibrios from faeces. High (8.5) pH and potassium tellurite, in this medium, are inhibitory to most enterobacteria (except *Proteus*) and Gram-positive bacteria. After 24 hours incubation, vibrios produce small (1–2 mm) translucent colonies with greyish-black centre and a turbid halo, due to hydrolysis and denaturation of gelatin.
- **Thiosulphate citrate bile sucrose (TCBS) agar:** This is most widely used selective plating medium for isolation of vibrios. This medium resembles DCA except that it has the high pH value of 8.6 and contains sucrose instead of lactose. Sucrose-fermenting vibrios such as *V. cholerae* form yellow colonies and non-sucrose-fermenters such as *V. parahaemolyticus* produce blue green colonies.

Biochemical Reactions

V. cholerae is strongly indole positive and reduces nitrates to nitrites. These two properties contribute to the '**cholera red reaction**', the development of a red colour when concentrated sulphuric acid is added to a 4-day-old culture at 37°C in peptone water. It is due to the formation of **nitrosoindole** which is red in colour. It ferments glucose, sucrose, mannitol, maltose and mannose with the production of acid but no gas and ferments lactose only after several days (late lactose-fermenter). Arabinose and dulcitol are not fermented.

It is catalase and oxidase-positive, methyl red and urease negative and liquefies gelatin. Voges-Proskauer reaction and haemolysis of sheep RBCs are positive in El Tor biotype and both these reactions are negative in classical biotype. The differences between classical and El Tor biotypes of *V. cholerae* are shown in Table 24.1.

Susceptibility to Physical and Chemical Agents

Vibrios are killed by heating at 56°C for 30 minutes. They are sensitive to common disinfectants, drying and a pH less than 5. They die within minutes when exposed to normal gastric juices. They survive for 1–2 weeks in clean, non-acid, fresh or sea water. In grossly contaminated water, such as the Ganges water in India, the vibrios do not survive for any length of time. This is perhaps

TABLE 24.1: Differences between classical and El Tor biotypes of *Vibrio cholerae*

Property	Biotype	
	Classical	**El Tor**
Voges-Proskauer test	–	+
Agglutination of fowl RBCs	–	+
Haemolysis of sheep RBCs	–	+
Sensitivity to:		
• Polymyxin B	+	–
• Mukherjee's group IV phage	+	–
• Basu and Mukherjee's group V phage	–	+

due to the presence of a large number of vibriophages in this water. They survive in clean tap water for 30 days. On fruits, they survive for 1–5 days at room temperature and for a week in the refrigerator. In general, the El Tor vibrio has been found to be hardier and more capable of surviving in the environment.

Antigenic Structure

V. cholerae possesses at least 139 different O antigens on the basis of which it has been divided into corresponding number of serogroups or serovars. All strains share a common, heat-labile flagellar (H) antigen. Epidemic cholera is caused by *V. cholerae* serogroup O1 and *V. cholerae* O139 Bengal. Both classical and El Tor biotypes, belong to serogroup O1. They are agglutinated by *V. cholerae* O1 antiserum.

Two recognized serogroups of *V. cholerae* which are choleragenic are serogroups O1 and O139. The serogruops O2–O138 are known as non-O1 vibrios, non-cholera vibrios (NCV) or non-agglutinable (NAG) vibrios because they are not agglutinated by O1 antiserum. However, they are readily agglutinated by their own antisera. From time to time, they have been associated with outbreaks of diarrhoeal or choleraic disease. Both *V. cholerae* O1 and O139 produce enterotoxin (cholera toxin). Some strains of NCV also produce an enterotoxin similar to the cholera toxin.

O1 serogroup can be further subdivided into three subtypes, Ogawa, Inaba and Hikojima. This is on the basis of differences in minor O antigens (A, B and C). Antigen A is present in all the three subtypes. O antigens present in Ogawa, Inaba and Hikojima are A and B, A and C, and A, B and C respectively (Table 24.2). Ogawa and Inaba strains agglutinate with their specific absorbed antisera, while Hikojima strains which are rare are agglutinated by both Ogawa and Inaba antisera.

Pathogenesis

V. cholerae O1 causes an acute diarrhoeal disease known as **cholera**. It occurs only in man. The vibrios enter orally by the ingestion of faecally contaminated food or drink. After passing

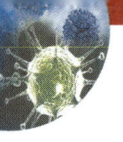

TABLE 24.2: Subtypes of *Vibrio cholerae* O1

Subtypes	Antigens
Ogawa	A and B
Inaba	A and C
Hikojima	A, B and C

the acid barrier of the stomach, they multiply in the alkaline contents of the small intestine and produce a potent toxin known as cholera toxin (CT), cholera enterotoxin or choleragen. It resembles heat-labile toxin-I (LT-I) of *Escherichia coli* chemically, antigenically and in its mode of action.

CT is a heat-labile multimeric protein, inactivated by heating at 56°C for 30 minutes. It has a molecular weight of 85,600. It consists of a single A (active) subunit of molecular weight 27,215 and five B (binding) subunits each of molecular weight 11,677.

The B subunit binds specifically to the Gm_1 ganglioside receptor on the cell lining of the villi and crypts of the small intestine. The active subunit is cleaved to subunits A1 and A2. The A2 subunit links the active A1 to the B subunits. The A2 subunit then facilitates the entrance of the A1 subunit. Once inside the cell, the active A1 subunit stimulates the production of adenyl cyclase. This leads to accumulation of cyclic adenosine monophosphate (cAMP) along the cell membrane, which stimulates hypersecretion of the electrolytes (Na^+, K^+, HCO) and water out of the cell and into the lumen of intestine, resulting in the massive outpouring of watery stools.

Laboratory Diagnosis

Collection of Specimen

- Fresh faecal material should be collected as early in the disease process as possible before the administration of antibiotics. It is best collected by inserting a sterile soft rubber catheter (No. 24–26) and letting the liquid stool flow directly into a sterile screw-capped container.
- A rectal swab may also be collected. It is particularly useful for collecting specimen from a convalescent who no longer has watery diarrhoea. Collection of stool from a bedpan should be avoided because of the risk of contamination or the presence of disinfectants.
- Culture of vomitus may yield the growth of the organisms particularly in the early stages of disease.

Transportation and Enrichment

The cultures should be put up immediately. If it is not possible, then the specimen should be preserved in a suitable transport (holding) medium such as VR medium or Cary-Blair medium for long periods. If the specimen can reach the laboratory within a few hours, it may be transported in enrichment media such as APW or Monsur's taurocholate tellurite peptone water, thus saving the time required for isolation. As discussed above,

if transport media are not available, a 5 × 1.5 cm strip of thick blotting paper can be soaked in the watery stool and sent to the laboratory packed in a plastic envelope.

Culture

In the laboratory, the sample should be plated both directly and after enrichment culture, onto suitable solid media. Early in the choleraic infection, *V. cholerae* are present in very large numbers (10^7–10^9/ml) in the diarrhoeal stool, so direct plating on non-selective media might well be sufficient for the isolation of these organisms. At later stage of infection, and if antibiotics have been given, the number of *V. cholerae* in the stools will be relatively less, therefore, both enrichment and selective plating media should be used to prevent overgrowth by other intestinal bacteria.

- Inoculate 2 g faeces in 20 ml APW. Also inoculate non-selective culture media like 5% sheep blood agar and MacConkey agar and a selective medium like TCBS or GTTA. Incubate these media at 37°C.
- After 3–6 hours incubation, subculture a loopful from the surface of the APW onto a second plate of selective medium. The inoculated plates are examined after overnight incubation at 37°C. On MacConkey medium, they form translucent colonies, on GTTA medium they form translucent colonies with greyish-black centre and a turbid halo and on TCBS, they form yellow colonies. Do the Gram staining from the suspected colonies and look for Gram-negative curved or comma-shaped rods. Perform motility and oxidase tests. Cholera vibrios show characteristic motility and are oxidase-positive.
- Pick up oxidase-positive colonies with a straight wire and test by slide agglutination with *V. cholerae* O1 antiserum. If positive, the test is repeated using monospecific Ogawa and Inaba antisera. Hikojima strains will agglutinate well with both Ogawa and Inaba antisera. If agglutination is negative with one colony, repeat the test with at least five more colonies as O1 and non-O1 vibrios may co-exist in the same specimen. When the isolated strain is not agglutinated by *V. cholerae* O1 antiserum, it should be tested for agglutination with *V. cholerae* H antiserum. Any vibrio which is agglutinated by H antiserum and not by O1 antiserum is considered to be serogroup O2–O138, because H antigen is shared by all serogroups of *V. cholerae*. It should then be tested with other O antisera to establish their identity as belonging to one of O2–O138 serogroups.
- For determination of the biotype of the O1 isolate, do VP test, agglutination of fowl RBCs, haemolysis of sheep RBCs, and sensitivity to polymyxin B, Mukherjee phages IV and V (Table 24.1).

Rapid Diagnosis

For rapid diagnosis, the characteristic motility of the vibrio and its inhibition by antiserum can be demonstrated under the dark-

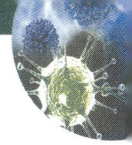

field or phase-contrast microscope, using stool from acute cases or more reliably after enrichment for 6 hours.

Treatment

Oral Rehydration Therapy

Death in cholera is caused by loss of fluids. Therefore, the mortality rate of cholera can be reduced to less than 1% by the adequate replacement of fluids and electrolytes. The more serious cases require immediate intravenous rehydration, but otherwise **oral rehydration therapy (ORT)** will suffice.

Antibiotics

Antibiotics, particularly tetracycline, which reduce the number of intestinal vibrios should be used along with fluid replacement. Administration of 500 mg of tetracycline six hourly for three days to an adult patient, curtails excretion of live vibrios and reduces the carrier rate.

Prophylaxis

General Measures

General measures for control of cholera are:
- Provision of safe water supply.
- Proper disposal of human faeces.
- Handling of food hygienically.
- Periodic examination of food handlers that they are not carriers.
- Improvement of the nutrition of the inhabitants of cholera-prone regions. (This decreases susceptibility to infection by ensuring a more frequent secretion of gastric acid and offers a greater resistance to the disease process among those who become infected.)

Vaccines

Following vaccines are available:

Killed Whole Organism Vaccine

It is killed suspension containing 8000 million *V. cholerae* per ml, composed of equal numbers of Ogawa and Inaba serotypes. In order to improve the antigenic stimulus, the number of organisms in the vaccine may be increased to 12,000 million per ml. Two injections are given at an interval of four weeks.

Non-living Oral B Subunit-whole Cell (BS-WC) Vaccine

This vaccine contains CT subunit B, 2.5×10^{10} heat killed vibrios each of Ogawa and Inaba serotypes of classical biotype and equal number of formalin killed vibrios each of Ogawa and Inaba serotypes of El Tor biotype.

Live Vaccine

Recombinant DNA vaccine with expression of *V. cholerae* O1 in attenuated strain of *S.* serotype Typhi Ty21a as a carrier bacterium has been developed. The live salmonellae colonize the Peyer's patches of the small intestine and induce IgA response by local immune system of the gut. Live attenuated oral vaccine against *V. cholerae* O139 is also available in some countries.

V. CHOLERAE NON-O1

V. cholerae serogroups O2–O138 are known as *V. cholerae* non-O1, NCV or NAG vibrios. They resemble *V. cholerae* O1 biochemically and genetically. They occur widely in aquatic environments. They may produce enterotoxins, cytotoxins, haemolysins and colonizing factors. Exposure to saline environments or consumption of seafoods may lead to infection with these organisms. They may cause mild to severe diarrhoeal disease resembling cholera. Occasionally, they may lead to bloody diarrhoea, accompanied by abdominal cramps. In addition, they may cause extraintestinal infections such as wound infections, septicaemia and meningitis.

HALOPHILIC VIBRIOS

Vibrios that grow best in media with about 3% sodium chloride, can grow in media containing up to 7–10% sodium chloride and cannot grow in media lacking sodium chloride are known as halophilic vibrios. Their natural habitat is sea water and marine life. V. parahaemolyticus, V. alginolyticus and V. vulnificus are three important species of halophilic vibrios.

Key Points

- Vibrios are small **comma-shaped, Gram-negative, oxidase-positive** bacteria that prefer an alkaline growth environment.
- *Vibrio cholerae* is the major pathogen in the genus and is **responsible for cholera epidemics**, especially in the developing world.
- *V. cholerae* adheres to enterocytes and produces cholera enterotoxin.
- **Epidemic cholera** is caused by *V. cholerae* serogroup O1 and *V. cholerae* O139 Bengal.

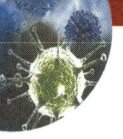

? ASSESS YOURSELF

LONG ANSWER QUESTIONS

1. Discuss various culture media for the isolation of *Vibrio cholerae*.
2. Discuss the antigenic structure of *Vibrio cholerae*.
3. Discuss pathogenesis of cholera.

MULTIPLE CHOICE QUESTIONS

1. Which of the following media can serve as transport medium for *Vibrio cholerae*?
   - (a) Selenite F broth
   - (b) Tetrathionate broth
   - (c) Venkatraman-Ramakrishnan medium
   - (d) Nutrient broth

2. The colonies of *Vibrio cholerae* and *V. parahaemolyticus* can be differentiated on:
   - (a) Thiosulphate citrate bile sucrose agar
   - (b) Alkaline bile salt agar
   - (c) MacConkey medium
   - (d) Lowenstein-Jensen medium

3. Cholera toxin resembles which of the following toxins?
   - (a) Labile toxin-1 of *Escherichia coli*
   - (b) Stable toxin of *E. coli*
   - (c) Diphtheria toxin
   - (d) Tetanus toxin

4. Stools from suspected cholera cases can be transported to the laboratory in:
   - (a) Venkatraman-Ramakrishnan medium
   - (b) Cary-Blair medium
   - (c) Thick blotting paper
   - (d) All of the above

5. On the basis of which of the following antigens *Vibrio cholerae* is divided into various serogroups or serovars?
   - (a) O antigen
   - (b) H antigen
   - (c) Vi antigen
   - (d) K antigen

ANSWERS TO MCQs

1. c   **2.** a   **3.** a   **4.** d   **5.** a

Chapter 25

Pseudomonas

PSEUDOMONAS AERUGINOSA

Morphology

It is a slender, Gram-negative bacillus, 1.5–3.0 × 0.5 μm, actively motile by a polar flagellum. Occasional strains have two or three flagella. Clinical isolates often possess pili. It is non-capsulated but many strains have a mucoid slime layer. Mucoid strains, particularly isolates from cystic fibrosis patients, have an abundance of polysaccharide composed of alginate polymer. This forms a loose capsule in which microcolonies of the bacillus are enmeshed and protected from host defences.

Cultural Characteristics

It is a strict aerobe and grows well on ordinary media. It can grow over a temperature range of 5–42°C, the optimum temperature being 37°C.

Nutrient Agar

After aerobic incubation on nutrient agar at 37°C for 24 hours, the colonies are large, 2–3 mm in diameter, smooth, translucent, irregularly round and emit a characteristic fruity odour.

MacConkey Medium

It forms non-lactose fermenting colonies.

Blood Agar

Many strains are haemolytic on blood agar medium.

Nutrient Broth

It produces a dense turbidity and surface pellicle.

Pigment Production

P. aeruginosa produces at least 4 distinct pigments:
1. **Pyocyanin:** It is a bluish-green phenazine pigment soluble in chloroform and water. It diffuses into the surrounding medium. This pigment is not produced by other species of this genus, therefore, its detection is diagnostic of *P. aeruginosa*.
2. **Pyoverdin (fluorescein):** It imparts a yellowish tinge to cultures.
3. **Pyorubrin:** It is a bright red water soluble pigment.
4. **Pyomelanin:** It is a brown to black pigment.

Biochemical Reactions

P. aeruginosa derives energy from carbohydrates by an oxidative rather than a fermentative metabolism. Because the amount of acid produced by oxidative pathways is less than that produced by fermentation, special media such as the O-F medium of Hugh and Leifson must be used for diagnostic tests. It utilizes glucose oxidatively with the production of acid only. Lactose and maltose are not utilized. Indole, MR, VP and H_2S tests are negative. All strains are **oxidase-positive within 30 seconds**. This is a useful preliminary test for identification of non-pigmented strains. None of the other oxidase-positive, Gram-negative bacilli reacts as swiftly as *P. aeruginosa*. It reduces nitrates to nitrites and further to gaseous nitrogen. It is catalase, arginine dihydrolase and gelatinase positive and lysine decarboxylase and aesculin hydrolysis negative.

Sensitivity to Physical and Chemical Agents

P. aeruginosa is killed by heating at 55°C for one hour. It is very resistant to chemical disinfectants and can even grow in certain types of quaternary ammonium compounds, hexachlorophene soaps and iodine solutions. Therefore, dettol and cetrimide can be incorporated in selective media for isolation of *Pseudomonas*. It is sensitive to a 2% aqueous alkaline solution of glutaraldehyde (cidex).

Bacteriocin (Pyocin) Typing

Typing of *P. aeruginosa* based on pyocin production is the most popular method for typing *P. aeruginosa*. The most widely used method is the one described by Gillies and Govan (1966) and later modified by Govan and Gillies (1969). The test strain is inoculated as a one cm wide band across the tryptone soya blood agar plate, incubated overnight at 32°C for pyocin production. The resultant growth is removed by scraping with a sterile glass slide. The residual growth is killed by exposure to chloroform

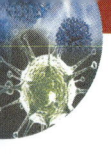

vapours and eight indicator strains (numbers 1–8) are cross-streaked in parallel lines at right angles to the original inoculum followed by incubation at 37°C for 24 hours.

The pattern of inhibition of the indicator strains determines the type of the strain. Further discrimination among the members of the more frequent types (1, 3, 5, 10 and untypable) can be obtained by subtyping with five additional indicator (A–E) strains. Pyocin typing is easy to perform, results are available by the third day and has a reasonable reproducibility and good discrimination.

Pathogenesis

P. aeruginosa causes:

- Urinary tract infection when it is mechanically placed into the urinary tract during catheterization.
- Acute purulent meningitis when it is mechanically placed into the meninges during a lumbar puncture or after cranial injury.
- It is able to multiply on respiratory ventilators and deliver large numbers of organisms directly into the lungs of an already debilitated person leading to respiratory infections like necrotizing pneumonia.
- Septicaemia may develop in persons with leukaemia or persons receiving immunosuppressive drugs and in newborn babies and old debilitated persons.

- In drug addicts, it may cause endocarditis and septic arthritis.
- In addition, it may cause wound and burn infection, chronic otitis media and otitis externa, and eye infection.

Laboratory Diagnosis

Specimens

The specimens to be collected include pus, wound swab, urine, sputum, CSF or blood. The specimens may be inoculated on MacConkey agar and blood agar. It may be necessary to use selective media such as cetrimide agar for isolation of *P. aeruginosa* from faeces or other samples with mixed flora such as wound swab. The isolates are identified by their colonial morphology and biochemical characters. The typing of the organisms may be carried out by pyocin typing.

Treatment

P. aeruginosa is intrinsically resistant to most commonly employed antimicrobial agents. Many strains are, however, susceptible to carbenicillin, azlocillin, ticarcillin, cefotaxime, ceftazidime, gentamicin and tobramycin. Ciprofloxacin exhibits good activity against *P. aeruginosa* and penetrates well into most tissues. Since this can be given orally, therefore, it may be used if therapy has to be prolonged. However, resistance to ciprofloxacin may sometimes develop during therapy.

Key Points

- *Pseudomonas aeruginosa* differs from members of the family Enterobacteriaceae by deriving energy from carbohydrates by an **oxidative rather than a fermentative metabolism**.
- *Pseudomonas aeruginosa* causes urinary tract infection, acute purulent meningitis, respiratory infections, and wound and burn infection.

? ASSESS YOURSELF

SHORT ANSWER QUESTION

Write short notes on:

    (a) Pathogenicity of *Pseudomonas aeruginosa*

    (b) Bacteriocin (pyocin) typing of *Pseudomonas aeruginosa*

MULTIPLE CHOICE QUESTIONS

1. Which of the following pigments is diagnostic of *Pseudomonas aeruginosa*?

    (a) Pyocyanin

    (c) Pyomelanin

    (b) Pyoverdin

    (d) Pyorubrin

Contd...

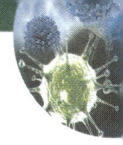

? ASSESS YOURSELF

2. Which is the most popular method for typing of *Pseudomonas aeruginosa*?

(a) Pyocin typing

(b) Serotyping

(c) Bacteriophage typing

(d) Antibiogram typing

3. Which of the following infections can be caused by *Pseudomonas aeruginosa*?

(a) Urinary tract infection

(h) Wound and burn infection

(c) Respiratory tract infection

(d) All of the above

4. Many strains of *Pseudomonas aeruginosa* are susceptible to:

(a) Ceftazidime

(b) Tobramycin

(c) Ticarcillin

(d) All of the above

ANSWERS TO MCQs

1. a   **2.** a   **3.** d   **4.** d

Haemophilus influenzae and Bordetella pertussis

HAEMOPHILUS INFLUENZAE

Morphology

H. influenzae is a slender, short, (1.5 × 0.3 μm) non-motile, non-sporing, non-acid-fast, Gram-negative rod or coccobacillus. In some cultures and occasionally in clinical material, longer filamentous forms may be seen often in association with large, spherical or fusiform bodies, 2–3 μm in diameter. A few more virulent strains possess capsule. It can be demonstrated by **India ink wet films** and by **Quellung reaction** with type-specific antiserum. In Gram-stained direct smear the capsule appears as clear, **nonstaining area (halo) surrounding the organism** in purulent secretions.

Cultural Characteristics

H. influenzae grows better in aerobic than in anaerobic conditions. Some strains require extra (5–10%) CO_2. The temperature range for growth is 20–42°C, the optimum temperature being 35–37°C. It has fastidious growth requirements. Accessory growth factors known as X and V, present in blood, are essential for its growth. Therefore, it can grow on blood agar and not on nutrient agar which lacks sufficient amount of them.

- **X factor:**
  It is heat-stable porphyrin IX, haemin or other iron-containing porphyrin. It is necessary for the synthesis of cytochrome and other haem enzymes such as catalase and peroxidase involved in aerobic respiration.

- **V factor:**
  V factor is a heat-labile (at 121°C for 30 minutes) factor present in red blood cells and in many other animal and plant cells. It is synthesized by most bacterial species other than *H. influenzae*. It is either nicotinamide adenine dinucleotide (NAD, coenzyme I) or NAD phosphate (NADP, coenzyme II) or certain unidentified precursors of these compounds. It is essential for the oxidation-reduction processes in the growing bacterial cell.

Both X and V factors are found within red blood cells including the sheep erythrocytes in sheep blood agar used in clinical laboratories. Sheep blood also contains NADase activity that slowly hydrolyses V factor. Therefore, ordinary blood agar is not suitable for the growth of *H. influenzae* where it forms only pinpoint colonies. Heating blood agar at 80–90°C until it acquires a chocolate colour, results in lysis of erythrocytes, liberation of both X and V factors and inactivation of NADase enzyme that hydrolyses V factor. Most laboratories rely on chocolate agar for the recovery of *Haemophilus* species from clinical specimens.

When an organism, such as *Staphylococcus aureus* is streaked across a plate of blood agar on which a specimen containing *H. influenzae* has been inoculated, after overnight incubation, the colonies of *H. influenzae* will be large and well developed alongside the streak of *S. aureus*, and smaller farther away (Fig. 26.1). This phenomenon is known as **satellitism**. The lysed erythrocytes in the agar surrounding the *S. aureus* streak provide X factor, and staphylococcal cells themselves secrete V factor during logarithmic growth. The 'Staphylococcus streak' technique can be used to recover *Haemophilus* species from clinical specimens.

Good growth is also obtained on certain transparent media where red cells have been disrupted and NADase enzyme inactivated either by peptic digest (Fildes' agar) or heat (Levinthal's agar). These media are useful for demonstrating capsulated strain, colonies of which are iridescent when viewed obliquely with transmitted light. Type b capsulavted strains can also be detected by the presence of precipitin haloes on transparent media containing hyperimmune *H. influenzae* type b antiserum.

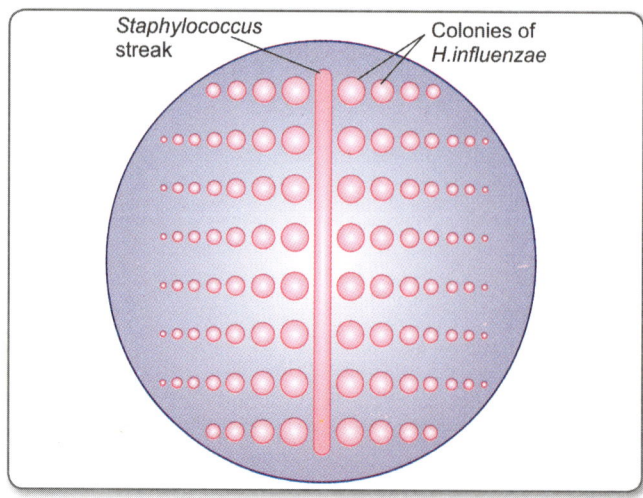

Fig. 26.1: Satellite growth of *Haemophilus influenzae*.

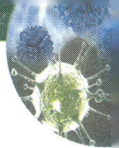

Biochemical Reactions

H. influenzae is catalase-positive, oxidase-positive, reduces nitrate to nitrite and ferments glucose and galactose. It does not ferment sucrose, lactose and mannitol.

Antigenic Structure

Three major surface antigens are present in *H. influenzae* – capsular polysaccharide, outer membrane protein (OMP) and lipooligosaccharide (LOS). Capsular polysaccharide antigen is the major antigenic determinant of capsulated *H. influenzae*, on the basis of which strains of *H. influenzae* have been classified by Pittman into six capsular types – a to f. Most infections are caused by *H. influenzae* strains belonging to capsular serotype b (Hib). These strains are associated with rapidly progressive and even life-threatening infections. The type b capsular serotype is a polymer of ribose, ribitol and phosphate, or polyribosyl-ribitol-phosphate (PRP).

The OMP antigen shows considerable variation. These antigens of Hib have been classified into at least 13 subtypes. *H. influenzae* lipooligosaccharides are antigenically complex.

Serotyping of *H. influenzae* is done by agglutination or Quellung reaction (swelling of capsule) with type-specific antisera.

Sensitivity to Physical and Chemical Agents

H. influenzae is a delicate organism. It is readily killed by moist heat (at 55°C in 30 minutes), refrigeration (4°C), drying and disinfectants. It also dies in 1–48 hours in dried secretions and airborne droplet-nuclei.

Pathogenesis

H. influenzae is an obligate human parasite. Twenty five to eighty per cent of healthy adults harbour non-capsulate organisms in the nasopharynx and oropharynx. Colonization by capsulate strains is seen in 5–10%, of which capsular type b strains are found in 1–5%. *H. influenzae* causes invasive and non-invasive infections. The former are caused by capsulate strains, type b accounting for the most cases, and the latter by non-capsulate strains.

Invasive Infections

Meningitis

Hib is a common cause of paediatric meningitis with case fatality rate of about 90% in the untreated. It tends to occur in children of 2 months to 2 years of age. Prior nasopharyngeal colonization in a susceptible host leads to invasion of the blood stream and subsequent seeding of the meninges. Onset of meningeal symptoms may be abrupt or more commonly insidious.

Epiglottitis

Hib is the most common cause of epiglottitis. It tends to occur in slightly older children, having a peak incidence between 2 and 4 years of age. In this case, an apparently healthy child develops acute obstructive laryngeal oedema which may need immediate tracheostomy and vigorous administration of antimicrobial and supportive therapy. The epiglottis is usually markedly swollen, red and oedematous. This condition is always associated with bacteraemia and Hib can be recovered from blood cultures in more than 97% of cases.

Pneumonia

Haemophilus pneumonia typically occurs in infants and is accompanied by empyema and sometimes meningitis. It is caused by capsulate strains.

Septic Arthritis

The bacteraemic spread of Hib is the most common cause of arthritis seen in children younger than 2 years of age.

Non-invasive Infections

H. influenzae produces a number of local infections which are usually associated with some underlying anatomical or physiological abnormality. These include otitis media, sinusitis, chronic bronchitis and bronchiectasis.

Laboratory Diagnosis

Specimen Collection and Transportation

Depending upon the type of lesion, *H. influenzae* can be detected in cerebrospinal fluid (CSF), blood, throat swab, sputum, pus, aspirates from joints, middle ears or sinuses, etc. *As haemophili are poorly viable in clinical specimens particularly at 4°C, therefore, the specimens should never be refrigerated. For optimal yield, specimens should be transported to the laboratory and seeded onto appropriate culture media without delay.*

Direct Examination

- **Gram-stained smear** of clinical material showing poorly stained Gram-negative coccobacilli and occasionally slender filamentous forms should arouse the suspicion of *H. influenzae* infection.
- **Immunofluorescence** and **Quellung reaction** can be employed for direct demonstration of *H. influenzae* after mixing with specific rabbit antiserum type b.
- **Type b capsular antigen** can be detected in patient serum, urine, CSF or pus by:
  - **Agglutination of latex particles** (LA) coated with rabbit antibody to type b antigen.

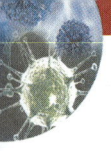

SECTION IV • PATHOGENIC ORGANISMS-I BACTERIA

- ■ **Coagglutination (COA) of** *S. aureus* **coated with antibody to type b antigen**.
- ■ **Counterimmunoelectrophoresis (CIE)** with specific antiserum.

CSF Culture

CSF should be promptly plated on blood agar or chocolate agar. A strain of *S. aureus* should be streaked across the plate. It is then incubated at 35–37°C in air with 5–10% CO_2, overnight. The isolate is identified by its colonial morphology, phenomenon of satellitism, Gram staining, biochemical reactions and serotyping. Culture may also be done on Leventhal's agar and Fildes' agar.

Blood Culture

Blood culture is usually positive in cases of epiglottitis and pneumonia. Culture may be done in nutrient broth, as it will be enriched with X and V factors from the blood sample itself. For early results culture may be examined after 4–5 hours by Quellung reaction. After overnight incubation, subculture is made on chocolate agar and processed further as above.

Throat Swab and Sputum Culture

For the isolation of *H. influenzae* from throat swab and sputum, antibiotics like penicillin, bacitracin and cloxacillin may be added to the medium to inhibit the growth of normal respiratory tract flora. Sputum should be homogenized by treatment with pancreatin or by shaking with sterile water and glass beads for 10–15 minutes.

Prophylaxis

- A purified type b capsular polysaccharide vaccine (Hib PRP vaccine) has shown to stimulate the formation of protective antibodies in children older than 18 months of age.
- PRP is poorly immunogenic in children below two years. Its immunogenicity can be enhanced by coupling with protein carriers like diphtheria and tetanus toxoids or *Neisseria meningitidis* outer membrane protein. Such conjugate Hib PRP are available for use in young children.

BORDETELLA PERTUSSIS

Morphology

B. pertussis is a small, Gram-negative, coccobacillus, measuring $0.5–2.0 \times 0.3–0.5$ µm, arranged singly, in pairs or in small groups. It is non-motile and non-sporing.

Cultural Characteristics

It is an obligate aerobe. No growth occurs anaerobically. The optimum temperature for growth is 35–36°C. It does not require X and V factors for its growth. The preferred medium used for isolation of *B. pertussis* is **charcoal blood agar** to which cephalexin has been added; the antibiotic inhibits other organisms commonly found in specimens and only minimally restricts the growth of *Bordetella* species. This medium is superior to Bordet-Gengou medium in that it supports a heavier growth of the organism on primary isolation, and the colonies are larger. The inoculated medium is incubated at 35–36°C in a humidified incubator. If it is not available, a bowl of water should be placed on the floor of incubator to provide humidity by evaporation.

Growth of *B. pertussis* is slow. After 3–5 days incubation at 35–36°C, the colonies are small (0.5 mm in diameter), dome-shaped, smooth, opaque, greyish-white with a shiny surface resembling **bisected pearls** or '**mercury drops**'.

Biochemical Reactions

B. pertussis is biochemically inactive. It does not ferment sugars, form indole, reduce nitrates, split urea or utilize citrate. It is weakly oxidase-positive.

Susceptibility to Physical and Chemical Agents

B. pertussis is a delicate organism. It can be killed by heating at 56°C for 30 minutes, drying and disinfectants. Outside the body it can survive for five days on glass, three days on cloth and a few hours on paper.

Pathogenesis

B. pertussis causes the syndrome called pertussis or '**whooping cough**'. All age groups are susceptible but 80% of clinical cases occur in children under the age of ten. *B. pertussis* is an obligate human parasite involving primarily the ciliated epithelial cells of bronchi and trachea. They cause damage to cilia and consequently initiate the irritation that induces increased secretion of mucus which acts as a stimulus for paroxysmal cough and bronchospasm. The source of infection is the patient in the early stage. There is no healthy carrier. The organism is acquired through droplet infection and is highly contagious, with an attack rate of more than 90% in nonimmunized individuals.

Laboratory Diagnosis

Nasopharyngeal aspirate, cough plate, pernasal swab and postnasal swab may be collected.
- **Nasopharyngeal aspirate**
  Nasopharyngeal aspirate collected through a soft catheter is the optimal diagnostic specimen.
- **Cough plate method**
  A culture plate is held about 10–15 cm in front of the patient's mouth during a bout of spontaneous or induced coughing. During the process of coughing, droplets of respiratory exudates are directly deposited on the medium.

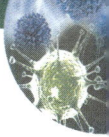

- **Pernasal swab**

  B. pertussis can be recovered readily from the nasopharynx by pernasal swab. A calcium alginate swab on a flexible nichrome wire is passed gently along the floor of the nasal cavity until stopped by the posterior wall of the naso-pharynx. The swab is left in place for 30 seconds to one minute to allow organisms to adsorb onto the swab. Cotton-tipped swab should not be used because cotton is inhibitory to the organisms. Pernasal swab has replaced 'cough plates' and postnasal swabs because of overgrowth by commensal bacteria. A pernasal swab acquires fewer commensals which can be suppressed by incorporation of methicillin or cephalexin in the medium.

- **Postnasal swab**

  A calcium alginate swab on a bent wire is employed to collect posterior pharyngeal wall secretions through oral cavity. West's postnasal swab may be conveniently employed. Contamination with saliva should be avoided for better results. Nasopharyngeal aspirate collected through a soft catheter is a better source. It can be used for polymerase chain reaction also.

The specimen is inoculated immediately on charcoal blood agar to which cephalexin has been added and incubated in high humidity at 35–36°C for at least seven days before being discarded as negative. If cough plate has been collected, it should also be incubated in high humidity at 35–36°C. The colonies are identified by microscopy, biochemical characters and slide agglutination. If delay in transport is unavoidable, then the specimen may be transported in Regan-Lowe transport medium. The use of transport medium reduces the isolation rate. *B. pertussis* in nasopharyngeal secretions and organisms growing on culture plates may be identified by **direct fluorescent antibody test**.

Serology

Bordetella antibody can be detected in the patient serum by direct agglutination, indirect haemagglutination, complement fixation test and ELISA. However, a negative result does not exclude pertussis because the serological response is often slow and weak especially in very young children.

Polymerase Chain Reaction (PCR)

PCR is the preferred method for the direct detection of *B. pertussis* and *B. parapertussis* from a nasopharyngeal swab or a nasopharyngeal aspirate.

Prevention

The incidence of whooping cough has been markedly reduced by the introduction of an effective vaccine. It consists of heat-killed or thiomersal-treated phase I organisms that are usually incorporated with diphtheria and tetanus toxoids (commonly called DPT). Three deep intramuscular injections at intervals of 4 weeks should be given from 1½ months of age followed by one injection each of DPT and DT at the age of 16–24 months and 5–6 years, respectively.

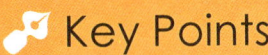

Key Points

- *Bordetella pertussis* **does not require X and V factors** for its growth.
- It causes the syndrome called **pertussis** or **'whooping cough'**.
- **'Whooping cough'** *is preventable by the whole cell vaccine incorporated in the childhood DPT vaccination programme.*

? ASSESS YOURSELF

LONG AND SHORT ANSWER QUESTIONS

1. Discuss pathogenesis and laboratory diagnosis of infections caused by *Haemophilus influenzae*.
2. Write short notes on:
   - (a) Antigenic structure of *Haemophilus influenzae*
   - (b) Pathogenesis and laboratory diagnosis of pertussis

MULTIPLE CHOICE QUESTIONS

1. Which of the following infections is/are caused by *Haemophilus influenzae*?
   - (a) Meningitis
   - (b) Epiglottitis
   - (c) Pneumonia
   - (d) All of the above

Contd...

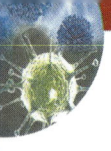

SECTION IV • PATHOGENIC ORGANISMS-I BACTERIA

2. For growth, *Haemophilus influenzae* requires:

   (a) X factor alone
   (b) V factor alone
   (c) Both X and V factors
   (d) Neither X nor V factor

3. *Haemophilus influenzae* shows the phenomenon of satellitism on:

   (a) Blood agar
   (b) Loeffler's serum slope
   (c) Nutrient agar
   (d) Dorset egg medium

4. Which of the following species of *Bordetella* is the most important human pathogen?

   (a) *B. pertussis*
   (b) *B. parapertussis*
   (c) *B. bronchiseptica*
   (d) *B. avium*

5. Which of the following media is employed most frequently for the isolation of *Bordetella pertussis*?

   (a) Blood agar
   (b) Chocolate agar
   (c) Charcoal blood agar
   (d) Nutrient agar

ANSWERS TO MCQS

1. d   **2.** c   **3.** a   **4.** a   **5.** c

Chapter 27

Brucella

Genus *Brucella* has six species:
- *B. melitensis,*
- *B. abortus,*
- *B. suis,*
- *B. canis,*
- *B. ovis,* and
- *B. neotomae.*

B. ovis and *B. neotomae* do not cause disease in man.

MORPHOLOGY

Brucellae are small, Gram-negative, coccobacilli measuring 0.6–1.5 µm in length and 0.5–0.7 µm in width. They are arranged singly, sometimes in end-to-end pairs, small clusters or short chains of 4–6 bacteria. They are non-motile, non-sporing, non-capsulated and non-acid-fast.

CULTURAL CHARACTERISTICS

Brucellae are strict aerobes and many strains of *B. abortus* and nearly all of *B. ovis* are capnophilic, requiring 5–10% CO_2 for growth. The optimum temperature for growth is 37°C (range 20–40°C). The optimum pH for growth is 6.6–7.4. They may grow on nutrient agar, though the growth tends to be slow and colony size small. Growth is improved by the addition of blood, serum and tissue extracts. Trypticase soy agar, serum dextrose agar, serum potato infusion agar and tryptose agar are employed for cultivation of brucellae. Addition of bacitracin, polymyxin and cycloheximide to the above media makes them selective. These can be used for isolation of brucellae from contaminated material. Erythritol has a stimulatory effect on the growth of brucellae.

On solid media they produce small, low convex, circular, smooth, transparent colonies 0.5–1 mm in diameter, after incubation at 37°C for 48 hours. Less fastidious strains, especially of *B. melitensis* and *B. suis* can grow on bile salt media producing non-lactose-fermenting colonies. In liquid media growth is uniform. A powdery or viscous deposit is formed in old cultures.

SUSCEPTIBILITY TO PHYSICAL AND CHEMICAL AGENTS

Brucellae are destroyed by heat at 60°C for 10 minutes, hence in milk they are readily destroyed by pasteurization. They are sensitive to acid and die out in butter and cheese involving lactic acid fermentation. They can survive for three weeks in meat. *B. melitensis* may survive for six days in urine, six weeks in dust and ten weeks in water or soil. *B. abortus* may survive for 75 days in aborted foetuses. They can be killed by 1.0% phenol in 15 minutes.

BIOCHEMICAL REACTIONS

Brucellae are catalase-positive, urease-positive (variable in *B. melitensis*) and usually oxidase-positive but *B. neotomae*, *B. ovis* and some strains of *B. abortus* are oxidase-negative. Most *Brucella* strains reduce nitrates to nitrites.

PATHOGENESIS

Brucellae are capable of causing infection in a wide range of host species, including man. *B. melitensis* is the most pathogenic species for man followed by *B. suis*, *B. abortus* and *B. canis*.

Brucellosis is a **zoonosis**. Man acquires infection by:
- Direct contact with animal tissues. Therefore, farmers, dairy workers, abattoir workers, butchers, live stock producers and veterinarians are particularly at risk.
- Ingestion of contaminated meat, raw infected milk or milk products.
- Inhalation of aerosolized organisms.
- In the laboratory, brucellae may be acquired as a result of accidental ingestion, inhalation, injection, and mucosal and skin contamination.

After entering into the body, brucellae enter into the lymphatics and lymph nodes, leading to **lymphadenopathy** and subsequent blood stream invasion. From the blood, the organisms are localized in the reticuloendothelial system particularly in liver sinusoids, spleen and bone marrow. However, they may also localize in many other sites like joints, heart, kidneys, central nervous system and genital tract. Intracellular organisms are protected from antibodies and antibiotics. Cellular immune defence mechanisms are required to contain the intracellular bacteria. Infected tissues may have granulomas, microabscesses and unusually caseation.

Following an incubation period of about three weeks (with a range from one week to six months), the onset of symptoms may be acute or insidious.

Acute Brucellosis

Acute brucellosis is characterized by an intermittent fever with a maximum temperature varying from 38–41°C and sometimes higher. The body temperature is usually near normal during the early part of the day but rises sharply during evening. This is accompanied by chills, shivering, malaise, night sweats, severe headache, myalgias and arthralgias. After reaching its peak the temperature shows a rapid fall, accompanied by profuse sweating.

Chronic Brucellosis

When the disease persists for 6 months or more it is regarded as chronic. It is usually non-bacteraemic low-grade infection with periodic exacerbations. The common manifestations are sweating, lassitude and joint pain with minimal or no pyrexia. The illness lasts for years.

The name '**undulant fever**' has been given to brucellosis because of the periodic noctural fever that may occur over weeks, months or years particularly in untreated cases. Lympha-denopathy, splenomegaly and hepatomegaly may also be present.

LABORATORY DIAGNOSIS

Culture of Brucellae

Five to 10 ml of blood should be inoculated into a bottle of **trypticase soy broth or serum dextrose broth** and incubated at 37°C in an atmosphere containing 5–10% carbon dioxide. Other materials such as **bone marrow, solid tissue samples or exudates** are also suitable for culture. Bone marrow cultures yield a higher rate of isolation and remain positive long after blood culture has become negative.

Subcultures are made every 3–5 days for eight weeks on trypticase soy agar or serum dextrose agar before being discarded as negative. *B. melitensis* and *B. suis* are more frequently isolated from blood than are *B. abortus* or *B. canis*.

The need for frequent subculture can be avoided by use of a two-phase system or **Castaneda method** of blood culture. In this method, both liquid serum dextrose broth and solid serum dextrose agar media are contained within the same bottle (Fig. 27.1). The blood is inoculated into the broth and the bottle incubated in the upright position. For subculture, the bottle is tilted so that the broth flows over the surface of the agar slant. It is again incubated in upright position. In positive cases, colonies

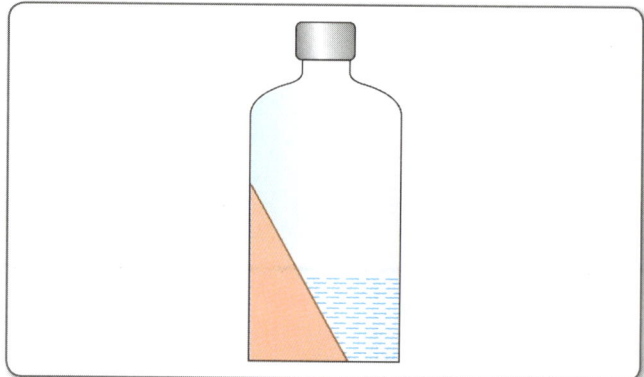

Fig. 27.1: Castaneda blood culture medium.

appear on the slant. This technique reduces the chances of contamination and risk of infection to laboratory personnel.

BACTEC and BacT are rapid methods for blood culture and the positive culture may be obtained within 7 days.

Serological Tests

Brucella antibodies can be detected by a variety of serological tests. The most useful are:

- standard tube agglutination test (SAT),
- 2-mercaptoethanol (2ME) agglutination test,
- complement fixation test,
- anti-human globulin (Coombs') test,
- enzyme-linked immunosorbent assay (ELISA), and
- radioimmunoassay (RIA).

The most widely used procedure is SAT. This is a tube agglutination test in which equal volumes of serial two-fold dilutions of (uninactivated) patient serum from 1 in 20 to 1 in 640 and the standardized antigen (heat-killed smooth *Brucella* cells in saline containing phenol 0.5%) are mixed, and incubated at 37°C for 24 hours. Most patients with acute brucellosis develop agglutinin titres of 640 or more by the end of the third or fourth week of illness. Thereafter the titre falls. A single titre greater than 1 in 160 by SAT is presumptive evidence of recent *Brucella* infection.

ELISA and **RIA** are very sensitive tests and can distinguish IgM, IgG and IgA *Brucella* antibodies. Therefore, these tests are helpful to distinguish acute and chronic brucellosis.

Rose Bengal plate test is a rapid slide agglutination test with a buffered stained antigen. It is widely used as a screening test in farm animals, but also gives good results in human brucellosis. It is not affected by prozones or immunoglobulin switching.

Polymerase Chain Reaction

Polymerase chain reaction with primers specific for the *omp 2*, *omp 25* and *rrs-rrl* genes can detect *Brucella* specifically and also give an indication of species and biovar. Promising results have been obtained in clinical studies.

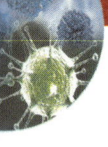

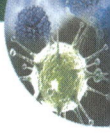

TREATMENT

Brucella infections respond to a combination of rifampicin and doxycycline. Treatment should be continued for 6 weeks. Co-trimoxazole and rifampicin can be used in children.

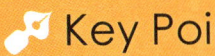

Key Points

- Brucellosis is a **zoonosis**; man acquires infection by direct contact with animal tissues, ingestion of contaminated meat, raw infected milk or milk products, and by inhalation of aerosolized organisms.
- Cellular immune defence mechanisms are required to contain the **intracellular brucellae**.
- Blood culture is the most definitive method for the diagnosis of brucellosis, however, it is positive in only 30–50% of the cases.
- The most useful investigation for serodiagnosis of brucellosis is the **standard tube agglutination test**.
- For the treatment of brucellosis, prolonged use of antibiotics is essential.

Assess Yourself

Long Answer Questions

1. Discuss pathogenesis of brucellosis.
2. Discuss laboratory diagnosis of brucellosis.

Multiple Choice Questions

1. Common reservoir hosts of *Brucella melitensis* are:
   - (a) Sheep and goats
   - (b) Cattle
   - (c) Pigs
   - (d) Rats

2. Which of the following *Brucella* spp. is most pathogenic for man?
   - (a) *B. melitensis*
   - (b) *B. abortus*
   - (c) *B. suis*
   - (d) *B. canis*

3. Brucellae are transmitted to humans by:
   - (a) Direct contact with animal tissues
   - (b) Ingestion of contaminated meat
   - (c) Ingestion of raw infected milk
   - (d) All of the above

ANSWERS TO MCQs

1. a   **2.** a   **3.** d

28 Chapter

Mycoplasma and Ureaplasma

MORPHOLOGY AND GENERAL CHARACTERS

- Mycoplasmas and ureaplasmas are smallest free-living bacteria. They measure 0.2–0.3 µm in diameter. Therefore, they can pass through the bacterial filters.
- Mycoplasma cell contains minimum set of organelles essential for growth and replication – a plasma membrane, ribosomes, and a genome consisting of a double-stranded circular DNA molecule.
- They differ from other bacteria in that they **lack a rigid cell wall** and their cell membrane contains sterols. In contrast, other cell wall-deficient bacteria (called **L forms**) do not have sterols in their cell membrane and can form cell walls under appropriate growth conditions.
- **They cannot synthesize their own cholesterol** and require it as a growth factor in the culture medium.
- Because they lack a rigid cell wall, they are **extremely pleomorphic** varying in shape from coccoid to filamentous and other bizarre forms.
- Also because of the lack of bacterial cell wall containing peptidoglycan, these organisms are **insensitive to cell wall-active antibiotics** such as penicillins and cephalosporins. The mycoplasmas are susceptible to antibiotics, such as tetracyclines and chloramphenicol, that inhibit protein synthesis on prokaryotic ribosomes.
- They possess a **small genome** (molecular weight 5–10 × 10^8 daltons). Therefore, these organisms have limited biosynthetic capabilities.
- They **multiply by binary fission** (typical of all bacteria), grow on artificial cell-free media and contain both RNA and DNA. Cytoplasmic division may lag behind genome replication. This results in the formation of multinucleate filaments and other shapes.
- They **do not possess flagella or pili**, but some myco-plasmas including *M. pneumoniae*, exhibit gliding motility on liquid-covered surfaces. This is attributed to specialized tip structures that also help the organisms in the attachment to the host cell.
- They stain poorly by Gram stain and are Gram-negative. They stain well with Giemsa and Dienes stain.
- The organisms of the genus *Ureaplasma* can hydrolyse urea while other genera cannot do so.
- Most species, on solid media, form characteristic small **'fried egg'** colonies.

CULTURAL CHARACTERISTICS

With the exception of *Anaeroplasma*, the organisms of the order Mycoplasmatales are aerobes and facultative anaerobes. However, for primary isolation, an atmosphere of 95% N_2 and 5% CO_2 is preferred. They can grow within a temperature range of 22–41°C, the parasitic species growing optimally at 35–37°C.

A medium widely used for the isolation of mycoplasmas consists of bovine heart infusion broth (PPLO broth) to which are added 20% horse serum and 10% fresh yeast extract along with glucose and phenol red as a pH indicator. High concentration of serum is necessary as a source of cholesterol and other lipids. Growth of *M. pneumoniae* is detected by turbidity and colour change (red to yellow) of phenol red indicator due to fermentation of glucose.

Ureaplasma and other mycoplasmas which do not ferment glucose show only turbidity. This medium can be solidified by the addition of agar. Penicillin and polymyxin B may be added to the medium to inhibit contaminating bacteria and amphotericin B to inhibit contaminating fungi. Since thallium acetate is inhibitory for *U. urealyticum* and *M. genitalium*, and highly poisonous for humans, therefore, it should not be added to the medium. A diphasic medium in screw-capped bottle containing an agar phase that is overlain with broth medium of similar composition may also be used.

Colonies usually appear after incubation for 2–3 days. However, media for isolation of genital mycoplasmas and *M. pneumoniae* should be incubated for 1 and 4 weeks respectively, before a final culture report is made. Initially, the mycoplasma cells multiply within the agar to form an opaque ball-shaped colony that grows up to the surface of the agar and spreads around it forming a translucent peripheral zone. Such a colony presents a **'fried egg'** appearance (Fig. 28.1). Colony size varies from 200–500 µm for 'large colony' mycoplasmas to 15–60 µm for the ureaplasmas. The small colonies of the latter usually lack the peripheral zone.

Colonies may be seen with a hand lens. However, visualization of colonial morphology is facilitated by application

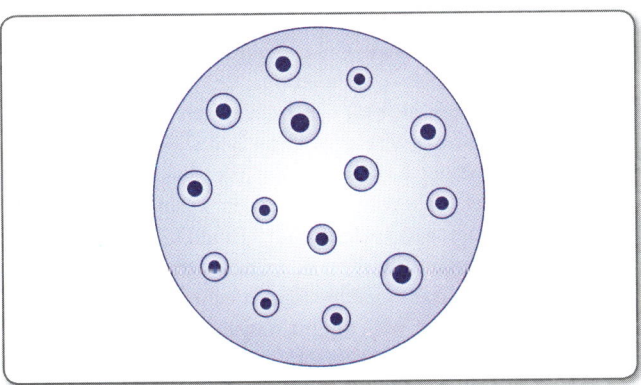

Fig. 28.1: Colonies of *Mycoplasma* on agar, showing 'fried egg' appearance.

of **Dienes stain** directly to the agar surface. For this a block of agar containing the colony is cut and placed on a slide. It is covered with a coverslip on which an alcoholic solution of methylene blue azure has been dried.

Mycoplasmas with the fried egg colony morphology appear highly granular and stain with a dark blue centre and a light blue periphery. The agar background appears clear or slightly violet. Mycoplasmas other than *M. pneumoniae* remain stained, but *M. pneumoniae* reduces the methylene blue after a period of time and becomes colourless.

BIOCHEMICAL REACTIONS

Most species utilize glucose or arginine as the major source of energy. Urea is not hydrolysed, except by ureaplasmas. They are, generally, not proteolytic.

PATHOGENICITY

Mycoplasmas are **opportunistic infectious agents**. Therefore, the infections caused by these organisms occur more frequently in patients with hypogammaglobulinaemia, Hodgkin's disease, lymphoma, leukaemia, organ transplant and AIDS.

Mycoplasma pneumoniae

- *M. pneumoniae* (also called **Eaton agent** after the investigator who originally isolated it) commonly causes tracheo-bronchitis, pharyngitis, sinusitis and **primary atypical pneumonia (PAP)** accompanied by formation of (i) cold haemagglutinins that **agglutinate** human red cells in cold, (ii) *Streptococcus* MG agglutinins, and (iii) antibodies giving biological false positive Wasserman reaction. Penicillin has no effect on PAP which has served to differentiate PAP from typical pneumonias.
- *M. pneumoniae* has been shown to produce an exotoxin that is believed to play a major role in the damage to the respiratory epithelium that occurs during acute infection.

- In addition, *M. pneumoniae* may also cause extrapulmonary lesions such as arthritis, hepatitis, meningoencephalitis, cerebral ataxia, transverse myelitis, Guillain-Barré syndrome, haemolytic anaemia, myocarditis and pericarditis.

M. pneumoniae is transmitted from person-to-person through airborne transfer of droplets containing the organisms. They attach to epithelial cells in the respiratory tract and multiply.

Incubation period is 1–3 weeks. The onset is gradual. Patient develops fever with chills, malaise, headache, sore throat, nasal congestion and nonproductive cough. The disease is self-limited, recovery occurring in 3–10 days without antimicrobial therapy.

Ureaplasma urealyticum

- *U. urealyticum* may cause nonchlamydial, non-gonococcal urethritis (NGU), epididymitis, vaginitis and cervicitis.
- Ureaplasmas may cause prematurity, postpartum endometritis, chronic lung disease of the premature infant and infection of wounds and soft tissues.
- Ureaplasmas are the commonest organisms isolated from the CNS or lower respiratory tract of sick premature or newborn infants.
- Ureaplasmas have also been blamed to cause male and female infertility and low birth weight but there are conflicting reports.

Mycoplasma hominis

- *M. hominis* may cause salpingitis, tubo-ovarian abscess, pelvic abscess, septic abortion, puerperal infection, septic arthritis, septic thrombophlebitis, peritonitis and brain abscess.
- It may cause PAP similar to that caused by *M. pneumoniae* and meningitis in newborn.

Mycoplasma genitalium

M. genitalium has been associated with some cases of non-gonococcal urethritis and pelvic inflammatory disease. Its prevalence is not known.

LABORATORY DIAGNOSIS

Laboratory diagnosis of *Mycoplasma* and *Ureaplasma* infections may be carried out by (i) culture and (ii) serological tests.

I. Culture

M. pneumoniae may be recovered from throat swabs, nasopharyngeal swabs, sputum, throat washings, bronchoalveolar lavage, tracheal aspirate and lung tissue specimens. Genital mycoplasmas may be isolated from urethral, vaginal and cervical swabs, semen, prostatic secretions, urine, blood, CSF, amniotic fluid, respiratory tract secretions, synovial fluid, pericardial fluid, and biopsy specimens from endometrium, fallopian tubes, placenta and aborted foetus.

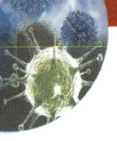

Because of the fastidious nature of these bacteria, the culture media should be inoculated as soon after collection as possible. Standard *Mycoplasma* broth medium dispensed into small vials may be used for transport of swab specimens, while other specimens may be transported in sterile screw-capped containers. In the laboratory, if inoculation is not possible immediately, then the specimen may be held up to 24 hours at 4°C. If delay more than 24 hours is expected, then the specimen should be frozen at –70°C. Urine specimen should be centrifuged and deposit inoculated into the culture medium. If inoculation is not immediately possible, then urine deposit should be diluted with equal volume of transport medium and frozen.

Mycoplasma broth medium, containing penicillin, polymyxin B, amphotericin B, glucose and phenol red as a pH indicator is inoculated with the specimen and incubated at 37°C preferably in an atmosphere of 95% N_2 and 5% CO_2. If specimen contains *M. pneumoniae*, its growth is revealed by turbidity and a colour change (red to yellow) of phenol red, due to fermentation of glucose. It usually occurs in 4–28 days. Ureaplasmas and other mycoplasmas which do not ferment glucose will show only turbidity. It is then subcultured on agar medium and incubated in air for 5–7 days. *M. pneumoniae* form large (200–500 μm) colonies with a characteristic 'fried egg' appearance, while colonies of ureaplasmas are small, 15–60 μm in diameter and usually lack peripheral zone. Colonies of *M. pneumoniae* may be identified by:

- *Haemadsorption test:* Colonies growing on the surface of the agar are flooded with 2 ml of 0.2–0.4% suspension of washed guinea pig erythrocytes suspended in *Mycoplasma* broth medium. The plate is then incubated at 35°C for 30 minutes. It is occasionally rotated during this time. It is then washed with 3 ml of *Mycoplasma* broth medium by gently rotating the plate. Wash fluid is removed by aspiration with a pipette and colonies examined under 50× to 100× magnification. Colonies of *M. pneumoniae* adsorb the erythrocytes to their surface. This is due to binding of the *Mycoplasma* to sialic acid-containing oligo-saccharides present on the surface of erythrocytes. However, colonies of *M. genitalium* also share this property.
- *Tetrazolium reduction test:* Colonies of *M. pneumoniae* appear red when these are flooded with solution of tetrazolium compound which is colourless. *M. pneumoniae* reduces tetrazolium (colourless) to red-coloured compound.
- *Serological techniques:* These include inhibition of colony development around discs impregnated with specific antiserum, or the fluorescence of colonies treated with such antiserum labelled with a fluorochrome.

II. Serological Tests

These are of two types—(a) detection of antigen, and (b) detection of antibody.

(a) *Detection of antigen:* Detection of antigen in respiratory exudates by direct immunofluorescence, counterimmuno-electrophoresis, immunoblotting with monoclonal anti-bodies and enzyme immunoassay.

(b) *Detection of antibody:*
1. **Cold agglutinins:** Cold agglutinins (IgM antibodies that bind the I antigen on the surface of human erythrocytes at 4°C) can be detected by agglutination of O Rh-negative erythrocytes at 4°C. Cold agglutinins appear about one week after infection with a peak at 4–5 weeks. Thereafter, titre declines rapidly and the test becomes negative after about 5 months. A four-fold rise in cold agglutinin titres or a single titre of 64 or more is suggestive of *M. pneumoniae* infection.
2. *Streptococcus* **MG agglutination test:** In this test, a heat-killed suspension of *Streptococcus* MG is mixed with serial dilutions of patient's unheated serum. The agglutination is observed after overnight incubation at 37°C. An antibody titre of 1 : 20 or more is suggestive of *M. pneumoniae* infection.
3. **Complement fixation test:** This is the most widely used serological test for diagnosis of *M. pneumoniae* infection. The antigen used is a glycolipid from the organism that is extracted by chloroform-methanol. A recent infection is indicated by four-fold or more rise in antibody titre or a single titre of 64 or more. Comple-ment fixing antibodies appear 7–10 days after infection with the organism and reach peak titre after 4–6 weeks. Such results are obtained in about 80% of cases.
4. **Enzyme immunoassay:** This is more sensitive test than complement fixation test. It can be used to detect specific IgM, IgG and IgA antibodies against *M. pneumoniae*.

III. Detection of Specific DNA

Detection of specific DNA by dot blot hybridization and PCR in respiratory exudate.

TREATMENT

Mycoplasmas and ureaplasmas are resistant to penicillins and cephalosporins which act on the cell wall and are sensitive to tetracyclines and erythromycin which inhibit protein synthesis. Therefore, tetracyclines and erythromycin are drugs of choice for the treatment of *Mycoplasma* and *Ureaplasma* infections. However, *M. pneumoniae* is more sensitive to erythromycin than some other mycoplasmas of human origin. The genital mycoplasmas are more variable in their antimicrobial susceptibility patterns and their resistance to both these antibiotics is fairly common.

PROPHYLAXIS

The best prophylaxis is to avoid contact with person suspected of having the disease. Tetracyclines or erythromycin may be administered prophylactically to prevent the spread of infection to the contacts. At present, no vaccine against *Mycoplasma* and *Ureaplasma* is available.

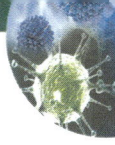

Atypical pneumonia

Around the turn of century, any patient who presented with a sudden onset of fever with shaking chills, pleuritic pain and the production of rust-coloured sputum was thought to have typical pneumonia attributable to *Streptococcus pneumoniae*. All other patients who did not show this characteristic picture were referred to as patients with 'atypical pneumonia'. *M. pneumoniae*, *Legionella pneumophila* and *C. pneumoniae* are three atypical pathogens responsible for community acquired pneumonia (CAP). The only thing 'atypical' about these pathogens is that they are not recovered on routine sputum cultures.

Atypical pathogens do not respond to β-lactam antibiotics and their presence is often overlooked untill patients fail to respond to standard penicillin or cephalosporin therapy. β-lactam antibiotics act by inhibiting cell wall synthesis. This makes them ineffective against *Mycoplasma*. Neither penicillin nor cephalosporins have good intracellular penetration. Hence they are also ineffective against *Chlamydia* and *Legionella*.

✦ Key Points

- Mycoplasmas are **smallest prokaryotes** capable of binary fission, and exist as pleomorphic morphologic forms as they lack peptidoglycan cell wall.
- *Mycoplasma pneumoniae is an important human pathogen and causes primary atypical pneumonia, haemolytic anaemia, and skin rashes and ulcerations of oral and vaginal mucosa.*

❓ ASSESS YOURSELF

LONG ANSWER QUESTIONS

1. Discuss laboratory diagnosis of *Mycoplasma* and *Ureaplasma* infections.
2. Discuss pathogenicity of *Mycoplasma* and *Ureaplasma*.

MULTIPLE CHOICE QUESTIONS

1. Which of the following genera can hydrolyse urea?
   - (a) *Mycoplasma*
   - (b) *Ureaplasma*
   - (c) *Acholeplasma*
   - (d) All of the above

2. Colonies with 'fried egg' appearance are seen in:
   - (a) *Mycoplasma*
   - (b) *Pseudomonas*
   - (c) *Haemophilus*
   - (d) *Bordetella*

3. Cell wall is lacking in:
   - (a) *Mycoplasma*
   - (b) *Actinomyces*
   - (c) *Corynebacterium*
   - (d) *Brucella*

4. Colonies of *Mycoplasma pneumoniae* can be identified by:
   - (a) Haemadsorption test
   - (b) Tetrazolium reduction test
   - (c) Fluorescence of colonies treated with specific antiserum labelled with a fluorochrome
   - (d) All of the above

ANSWERS TO MCQs

1. b   2. a   3. a   4. d

Rickettsia, Orientia, Ehrlichia, Anaplasma, Neorickettsia, Coxiella and Bartonella

RICKETTSIA

General Characters of Rickettsia and Orientia

- The organisms of these genera are small (0.3–0.5 × 0.8–2.0 μm) Gram-negative bacilli. The stains commonly used for staining these organisms are Gimenez, Macchiavello and Giemsa. They appear deep red with Gimenez and Macchiavello and purple with Giemsa stain.
- They are **obligate intracellular parasites**.
- They require an arthropod vector as part of their natural cycle and are **transmitted to man by blood sucking arthropods**. The species that are pathogenic for humans parasitize endothelial cells almost exclusively.
- They multiply by binary fission.
- They possess a trilaminar cytoplasmic membrane and cell wall of bacterial type.
- They are sensitive to lysozyme and antibiotics.
- They possess both RNA and DNA.
- They are large enough to be seen under the light microscope and are held back by bacterial filters.
- Scrub typhus rickettsiae appear to be fundamentally different and have been placed in a separate genus as *Orientia tsutsugamushi*.

Cultural Characteristics

Rickettsiae are **unable to grow on cell-free media**. Growth generally takes place in the cytoplasm of infected cells, but in the case of spotted fever rickettsiae, growth may take place in the nucleus as well. **Embryonated hens' eggs, inoculated in the yolk sac** during the 5th or 6th day of development, are highly susceptible to infection. Rickettsiae grow in the cells of the membrane surrounding the yolk.

The inoculated eggs are incubated for eight days. Optimum temperature of incubation for most rickettsiae is 35°C and for those of the spotted fever group is 33°C. After incubation, the eggs are harvested and the yolk sac membrane is removed. It serves as an excellent source of organisms for diagnostic antigens and vaccines. Limited growth occurs on the chorioallantoic membrane also.

They can also grow on **mouse fibroblasts, HeLa, HEp-2, Detroit 6 and other continuous cell lines**, but cell cultures are not satisfactory for primary isolation of rickettsiae from the patient. They may also be propagated in **arthropods**. **The guinea pig and mice** are commonly used laboratory animals for isolation of *Rickettsia* from patients.

Susceptibility to Physical and Chemical Agents

Rickettsiae are readily inactivated by physical and chemical agents. They are unstable extracellularly under ordinary environmental conditions. However, in the dried faeces of infected lice, they remain infective for months at room temperature.

Pathogenesis

Rickettsiae are transmitted to man by the bite or faeces of an infected arthropod vector. On entry into human body, they multiply locally and enter the blood stream followed by multiplication of the organisms in the endothelial cells lining the small blood vessels. This leads to endothelial proliferation and perivascular infiltration which results in thrombosis of the vessel leading to rupture and necrosis.

Diseases caused by various species of *Rickettsia* include typhus fevers, spotted fevers and scrub typhus (Table 29.1).

Typhus Fevers

This group consists of epidemic (classical) typhus and its recrudescent infection (Brill-Zinsser disease), and endemic (murine) typhus.

Epidemic (Classical) Typhus

Epidemic typhus is caused by *R. prowazekii*. Human body louse (*Pediculus corporis*) is the vector. Head louse (*Pediculus capitis*) may also transmit the infection but not pubic louse. Lice become

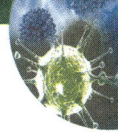

TABLE 29.1: Rickettsial diseases of man

Group	Disease	Causative agent	Insect vector	Mode of transmission
Typhus fevers	• Epidemic typhus	*R. prowazekii*	Human body louse	Louse faeces scratched into skin
	• Recrudescent typhus (Brill-Zinsser disease)	*R. prowazekii*	—	—
	• Murine typhus	*R. typhi* (syn. *R. mooseri*)	Rat flea	Rat flea faeces scratched into skin
Spotted fevers	• Rocky Mountain spotted fever	*R. rickettsii*	Ixodid ticks	Tick bite
	• Boutonneuse fever	*R. conorii*	Ixodid ticks	Tick bite
	• Australian tick typhus	*R. australis*	Ixodid ticks	Tick bite
	• Siberian tick typhus	*R. sibirica*	Ixodid ticks	Tick bite
	• Rickettsialpox	*R. akari*	Mites	Mite bite
Scrub typhus	• Scrub typhus	*O. tsutsugamushi*	Trombiculid mites	Mite bite

infected by ingesting the blood from a rickettsiaemic human. The rickettsiae multiply in the gut of lice and appear in the faeces after about a week. Lice do not transmit *R. prowazekii* to their progeny but succumb to the infection within 2–4 weeks, remaining infective till they die. Lice are sensitive to temperature. They abandon a host with a body temperature of 40°C or more or the cooling carcass and parasitize other persons.

Lice defaecate while feeding. The feeding process is irritating and scratching by the host produces minute abrasions that function as portal of entry for the rickettsiae in the louse faeces. Occasionally, infection may also be transmitted by inhalation of dried louse faeces containing viable rickettsiae or through the conjunctiva. *R. prowazekii* has been demonstrated in flying squirrels in the United States and a small number of associated human infections have occurred. Therefore, flying squirrels may act as a non-human reservoir of *R. prowazekii*.

After an **incubation period of 5–21 days**, patient develops severe headache, chills, generalized myalgia, high fever (39–41°C) and vomiting. Four to seven days after the onset of illness, a macular rash appears first on the trunk and then spreads to the limbs but sparing face, palms and soles. In the second and third weeks, the patient may become comatosed or delirious. Patient may also develop patchy pneumonia and gangrene of toes, feet, tips of fingers, ear lobes, nose, penis, scrotum or vulva. Mortality rate varies from 10–40% and increases with age.

Brill-Zinsser Disease (Recrudescent Typhus)

In some individuals who recover from epidemic typhus, **the rickettsiae may remain latent in the lymphoid tissues or organs for years**. Such latent infection may be reactivated, many years later, leading to recrudescent typhus. Lice that feed on a patient with recrudescent typhus can become infected and if conditions are favourable for louse-human-louse transmission, an outbreak of epidemic typhus may result. Therefore, latent human infections, act as a reservoir of *R. prowazekii*.

Brill-Zinsser disease is a milder illness. The duration of disease is shorter (less than two weeks), skin rash is rare, fever is erratic and case fatality rate is lower. Patient develops severe headache, malaise and myalgia. The disease was first noticed by Brill in 1898, and Zinsser (1934) isolated *R. prowazekii* from such cases. Hence the disease is called Brill-Zinsser's disease.

Endemic (Murine) Typhus

It is a milder disease than epidemic typhus. It is caused by *R. typhi* (syn. *R. mooseri*). Rat acts as a reservoir and the rickettsiae are passed from rat-to-rat by the rat flea (*Xenopsylla cheopis*). Rat flea acquires infection by feeding upon a rickettsiaemic rat. The rickettsiae multiply in the gut of the flea. It may infect other susceptible rats and thus a natural cycle of flea-rat-flea infection may become established. The flea is not incapacitated and goes on excreting rickettsiae in its faeces for long periods. Infection in flea is not transmitted transovarially.

Man acquires the infection usually through the bite of infected fleas. When infected flea takes a blood meal, it defaecates on the host. The latter rubs the infected faeces into minute abrasions (produced by scratching) that function as portal of entry for rickettsiae in the infected faeces. Infection may also be transmitted by:

- Ingestion of food contaminated with infected rat urine or flea faeces,
- Inhalation of dried flea faeces, and
- Contamination of respiratory tract or conjunctiva, with infective flea faeces.

Man-to-man transmission does not occur. *R. typhi* can be differentiated from *R. prowazekii* by the following tests:

- *Neil-Mooser or tunica reaction:* When a male guinea pig is inoculated intraperitoneally with blood from a case of endemic typhus or with a culture of *R. typhi*, it develops fever and a characteristic scrotal inflammation. The scrotum becomes enlarged and the testes cannot be pushed back into the abdomen because of inflammatory adhesions between

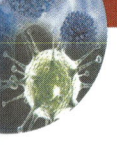

the layers of the tunica vaginalis. This is known as **Neil-Mooser** or **tunica reaction**. This reaction is negative with *R. prowazekii*.

Clinically, endemic typhus resembles epidemic typhus but it is usually a mild illness of shorter duration, has fewer complications and has a case fatality rate of less than 1%. Patient develops fever, headache, malaise and myalgia. Macular rash appears on third to fifth day on trunk and spreads to the extremities. As in epidemic typhus, the involvement of palms, soles and face is rare. Untreated, the illness may last up to two weeks.

Spotted Fevers

These diseases include **Rocky Mountain spotted fever (RMSF), boutonneuse fever, Australian tick typhus, Siberian tick typhus and rickettsialpox**. The infection is transmitted by ticks except in case of rickettsialpox, in which mite is the vector. **Rickettsiae are transmitted transovarially in ticks and mites which act both as vectors and reservoirs**. Human infection occurs by the bite of an infected tick or mite or by ingestion of food contaminated with their faeces. Rickettsiae do not harm ticks and mites. An eschar frequently develops at the site of tick bite in spotted fevers except RMSF.

Scrub Typhus

It is caused by *O. tsutsugamushi*. Scrub typhus normally occurs in a range of mammals, particularly field mice and rats and also birds including migratory birds, all of which can act as host reservoirs. Migratory birds may act as transporters of the disease agent over long distances. The infection is transmitted by the larval forms the trombiculid mites (chiggers).

After 1–3 weeks of chigger bite, patient abruptly develops severe headache, chills, fever, conjunctivitis, deafness and a characteristic eschar at the site of chigger bite. Spleen, and lymph nodes proximal to eschar enlarge. About one week after the onset of fever, a maculopapular rash appears on the trunk which later becomes generalized. This may be accompanied by stupor and prostration. Case fatality rate varies from 10–60%.

Laboratory Diagnosis

It may be carried out by:
- Isolation of rickettsiae in laboratory animals, fertile hen's eggs and cell cultures,
- Direct detection of the organisms and their antigens in clinical specimens, and
- Serology.

Isolation of Rickettsiae

Blood clot ground in skimmed milk or brain heart infusion broth is inoculated intraperitoneally in male guinea pigs or mice. The inoculated animals are observed for 3–4 weeks. The response of animals to different rickettsial infections vary:

- In RMSF, guinea pigs develop fever, scrotal necrosis and may even die due to overwhelming infection of *R. rickettsii*.
- In *R. typhi*, *R. conorii* and *R. akari* infection, guinea pigs develop fever and tunica reaction.
- In *R. prowazekii* infection, the animals develop fever without any testicular inflammation.
- For isolation of *O. tsutsugamushi*, mice are preferred over guinea pigs. The infected animals become ill and develop ascites.
- Smears from peritoneum, tunica and spleen of infected animals may be stained by Giemsa or Gimenez methods to demonstrate the rickettsiae.
- Rickettsiae can also be grown in the yolk sac of embryonated hens' eggs and cell cultures.

Direct Detection of the Organisms and their Antigens

Biopsy specimens from the rash of spotted fever and chronic hepatitis, impression smears from the organs of infected animals, and endolymph from ticks may be stained with Giemsa, Macchiavello or Gimenez stains, and with direct and indirect immunofluorescence techniques. In tissue smears, rickettsiae are usually seen as bipolar rods occurring near cells or free in the cytoplasm. *R. rickettsii* may also be seen within the nuclei of infected cells.

Immunofluorescence technique has the benefits of greater sensitivity and specificity as compared with classical staining methods. The sensitivity of the procedure in the detection of antigens of *R. rickettsii* is approximately 70% and the specificity approaches 100%. By immunofluorescence technique, antigens can also be demonstrated in paraffin-embedded, formalin fixed specimens if the section is treated first with trypsin to unmask antigens.

Molecular Methods

Primers and probes for unique sequences in the genome of the rickettsiae or its plasmids have been synthesized and the sequences amplified by PCR.

Serological Diagnosis of Rickettsial Diseases

Serological diagnosis of rickettsial diseases may be done by **Weil-Felix (WF) reaction** or by specific tests using rickettsial antigens. The latter include:
- Complement fixation test with purified antigens,
- Immunofluorescence on microdots of purified rickettsiae,
- Enzyme immunoassay with particulate or extracted antigens, and
- Latex agglutination test.

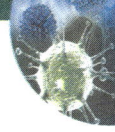

TABLE 29.2: Weil-Felix reaction in rickettsial disease

Disease	Agglutination with		
	OX19	OX2	OXK
Epidemic typhus	++++	+	–
Brill-Zinsser disease	± / –	–	–
Endemic typhus	++++	+	–
Spotted typhus	++++ to +	+ to ++++	–
Scrub typhus	–	–	+++

Weil Felix Reaction

Weil-Felix reaction is an agglutination test which detects anti-rickettsial antibodies that cross react with certain strains of *Proteus*. The basis of this test is the sharing of an alkali-stable carbohydrate antigen of some rickettsiae with O antigen of certain non-motile strains of *Proteus*, *P. vulgaris* OX19 and OX2, and *P. mirabilis* OXK. The test may be performed as a microagglutination reaction in microtitre plates with round bottomed wells with haematoxylin-stained antigen or as a tube agglutination test.

Sera from patients with epidemic and endemic typhus strongly agglutinate OX19 and weakly agglutinate OX2. In Brill-Zinsser disease, the test is negative or weakly reactive. In spotted fevers both OX19 and OX2 are agglutinated. OXK agglutinins are present only in scrub typhus (Table 29.2). However, this test is both insensitive and nonspecific.

COXIELLA BURNETII

Coxiella burnetii is also an obligate intracellular pathogen. It is a pleomorphic, coccobacillary bacterium measuring 1.0 × 0.3 μm in size. It has a Gram-negative cell wall. It grows within the phagolysosome of macrophages of the vertebrate host. It is more resistant to heat and drying than many non-sporing microorganisms. **It survives holder method (63°C for 30 minutes) of pasteurization of milk and is at borderline of inactivation in the flash method** (72°C for 20 seconds) of pasteurization. It can remain infectious for months in milk, tap water, soil, dried blood and on wool. Therefore, it can survive in dust and aerosols and can be transmitted as an airborne infection. It can be inactivated by 2% formaldehyde, 1% lysol and 5% hydrogen peroxide.

Pathogenesis

C. burnetii causes **Q fever** which has a worldwide distribution. In nature, there are two cycles of infection with this organism, one in wild animals with their ticks, and the other in domestic animals (cattle, sheep and goats). The latter cycle is not dependent on arthropod transmission, but is maintained primarily through airborne transmission. Infected domestic animals do not appear ill, but shed large numbers of infectious organisms in their milk, urine, faeces and particularly in their placental product.

Infectious organisms in placental products become aerosolized after parturition which contaminate the surrounding area. Dust in sheep or cattle sheds may become heavily contaminated and function as a source of infection for susceptible animals and man.

Human infections have been traced to:
- consumption of infected milk,
- handling of infected wool or hides,
- soil contaminated with faeces of infected animals,
- infected straw, and
- contaminated clothing.

Man-to-man transmission of Q fever can also occur. Ticks do not play any significant role in transmitting the infection to man. After an incubation period of 2–4 weeks, patient develops fever, chills, headache, malaise, myalgia, pneumonia, hepatitis, endocarditis and meningoencephalitis. Unlike most other rickettsial diseases, no skin rash occurs in Q fever. The rickettsia may remain latent in the tissues of patients for months or years and latent infection may become activated naturally or by use of X-ray treatment or multiple cortisone injections.

Laboratory Diagnosis

C. burnetii can be isolated from clinical specimens by intraperitoneal inoculation of guinea pigs and mice, and yolk sac of embryonated hen's eggs. **However, unless special facilities are available, isolations should not be attempted**. Therefore, diagnosis mainly relies on the demonstration of specific antibodies by complement fixation test and indirect immuno-fluorescence assay. Weil-Felix test is negative in Q fever.

NEORICKETTSIA SENNETSU

It produces **sennetsu ehrlichiosis**, an illness resembling glandular fever (sennetsu means glandular fever). Patient develops lymphoid hyperplasia and atypical lymphocytosis. It is suspected to be ingested with raw fish. It occurs in Japan and Malaysia.

EHRLICHIA CHAFFEENSIS

It infects human monocytic cells and causes **human monocystic ehrlichiosis.** It produces febrile illness with leucopenia, thrombocytopenia, perivascular lymphohistiocytic infiltrates in many organs and non-necrotizing granulomata in bone marrow and liver. It is transmitted to humans by ticks (*Amblyomma americanum*). It occurs in the USA, Europe and Africa.

ANAPLASMA PHAGOCYTOPHILA

It infects human granulocytic cells and causes **human granulocystic anaplasmosis.** It produces febrile illness with leucopenia and thrombocytopenia. Like, *E. chaffeensis* it is also transmitted to humans by *Ixodes ricinus*-like ticks. It occurs in the USA and Europe.

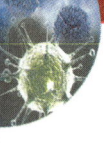

Laboratory Diagnosis

- Human granulocytic anaplasmasis may be diagnosed by demonstration of **bluish intracytoplasmic inclusion (morula)** in Giemsa-stained peripheral blood neutrophils.
- Diagnosis may be established by demonstration of **specific antibodies** by indirect immunofluorescent methods using cell culture-propagated organisms.
- *E. chaffeensis* and *A. phagocytophila* infections have also been diagnosed by **PCR**.

BARTONELLA BACILLIFORMIS

B. bacilliformis is small, Gram-negative coccobacillus (0.3–1.5 × 0.2–0.5 μm). The organisms occur singly, in pairs, chains or clumps. They are motile by means of 10 flagella situated at one end of the bacterium. They are strict aerobes, optimum pH and temperature for growth are 7.8 and 25–28°C respectively. They can grow in semisolid nutrient agar containing rabbit serum and haemoglobin. Growth is slow and becomes visible after 10 days incubation.

Pathogenesis

B. bacilliformis causes **Oroya fever**, spread by sandflies. After the bite, the bacteria reach blood circulation, multiply and invade RBCs. This causes an increase in the fragility of the RBCs, thereby facilitating their removal by the reticuloendothelial cells of the spleen, thus leading to severe anaemia. After an incubation period of 3 weeks to 3 months patient develops fever, severe headache and chills, followed by severe anaemia. Patient may also develop enlargement of spleen and liver, and haemorrhages into the lymph nodes. Case fatality rate may be up to 40%.

Several weeks after recovery, or even without the initial attack of Oroya fever, patient may develop nodular lesions on skin usually of exposed parts of the body, on mucous membranes or in internal organs. These may become secondarily infected producing ulcers and haemorrhagic lesions. This condition is known as **verruga peruana**.

Laboratory Diagnosis

- *B. bacilliformis* can be demonstrated in blood smears stained by Giemsa. Organisms are seen in the cytoplasm of erythrocytes as well as adhering to the cell surfaces.
- Organisms may be isolated from the blood, in semisolid medium containing rabbit serum and haemoglobin.
- Guinea pig inoculation leads to verruga peruana but not Oroya fever.

BARTONELLA QUINTANA

B. quintana (formerly *Rochalimaea quintana*) is a small, Gram-negative bacillus measuring 0.3–0.5 × 1.0–1.7 μm. It does not possess flagella, although it may exhibit twitching movement caused by fimbriae. It grows slowly on rabbit or sheep blood agar at 35°C in 5% CO_2 in air. Colonies appear after two weeks in primary culture, and 3–5 days in subsequent passages. It proliferates in an extracellular environment in the arthropod host, in the lumen of the gut rather than within the intestinal epithelial cells. Besides man and louse, only rhesus monkeys can be infected.

Pathogenesis

B. quintana causes **trench fever** which was first recognized in the First World War as a **five-day fever** in men engaged in trench warfare in Europe. The disease is spread from human-to-human by the body louse in a human-louse-human cycle of infection. The faeces of the lice become infectious 5–9 days after feeding on a trench fever patient. Infection is acquired when infected lice faeces are scratched into the skin. The lice are unharmed and remain infectious for life. Vertical transmission does not occur in lice.

Clinically, after an incubation period of 14–30 days patient develops headache, malaise, fever, chills, severe pain in the back and legs and a roseolar rash on the chest, abdomen or back. Recovery is frequently followed by relapses occurring at five day intervals (hence the species name, *quintana*). The infection is mild, recovery is slow and fatalities are rare.

Laboratory Diagnosis

B. quintana can be isolated by allowing healthy lice to feed upon the patient and the bartonellae may be detected in the gut of these lice. It can also be cultivated from patient's blood on rabbit or sheep blood agar. **Weil-Felix reaction, in trench fever, is negative**.

BARTONELLA HENSELAE

B. henselae is a small, slightly curved Gram-negative bacillus measuring about 2.0–2.5 × 0.5–0.6 μm. It displays twitching motility. It can be grown on chocolate agar, columbia agar with 5% sheep or rabbit blood and blood-supplemented brain heart infusion agar. Growth appears after 5–15 days incubation at 35–37°C in 5% CO_2. Colonies of *B. henselae* are white, dry, adherent, cauliflower-like and embedded in the agar.

B. henselae causes **cat-scratch disease**, a severe condition of regional lymphadenopathy and fever resulting from contact, scratch or bite of an infected cat. It occurs throughout the world. It most frequently involves cervical and axillary lymph nodes, although other sites may be involved as well. In AIDS patients, as a result of immunosuppression, *B. henselae* may lead to **bacillary angiomatosis**, a condition resembling Kaposi's sarcoma.

Diagnosis can be established by:
- Demonstration of clusters of bacillary organisms in sections of lymph node biopsies stained with the Warthin-Starry silver impregnation stain.
- *B. henselae* can be isolated by inoculation of clinical specimens on chocolate agar or columbia agar with 5% sheep or rabbit blood.
- ELISA with various protein antigens, is the most useful serological test.

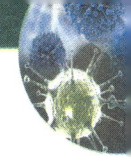

Key Points

- Rickettsiae are **obligate intracellular Gram-negative bacilli**.
- All members of the genus *Rickettsia* **are transmitted** to humans **by bites** of infected **arthropods**.
- Rickettsiae *are transmitted transovarially in ticks and mites* which act both as *vectors and reservoirs*.
- *Coxiella burnetti*, an organism closely resembling rickettsiae, causes **Q fever**, a typhus-like illness.
- *Coxiella burnetti* **survives holder method of pasteurization of milk** and is at borderline of inactivation of the flash method.
- *Bartonella bacilliformis, B. quintana* and *B. henselae* cause **Oroya fever, trench fever or five day fever**, and **cat scratch disease, respectively**.

? ASSESS YOURSELF

LONG AND SHORT ANSWER QUESTIONS

1. Write short notes on:
   - (a) General characters of rickettsiae
   - (b) Typhus fevers
   - (c) Spotted fevers
   - (d) Scrub typhus
   - (e) Trench fever
2. Discuss laboratory diagnosis of rickettsial infections.

MULTIPLE CHOICE QUESTIONS

1. Which of the following bacteria **does not** require an arthropod vector for its transmission?
   - (a) *Coxiella burnetii*
   - (b) *Rickettsia akari*
   - (c) *R. prowazekii*
   - (d) *Bartonella quintana*

2. The causative agent of Q fever is:
   - (a) *Rickettsia prowazekii*
   - (b) *R. akari*
   - (c) *Coxiella burnetti*
   - (d) *Orientia tsutsugamushi*

3. The causative agent of epidemic typhus is:
   - (a) *Rickettsia prowazekii*
   - (b) *R. rickettsii*
   - (c) *R. akari*
   - (d) *Coxiella burnetii*

4. Which of the following bacteria can be grown on artificial media?
   - (a) *Bartonella quintana*
   - (b) *Coxiella burnetii*
   - (c) *Rickettsia prowazekii*
   - (d) *R. typhi*

5. Human infections due to *Coxiella* can be acquired by:
   - (a) Consumption of infected milk
   - (b) Handling of infected wool or hides
   - (c) Soil contaminated with faeces of infected animals
   - (d) All of the above

6. Weil-Felix test is negative in:
   - (a) Epidemic typhus
   - (b) Endemic typhus
   - (c) Spotted fevers
   - (d) Q fever

ANSWERS TO MCQs

1. a **2.** c **3.** a **4.** a **5.** d **6.** d

30 Chapter

Chlamydia and Chlamydophila

Family Chlamydiaceae consists of two genera—*Chlamydia* and *Chlamydophila*. The genus *Chlamydia* has one species—*C. trachomatis* and the genus *Chlamydophila* has three species—*C. psittaci, C. pneumoniae* and *C. picorum*.

GENERAL CHARACTERS OF FAMILY CHLAMYIACEAE

- They are small, **obligate intracellular, Gram-negative bacteria**.
- They possess both RNA and DNA, ribosomes and cell wall similar to that of Gram-negative bacteria. However, they differ from most true bacteria in that they do not have peptidoglycan.
- They lack the ability to produce their own ATP, therefore, they use host's ATP (**energy parasites**).
- They multiply by binary fission.
- They are non-motile and stain poorly with Gram, but readily with Giemsa, Castaneda, Gimenez and Macchiavello methods. They stain blue by Castaneda and red by Macchiavello and Gimenez techniques. Giemsa staining is preferable for staining inclusions in cell culture. Inclusion bodies of Chlamydiaceae are basophilic in nature. Mature inclusions of *C. trachomatis* possess glycogen matrix, therefore, iodine stains them coppery brown.
- They can also be demonstrated by direct immunofluorescence staining.
- They multiply in the cytoplasm of the host cell forming microcolonies or inclusion bodies which drape around the nucleus like a cloak or mantle (*chlamys* means mantle).
- Like Gram-negative bacteria, the outer membrane of various chlamydiaceae possesses several proteins of which major outer membrane protein (MOMP) has species-specific epitopes.
- They possess a genus-specific lipopolysaccharide-protein complex antigen.
- They infect a wide spectrum of vertebrate hosts including birds, mammals and humans.
- They are susceptible to a wide range of antibiotics such as tetracyclines, erythromycin, macrolides and rifampicin. *C. trachomatis* is sensitive to sulphonamides, but *C. psittaci* and *C. pneumoniae* are not.

Morphology

There are two morphologically distinct forms of Chlamydiaceae, namely **elementary body (EB)** and **reticulate body (RB)**.

- The EB is the extracellular infectious particle. It is a small (200–300 nm in diameter), spherical body in case of *C. trachomatis* and *C. psittaci,* and pear-shaped in case of *C. pneumoniae*. It has an irregular electron-dense central nucleoid and a rigid trilaminar cell wall similar to the cell walls of Gram-negative bacteria.
- The RB is the intracellular, metabolically active form that divides by binary fission to form EBs. It is 500–1000 nm in diameter and its cell wall is fragile and pliable, leading to pleomorphism.

Developmental Cycle

- Infection is initiated by the attachment of infectious EB to the susceptible host cell (Fig. 30.1).
- After attachment, organism enters the host cell within a vesicle.
- By 9 hours after infection, the EB within the vesicle increases in size and differentiates into RB.
- By 18 hours, within the enlarging vesicle, the RB divides by binary fission to yield pleomorphic organisms, and genus-specific antigens become associated with the host cell surface.
- By 24 hours new EBs develop within the vesicle. The developing chlamydiaceal microcolony, within the vesicle, is termed as **inclusion body** which is typically perinuclear and may contain 100–500 EBs.
- By 40–70 hours, infectious EBs are released from the cell by rupture of the inclusion which may infect new cells.

PATHOGENICITY

Chlamydiaceae produce infections of eye, and genital and respiratory tracts of man (Table 30.1).

Trachoma

It is a communicable chronic keratoconjunctivitis characterized by follicles, papillary hyperplasia, pannus formation and in late stages, cicatrization. It occurs only in humans. It is caused by

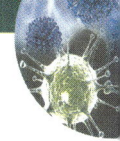

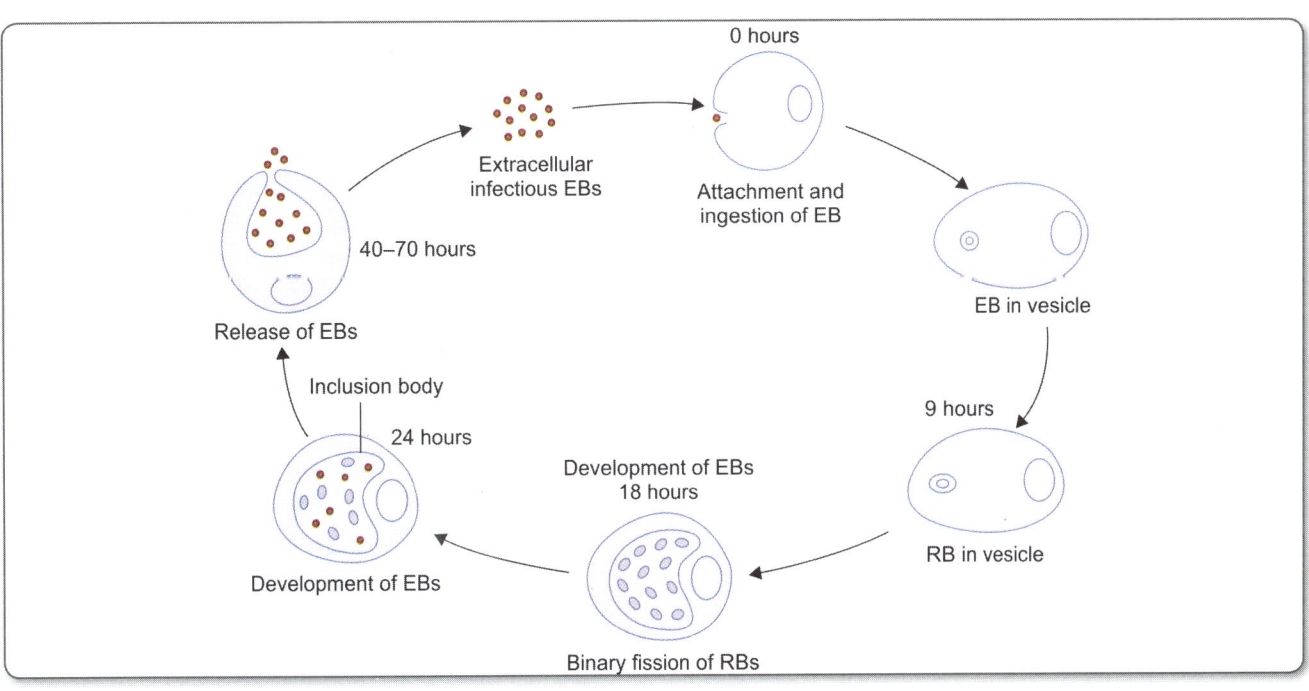

Fig. 30.1: The developmental cycle of Chlamydiaceae.

TABLE 30.1: Chlamydiaceal infections of man

Site of infection	Disease	Organism	Biovar	Serovar
Eye	• Trachoma	*C. trachomatis*	TRIC	A, B, Ba, C
	• Inclusion conjunctivitis	*C. trachomatis*	TRIC	D–K
	• Ophthalmia neonatorum	*C. trachomatis*	TRIC	D–K
Genital tract				
Male	• Urethritis, epididymitis, proctitis	*C. trachomatis*	TRIC	D–K
Female	• Urethritis, cervicitis, salpingitis, infertility, perihepatitis, periappendicitis, proctitis	*C. trachomatis*	TRIC	D–K
	• Abortion, stillbirth (ovine strains)	*C. psittaci*	—	—
Male and female	• Lymphogranuloma venereum	*C. trachomatis*	LGV	L1–L3
Respiratory tract	• Pneumonitis of infant	*C. trachomatis*	TRIC	D–K
	• Pharyngitis, pneumonia	*C. pneumoniae*	—	—
	• Psittacosis	*C. psittaci*	—	—

C. trachomatis biovar TRIC and serovars A, B, Ba and C. The infection is transmitted from eye to eye by direct contact with fingers or contaminated towels and clothing. Flies may also transmit the infection mechanically. Incubation period of the disease appears to be 7–14 days.

Inclusion Conjunctivitis

It is caused by *C. trachomatis* biovar TRIC serovars D–K, natural habitat of which is genital tract of both sexes. It is most prevalent in sexually active young people and is spread from genitalia to eye. The incubation period is 1–2 weeks. The onset is acute, with intense hyperaemia, mucopurulent discharge and follicular hyperplasia. Unlike trachoma, lesions are most pronounced in the lower than in the upper lid. Some patients may develop scarring, corneal lesions or pannus formation. Genital symptoms are minimal or absent particularly in women. Disease is usually self-limiting and does not lead to blindness.

Ophthalmia neonatorum (Inclusion blennorrhoea)

It is the neonatal form of inclusion conjunctivitis. It develops when the infant acquires infection from the birth canal. About 5–12% of all pregnant women have a chlamydial infection of the cervix and 50% of infants born to such mothers develop conjunctivitis. Five to 21 days after birth the neonate develops swelling of the eyelids, hyperaemia and a purulent infiltration of the conjunctiva. A proportion of untreated neonates develop pneumonia.

Genital Infections

Genital infection due to *C. trachomatis* is the most prevalent among the bacterial sexually transmitted diseases. *C. trachomatis* infection, if undiagnosed and untreated, can result in pelvic inflammatory disease, epidydimitis, etc., finally damaging the human reproductive tract irreversibly.

Males

C. trachomatis biovar TRIC serovars D–K account for at least 30% of cases of non-gonococcal urethritis (NGU). This condition develops 7–14 days after sexual intercourse. A minority of cases of NGU are caused by *Ureaplasma urealyticum*. *C. trachomatis* is also responsible for 50% cases of epididymitis in men under 35 years and 15% in men above this age. It may also cause proctitis in homosexual males.

Females

C. trachomatis biovar TRIC serovars D–K may cause urethritis, mucopurulent cervicitis, vaginitis and vaginal discharge, endometritis, salpingitis, infertility, perihepatitis and peri-appendicitis.

Lymphogranuloma Venereum

C. trachomatis biovar TRIC serovars L1–L3 can cause lympho-granuloma venereum in both males and females. Usually 1–3 weeks after sexual contact, male patient develops a small (5–8 mm) painless papule or ulcer on the penis. Rectal infections occur in homosexuals. In women, the commonest site is the fourchette. In both sexes, the primary lesions may pass unnoticed. Primary lesions may occasionally occur on extra genital sites such as fingers or tongue. The primary lesion soon heals but after 1–2 months, the regional lymph nodes (inguinal in males and intrapelvic and pararectal in females) become enlarged and tender, and may break open with the formation of sinuses. These enlarged lymph nodes are called **bubos**.

Respiratory Tract Infections

Chlamydophila pneumoniae causes an acute infection of lower respiratory tract in man. Infection seems to spread from person-to-person without the intervention of an avian host. **Psittacosis** is a disease of the birds of the psittacine (parrot) family, transmissible to man. Similar organisms are also present in a great variety of non-psittacine birds including pigeons, ducks and domestic fowl. The disease acquired by contact with non-psittacine birds is known as **ornithosis**.

Man acquires infection by the inhalation of dried infected faeces of birds. After an incubation period of 1–2 weeks, patient develops clinical disease which may vary from a mild 'influenza-like' syndrome with general malaise, fever, anorexia, rigors, sore throat, headache and photophobia to severe illness with pneumonia, septicaemia, meningoencephalitis, pericarditis, myocarditis, endocarditis, arthritis or a typhoid-like syndrome with enlarged liver and spleen, and a rash.

LABORATORY DIAGNOSIS OF CHLAMYDIACEAL INFECTIONS

- **Direct detection of Chlamydiaceal antigens:**
  - *Light microscopy:* *C. trachomatis* infection of conjunctiva, may be diagnosed by demonstrating typical **reniform inclusion bodies** surrounding the nucleus (Figs 30.2 and 30.3), in the conjunctival smear stained with Giemsa, Castaneda or Macchiavello methods and seen under light microscope. Because the inclusion bodies possess a glycogen matrix, therefore, they may be stained with iodine solution also. This method has a low sensitivity.
  - *Immunofluorescence (IF)*
  - *ELISA for detection of chlamydiaceal antigens*
  - *DNA probes*
- **Isolation of chlamydiaceae:** Chlamydiaceae may be isolated in mice, yolk sac of 6–8-day-old chick embryo and in cell cultures.

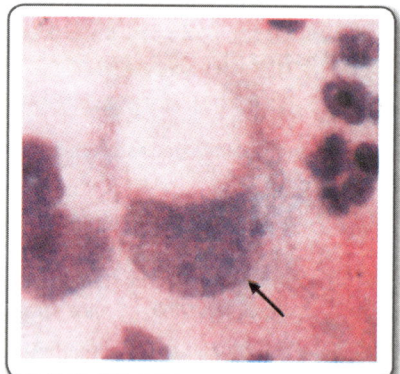

Fig. 30.2: Perinuclear inclusion body of *Chlamydia* (Giema stain, × 400).

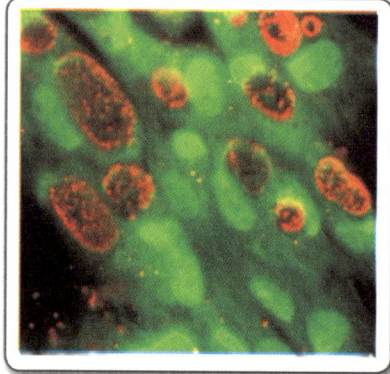

Fig. 30.3: Inclusion body of *Chlamydia* under fluorescence microscope (× 400).

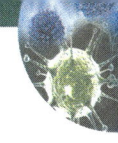

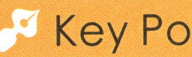

Key Points

- Chlamydiaceae are small obligate intracellular Gram-negative bacteria.
- *Chlamydia trachomatis* causes ocular, genital and respiratory tract infections.

? ASSESS YOURSELF

SHORT ANSWER QUESTION

1. Write short notes on:
   - (a) Developmental cycle of chlamydiaceae
   - (b) Pathogenicity of *Chlamydia* and *Chlamydophila*
   - (c) Laboratory diagnosis of chlamydiaceal infections

Actinomycetes

ACTINOMYCES

Actinomyces are Gram-positive, non-motile, non-sporing, non-acid-fast, 0.5–1 μm in diameter. They often grow in mycelial forms and break up into coccoid and bacillary forms. Most show true branching.

Cultural Characteristics

They grow best under anaerobic or microaerophilic conditions with the addition of 5–10% CO_2. The optimum temperature for growth is 35–37°C. They can be grown on brain heart infusion agar and blood agar. Most species show good growth after 3–4 days' incubation, however, *A. israelii* may take 7–14 days.

Pathogenesis

The *Actinomyces* causes the disease known as actinomycosis. In man, it is usually caused by *A. israelii*. The other species – *A. naeslundii, A. meyeri, A. odontolyticus* and *A. viscosus*, are very rare cause of actinomycosis. All these species are commensals of the mouth, therefore, endogenous cause of disease.

Actinomycosis is a chronic suppurative disease characterized by peripheral spread to contiguous tissues, rare haematogenous spread, formation of sinus tracts which drain suppurative lesions and presence in the pus of colonies of *Actinomyces*. These colonies are 0.25–2 mm in diameter, white to yellowish and are known as '**sulphur granules**'. There are four important sites of primary infection in actinomycosis—cervicofacial, thoracic, abdominal and pelvic.

Laboratory Diagnosis

Specimens

Pus, sinus discharge, bronchial secretions, sputum or infected tissues are collected aseptically. These specimens may contain innumerable 'sulphur granules'. The granules may also be present on dressings removed from a draining sinus tract.

Microscopy

Pus from suspected cases is shaken with sterile water in a tube. '**Sulphur granules**' settle to the bottom. These are removed with a pasteur pipette. Granules are crushed between two slides and stained with Gram and Ziehl-Neelsen staining using 1% sulphuric acid for decolourization. The granules are seen to consist of **Gram-positive hyphal fragments** 0.5–1 μm in diameter, sometimes remaining as intact hyphae several micrometers long and rarely with branches, surrounded by a peripheral zone of swollen radiating club-shaped structures presenting a **sun ray appearance**. These clubs are Gram-negative and are believed to be antigen-antibody complexes. 'Sulphur granules' and mycelia in tissue sections can also be identified by **direct fluorescence microscopy**.

Culture

'Sulphur granules' are washed thoroughly in sterile normal saline in a Petri dish or tube and crushed in a drop of saline with a glass rod. It is then inoculated on brain heart infusion agar, blood agar and in thioglycollate broth, and incubated both anaerobically and under microaerophilic condition with 5–10% CO_2 at 35–37°C for up to 14 days. The colonies of *A. israelii* are 0.5–2 mm in diameter, white to grey-white, smooth, entire or lobulated resembling molar teeth (Fig. 31.1).

Biopsy

In haematoxylin and eosin stained sections, the 'sulphur granules' are deeply stained with haematoxylin except in the periphery which is stained by eosin, which shows short, radiate, club-like

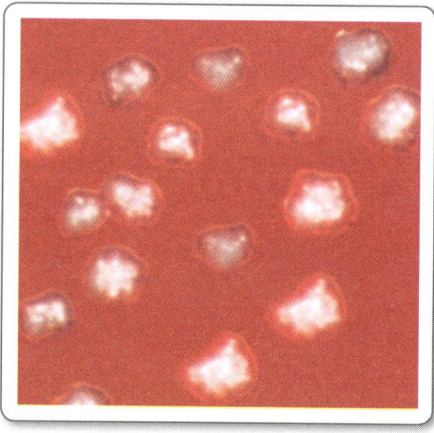

Fig. 31.1: Colonies of *Actinomyces israelii* on blood agar medium. These resemble molar teeth.

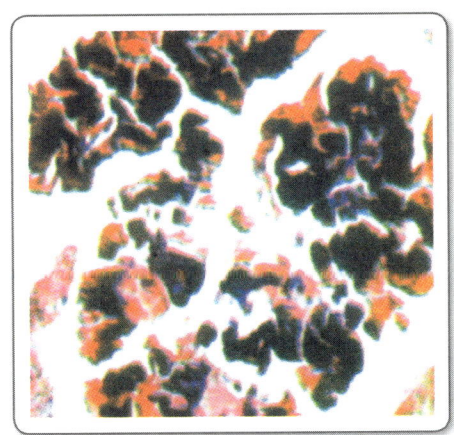

Fig. 31.2: Actinomycosis showing a grain of *Actinomyces israelii*. It is deeply stained with haematoxylin except in the periphery which is stained with eosin (H & E stain × 400).

structures (Fig. 31.2). On Gram staining, the filaments are Gram-positive and periphery Gram-negative. The tissue reaction is a chronic suppurative, fibrosing, inflammatory process.

NOCARDIA, STREPTOMYCES AND ACTINOMADURA

Nocardiae are strictly aerobic, non-motile, Gram-positive bacteria. They form hyphae that often fragment into rod-shaped or coccoid elements. They are acid-fast when decolourized with 1% sulphuric acid. *Streptomyces* and *Actinomadura* are strictly aerobic and non-acid-fast.

Cultural Characteristics

Nocardiae readily grow on nutrient agar, Sabouraud dextrose agar and brain heart infusion agar. The inoculated plates should be incubated at 36°C for up to 3 weeks and examined both macroscopically and microscopically for growth every few days. Nocardiae form white, yellow, pink or brown colonies. *A. madurae* produces waxy, heaped, folded, membranous and tough colony. It may be white, tan, pale orange, pink or red in colour.

A. pelletieri produces heaped, irregular, waxy, and granular colony. It possesses areas of bright and dark red, sparse aerial hyphae. Colonies of *Streptomyces* are usually highly filamentous with dense aerial hyphae.

Pathogenicity

N. asteroides and sometimes *N. farcinica*, *N. nova*, *N. brasiliensis* and *N. otitidiscaviarum* produce opportunistic pulmonary disease known as nocardiosis in usually, but not always, immunocompromised individuals including those receiving immunosuppressive therapy and those with AIDS. Soil and composting matter is known to be the natural habitat of *Nocardia*. It is, therefore, believed that man and animals acquire infection by inhalation of the organism from environmental sources.

Nocardiosis is a systemic bacterial disease. It generally originates as a pulmonary infection, varying in its course from mild and slowly progressive to fulminant and fatal. It may be characterized by single or multiple nodules, miliary pattern, scattered infiltrations, bronchopneumonia, abscesses, masses with central cavitation, pleural effusions and empyema. Dissemination from the primary focus of infection may occur through pleural extension, lymphohaematogenous spread or invasion of blood vessels with bacteraemia. Although, every organ of the body may be affected, involvement of brain, meninges and spinal cord is said to be commoner than that of other parts such as skin, subcutaneous tissues, eye, liver, lymph node, etc.

Laboratory Diagnosis

Microscopy

Pus or purulent blood-flecked sputum is spread on a slide by crushing between two slides. The smears are stained by Gram and Ziehl-Neelsen techniques and examined under oil-immersion lens. Granules may be seen in specimens from cutaneous infection. Sampled tissue and pus from the draining sinuses are the specimens of choice for direct examination. The granules may be visualized by separating them from the pus with an inoculating needle and then washing in sterile saline. These may be crushed between two glass slides which are then used for Gram and Ziehl-Neelsen staining.

Culture

Pus, sputum or the granules are then inoculated on nutrient agar, Sabouraud dextrose agar and brain heart infusion agar, and incubated at 36°C for 3 weeks. Culture media are examined both macroscopically and microscopically every few days for identification of the isolate.

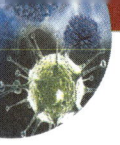

Key Points

- *Actinomyces* spp. are **potentially pathogenic commensals** of the mouth in humans and animals
- An association between **root surface caries** of teeth and *Actinomyces* has been described.
- *Actinomyces* spp. cause **cervicofacial, thoracic, abdominal** and **pelvic actinomycosis**, which are essentially **chronic granulomatous infections.**

ASSESS YOURSELF

SHORT ANSWER QUESTIONS

1. Write short notes on:
   - (a) Actinomycosis
   - (b) Nocardiosis
   - (c) Laboratory diagnosis of actinomycosis

MULTIPLE CHOICE QUESTIONS

1. Which of the following bacteria is acid-fast to 1% sulphuric acid:
   - (a) *Actinomyces*
   - (b) *Nocardia*
   - (c) *Streptomyces*
   - (d) *Corynebacterium*
2. Which of the following bacteria is the commonest cause of cervicofacial actinomycosis?
   - (a) *Actinomyces israelii.*
   - (b) *A. naeslundii*
   - (c) *A. viscosus*
   - (d) *A. meyeri*

ANSWERS TO MCQs

1. b   2. a

Pathogenic Organisms-II
Viruses

Section Summary

Chapter 32

General Properties of Viruses

Viruses are the smallest known infective agents. They are obligate intracellular parasites. The extracellular infectious virus particle is known as virion. Three main properties distinguish viruses from other microorganisms:

- **Small size:** Viruses are smaller than other organisms. They vary in size from 10–300 nm. Therefore, they can pass through bacterial filters and they cannot be seen by light microscope. However, the poxviruses which are the largest members of the virus family and are very similar in size to the smallest bacteria, are close to the resolution of light microscope. For visualization of all other viruses an electron microscope is necessary.
- **Genome:** A virus carries its own genetic information in the form of either RNA or DNA, but not both. The genome may be single-stranded or double-stranded, circular or linear, and segmented or unsegmented.
- **Metabolically inert:** Viruses have no metabolic activity outside susceptible host cells. They do not possess ribosomes or protein-synthesizing apparatus. Viruses, therefore, cannot multiply in inanimate media but only inside living cells. Inside the living cells the virus genome is capable of replicating new virus particles.

STRUCTURE OF THE VIRUSES

Viruses consist of nucleic acid core surrounded by a protein coat called **capsid**. It is composed of capsomers. The capsid with the enclosed nucleic acid is known as **nucleocapsid**.

Virus Symmetry

Capsid of the virus particles shows three types of symmetry. It is determined by the arrangement of the capsomers around the nucleic acid.

- **Icosahedral symmetry:** The capsomers are arranged as if they lay on the faces of an icosahedron which has 20 equilateral triangular faces and 12 corners or apices (Fig. 32.1).
- **Helical symmetry:** The nucleic acid and the capsomers are wound together in the form of a helix or spiral.
- **Complex symmetry:** Viruses (e.g. poxviruses) which do not show either icosahedral or helical symmetry due to

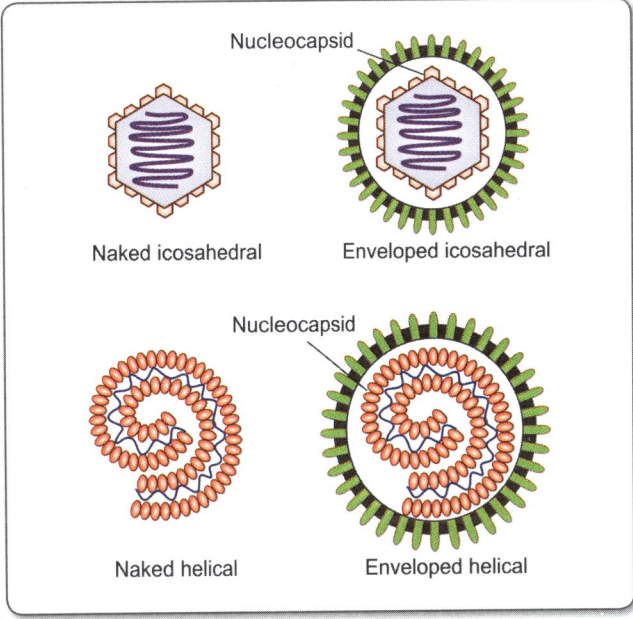

Fig. 32.1: Symmetry of viruses.

complexity of their structure are referred to have complex symmetry.

Envelope

Generally, DNA viruses replicate and are assembled in the nucleus and RNA viruses are assembled in the cytoplasm. The final assembly of some viruses occurs at the nuclear or cytoplasmic membrane. As the virus particle moves from the nucleus to the cytoplasm or passes from the cytoplasm to the extracellular space, an external lipid-containing envelope (host origin) with virus-coded polypeptides or virus-specified glycoproteins is added to the nucleocapsid. In mature virus particle the glycoproteins often appear as projecting spikes on the outer surface of the envelope. These are known as **peplomers**.

REPLICATION OF VIRUSES

The genetic information necessary for viral multiplication is contained in the viral nucleic acid but the biosynthetic enzymes

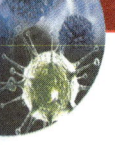

are lacking. They replicate by taking over the biochemical machinery of the host cell and redirecting it to the manufacture of virus components. The viral replication is divided into six stages:

Adsorption

The first event in the infection of a cell by a virus is the attachment of the virus particle to the cell surface.

Entry into the Host Cells

After attachment nonenveloped viruses are engulfed by a mechanism resembling phagocytosis, a process known as **viropexis**. In case of enveloped viruses, the envelope fuses with the plasma membrane of the host cell and releases the nucleocapsid into the cytoplasm.

Uncoating

This is the process of stripping the virus of its capsid so that nucleic acid is released into the cell.

Biosynthesis

This phase includes synthesis of:
- The viral nucleic acid.
- Capsid protein.
- Enzymes necessary in the various stages of viral synthesis, assembly and release.
- Certain regulatory proteins which serve to shut down the normal cellular metabolism and direct the sequential production of viral components.

Virion Assembly

Assembly of the various viral components into virions occurs shortly after the replication of the viral nucleic acid and may take place in either the nucleus (herpesviruses and adenoviruses) or cytoplasm (picornaviruses and poxviruses). In case of enveloped viruses, the envelope is derived from the nuclear membrane if they assemble in the nucleus (herpesviruses), and from plasma membrane, if they assemble in the cytoplasm of the host cell (orthomyxoviruses, paramyxoviruses and retroviruses). However, in this envelope virus encoded peplomers are also embedded.

Release

Release of completed viruses is the final step in virus multiplication. Viruses that exist as **naked nucleocapsids** may be released by the lysis of the host cell (polioviruses) or they may be extruded by a process which may be called reverse phagocytosis. **Enveloped viruses** are released by a process of budding through special areas of host cell membrane (cytoplasmic or nuclear), where virus-specified transmembrane glycoproteins (peplomers) have been embedded.

VIRUS ISOLATION

Viruses can replicate only in living cells, therefore, they cannot be grown on any of the inanimate culture media. Most of the viruses can be cultivated in laboratory animals, chick embryos or cell cultures.

Laboratory Animals

Suckling mice less than 24-hour-old are used in the isolation of arboviruses, rabies virus and some of the group A coxsackieviruses. These are inoculated intracerebrally and/or intraperitoneally, then observed for up to 2 weeks for the development of pathognomonic signs before sacrificing the animal for histological examination of affected organs.

Chick Embryos

Embryonated eggs offer several sites for the cultivation of viruses. Chorioallantoic membrane (CAM), allantoic cavity, amniotic cavity and yolk sac (Fig. 32.2) of 8–11-day-old eggs are inoculated and incubated for 2–9 days. The duration of incubation depends on the virus type and route of inoculation. Viruses may kill the embryo or may produce visible lesions like pocks on CAM, and haemagglutinating activity in the harvested amniotic and allantoic fluid. These effects help in the identification of the virus.

The chorioallantoic membrane method is used mainly for poxviruses. The amniotic route of inoculation is used mainly for primary isolation of influenza viruses, and the allantoic route for serial passages and for obtaining large quantities of virus for vaccine production.

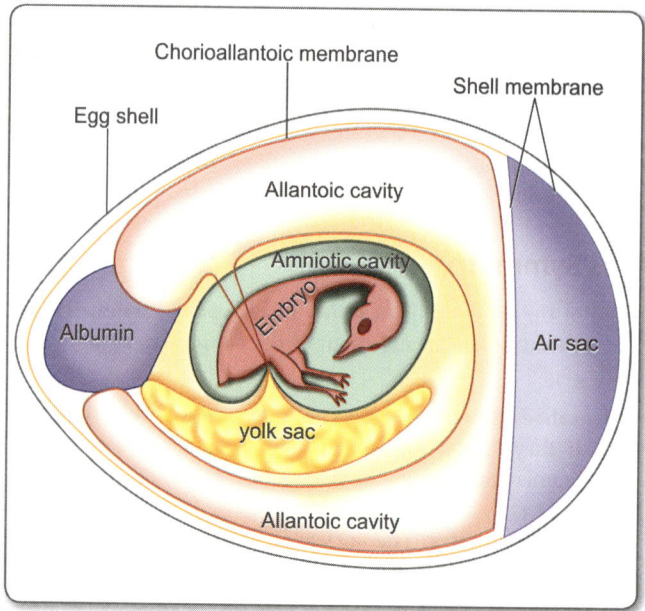

Fig. 32.2: Cross-section of an embryonated hen's egg.

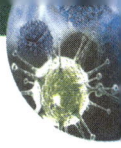

Cell Culture

This is the type of culture routinely employed for diagnostic virology and for studying virus-cell interactions.

Primary Cell Culture

These are normal cells freshly taken from the body and cultured. They are capable of very limited growth *in vitro* perhaps 5–10 divisions at the most.

Finite (diploid) Cell Cultures

These are cells of a single type, usually fibroblasts, that retain their original diploid chromosome number and karyotype. They can be subcultured for about 50 passages before the cells die off.

Continuous Cell Lines

These are cells of a single type that are capable of indefinite propagation *in vitro*. Therefore, they are known as continuous cell lines. They have been derived from diploid cell lines or from malignant tissues. Continuous cell lines such as HeLa, HEp-2 and KB derived from human carcinoma of cervix, human epithelioma of larynx, and human carcinoma of nasopharynx respectively, support the growth of a number of viruses.

Detection of Virus Growth in Cell Culture

Virus growth in cell culture can be detected by the following methods:

Cytopathic Effect

Many viruses produce morphological changes in the cultured cells in which they grow. These changes are known as **cytopathic effects (CPE)** and viruses causing CPE are known as **cytopathogenic viruses**. Following are the main types of CPE:

- **Rounding of cells:** Viral replication may lead to nuclear pyknosis, rounding, refractility, degeneration and eventually complete or partial detachment of infected cells from the glass. This is seen in picornaviruses.
- **Rounding and aggregation:** Some viruses may lead to cell rounding and aggregation into grape-like clusters which detach from the glass, leaving clear areas. It is seen in adenoviruses.
- **Syncytium formation:** Some viruses (measles virus, respiratory syncytial virus and HIV) lead to syncytium formation in which infected cells fuse with neighbouring infected or uninfected cells to form giant cells containing several (up to 100) nuclei.
- **Inclusion bodies:** These are intranuclear or intra-cytoplasmic aggregates of products of viral replication such as virus particles ready for release, overproduction of a particular viral protein or some aberrant cellular structure

such as clumped chromatin. They can be seen in stained preparations under a light microscope. They may be present in the cytoplasm or in the nucleus, or both of infected cells and may be acidophilic or basophilic, single or multiple, large or small and round or irregular. Vaccinia and rabies viruses produce intracytoplasmic inclusion bodies, and adenoviruses and herpesviruses produce intranuclear inclusions. Inclusion bodies of measles virus are seen in both the locations.

Haemadsorption

Orthomyxoviruses (influenza) and paramyxoviruses (para-influenza, measles and mumps) code for red cell agglutinins which are incorporated into the cell membrane during infection, so that guinea pig erythrocytes adhere to the infected cells. This adherence of erythrocytes to the infected cells is known as haemadsorption. It can be used to recognize infection with non-cytocidal viruses, as well as the early stage of cytocidal viruses. Sometimes virus can be detected by haemagglutination in the medium (culture fluid).

Interference

The multiplication of one virus in a cell usually inhibits the multiplication of a second virus, called the challenge virus, when it is added to the culture. This is because the first virus interferes with the replicative process of the challenge virus and is known as **interference challenge test**. This can be used for the detection of the growth of a non-cytopathogenic virus in cell culture.

Transformation

Tumour-forming (oncogenic) viruses induce cell transformation and loss of normal contact inhibition, so that growth appears in a piled-up fashion producing microtumours.

Fluorescent Antibody Testing

Cells from virus infected cultures can be stained with fluorescein-conjugated antiserum and seen under fluorescence microscope for virus antigens.

Detection of Enzymes

The virus isolate can be identified by detection of viral enzymes, such as reverse transcriptase in retroviruses, in the culture fluid.

Electron Microscopy

Viruses have distinctive appearances and can be detected by electron microscopy of ultra-thin sections of infected cells.

CLASSIFICATION OF VIRUSES

Viruses are broadly classified into DNA and RNA viruses and then further divided into families, subfamilies, genera and species.

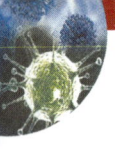

LABORATORY DIAGNOSIS OF VIRAL INFECTIONS

Direct Detection of Virus, Viral Antigen or Viral Genomev

Electron Microscopy

Electron microscopy (EM) is one of the most useful tools for the direct demonstration of viruses in clinical specimens.

Immunoelectron Microscopy

EM as a diagnostic tool has low sensitivity. The sensitivity of electron microscopy can be increased by mixing specific antibody with the specimen to aggregate the virus particles. These aggregates can be sedimented by centrifugation, negatively stained and observed under EM.

Fluorescence Microscopy

Virions or viral antigens can be detected in frozen tissue sections, acetone-fixed cell smears, cells from virus infected cultures or vesicle fluid by direct or indirect fluorescent antibody technique. Fluorescence microscopy of brain biopsy can be used for the diagnosis of herpes simplex encephalitis, subacute sclerosing panencephalitis (a late sequelae of measles), for the verification of rabies in the brain of animals suspected to be rabid. This method is also useful for the rapid diagnosis of respiratory infections caused by paramyxoviruses, orthomyxoviruses, adenoviruses and herpesviruses.

Light Microscopy

Inclusion bodies in tissue section may be detected by light microscopy, e.g. demonstration of Negari bodies in the brain cells of animals is a useful method for presumptive diagnosis rabies. Viral antigens in infected cells can be detected by immunoperoxidase staining.

Viral Antigens

These may be detected by direct and indirect ELISA, radioimmunoassay and latex agglutination.

Nucleic Acid Probes

- Enzyme-labelled or radiolabelled nucleic acid (DNA or RNA) sequences complementary to unique regions in nucleic acid sequences of most viruses are now manufactured commercially. These labelled complementary sequences are known as nucleic acid probes. Two strands of the target DNA molecule in the clinical specimens are first separated by boiling, then, following cooling, allowed to hybridize with a labelled single-stranded DNA or RNA probe present in excess. Depending on the type of label attached to the probe, hybridized-labelled probe can be detected by radiography, gamma counting or by a simple colourimetric evaluation (dot-blot hybridization).
- By use of nucleic acid probes cytomegalovirus, papillomavirus and Epstein-Barr virus have been identified.
- **In situ hybridization** may be used to detect integrated or nonintegrated copies of viral genome in persistent infections or viral cancers.
- **Southern blot hybridization and northern blot hybridization** can be used for detection of DNA and RNA respectively.

Polymerase Chain Reaction (PCR)

It is a DNA amplification system that allows molecular biologists to produce microgram quantities of DNA from picogram amounts of starting material. It is based on repeated cycles of high temperature template denaturation, oligonucleotide primer annealing and polymerase mediated extension. With the revolutionary PCR technique, a target DNA sequence can be amplified at least 100,000 folds in just a few hours, a sharp contrast to the days required for conventional amplification method (culture). Thus, viral DNA extracted from a very small number of virions or infected cells can be amplified to the point where it can readily be identified using labelled probes in a hybridization assay. For the detection of viral RNA, it is first converted into DNA by reverse transcriptase.

PCR can be used for the diagnosis of infections caused by HIV-1, HIV-2, HTLV-1, cytomegalovirus, human *Papillomavirus*, herpes simplex viruses, HBV, HCV, HDV, HEV, rubella virus, Epstein-Barr virus, varicella-zoster virus, human herpesvirus 6 and 7, *Parvovirus* B19, enteroviruses, coxsackieviruses, echoviruses, rhinoviruses, measles virus and *Rotavirus*.

Virus Isolation

Most of the viruses can be cultivated in laboratory animals, chick embryos and cell cultures.

Detection of Specific Antiviral Antibodies

Using panels of known antigens, a number of serological techniques may be used to detect specific viral antibodies. Paired sera should be collected from the patient, the 'acute-phase' serum sample collected as early as possible in the illness and the 'convalescent-phase' sample collected at least 2 weeks later. Antibodies in the serum samples can be detected by ELISA, RIA, western blot, latex agglutination, virus neutralization, haemagglutination inhibition, immunofluorescence, immunodiffusion and complement fixation tests.

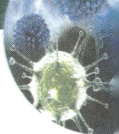

Cytological or Histological Examination of Cells from the Site of Infection

Virus-induced histopathology (multinucleate giant cells and inclusion bodies) may be recognized by light microscopy. For example, demonstration of Negri bodies in the brain cells of animals is a useful method for presumptive diagnosis of rabies.

 ## Key Points

- **Viruses** are **obligate intracellular parasites**, which are metabolically inert, and can replicate only within living cells.
- The virus **genome** has either **DNA** or **RNA** but never both.
- The genome is protected by an **outer protein coat (capsid)** composed of **capsomers**; the **nucleocapsid** is the term given to the **protein and the viral genome** complex.
- The nucleocapsid of viruses is arranged in one of three spatial configurations – **icosahedral**, **helical** or **complex symmetry**.
- The stages of **viral replication** are **adsorption**, **entry into host cells**, **uncoating**, **biosynthesis**, **virion assembly** and **release**.

ASSESS YOURSELF

LONG AND SHORT ANSWER QUESTIONS

1. Write short notes on:
   - (a) Viral capsid
   - (b) Viral envelope
2. Discuss replication of viruses.
3. Discuss various methods of detecting viral growth in cell cultures.
4. Describe laboratory diagnosis of viral infections.

MULTIPLE CHOICE QUESTIONS

1. The function/s of a viral capsid is/are:
   - (a) it protects the viral genome from physical and enzymatic destruction
   - (b) it provides binding sites that enable the virus to attach to specific receptor sites on the host cell
   - (c) it serves as a vehicle of transmission from one host to another
   - (d) All of the above

2. Which of the following viruses is/are enveloped?
   - (a) Herpes
   - (b) Polio.
   - (c) Adeno
   - (d) All of the above

3. Lesions on chorioallantoic membrane are produced by which of the following viruses?
   - (a) Vaccinia virus
   - (b) Herpes simplex virus
   - (c) Herpes B virus
   - (d) All of the above

4. Haemadsorption of infected cells is observed with:
   - (a) Parainfluenza viruses
   - (b) Measles virus
   - (c) Mumps virus
   - (d) All of the above

5. Which of the following viruses show/s transformation of infected cells?
   - (a) Hepatitis B virus
   - (b) Human T cell lymphotropic virus type 1
   - (c) Epstein-Barr virus
   - (d) All of the above

6. Which of the following viruses belong/s to the family Hepadnaviridae?
   - (a) Hepatitis A virus
   - (b) Hepatitis B virus
   - (c) Hepatitis D virus
   - (d) All of the above

Contd...

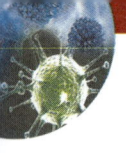

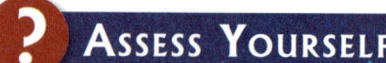

❓ ASSESS YOURSELF

7. Which of the following viruses belong/s to family Caliciviridae?
   - (a) Hepatitis B virus
   - (b) Hepatitis D virus.
   - (c) Hepatitis E virus
   - (d) All of the above

8. Which of the following is RNA virus?
   - (a) Papilloma virus
   - (b) Influenza virus
   - (c) Hepatitis B virus
   - (d) Epstein-Barr virus

9. Which of the following is DNA virus?
   - (a) Polio virus
   - (b) Rubella virus
   - (c) Vaccinia virus
   - (d) Human immunodeficiency virus

10. Which of the following is **not** RNA virus?
    - (a) Retrovirus
    - (b) Enterovirus
    - (c) Rhabdovirus
    - (d) Adenovirus

ANSWERS TO MCQs

1. d   **2.** a   **3.** d   **4.** d   **5.** d   **6.** b   **7.** c   **8.** b   **9.** c   **10.** d

Chapter 33

Smallpox and Herpesviruses

SMALLPOX

Morphology

Smallpox virus is brick-shaped with rounded corners, measuring $250 \times 200 \times 200$ nm in size (Fig. 33.1). Nucleocapsid of this virus does not conform to either of two types of symmetry found in most other viruses, hence, it is known as complex virus. It has a biconcave dumbbell-shaped DNA core and two lateral bodies enclosed in a protein shell about 12 nm thick. It is known as outer membrane, surface of which consists of irregularly arranged tubules. Virions released from the cell are enclosed within an envelope which consists of host cell lipids and several virus-specified polypeptides, including the haemagglutinin. The virus can be cultured on chorioallantoic membrane, HeLa and chick embryo cell cultures.

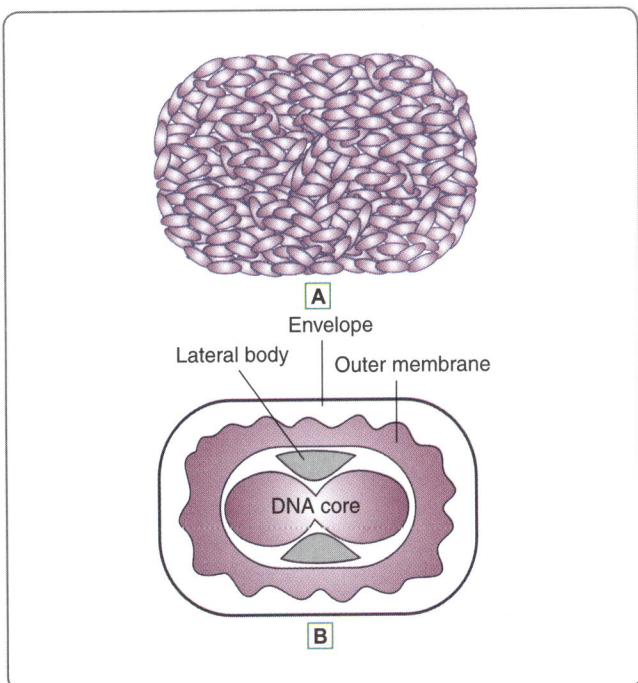

Fig. 33.1: Structure of smallpox virus: (A) surface structure, (B) section of virus.

Eradication

In 1967 the World Health Organization (WHO) embarked on a Smallpox Eradication Campaign. The world's last naturally occurring case of smallpox was recorded in Merca, Southern Somalia, in October, 1977. On May 8, 1980, the WHO formally announced the **global eradication of smallpox**. Eradication of smallpox could be achieved because of:

- Its low communicability.
- No subclinical infection or carrier state.
- A single serotype virus which induced good immunity.
- An effective vaccine (originally discovered by Jenner in 1796).
- No animal reservoir.
- Aggressive surveillance containment measures.

VACCINIA

Origin of vaccinia virus is not known. It may have evolved from cowpox or smallpox virus. In the past, this virus was used for smallpox vaccination. Strains of recombinant vaccinia virus as vectors incorporating genes for protective antigens for several different pathogens are being developed. Because the large vaccinia genome can accommodate at least a dozen foreign genes, it is theoretically possible to construct a single recombinant virus as a vaccine capable of protecting against most of the common viral and nonviral infectious diseases of childhood.

HERPESVIRUSES

Morphology

Herpesviruses are 120–200 nm in diameter. They comprise of four distinct structural elements – envelope, tegument, capsid and core (Fig. 33.2). Envelope is the outermost, it is composed of lipid with numerous small glycoprotein peplomers. Tegument is the electron-dense material present between envelope and capsid. It contains several proteins. Inner to the tegument is icosahedral capsid of 100 nm diameter. It has a total of 162 capsomers. Core, inside the capsid, consists of double-stranded, 124–235 kb DNA.

Essentials of Applied Microbiology for BSc Nursing

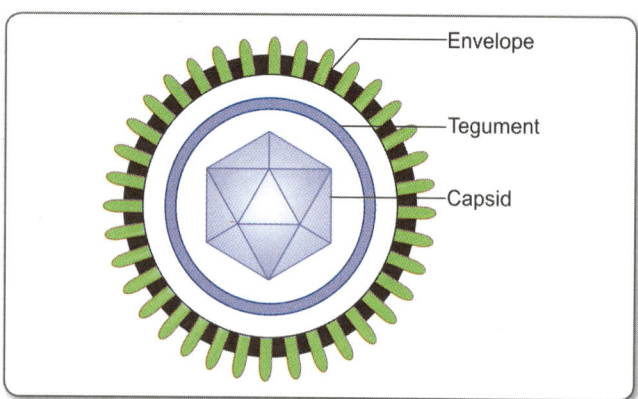

Fig. 33.2: Herpesvirus.

Cultivation

Members of Herpesviridae can be cultivated in cell culture.

Herpes Simplex Virus (HSV)

There are two types of herpes simplex virus – type 1 virus (HSV-1) and type 2 virus (HSV-2). Both these viruses share many characteristics, including DNA homology, antigen determinants, tissue tropism, and disease signs.

Pathogenesis

HSV-1 infects primarily the mouth, the eye and the central nervous system (regions of the body above the waist), but it is also responsible for a proportion of cases of genital herpes. HSV-2 infects genital and anal regions. The infections caused by herpes simplex viruses can be divided into primary infection, latent infection, reactivation and recrudescence.

Primary Infections

HSV is transmitted only by contact. The portal of entry in primary infection is the damaged skin or mucosa and the classic lesion is a vesicle beneath the keratinized squamous epithelial cells.

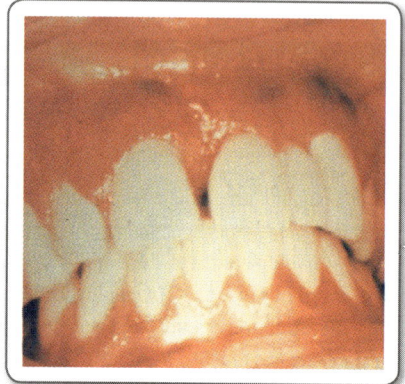

Fig. 33.3: Herpetic gingivostomatitis.

HSV-1

Infections caused by HSV-1

- Acute gingivostomatitis (Fig. 33.3).
- Herpetic whitlow.
- Keratoconjunctivitis.
- Eczema herpeticum.
- Encephalitis.
- Generalized infection.

HSV-2

Infections caused by HSV-2

- Genital herpes.
- Aseptic meningitis.
- Neonatal infection.

It may rarely cause head and neck infections.

Latent Infection

During primary infection, the virus travels from the site of infection in the mouth to the trigeminal and probably other cranial and cervical ganglia. In genital herpes, HSV-2 travels to sacral ganglia. Within the sensory ganglia, viral DNA exists as a free circular episome perhaps about 20 copies per infected cells.

Reactivation and Recrudescence

Reactivation of the virus is provoked by various stimuli such as common cold, fever, pneumonia, menstruation, exposure to sunlight, stress, etc. Infectious virions migrate along the nerve axon back to the nerve endings, where infection of epithelial cells may result in cluster of vesicles at the mucocutaneous junctions of the lips, in the nose, or eyes or on areas of skin that have experienced a primary infection. Reactivation recurs sporadically, sometimes often, throughout life.

Laboratory Diagnosis

Specimens

Specimens include vesicle fluid, skin swab, saliva, conjunctival fluid, corneal scrapings, brain biopsy and CSF.

Microscopy

Diagnosis of HSV infection can be made by direct examination of clinical specimens by electron microscopy (EM), fluorescence

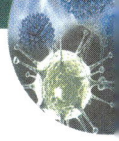

microscopy (FM) and light microscopy (LM). Herpes virions may be demonstrated in the negatively stained smear of the specimen by EM. Viral antigens can be detected by FM in the cells scraped from the base of the lesions and tissue preparations stained by immunofluorescent staining. By LM, infected cell may be identified by characteristic changes, which include ballooning of cells, ground glass nuclei, **eosinophilic intranuclear inclusions and multinucleated giant cells**.

Virus Isolation

HSV can be isolated on human fibroblast, Vero cells, human amnion and HeLa cells. Within 1–5 days distinctive foci of swollen, rounded cells appear. Some virus strains (particularly HSV-2 strains) may give rise to fusion of infected cells leading to **syncytium formation**. Diagnosis can be confirmed within 24 hours by **immunofluorescent staining** of infected cell culture. Differentiation of HSV-1 and HSV-2 can be made by use of monoclonal antibodies in immunofluorescent staining or by **neutralization test** with specific antiserum.

Serology

Primary infections can be diagnosed serologically by detection of virus-specific IgM or of a rising IgG titre by complement fixation, neutralization, immunofluorescence, ELISA or RIA. However, serology is not widely used.

Polymerase Chain Reaction

Polymerase chain reaction may be used for detection of HSV DNA in CSF.

Chemotherapy

HSV infection can be successfully treated with acyclovir (acycloguanosine). For the treatment of ophthalmic herpes simplex infection, it may be used in the form of ointment.

Varicella-Zoster Virus (VZV)

VZV causes varicella (chickenpox) in children and herpes zoster (shingles) in adults and immunocompromised patients. **Varicella follows primary infection in a nonimmune individual while herpes zoster is a reactivation of latent virus when immunity has fallen to ineffective levels.** A child can catch varicella from an elderly patient with herpes zoster, but the latter occurs only if the elderly or immunocompromised person had suffered from variccla in carly part of his life.

Varicella

It is one of the common childhood exanthemata. Portal of entry of the virus is respiratory tract. Incubation period is about 2 weeks. The earliest manifestation is a **maculopapular rash** that progresses within a few hours to the vesicular stage. Vesicles

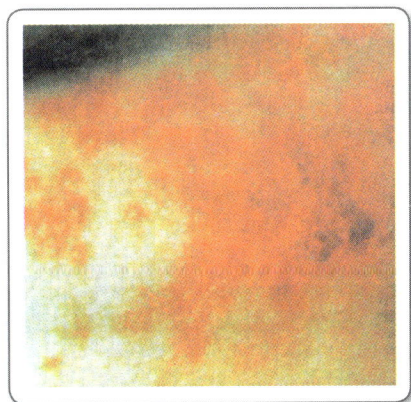

Fig. 33.4: Vesicles of varicella zoster infection on the left shoulder and neck.

characteristically are surrounded by a red rim. The lesions then rupture and crust or may become secondarily infected and pustular before healing.

Herpes Zoster

Herpes zoster or shingles is an **endogenous reactivation of virus** which has remained latent in one or more sensory ganglia following primary varicella many years earlier. Virus travels down the sensory nerves to produce painful vesicles in the area of skin (dermatome) enervated from the affected ganglion (Fig. 33.4). Thoracic nerves supplying the chest wall are most often affected. When the ophthalmic nerve of trigeminal ganglion is affected, the rash is distributed on the scalp and forehead. In about half of the patients, the eye is affected leading to corneal ulceration, stromal keratitis and anterior uveitis.

Laboratory Diagnosis

- Direct examination of vesicle fluid by **electron microscopy** may reveal herpes virus particles.
- Stained smears from the base of the lesion or sections from biopsy tissue show **multinucleated giant cells containing acidophilic intranuclear inclusion bodies**.
- Rapid diagnosis is possible by using **monoclonal fluorescent antibody technique**.
- VZV antigens can be detected in vesicle fluid by **ELISA**.
- DNA can be extracted from virions in vesicle fluid, CSF, aqueous humour, and amplified by **PCR** and detected by nucleic acid hybridization.
- The virus can be **isolated** from vesicle fluid in human embryonic lung fibroblasts, human amnion, HeLa or Vero cells. Cytopathic effect is focal with refractile ballooned cells. It develops slowly over a period of 2 or more weeks. However, VZV antigen can be demonstrated in nuclear inclusions by immunofluorescence with monoclonal antibody before the end of first week.

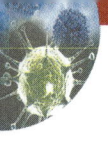

SECTION V • PATHOGENIC ORGANISMS–II VIRUSES

- Recent infection can be diagnosed by **ELISA test** for varicella-zoster specific IgM antibody in patient serum.

Treatment

Acyclovir and vidarabine given intravenously are effective in the treatment of severe varicella and herpes zoster (e.g. in the immunocompromised patients).

EPSTEIN-BARR VIRUS (EBV)

EBV has been named after the virologists (Epstein and Barr) who first observed it under electron microscope in cultures of lymphoblasts from Burkitt's lymphoma. EBV replicates in epithelial cells of nasopharynx and salivary glands. Most shedding of virus takes place in the oral cavity, therefore, transmission of virus requires salivary contact, either through kissing or contaminated eating utensils. Most infections are symptomless, especially when acquired during childhood. However, in adolescents it may cause infectious mononucleosis or glandular fever, infections in immunocompromised hosts and when EBV exerts its oncogenic potential, it may cause Burkitt's lymphoma, B cell lymphoma and nasopharyngeal carcinoma. In HIV-infected individuals, it may cause hairy leukoplakia and lymphocytic interstitial pneumonitis.

Infectious Mononucleosis (Glandular Fever)

It is a primary EBV infection seen mainly in the 15–25 years age group. EBV is commonly transmitted by infected saliva and initiates infection in the oropharynx. Viral replication occurs in epithelial cells of the pharynx and salivary glands.

After an incubation period of 4–7 weeks, patient presents with sore throat due to exudative tonsillitis, generalized lymph-adenopathy, fever, malaise, headache, sweating, fatigue and gastrointestinal discomfort. In some cases spleen and liver are often enlarged. A faint transient morbilliform rash may be seen. A maculopapular rash may appear, especially following treatment with ampicillin due to immune complexes with antibody to ampicillin. The disease usually lasts for 2–3 weeks. However, some patients develop complications such as Guillain-Barré syndrome, Bell's palsy, meningoencephalitis, transverse myelitis, haemolytic anaemia, thrombocytopenia, carditis, nephritis, pneumonia and splenic rupture.

EBV-associated Malignancies

1. Burkitt's Lymphoma

This lymphoma is a **malignant B cell lymphoma** (a tumour of the jaw) seen in regions of equatorial Africa and New Guinea where malaria is hyperendemic. EBV infection is acquired early in life. Malaria being immunosuppressive, may act as a co-factor by interfering with the immune responses that normally prevent reactivation of EBV from B cells thus enabling its full oncogenic potential to be expressed. The EBV genomic DNA is present in multiple copies, in the form of circular episomes, in each cell of most African Burkitt's lymphomas, but the cells do not produce virus unless induced to do so following cultivation *in vitro*. Tumour cells express viral antigens and sera from such patients contain elevated levels of antibody to virus-specific antigens.

2. B Cell Lymphoma

Immunodeficient patients, e.g. recipients of transplants and HIV-infected patients may develop EBV associated B cell lymphoma.

3. Nasopharyngeal Carcinoma

It is also associated with EBV and viral DNA is regularly present in the malignant epithelial cells of the tumour. The patients have high levels of antibody to EBV. It shows a striking geographical and probably racial distribution, for example, the disease is common in people from Southern China, and in Eskimos and Greenlanders.

Oral Hairy Leukoplakia

This lesion is a wart-like growth that develops on the tongue in some HIV-infected patients and recipients of transplant (Fig. 33.5). It is an epithelial focus of EBV replication.

Lymphocytic Interstitial Pneumonitis

EBV has also been associated with lymphocytic interstitial pneumonitis in HIV-infected children.

Laboratory Diagnosis of Infectious Mononucleosis

1. Differential White Blood Cell Count

By the second week of the illness patient develops leucocytosis (10,000–20,000/μl or more). Lymphocytes and monocytes account for 60–80%. Of these, 20% or more are **'atypical lymphocytes'**.

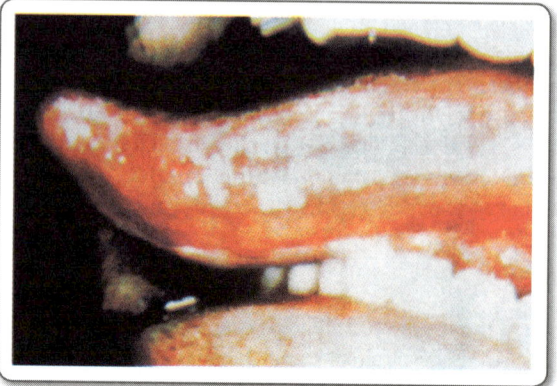

Fig. 33.5: Oral hairy leukoplakia in an AIDs patient.

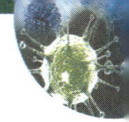

The latter are large pleomorphic blasts with deeply basophilic vacuolated cytoplasm and lobulated nuclei. They persist for 2 weeks to several months.

2. Paul-Bunnell Heterophile Antibodies

Infectious mononucleosis is accompanied by production of **heterophile agglutinins**. These are heterophile IgM antibodies elicited by EBV infection. These antibodies appear in 85–90% of patients' sera during the acute phase of illness, reaching peak levels 2 weeks after the onset. Their titre decreases rapidly after fourth week and are not detectable after 3 months. Heterophile antibodies may be readily detected by a rapid slide agglutination test or Paul-Bunnell test. Agglutination of sheep or horse red cells by patient serum, adsorbed with guinea pig kidney cells, to remove Forssman antibody, is the basis of this test.

3. EBV-specific Antibodies

More reliable indicator of EBV infection is the demonstration of IgM antibody to the EBV viral capsid antigen by ELISA or indirect immunofluorescence. This antibody becomes detectable within 4 weeks and declines rapidly over the next 3 months or so.

4. Virus Isolation

Saliva or throat washing and peripheral blood leucocytes can be inoculated onto umbilical cord lymphocytes. If the specimen contains EBV, it leads to immortalization of the cells to produce a lymphoblastoid cell line.

5. PCR and DNA Hybridization

EBV can also be detected by PCR and DNA hybridization.

CYTOMEGALOVIRUS (CMV)

CMV is the largest virus in the family Herpesviridae, being 150–200 nm in size. The virus exhibits strict host-specificity. *In vivo*, CMV replicates in epithelial cells in salivary glands, kidneys and respiratory epithelium. The infected cells are enlarged and possess inclusions in both the nuclei and cytoplasm. *In vitro*, they can be isolated on human fibroblast cells. An individual infected with CMV carries the virus for life and may shed it intermittently in saliva, urine, semen, cervical secretions and breast milk. Infection is transmitted by close contact between individuals and blood transfusion. It may be acquired at any time, i.e. prenatal, perinatal and postnatal.

Prenatal (Intrauterine) Infection

CMV is the most common agent to cause intrauterine infection and prenatal damage to foetus leading to congenital abnormalities. Approximately 1% of all babies become infected *in utero*. Maternal viraemia following primary CMV infection or a reactivation during pregnancy may result in foetal infection.

Majority (95%) of these are without obvious symptoms at the time of birth and 5% symptomatic infants have cytomegalic inclusion body disease. These infants show signs of growth retardation, hepatosplenomegaly, jaundice, thrombocytopenia, microcephaly, encephalitis and chorioretinitis. Of the remaining 95%, about 15% develop deafness and mental retardation.

Perinatal Infection

This is acquired from infected maternal genital secretions or from breast feeding.

Postnatal Infection

This may be acquired by kissing (from saliva), sexual intercourse or artificial insemination (from semen), blood transfusion and organ transplantation.

Infection acquired after birth is generally subclinical. However, it may cause hepatitis in young children. In adults and older children, it may cause a syndrome resembling EBV infectious mononucleosis, but with a negative Paul-Bunnell test and no pharyngitis or lymphadenopathy. CMV may cause widely disseminated infection in immunocompromised individuals such as graft recipients and AIDS patients leading to interstitial pneumonia, chorioretinitis, hepatitis, arthritis, chronic gastro-intestinal infection, encephalitis, Guillain-Barré syndrome and transverse myelitis.

Laboratory Diagnosis

1. Specimens

CMV can be isolated from urine, saliva, stool, breast milk, semen, cervical secretions and blood leucocytes.

2. Demonstration of Cytomegalic Cells

Cytomegalic cells can be demonstrated in centrifuged deposits of urine or saliva.

3. Isolation of Virus

The specimens are inoculated on cultured human fibroblasts. The virus replicates very slowly, therefore, characteristic CPE of foci of swollen refractile cells with cytoplasmic granules may take 2–3 weeks to appear. When stained, these cells are **multinucleated giant cells containing acidophilic inclusions with perinuclear halo (owl's eye appearance) in the nuclei and cytoplasm** (Fig. 33.6). For precise identification, the cell line may be stained by immunofluorescence or immunoperoxidase technique using monoclonal antibody.

4. Polymerase Chain Reaction (PCR)

CMV DNA, in the specimen, can be amplified by PCR.

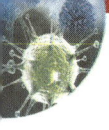

5. Serology

CMV-specific IgM can be detected in the patient serum by ELISA.

Treatment

For the treatment of severe CMV infections such as pneumonia, chorioretinitis and colitis in AIDS patients or in other immunocompromised patients, ganciclovir is the drug of choice.

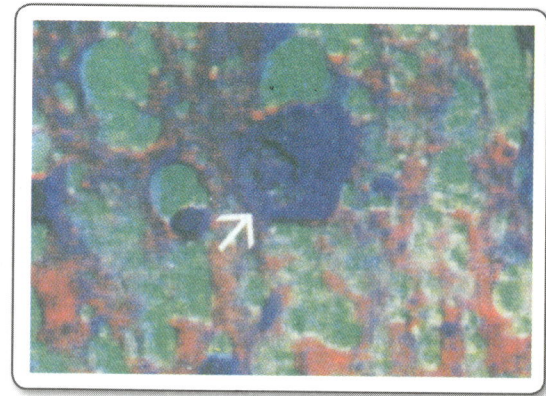

Fig. 33.6: Cytomegalovirus infection showing intranuclear inclusion bodies with perinuclear halo (owl's eye appearance).

Key Points

- *Herpes simplex* and *varicella-zoster* viruses cause **primary** and **reactivation infection**.
- In general, *herpes simplex* viruses HSV types 1 and 2 cause infections **above and below the belt**, respectively (i.e. oral and genital infections respectively).

ASSESS YOURSELF

LONG ANSWER QUESTION

1. Name various viruses of the family Herpesviridae and discuss various infections caused by herpes simplex virus types 1 and 2.

MULTIPLE CHOICE QUESTIONS

1. Which of the following infection/s is/are caused by herpes simplex virus type 1?
   - (a) Acute gingivostomatitis
   - (b) Keratoconjunctivitis
   - (c) Encephalitis
   - (d) All of the above

2. Which of the following drugs can be used for the treatment of herpes simplex virus infections?
   - (a) Acyclovir
   - (b) Azidothymidine
   - (c) Ribavirin
   - (d) All of the above

3. Shingles is caused by:
   - (a) varicella-zoster virus
   - (b) cytomegalovirus
   - (c) Epstein-Barr virus
   - (d) herpes simplex virus type 1

4. Viruses that can remain latent in ganglia for many years are:
   - (a) rhinoviruses
   - (b) retroviruses
   - (c) enteroviruses
   - (d) herpesviruses

ANSWERS TO MCQs

1. d   **2.** a   **3.** a   **4.** d

Chapter 34

Polioviruses and Rhinoviruses

POLIOVIRUSES

Morphology

The virion is 27–30 nm in diameter. Capsid is composed of 60 capsomers arranged in icosahedral symmetry. The genome is a single strand of positive sense RNA.

Resistance

- Poliovirus is resistant to ether, chloroform, bile, proteolytic enzymes of intestinal contents and detergents.
- In faeces, it can survive for months at 4°C and years at −20°C.
- It is readily inactivated by heat at 55°C for 30 minutes.
- Formaldehyde and oxidising disinfectants destroy the virus.
- Chlorination destroys the virus in water, but the presence of organic matter delays inactivation.
- Poliovirus does not survive lyophilization.

Antigenic Properties

On the basis of neutralization tests, polioviruses can be divided into three serotypes (1, 2 and 3).

Pathogenesis

Natural infection occurs only in man. The virus is spread from man-to-man by faecal-oral route.

On entering the body of a new host the virus multiplies in the tonsils and Peyer's patches of the ileum. Spread to regional lymph nodes (cervical and mesenteric) leads to a viraemia, enabling the virus to become disseminated throughout the body including spinal cord and brain.

In the central nervous system, the virus multiplies selectively in the neurons and destroys them. The lesions are mostly in the anterior horns of the spinal cord, causing flaccid paralysis, but posterior horns and intermediate columns may also be involved to some extent. In some cases encephalitis occurs, primarily involving the brain stem but extending upto the motor and premotor areas of the cerebral cortex.

Clinical Features

There are four types of poliovirus infection:
- **Asymptomatic illness:** Patient does not have any symptom but the virus may be isolated from stool or throat or both. This is seen in 90–95% individuals.
- **Minor illness:** Patient develops mild, transient 'influenza-like' illness. This is seen in 4–8% cases.
- **Non-paralytic poliomyelitis or aseptic meningitis:** In addition to 'influenza-like' illness patient also develops headache, neck stiffness and back pain that may indicate some degree of aseptic meningitis. The illness lasts 2–10 days with rapid and complete recovery. This is seen in 1–2% individuals.
- **Paralytic poliomyelitis or the major illness:** Patient develops paralysis during the course of the illness. It is uncommon, occurring in 0.1–2% poliovirus infections. On the basis of the site of involvement the paralysis may be spinal, bulbar or bulbospinal.

Laboratory Diagnosis

Specimens

Virus can be isolated from blood, faeces and throat swab taken early in the disease. It can seldom be isolated from CSF but can be obtained from the spinal cord and brain, postmortem.

Demonstration of Virus

Virus can be demonstrated in stool by electron microscopy and immunoelectron microscopy.

Virus Isolation

It can be cultivated on monkey kidney, human amnion, HeLa, HEp-2 and other cell cultures. A cytopathic effect is usually seen in the cells within 48 hours. It consists of cell retraction, increased refractivity, cytoplasmic granularity and nuclear pyknosis. The identification of the serotype is carried out by neutralization tests.

Prophylaxis

Two effective vaccines are available:

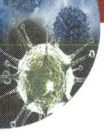

SECTION V • PATHOGENIC ORGANISMS-II VIRUSES

- Inactivated polio vaccine (Salk vaccine), and
- Live attenuated oral polio vaccine (Sabin vaccine).

Inactivated Polio Vaccine (IPV)

IPV (Salk vaccine) for parenteral injection was developed by Jonas Salk in 1956. The vaccine contains formalin inactivated strains of the three serotypes of virus grown in monkey kidney cell culture. The vaccine is given by deep subcutaneous or intramuscular injection. Three injections are given with intervals of 6–8 weeks between the first and second doses and 4–6 months between the second and third doses. IPV produces long-lasting immunity to all three poliovirus types. It is not associated with local or general reactions. The injection of this vaccine stimulates the production of IgG antibodies in the serum. It does not induce detectable levels of secretory IgA in the gut and, therefore, would not be expected to prevent alimentary tract infections. Following infection, a virulent virus is neutralized as it enters the blood stream, thus preventing involvement of the central nervous system. The absence of live virus makes it safe to administer to immunocompromised individuals.

Live Attenuated Oral Polio Vaccine (OPV)

OPV (Sabin vaccine) was developed by Albert Sabin in 1962. It contains live attenuated strains of the three serotypes of poliovirus grown either in cultures of monkey kidney cells or human diploid cells. The virus comprising the vaccine is unable to multiply in the cells of the central nervous system and, therefore, lacks neurovirulence. The vaccine is administered orally and parallels natural infection. It stimulates both local secretory IgA antibodies in the pharynx and alimentary tract, and humoral IgG antibodies. Virus is excreted in the faeces for several weeks, during which time the vaccine may spread to close contacts, inducing or boostering immunity in them.

At the age of 1½ months first dose of OPV is given along with DPT. Second, third and fourth doses of these vaccines are given at the ages of 2½, 3½ and 16–24 months, respectively.

Ideally, it is desirable to vaccinate all children aged 0–5 years in the whole community at one time so that natural dissemination is prevented. The strategy of administering the vaccine to all children in a region on the same day (**pulse immunization**) has been found to be useful in the developing countries. By global immunization with OPV it was considered possible to eradicate the disease by the year 2000. However, poor progress in immunization in many countries has been a setback to this objective. Following are the causes of poor response to OPV:

- Interference by other enteroviruses so common in the tropics;
- Frequent diarrhoeal diseases preventing colonization by the vaccine virus;
- Breast-feeding immediately before or after the vaccine is given (vaccine virus may be neutralized by antibodies in the breast milk); and
- Vaccine virus may also be neutralized by some other inhibitory agent in the saliva and intestinal secretions.

RHINOVIRUSES

Rhinoviruses are small RNA viruses. They are relatively stable in temperature range of 20–37°C and can survive on environmental surfaces such as door knobs for several days.

On the basis of a type-specific antigen in their capsid, rhinoviruses have been subdivided into more than 100 serotypes. They are fastidious, growing only at 33°C (temperature of the nose), instead of the usual 37°C, in human embryonic kidney cells, human embryonic nasal or tracheal epithelium, human diploid cell lines and HeLa cells without conspicuous CPE.

Pathogenesis

Rhinoviruses are the major cause of common cold accounting for about half of all colds. Rhinoviruses are transmitted by inhalation of droplets expelled from the nose of a patient during sneezing and coughing. After an incubation period of 2–4 days, patient develops profuse watery discharge (rhinorrhoea) with nasal obstruction, sneezing, sore throat, cough, headache, malaise and little or no fever. On an average, symptoms subside in about a week but in a proportion of the cases the symptoms may be prolonged for 2 weeks or longer. Sinusitis or otitis media may supervene, particularly if secondary bacterial infection occurs. The illness is generally worse in smokers. Recovery is mediated by endogenous interferons, locally synthesized IgA antibodies and serum IgG antibodies.

Laboratory Diagnosis

- Rhinoviruses may be isolated from nose and throat swabs or nasopharyngeal aspirate on human and monkey cell lines incubated at 33°C.
- Virus antigen, in nasal washings, may be demonstrated by ELISA.
- Virus RNA, in nasal washings, may be demonstrated by PCR.

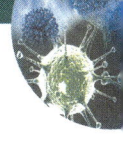

 # Key Points

- *Polioviruses*, agents of paralytic poliomyelitis, can be divided into **three serotypes**.
- Spread of poliovirus disease has been successfully checked through widespread immunization with either *inactivated polio vaccine* (*Salk vaccine*) or *live attenuated oral polio vaccine* (*Sabin vaccine*).
- *Rhinoviruses* are the major cause of **common cold** accounting for *about half of all colds*.

? ASSESS YOURSELF

LONG ANSWER QUESTIONS

1. Discuss pathogenesis and laboratory diagnosis of polioviruses.
2. Discuss prophylaxis against poliomyelitis.

MULTIPLE CHOICE QUESTIONS

1. Paralytic poliomyelitis is seen in:
   - (a) 90–95% of poliovirus infections
   - (b) 4–8% of poliovirus infections
   - (c) 3–5% of poliovirus infections
   - (d) 0.1–2% of poliovirus infections
2. Which of the following polio vaccines induce/s production of local secretory IgA antibodies?
   - (a) Salk vaccine
   - (b) Sabin vaccine
   - (c) Both of the above
   - (d) None of the above
3. How many serotypes of rhinoviruses are there?
   - (a) More than ten
   - (b) More than twenty
   - (c) More than sixty
   - (d) More than one hundred

ANSWERS TO MCQs

1. d   **2.** b   **3.** d

SECTION V • PATHOGENIC ORGANISMS-II VIRUSES

Rabies Virus

MORPHOLOGY

Rabies virus is bullet-shaped 180 × 75 nm, with one end rounded or conical and the other plane or concave (Fig. 35.1). **The core of the virion consists of a minus sense 11–12 kilobase, single-stranded RNA enclosed in a helically wound nucleocapsid.** RNA dependent RNA polymerase enzyme which is essential for the initiation of replication of the virus, is enclosed within the virion in association with the ribonucleoprotein core. The latter is surrounded by **matrix protein** (viral membrane) which may be invaginated at the plane end. The matrix protein, in turn, is surrounded by a **lipoprotein envelope** which carries glycoprotein peplomers (spikes). The spikes do not cover the plane end of the virion.

PATHOGENESIS

Rabies is a natural infection of dogs, foxes, wolves, skunks, cats and bats. The name 'rabies' comes from the Latin word *rabidus* meaning mad. Rabies virus is excreted in the saliva of affected animals. Man acquires infection by the bite of rabid dog or other animals. Rarely, infection can occur following licks on abraded skin and intact mucosa.

Infection by bite of rabid animal results in deposition of rabies-infected saliva in the wound (Fig. 35.2). The virus replicates in the muscles, connective tissue or nerves at the site of deposition. After it reaches a sufficient concentration, it infects peripheral nerves in the muscle or skin. Once within the nerve fibres, it is out of reach of any circulating antibody and it travels along the axon towards the central nervous system **at a speed of 3 mm per hour**. In the central nervous system, it multiplies and produces encephalitis. The virus then spreads outwards along the nerve trunks to various parts of the body including the salivary glands. **It multiplies in the salivary glands and is shed in the saliva.**

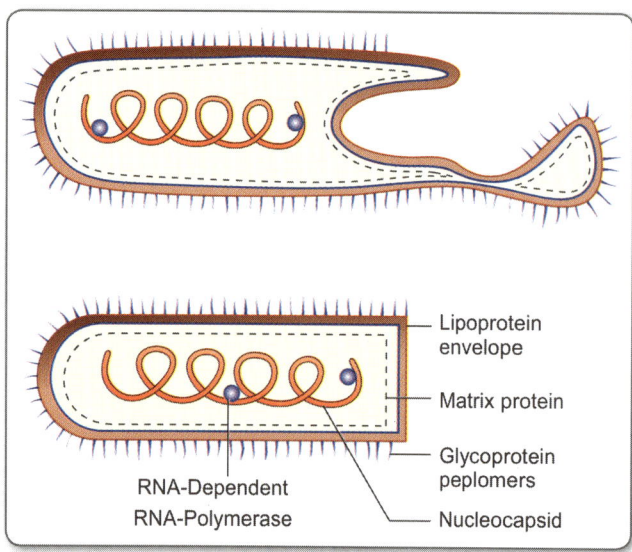

Lipoprotein envelope

Matrix protein

Glycoprotein peplomers

RNA-Dependent RNA-Polymerase

Nucleocapsid

Fig. 35.1: Rabies virus.

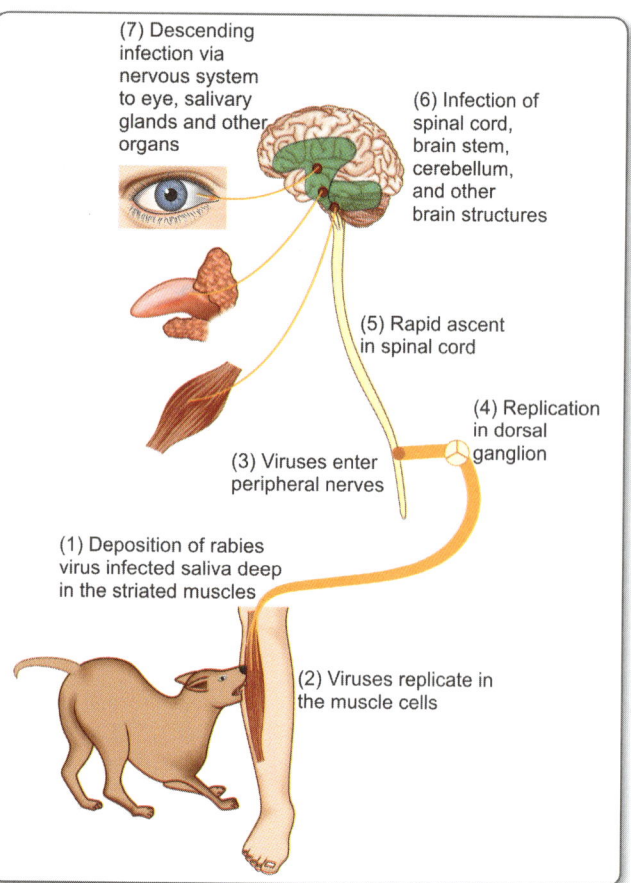

(7) Descending infection via nervous system to eye, salivary glands and other organs

(6) Infection of spinal cord, brain stem, cerebellum, and other brain structures

(5) Rapid ascent in spinal cord

(4) Replication in dorsal ganglion

(3) Viruses enter peripheral nerves

(1) Deposition of rabies virus infected saliva deep in the striated muscles

(2) Viruses replicate in the muscle cells

Fig. 35.2: Pathogenesis of rabies virus.

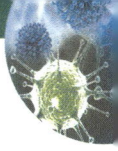

Clinical Features

Following the bite of a rabid animal, the incubation period is usually between 1 and 2 months. However, it may be as short as 9 days and rarely as long as a year or more. It is shorter in children than in adults and shorter in persons bitten on the face or head and longer in those bitten on the legs. This is related to the distance the virus has to travel to reach the brain.

After a prodromal phase of malaise, headache, fever and paraesthesia at and around the site of bite, muscles become hypertonic and the patient becomes anxious, with episodes of hyperactivity, aggression and convulsions. **Patient develops difficulty in drinking, together with intense thirst. Patient may be able to swallow dry solids but not liquids**. Attempts to drink bring on painful spasm of pharynx and larynx producing choking and gagging. Thereafter, mere sight or sound of water precipitates distressing muscular spasm leading to **hydrophobia** (fear of water). **The furious form of rabies, gradually subsides into delirium, convulsions, coma and death**.

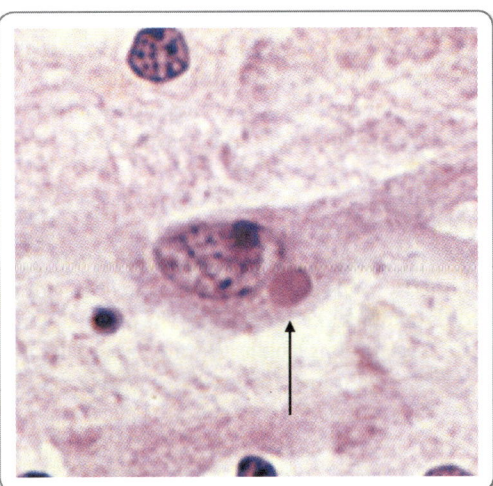

Fig. 35.3: Intracytoplasmic eosinophilic inclusion body in a cell infected with rabies virus (Negri bodies) (Seller's stain, × 400).

LABORATORY DIAGNOSIS

Demonstration of Negri Bodies

Sections or impression smears of brain stained by Seller's technique may reveal inclusion bodies, known as **Negri bodies**. These are intracytoplasmic, round or oval, purplish pink structures with basophilic inner granules (Fig. 35.3). Negri bodies vary in size, from 3 μm to 27 μm in diameter and are seen mainly in the pyramidal cells of Ammon's horn, in Purkinje cells of hippocampus, brain stem and cerebellum. Negri bodies may be absent in 20% of cases.

Demonstration of Rabies Antigen by Direct Immunofluorescence

Antemortem

In salivary, corneal or conjunctival smears or skin biopsy from the nape of the neck by direct immunofluorescence using antirabies serum tagged with fluorescein isothiocyanate.

Postmortem

In impression smears of the cut surface of the salivary gland, hippocampus, brain stem or cerebellum by direct immuno-fluorescence using antirabies serum tagged with fluorescein isothiocyanate.

Virus Isolation

Mouse inoculation

Rabies virus can be isolated by inoculation of suckling mice. The animals die in 7–21 days. However, they may be killed after five days and brain smears stained with fluorescent antibody.

Isolation in Cell Culture

Rabies virus can be grown in baby hamster kidney, mouse neuroblastoma, human diploid lung fibroblasts, chick embryo fibroblasts and Vero monkey kidney cells. No cytopathic changes are observed but rabies antigen can be detected by fluorescent antibody staining 18–24 hours after inoculation.

Detection of Rabies Antibodies

Rabies antibodies can be detected in the serum and CSF of the patient by ELISA. **High titre antibodies are present in the CSF in rabies but not after immunization**. Their demonstration can be used for the diagnosis.

POSTEXPOSURE TREATMENT AND PROPHYLAXIS

Postexposure treatment in a previously unvaccinated person consists of:

- **First-aid** treatment to eliminate virus from the site of infection by prompt cleansing of wound with plenty of soap and water or solutions of quaternary ammonium compounds (such as cetavlon). This is a very important step in the prevention of rabies as **soap and water, and quaternary ammonium compounds destroy the virus effectively**.
- **Human rabies immunoglobulin** 20 IU/kg body weight or heterologous (equine) antirabies serum 40 IU/kg body weight-up to half the dose should be administered intra-muscularly in the gluteal region and the remaining half should be infiltrated around the bite.
- **A potent cell culture vaccine** (see below): One ml of the vaccine should be given intramuscularly on days 0, 3, 7, 14, 30 and 90 in the deltoid region. The dose of cell culture vaccines is not age or body weight dependent.

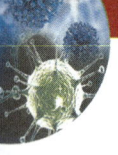

Rabies Vaccines

Rabies can be prevented by active immunization after infection, because a long incubation period of the disease allows time for immunity to develop before the onset of symptoms.

Neural Vaccines

Vaccination after exposure to rabies was introduced by Pasteur in 1885. He injected a young boy, bitten by a rabid dog, with ground-up spinal cords of rabies infected rabbits. The infected spinal cords had been dried for various lengths of time to partially inactivate the virus. After this came the vaccines (Table 35.1) which consisted of rabies-infected rabbit, sheep or goat brain in which virus was inactivated with phenol (at 22°C – Fermi vaccine and at 37°C – Semple vaccine) or beta-propiolactone (BPL vaccines). Fermi vaccine contains residual virus. The dose schedule of neural vaccines require repeated and painful injections and their potency is low. Moreover myelin component of the neural vaccines sensitizes 1 in 500 vaccinees leading to neuroparalytic accidents.

Since the brain tissues of newborn animals contain little myelin and they provide high yields of virus, therefore, a vaccine prepared from suckling mouse brain and inactivated with BPL was used, but was discontinued because of its poor immunogenicity.

Non-neural vaccines

Duck Egg Vaccine

Vaccine prepared from virus grown in duck embryos and inactivated with BPL was used for many years. It has been discontinued because of its poor immunogenicity.

Cell Culture Vaccines

- **Human diploid cell (HDC) vaccine:** This vaccine consists of fixed rabies virus grown on human diploid lung fibroblasts and inactivated with BPL or tris-*n*-butyl phosphate. It is highly antigenic and free from serious side effects but there may be local reaction in around 15% vaccinees. Because of the greater potency of HDC vaccine, quantity administered is much less than that of neural vaccines. Only five or six doses given intramuscularly in the **deltoid region** in 1.0 ml volumes on days 0, 3, 7, 14, 30 and 90 after exposure are recommended. The last dose is optional. *HDC vaccine should not be injected in gluteal region because high fat content in this region retards the absorption of vaccine.*
- **Purified chick embryo cell (PCEC) vaccine and purified Vero cell (PVC) vaccine:** Rabies vaccines with a similar potency to HDC vaccine have been produced in chick embryo fibroblasts and Vero cells. The vaccines produced in these cell cultures are known as purified chick embryo cell (PCEC) vaccine and purified Vero cell (PVC) vaccine, respectively. *No problems have arisen from a change of vaccine mid course and rabies antibody titres have been satisfactory in those people who were given more than one type of cell culture vaccine.*

TABLE 35.1: Rabies Vaccines

Neural vaccines
• Semple vaccine
• Beta-propiolactone (BPL) vaccine
• Suckling mouse brain vaccine
Non-neural vaccines
• Duck egg vaccine
• Cell culture vaccines
▪ Human diploid cell (HDC) vaccine
▪ Purified chick embryo cell (PCEC) vaccine
▪ Purified Vero cell (PVC) vaccine

🎵 Key Points

- **Rabies** is probably the most feared of all human diseases.
- *Rabies virus travels along the axon* towards the central nervous system at a speed of **3 mm per hour**.
- Rabies is the **only human disease** that can be prevented by *active immunization after infection*, because a long incubation period of the disease allows time for immunity to develop before the onset of symptoms.

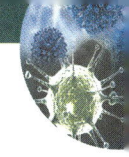

? ASSESS YOURSELF

LONG ANSWER QUESTIONS

1. Discuss the pathogenesis and clinical features of rabies.
2. Discuss laboratory diagnosis of rabies.
3. Describe the prophylaxis of rabies.

MULTIPLE CHOICE QUESTIONS

1. What is the shape of rabies virus?
   - (a) Spherical
   - (b) Polygonal
   - (c) Bullet-shaped
   - (d) Tubular

2. Negri bodies can be demonstrated in infection with:
   - (a) herpes simplex virus
   - (b) rabies virus
   - (c) hepatitis B virus
   - (d) vaccinia virus

3. Which of the following viral infections is associated with development of hydrophobia?
   - (a) Influenza
   - (b) Polio
   - (c) Rabies
   - (d) Hepatitis

4. Which of the following rabies vaccines is a cell culture vaccine?
   - (a) Duck egg vaccine
   - (b) Semple vaccine
   - (c) Suckling mouse brain vaccine
   - (d) Purified chick embryo cell vaccine

ANSWERS TO MCQS

1. c   2. b   3. c   4. d

36 Chapter

Orthomyxoviruses and Paramyxoviruses

ORTHOMYXOVIRUSES

Orthomyxoviruses are so named because of their affinity for mucins. They have three genera – *Influenzavirus A, B* and *C*.

Morphology

Influenzavirus A and *B* are morphologically similar, but *Influenza virus C* differs from them in certain aspects, particularly in having **only a single type of glycoprotein spike**. The virions are spherical, 80–120 nm in diameter, but larger pleomorphic and filamentous forms 1,000 nm or more in length may be abundant. The nucleocapsid (Fig. 36.1) has helical symmetry with a core of eight segments of single-stranded RNA of negative polarity and molecular weight of 5,000 kDa. The nucleocapsid is surrounded by a protein layer or **matrix protein M1**, which in turn is enclosed in host plasma membrane derived **lipid bilayer envelope**. The **M2 protein** projects through the envelope to form ion channels which allow pH changes in the endosome.

Attached to the lipid envelope of *Influenzavirus A* and *B* are two types of glycoprotein peplomers or spikes, the haemagglutinin (HA) and the neuraminidase (NA). HA peplomers exist as 500 tapered projections, 10 nm in length, with their broadest (5 nm) ends outermost and their narrow ends inserted in the lipid membrane. NA peplomers are 100 mushroom-shaped projections per virion measuring 9 nm in length. The virus particles bind to the host cell receptors (sialic acid) by haemagglutinin peplomers.

Antigenic Variation

Influenza virus is capable of undergoing antigenic variation due to frequent changes in the antigenicity of HA and NA. This is of great importance in the epidemiology of the disease.

Antigenic Drift

The gradual sequential change in the antigenic structure occurring regularly at frequent intervals is known as antigenic drift. It results from mutations in *HA* or *NA* genes. The new antigens acquired though different from the previous are yet related to them so that they can still react with antisera to the predecessor virus strain to some extent. Periodic epidemics of influenza are associated with antigenic drift.

Antigenic Shift

It is an abrupt, drastic, discontinuous variation in the antigenic structure resulting in a new virus strain unrelated antigenically to predecessor strain. It may involve HA or NA or both. Antibodies to predecessor virus strains do not neutralize the new variants, therefore, they can spread widely in the population leading to major epidemics and pandemics.

Pathogenesis

The route of entry of the virus is the respiratory tract. Very small doses, three viable particles or more can initiate infection. The viral neuraminidase facilitates infection by hydrolysing the mucus film lining the respiratory tract and exposing the cell surface receptors for virus adsorption. Ciliated epithelial cells of respiratory tract are the main sites of virus infection. The death and sloughing of these cells renders the respiratory tract vulnerable to secondary bacterial infection. Viraemic phase is extremely rare.

Incubation period is short varying from 1–4 days. The illness is characterized by a sudden onset of systemic symptoms such as

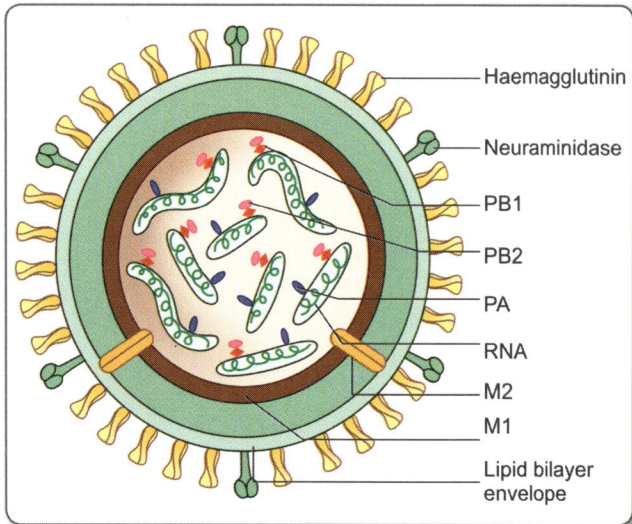

Fig. 36.1: Influenza virus.

Haemagglutinin

Neuraminidase

PB1

PB2

PA

RNA

M2

M1

Lipid bilayer envelope

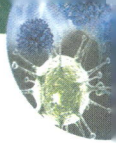

chills, fever, sore throat, nonproductive cough, myalgia, headache and malaise. The uncomplicated illness usually lasts for 3–7 days.

Laboratory Diagnosis

- **Demonstration of virus antigens**
  Smears of nasopharyngeal secretions and nasal swab or centrifuged deposit of throat garglings are stained with fluorescein-tagged influenza antiserum and seen under fluorescence microscope.

- **Virus isolation**
  Influenza viruses can be isolated during first 2–3 days of illness. Throat garglings are collected using suitable buffered salt solution. The specimen should be processed immediately. If short delay is expected then store it at 4°C and if long delay is expected then store it at –70°C. The specimen is treated with antibiotics to destroy bacteria and inoculated into amniotic cavity of chick embryos, primary monkey kidney or human embryo kidney cells or Madin-Darby canine kidney (MDCK) cells.

- **Serological tests**
  Serological diagnosis of influenza is based upon demonstrating a four-fold or higher increase in antibody titre between acute-phase and convalescent-phase sera. Complement fixation, haemagglutination inhibition and neutralization tests are done for this purpose. Since serological diagnosis is retrospective, therefore, it is of limited use.

Prophylaxis

Vaccination is the main method of preventing influenza, but major difficulty in immunoprophylaxis is the frequent change in the antigenic structure of influenza virus. Vaccines are of two types:

- **Inactivated vaccines**
  Influenza virus is grown in allantoic cavity of chick embryos. These are inactivated with formalin or β-propiolactone, then purified by zonal ultracentrifugation and disrupted with detergents. The resulting polyvalent inactivated vaccine is used every autumn. This vaccine can be further purified to contain only haemagglutinins and neuraminidases. This is known as subunit vaccine. Inactivated vaccines induce the formation of circulating antibodies. The level of antibodies in the respiratory mucosa is only a fraction of the serum level.

- **Live attenuated vaccines**
  Temperature-sensitive (ts) mutants of influenza virus may be used as live vaccine. They can grow at lower temperature of the nasopharyngeal mucosa (32–34°C) but not in lungs (37°C). Live vaccine is administered by aerosol spray or intranasally. It stimulates the production of local IgA antibodies. Circulating antibodies of IgM and IgG classes are not raised to the same extent as when killed vaccine is injected.

PARAMYXOVIRUSES

Morphology

Paramyxoviruses include parainfluenza, mumps and measles viruses. They are indistinguishable in the electron microscope. They range from 150–300 nm or more in diameter, occasionally there are filamentous forms and giant forms up to 800 nm in diameter. They are enclosed by a lipid envelope derived from plasma membrane of the host cell. It contains HN and F glycoprotein peplomers 12–14 nm long and 2–4 nm wide. The former carries both haemagglutinating and neuraminidase functions and latter causes fusion of cell membranes leading to the formation of syncytia. The spikes on the meales virus envelope carry a haemagglutinin but not neuraminidase. The inner surface of the envelope is lined by matrix (M) protein. Within the virion, there is a nucleocapsid of helical symmetry. It contains a single-stranded, negative sense RNA genome as a single piece (Fig. 36.2).

PARAINFLUENZA VIRUSES

There are four types of parainfluenza viruses, types 1, 2, 3 and 4.

Pathogenesis

- Parainfluenza viruses are highly transmissible and are acquired by droplets and by contact with respiratory secretions. **Incubation period varies from 2–6 days**. All parainfluenza viruses produce upper respiratory tract infections. In infants and children, these viruses may invade the lower respiratory tract, causing **pneumonia**. In older children (6 months to 5 years), parainfluenza virus type 1 and to some extent, type 2 may cause **laryngotracheobronchitis or croup**. The patient presents with fever, cough and respiratory distress that may need emergency tracheostomy. Type 3 infects infants within first year or two of life. Type 4 produces only mild illness.

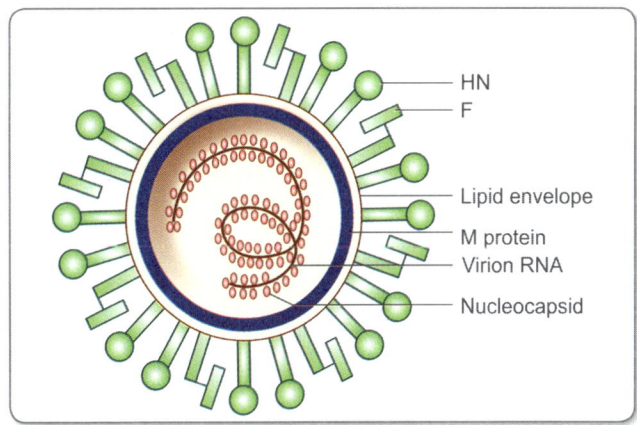

Fig. 36.2: Paramyxovirus.

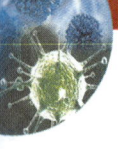

Laboratory Diagnosis

- Immunofluorescent staining of exfoliated cells aspirated from respiratory tract.
- Detection of free antigen in mucus by ELISA and RIA.
- Parainfluenza viruses may be isolated in primary human or monkey kidney cells or in continuous cell lines such as H292 derived from human lung mucoepidermoid carcinoma. They produce little cytopathic effect, except type 2 which induces syncytia. Viral growth can be detected by haemadsorption of guinea pig red cells or by use of specific immunofluorescent antibody.
- Type-specific antibody may be detected by haemadsorption inhibition, neutralization, ELISA and complement fixation test. A four-fold rise in titre is indicative of infection with a parainfluenza virus.

MUMPS

Pathogenesis

Mumps is predominantly a disease of childhood. The mumps virus is transmitted by way of respiratory and oral secretions and respiratory tract is the portal of entry. It multiplies in the upper respiratory tract and in local lymph nodes. The virus then enters the blood stream and the infection spreads to many organs of the body. The major manifestation is painful swelling of one or both parotid glands occurring 14–18 days after exposure. It may also cause meningoencephalitis, orchitis, oophoritis, pancreatitis, arthritis, myocarditis and renal dysfunction.

Laboratory Diagnosis

- Virus can be isolated from saliva from affected gland, throat swab, CSF and urine on primary monkey kidney cells, H292 and HEp-2 cells. It produces little cytopathic effect but virus can be detected by immunofluorescence and haemadsorption (of guinea pig or chicken red cells) which can be inhibited by specific antiserum.
- For rapid diagnosis, ELISA is useful for detecting mumps-specific IgM antibodies in the serum.

Prophylaxis

A live attenuated vaccine, derived by passage in chick fibroblasts, offers 95% protection which lasts for 12 years. It can be given by subcutaneous injection in combination with attenuated measles and rubella strains (MMR vaccine). This vaccine is administered to children of both sexes, aged 15 months.

MEASLES

Pathogenesis

Measles is the **commonest highly contagious childhood disease** spread by respiratory secretions. **After an incubation period of 10–12 days**, patient develops upper respiratory tract infection with high fever, rhinitis, cough and conjunctivitis. **Koplik's spots**, which are small, 1–3 mm in diameter, bluish white spots surrounded by erythema can be seen on the buccal mucosa during this stage and are pathognomonic of measles. After 1–2 days, the acute symptoms decline with the appearance of characteristic **maculopapular rash** which appears first on the neck and then spreads to the rest of the body. **The rash is due to type IV hypersensitivity to viral antigens**. In next 10–14 days, rash fades with considerable desquamation and sometimes by discolouration of the skin. There is only one antigenic type of measles virus. Infection confers lifelong immunity.

Since measles decreases the resistance of the respiratory epithelium, therefore, patient may develop secondary bacterial infections like sinusitis, otitis media, bronchitis, bronchiolitis, croup and bronchopneumonia. Giant cell pneumonia may occur most frequently in those with impaired cell-mediated immunity. In addition, acute postinfectious encephalitis and subacute sclerosing panencephalitis (SSPE) may occur in 1 in 1000 and 1 in 300,000 cases of measles respectively.

Laboratory Diagnosis

- The measles virus can be isolated, though with some difficulty, from throat washings, blood, urinary sediment, etc. on monkey kidney, primary human embryo kidney and human amnion cells. The appearance of multinucleated giant cells containing numerous acidophilic inclusions in cytoplasm and nuclei, in the cultured cells, suggests the presence of measles virus. For rapid diagnosis, both multinucleated giant cells and viral antigens can be detected in the cells aspirated from nasopharynx.
- Measles antibody in the patient serum can be detected by IgM capture ELISA. Complement fixation test can be carried out on acute and convalescent sera. A rise in antibody titre is diagnostic.

Prophylaxis

Children of the age of 15 months are given MMR vaccine, followed by a booster at the age of 4–6 years.

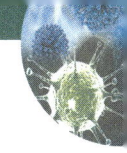

Key Points

- The nucleocapsid of influenza virus has **helical symmetry** with a core of **eight segments of single-stranded RNA** of negative polarity.
- Attached to the lipid envelope of *Influenzavirus A* and *Influenzavirus B* are two types of glycoprotein peplomers, the **haemagglutinin** (HA) and the **neuraminidase** (NA).
- Influenza virus is capable of undergoing **antigenic variation** by *antigenic drift* and *antigenic shift*.
- *Mumps virus* is the major agent of **parotitis**.
- *Measles is an acute febrile infection with an **exanthematous rash**; prodromal symptoms of measles include **Koplik's spots on the buccal mucosa**.*
- **MMR** vaccine prevents **measles**, **mumps** and **rubella**.

ASSESS YOURSELF

LONG AND SHORT ANSWER QUESTIONS

1. Discuss the morphology and pathogenesis of influenza virus infection.
2. Write short notes on:
   (a) Measles virus
   (b) Mumps virus

MULTIPLE CHOICE QUESTIONS

1. Which of the following genera is **not** included in family Orthomyxoviridae?
   (a) *Influenzavirus A*
   (b) *Influenzavirus B*
   (c) *Influenzavirus C*
   (d) *Parainfluenzavirus*

2. Measles virus belongs to which of the following genera?
   (a) Rubulavirus
   (b) Morbillivirus
   (c) Pneumovirus
   (d) Paramyxovirus

3. Koplik's spots are characteristic of which of the following infections?
   (a) Mumps
   (b) Measles
   (c) Herpes
   (d) Rubella

ANSWERS TO MCQS

1. d   **2.** b   **3.** b

37 Chapter

Rubella and Flaviviruses

RUBELLA (GERMAN MEASLES)

Morphology

Rubella virus (*Rubivirus*) is spherical, 50–70 nm in diameter and has an icosahedral capsid surrounded by a lipid envelope containing glycoprotein peplomers. The genome consists of a molecule of single-stranded positive sense RNA 11–12 kb in length.

Pathogenesis

Rubella or German measles is primarily a mild childhood fever. It may be acquired congenitally or postnatally. It is not transmitted by arthropods.

Postnatal Rubella

Rubella virus is excreted in oropharyngeal secretions and infection is acquired by inhalation. Virus multiplies locally in the upper respiratory tract and in the cervical lymph nodes, followed by dissemination throughout the body by the way of the blood stream. After an **incubation period of 2–3 weeks**, patient develops fine, pink, discrete macules of the erythematous rash which first appear on the face, then spread to the trunk and limbs. Fever is usually inconspicuous, but a characteristic feature is that postauricular, suboccipital and posterior cervical lymph nodes are enlarged and tender from very early in the illness.

The illness is of short duration and recovery is usually complete within 3–4 days after appearance of rash.

Congenital Rubella

Rubella virus can cross the placental barrier, particularly in early pregnancy, and infect the foetus, where it disseminates and grows in every foetal organ. It may result in a large variety of congenital abnormalities or death of the foetus. Congenital abnormalities may include total or partial neurosensory deafness, cataract, glaucoma, microphthalmia or retinopathy leading to blindness, congenital heart disease especially patent ductus arteriosus, sometimes accompanied by septal defects and pulmonary artery stenosis, microcephaly with mental retardation, thrombocytopenic purpura and hepatosplenomegaly. This is known as **congenital rubella syndrome (CRS)**.

Laboratory Diagnosis

- **Virus isolation**
  Rubella virus can be isolated from adult throat swab and from the throat, urine, CSF or leucocytes of a newborn infant with CRS on RK13 (rabbit kidney) and Vero cells. CPE is inconspicuous, therefore, rubella virus, in cell culture, is detected by **interference** with the CPE of a challenge virus (coxsackievirus A9) and by **immunofluorescence** or **immunoperoxidase staining** for detection of antigen in such cells.
- **Serology**
  Recent infection with rubella virus can be diagnosed by the demonstration of rubella IgM antibody in a single sample of blood by ELISA, radioimmunoassay and haemadsorption inhibition test. In case of rubella IgG antibody, four-fold or more rise in titre in paired sera has a diagnostic value.

In a newborn baby, demonstration of rubella IgM antibody is diagnostic of congenital rubella as IgM antibodies do not cross the placenta. However, many babies have rubella IgG antibodies, acquired transplacentally.

Prophylaxis

A live attenuated MMR vaccine is recommended for all infants in the second year of life, followed by a booster at the age of 4–6 years.

FLAVIVIRUSES

Morphology

Flaviviruses are spherical, 40–50 nm in diameter. They possess a molecule of single-stranded, positive sense RNA of 10.5–11 kb. Inner viral core is surrounded by a lipid bilayer envelope containing glycoprotein peplomers and a matrix or membrane protein.

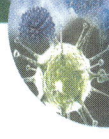

Dengue

Dengue virus has four serotypes – dengue 1, dengue 2, dengue 3 and dengue 4, all of which are endemic throughout the tropics. Considerable cross reactivity is observed among the different serotypes and recovery from an infection by one type does not provide complete immunity against infection by other types. Thus, individuals can have as many as 4 dengue infections in their life, one with each serotype. The virus is transmitted from person-to-person by several species of mosquitoes of the genus *Aedes* principally *A. aegypti*.

Clinical Features

Classic dengue usually affects older children and adults. After an incubation period of 5–8 days, patient develops fever of sudden onset and often biphasic with severe headache, chills, retrobulbar pain, conjunctivitis and severe pain in the back, muscles and joints (breakbone fever). A **maculopapular rash** generally appears on the trunk in 3–5 days of illness and spreads later to the face and extremities. Petechiae may sometimes be seen on the dorsum of the feet, legs, hands, axillae and palate. **The disease lasts for about 10 days after which recovery is generally complete**.

Dengue may also occur in more serious forms, with haemorrhagic manifestations. These are known as **dengue haemorrhagic fever** (DHF) and **dengue shock syndrome** (DSS).

Prophylaxis

Control measures include elimination of *Aedes* mosquitoes.

Japanese Encephalitis

Japanese encephalitis (JE) virus was first isolated from the brain of a fatal case of encephalitis in Tokyo, Japan. The mosquito, *Culex tritaeniorhynchus*, breeding in irrigated rice fields is the main vector. It transmits the virus to man from water birds and pigs, which act as amplifying hosts.

Clinical Features

Incubation period varies from 5–15 days. The disease has an abrupt onset with fever, headache and vomiting. After 1–6 days, signs of encephalitis set in with neck rigidity, convulsions, altered sensorium and coma. Residual neurological damage may persist in up to 50% of survivors.

Prophylaxis

Preventive measures include mosquito control and locating piggeries away from human dwellings. Inactivated vaccines prepared in mice and hamster kidney cell cultures and a live attenuated vaccine are available.

Laboratory Diagnosis of Flavivirus Infection

Virus Isolation

Virus can be isolated by intracerebral inoculation of newborn mice and by inoculation of cultured mosquito or vertebrate cells, from blood collected as early as possible during the course of dengue, from the brain in case of JE, and from the vectors. The viral isolates can be identified by immunofluorescence of the cultured cells, haemagglutination inhibition and neutralization tests.

Serology

In primary dengue infection, circulating IgM antibody to the viral coat proteins is detected 5–6 days after the onset of illness, and gradually decreases within 1–2 months of onset. IgG antibody to dengue virus is detected approximately 14 days after onset in primary infection, and by day 2 in secondary infection. In secondary infection, IgM antibody may reappear but gradually diminishes, while IgG antibody persists, often at high titre. These patterns of dengue antibody development permit serological differentiation of primary and secondary infections. Patients with secondary infection generally have higher IgG levels. Acute or recent infections are identified by a rise in antibody titre as well as high IgM levels. There is substantial cross reactivity among flaviviruses, due to the presence of common antigenic determinants. The four dengue serotypes cross react among themselves, but there are also unique determinants for each serotype.

CHIKUNGUNYA

Chikungunya virus was first isolated from patients and mosquitoes during an epidemic in the Newala district of Tanzania in 1952/53. It first appeared in India in 1963, when along with dengue, it caused very extensive epidemic in Kolkata, Chennai and other areas. The name 'Chikungunya' is derived from the native word for the disease in which the patient lies 'doubled up' due to severe joint pains. In Africa, a sylvatic transmission cycle occurs between wild primates and *Aedes* mosquitoes, while urban chikungunya epidemics in India and Southeast Asia causing hundreds-of-thousands of cases involve *Aedes aegypti* transmission in a human-mosquito-human cycle. It has frequently been isolated from humans and mosquitoes during epidemics in India, Southeast Asia, Southeast Africa and sub-Saharan Africa. Unlike dengue, which is endemic in many of the Asian cities, chikungunya disappears and reappears at regular intervals. The mechanism of virus maintenance during inter-epidemic periods or re-introduction is unknown.

After an **incubation period of 2–4 days**, patient develops fever, crippling joint pains, chills, flushed face, headache, myalgia, backache, photophobia, rash, anorexia and constipation with recovery in 5–7 days. Clinical picture resembles that of dengue fever, with which it is often confused.

Laboratory Diagnosis

Serodiagnosis is the most common approach.

- Using an IgM capture ELISA, serotype specific IgM antibody may be detected in the patient serum within 1–3 days after the onset of illness.
- The detection of a four-fold or greater rise of antibody titre by ELISA test on paired sera collected during the initial week and several days later also provides a good evidence of infection.

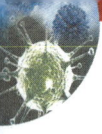

Key Points

- **Rubella** is a childhood fever resembling measles, except that it has a milder clinical course and shorter duration, however, if it is contracted in early pregnancy the virus can cause **severe congenital abnormalities and may cause the death of the foetus**.
- **MMR** vaccine prevents **measles**, **mumps** and **rubella**.
- Dengue virus causes **classic dengue**, **dengue haemorrhagic fever** and **dengue shock syndrome**.
- JE virus has a case fatality rate exceeding 20%. Residual neurological damage may persist in up to 50% of survivors.

? ASSESS YOURSELF

SHORT ANSWER QUESTION

Write short notes on:

    (a) Rubella   (b) Yellow fever

    (c) Dengue   (d) Japanese encephalitis

    (e) Chikungunia

MULTIPLE CHOICE QUESTIONS

1. Which of the following manifestations is/are characteristic of dengue?

    (a) Fever   (b) Pain in back, muscles and joints

    (c) Maculopapular rash   (d) All of the above

2. Which of the following mosquitoes act/s as vector for Japanese encephalitis virus?

    (a) Culex   (b) Aedes

    (c) Anopheles   (d) All of the above

3. Vaccine/s is/are available for:

    (a) Japanese encephalitis   (b) Rabies

    (c) Rubella   (d) All of the above

ANSWERS TO MCQs

1. d   **2.** a   **3.** d

Chapter 38

Human Immunodeficiency Virus

Morphology

Human immunodeficiency virus (HIV) is a spherical enveloped virus, about 80–120 nm in diameter with a three layer structure (Fig. 38.1). In the centre are two identical copies of ssRNA associated with reverse transcriptase and surrounded by structural proteins that form nucleocapsid, matrix protein shell and host cell membrane derived lipid bilayer envelope from which project 72 glycoprotein peplomers. Two antigenic types of HIV (HIV-1 and HIV-2) have been identified.

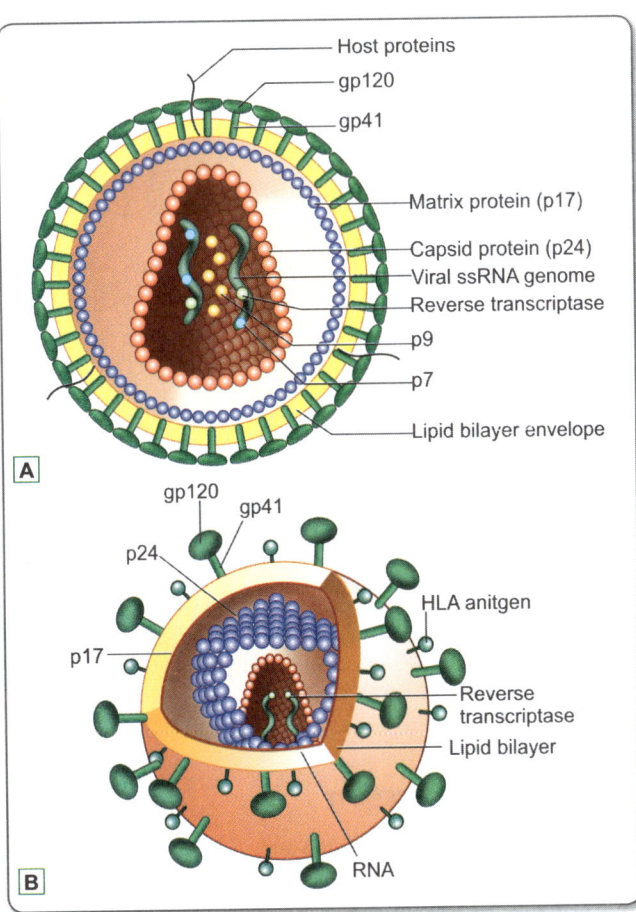

A

B

Fig. 38.1: HIV: (A) diagrammatic, and (B) 3-D view.

Host proteins
gp120
gp41
Matrix protein (p17)
Capsid protein (p24)
Viral ssRNA genome
Reverse transcriptase
p9
p7
Lipid bilayer envelope

gp120 gp41
p24
p17
HLA anitgen
Reverse transcriptase
Lipid bilayer
RNA

HIV-1 is divided into 3 groups (M, N and O). Group M (major) is responsible for global epidemic. Group O (outlier) is less common. It is mostly confined to West Africa. Group N (non-M, non-O) represents a few strains of HIV-1 isolated from Cameroon. Group M has been further divided into nine subtypes, or clades, designated A, B, C, D, F, G, H, J and K. Subtype A is most prevalent, being worldwide, while B is the most common in the Americas and Europe. **Subtype C is most prevalent in India and China.** The common subtypes in Africa are A, C and D. In Asia, the common subtypes are B, C and E. HIV-2 is divided into six subtypes (A–F).

Resistance

HIV is a delicate virus. It is thermolabile, being inactivated at 56°C in 30 minutes and in seconds at 100°C. It cannot survive outside the living host, however, the live virus has been reported to survive within blood up to 8 days. It is susceptible to common disinfectants.

Modes of Transmission of Virus

There are three modes of transmission of HIV – **sexual, parenteral** and **perinatal**. Of these, sexual mode of transmission is the most important. AIDS in 80% of the patients is due to sexual mode of trans-mission and in 10% each, it is due to parenteral and perinatal mode of transmission. During sexual intercourse virus gets transmitted from man-to-man, man-to-woman and woman-to-man.

Parenteral transmission may occur through blood transfusion. Therefore, each unit of blood should be tested for AIDS and if found positive, it should be incinerated. Transmission of HIV has been recorded in a few recipients of blood transfusion even when the blood transfused was found negative for HIV antibodies. This occurs when blood is collected in the '**window period**', i.e. the interval between the time of exposure to the virus and development of detectable levels of antibodies. This period varies from 1–3 months. Therefore, screening of blood is not 100% safe (How safe is safe?).

Infection can also be transmitted by blood products like plasma, serum and cells from HIV-positive individuals and AIDS cases. It can also be transmitted from the donors of bone marrow, semen and organs like cornea, kidney, heart, etc. Therefore, donors of various fluids and organs should be screened for AIDS before they donate them. AIDS can also be transmitted by sharing blood contaminated syringes. Therefore, HIV is more common in

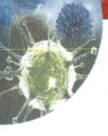

intravenous drug users who share syringes and needles. HIV can also be transmitted by the use of unsterile syringes and needles, needle-stick injury and through the barber's razor.

The third mode of transmission of infection is **perinatal, i.e. vertical transmission** from mother to the baby. Infection may be transmitted across the placenta before birth. Some of those who do not develop this infection before birth may develop it from the genital secretions during birth and from mother's milk after birth. In the absence of therapeutic intervention, the risk of mother-to-child transmission ranges from 15% to 30% and is further increased in the setting of breastfeeding. However, the risk can be significantly reduced to below 2% if antiretroviral therapy is administered to women during pregnancy and labour. Antiretroviral treatment of the mother and infant after birth can also significantly decrease the risk of HIV-1 infection in newborn.

Pathogenesis

AIDS is a unique sexually transmitted disease without local genital manifestations at any time during infection but with grave systemic manifestations. The first cells to become infected may be resident tissue macrophages or submucosal lymphocytes in the genital tract or rectum. The virus is then transported to the draining lymph nodes, where it replicates extensively. Two or three weeks after infection, most patients develop viraemia, fall in CD4+ T lymphocytes and glandular fever-like illness.

Since HIV infects cells expressing CD4 antigen, therefore, in the circulation the virus is found in CD4+ T lymphocytes and also in monocyte-macrophage cells, which may act as a reservoir for virus. Macrophages are also important in carrying the virus into the central nervous system across the blood-brain barrier. Virus is also present in the plasma. It is probably derived from the lysis of activated lymphocytes. Within one month or so, viraemia declines to a near undetectable level and illness subsides.

This is followed by a long asymptomatic period. For adults living in developing countries, the average length of time from HIV infection to the development of AIDS is about 10 years. About 20% develop AIDS within 5 years, and fewer than 5% have an asymptomatic infection for periods longer than 10 years. During this period, only a small number of circulating CD4+ cells are producing virus and only low titres of virus are present in the blood. However, many infected cells can be detected in the lymph nodes. Follicular hyperplasia develops in these and other lymphoid organs. When CD4+ T cell count falls below 400/μl, a large number of virions spill over from the degenerating lymph nodes into the blood and opportunistic infections with various microorganisms may develop. Cause of death is the opportunistic infections, and malignancy most common of which is Kaposi's Sarcoma (Fig. 38.2).

Clinical Features

The Centres for Disease Control in Atlanta, USA have classified the clinical course of HIV infection into 4 groups (Table 38.1).

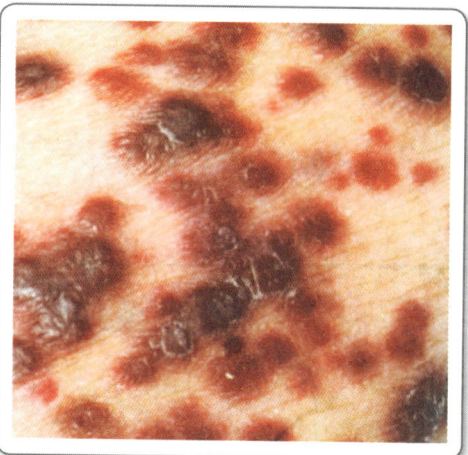

Fig. 38.2: Multiple lesions of papular cutaneous Kaposi's sarcoma on the back of an AIDS Patient

TABLE 38.1: Classification of HIV infection and AIDS (Centres for Disease Control, USA)

Group I	Acute HIV infection or HIV seroconversion illness
Group II	Asymptomatic infection
Group III	Persistent generalized lymphadenopathy
Group IV	
A	Constitutional disease
B	Neurological disease
C	Secondary infectious disease
D	Secondary cancer
E	Other conditions

Acute HIV Infection

Two to six weeks after infection, most patients develop acute-onset fever with or without night-sweats, malaise, headache, myalgia, arthralgia, lethargy, diarrhoea, depression, sore throat, lymphadenopathy, skin rash, mucocutaneous ulcerations and sometimes meningoencephalopathy. Spontaneous resolution occurs within one month. There is a temporary fall in CD4+ and CD8+ T cells, followed by CD8+ lymphocytosis. Virus, viral nucleic acid or viral p24 antigen may be detected during this illness. Tests for HIV antibodies are usually negative at the onset of the illness but become positive during its course. Therefore, acute HIV infection is also known as **seroconversion illness**.

Asymptomatic Infection

All persons infected with HIV, whether they develop sero-conversion illness or not, pass through a long asymptomatic period of 1–15 years (average 10 years). They show positive HIV antibody tests during this phase and are infectious.

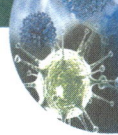

Persistent Generalized Lymphadenopathy (PGL)

Twenty five to thirty per cent of the patients who are otherwise asymptomatic develop enlarged lymph nodes, at least 1 cm in diameter, in two or more noncontiguous extrainguinal sites, that persist for at least three months. PGL must be distinguished from other causes of lymphadenopathy such as the lymphomas.

Symptomatic HIV Infection

Following features indicate disease progression:
- Downward trend of CD4+ T cells in successive samples.
- The ease of virus culture.
- The presence of p24 antigen in the plasma.
- The loss of antibody to p24 antigen.

When CD4+ T cells drop below 200/μl, their number generally begin to decline at an accelerated rate, the titre of virus in blood increases markedly and there is irreversible breakdown of immune defence mechanisms, leaving the patient a prey to progressive opportunistic infections and malignancies. Most of the patients with HIV disease die of infections other than HIV.

Laboratory Diagnosis

Laboratory diagnosis of HIV infection is generally based on the demonstration of anti-HIV antibodies, and in same cases, detection of viral antigen and RNA. Laboratory tests employed may be classified into three groups (Table 38.2).
- **Screening tests:** These are serological tests which are used to screen antibodies against HIV. These tests are of two types – ELISA and rapid (E/R) tests.
- **Supplemental tests:** These tests also detect antibodies against HIV. These tests are recommended for validation of the positive results of the screening tests. These include Western blot assay and immunofluorescence test.
- **Confirmatory tests:** These are the tests which confirm HIV infection in an individual who is either seropositive or has equivocal results from various serological tests. These include virus isolation, detection of p24 antigen and detection of viral nucleic acid.

Prophylaxis

- Do not have vaginal, anal or oral sex with prostitutes, male or female.

TABLE 38.2: Laboratory tests for the diagnosis of HIV infection

Screening (E/R) tests
• ELISA
• Rapid tests
▪ Dot blot assays
▪ Particle agglutination (gelatine, RBC, latex, microbeads)
▪ Dip stick and comb tests
▪ Immunochromatography based tests
Supplemental tests
• Western blot assay
• Immunofluorescence test
Confirmatory tests
• Virus isolation
• Detection of p24 antigen
• Detection of viral nucleic acid
▪ In situ hybridization
▪ Polymerase chain reaction

- Reduce the number of your sex partners if you have more than one. Practise abstinence before marriage and fidelity after marriage. Mutual monogamy should be the objective of all heterosexual partners.
- Men should always use condoms from start to finish and women should make sure their partners use them. Use of condom also protects from many other sexually transmitted diseases.
- Get all sexually transmitted diseases treated promptly.
- Sexually promiscuous and parenteral drug users should not donate blood.
- If you need blood transfusion, try to ensure that only screened blood is used.
- Screening of donors of blood, blood products such as factor VIII, bone marrow, cornea, kidney, heart, semen, and other organs and tissues should be carried out.
- Avoid injections unless absolutely necessary, use presterilized disposable syringes and needles.
- If you inject drugs, no matter what kind, never use anyone else's syringe.
- HIV- or AIDS-positive individuals should not donate blood.
- HIV- or AIDS-positive individuals should not allow anyone else to use their shaving kits.
- Do not let the barber use a razor during your haircut.
- Medical and laboratory personnel should follow strict standards of aseptic techniques in handling infectious material in the ward or laboratory.

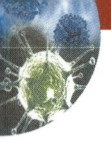

Key Points

- *Human immunodeficiency virus (HIV) is transmitted by sexual, parenteral and perinatal routes.*
- HIV infects CD4+ T lymphocytes.
- **Cause of death** in AIDS is the *opportunistic infections, malignancy and cachexia-like state.*
- Laboratory diagnosis of AIDS can be made by screening, supplemental and confirmatory tests.

? ASSESS YOURSELF

LONG ANSWER QUESTIONS

1. Discuss the modes of transmission of HIV.
2. Describe the laboratory diagnosis of HIV infection.
3. Discuss the pathogenesis and clinical features of HIV infection.

MULTIPLE CHOICE QUESTIONS

1. Which is the commonest mode of transmission of HIV?
   - (a) Sexual
   - (b) Parenteral
   - (c) Perinatal
   - (d) Oral

2. Which cells are infected by HIV most often?
   - (a) CD4+ T lymphocytes
   - (b) CD8+ T lymphocytes
   - (c) Null cells
   - (d) B cells

3. Which is the commonest opportunistic infection in AIDS patients in India?
   - (a) Tuberculosis
   - (b) Toxoplasmosis
   - (c) Cryptosporidiosis
   - (d) Cryptococcosis

ANSWERS TO MCQs

1. a   2. a   3. a

Chapter 39

Hepatitis Viruses

The term 'viral hepatitis' is reserved for infection of the liver caused by eight hepatitis viruses (Table 39.1) named hepatitis A virus (HAV), hepatitis B virus (HBV), hepatitis C virus (HCV), hepatitis D virus (HDV), hepatitis E virus (HEV) hepatitis G virus (HGV), SEN virus and transfusion-transmitted virus (TTE). HBV, TTV and SEN virus have DNA genome, other hepatitis viruses have RNA genome.

HEPATITIS A VIRUS (HAV)

Morphology

Hepatitis A virus is 27 nm, icosahedral, naked, single-stranded RNA virus, the sole member of the genus *Hepatovirus* in the family Picornaviridae (Table 39.1).

Pathogenesis

HAV is shed early in the stools of infected individuals, 1–2 weeks prior to the onset of symptoms, and persists for the first several days after the transaminase levels peak. There is very little virus in the serum and hardly any at all in other body fluids which explains the epidemiology of the disease as **faecal-oral enteric infection**. Transfusion-associated hepatitis A is exceedingly rare. It probably multiplies first in the intestinal epithelial cells and then spreads to the liver via the blood.

Clinical Features

Hepatitis A is an acute self-limiting disease with an incubation period of 2–6 weeks. The onset is abrupt with fever, malaise, anorexia, nausea and lethargy which comprise the prodromal (preicteric) stage. Hepatomegaly, due to cell necrosis, causes blockage of the biliary excretions resulting in jaundice. It may also produce pain in the right upper abdominal quadrant. Complete recovery occurs in 8–12 weeks.

The severity of the disease varies with age. Only 5% of the children under 3 years of age develop jaundice, while more than 50% of adults develop it. Fatality rate is also more in adults. **In contrast to hepatitis B, hepatitis A infection does not produce extrahepatic manifestations, no carrier state and is not associated with cirrhosis or hepatocellular carcinoma.**

Laboratory Diagnosis

Biochemical Tests

Serum levels of both alanine and aspartate aminotransferase are markedly raised.

Immunoelectron Microscopy

Virus particles can be demonstrated in faecal extracts by immunoelectron microscopy.

Serology

- Faecal HAV may be detected by ELISA.
- Detection of IgM anti-HAV by ELISA or RIA is the method of choice for the diagnosis of HAV infection. It is detectable in the serum for 2–6 months after the onset of symptoms. It is followed by the appearance of IgG anti-HAV which persists for many years and is a useful indicator of immunity.

Virus Culture

Virus, from the faeces, may be cultured on continuous lines of monkey kidney cells or human fibroblasts or hepatoma.

Polymerase Chain Reaction

Trace amounts of HAV in food or water can be detected by PCR.

Prophylaxis

- Proper collection, treatment and disposal of sewage.
- Bathing and cultivation of shellfish for human consumption should not be allowed near sewerage outlets.
- **Passive immunization** with normal human immuno-globulin (NIG) gives protection to seronegative individuals for a period of 4–6 months.
- Hepatitis A vaccine consisting of formalin inactivated preparation of virions grown in human fibroblasts or monkey kidney cell lines, adsorbed to alum as an adjuvant

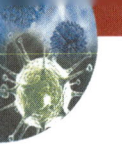

Essentials of Applied Microbiology for BSc Nursing

TABLE 39.1: Hepatitis viruses

Feature	Hepatitis A virus	Hepatitis B virus	Hepatitis C virus	Hepatitis D virus	Hepatitis E virus	Hepatitis G virus
Year of identification	1973	1965	1989	1977	1980	1995
Family	Picornaviridae	Hepadnaviridae	Flaviviridae	Unclassified	Hepeviridae	Flaviviridae
Genus	*Hepatovirus*	*Orthohepadnavirus*	*Hepacivirus*	*Deltavirus*	*Hepevirus*	*Hepacivirus*
Genome	ssRNA	dsDNA	ssRNA	ssRNA	ssRNA	ssRNA
Genome size	7.5 kb	3.2 kb	9.4 kb	1.7 kb	7.6 kb	9.4 kb
Virion	27 nm, icosahedral	42 nm, spherical	30–60 nm, spherical	36–38 nm, spherical	32–34 nm, icosahedral	?
Envelope	No	Yes (HBsAg)	Yes	Yes (HBsAg)	No	?
Stability	Heat- and acid-stable	Acid-stable	Ether- and acid-sensitive	Acid-sensitive	Heat-stable	?
Transmission	Faecal-oral	Parenteral, sexual	Parenteral, sexual	Parenteral, sexual	Faecal-oral	Parenteral, sexual
Vertical transmission						
• Intrauterine	No	Yes	Possible but rare	Possible but rare	Yes	?
• Perinatal	No	Yes	Yes	Yes	Yes	Yes
• Early postnatal infection	Possible but rare	Possible but rare	Possible	?	?	?
Incubation period	2–6 weeks	6 weeks – 6 months	6–8 weeks	6 weeks – 6 months	2–9 weeks	?
Onset	Acute	Insidious or acute	Insidious	Insidious or acute	Acute	?
Age preference	Children, young adults	Young adults, babies, toddlers	Any age but more common in adults	Any age	Young to middle-age adults	?
Antigens	HAV	HBsAg, HBcAg, HBeAg	HCV	HBsAg, HDAg	HEVAg	?
Antibodies	Anti-HAV	Anti-HBs, Anti-HBc, Anti-HBe	Anti-HCV	Anti-HBs, Anti-HD	Anti-HEV	?
Chronic carrier state	No	5–10%	50%	> 50%	No	?
Chronic hepatitis, cirrhosis	No	1–5%	20%	> 50%	No	?
Hepatocellular carcinoma	No	Yes	Yes	No	No	?

?, data not yet available.

can be used for active immunization. Two doses injected one month apart with or without a booster after 6 months elicit a good immune response in 99% of vaccinees lasting for some years.

HEPATITIS B VIRUS (HBV)

Hepatitis B virus is an enveloped partially double-stranded DIVA virus that belongs to the family Hepadnaviridae. Eight genotypes of HBV (A–H) have been identified.

Morphology

HBV or **Dane particle** is a complex 45 nm double-shelled particle (Fig. 39.1A and Table 39.1). The outer surface or envelope contains **hepatitis B surface antigen (HBsAg)**. It encloses an inner icosahedral 22 nm nucleocapsid (core). It contains **hepatitis B core antigen (HBcAg)**. Inside the core is the genome of HBV and a DNA-dependent DNA polymerase. The HBV genome consists of a 3.2 kilobase pair molecule of circular double-stranded DNA of most unusual structure. The plus strand is incomplete leaving 15–50% of the molecule single-stranded. The minus strand is complete.

From the core protein is derived hepatitis Be antigen (HBeAg). It is associated with the virion and is also found free in the plasma, especially when there is active viral replication.

Along with the mature virions (Fig. 39.1A), two subvirion morphological forms are formed in large excess (Fig. 39.1B and C) – (1) spherical particles with a diameter of 22 nm and (2) elongated tubules of similar diameter. Both these pleomorphic structures are composed of HBsAg, are devoid of HBcAg and nucleic acid. They are not infectious and consist solely of surplus virion envelope. They normally occur in large (100- to 1,000-fold) excess over the mature 45 nm virions.

Pathogenesis

There are three important modes of transmission of HBV infection – parenteral, perinatal and sexual.

- **Parenteral Transmission**
 HBV is present in the blood and in body fluids such as semen, vaginal secretions, menstrual discharge, saliva, colostrum and breast milk. The concentration of HBV in blood and body fluids is much greater than HIV. Less than 1 µl of blood contaminating a syringe or needle, can readily transmit hepatitis B from one individual to another. Transmission of infection may result from accidental inoculation of minute amounts of blood or fluid containing HBV during medical, surgical or dental procedures.

 Needlestick injuries, use of contaminated needles and syringes, intravenous and percutaneous drug abuse, ear and nose piercing, tattooing, acupuncture, sharing of shaving razor and kissing can transmit HBV infection.

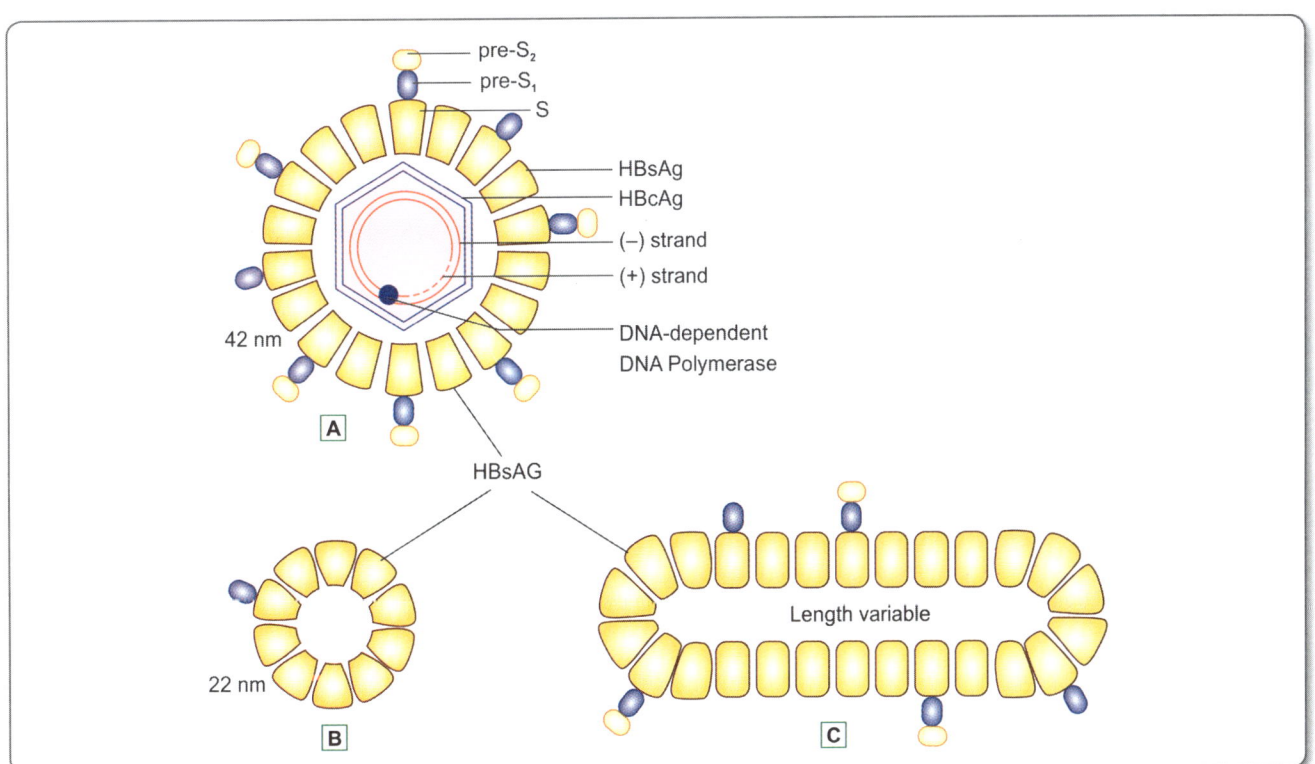

Fig. 39.1: Schematic diagram of hepatitis B virus particles: (A) Dane particle, (B) spherical particle, and (C) tubular particle.

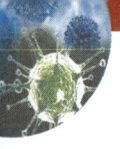

- **Perinatal Transmission**

  HBV can be transmitted from carrier mothers to their babies during the perinatal period. Transmission probably occurs when maternal blood contaminates the mucous membranes of the new born during birth. Infection may also result from haematogenous transplacental transmission, breast-feeding and close postnatal contact between infant and the infected parent.

- **Sexual Transmission**

  Since HBV is present in semen and vaginal secretions, therefore, it can be transmitted by sexual contact. Sexually promiscuous individuals particularly male homosexuals are at very high risk. Most of the HBV infections are subclinical, particularly in childhood.

  The course of acute HBV infection can be divided into three phases – preicteric, icteric and convalescent.

- **Preicteric (prodromal) phase**

  After an incubation period of 6 weeks to 6 months patient develops malaise, anorexia, weakness, myalgia, nausea, vomiting and pain in the right upper abdominal quadrant.

- **Icteric phase**

  Two days to two weeks following the initial symptoms patient develops jaundice, pale stools and dark urine (bilirubinuria). Hepatocellular damage is detectable biochemically before the onset of jaundice and persists after it has resolved.

- **Convalescent phase**

  This phase is long and drawn out with malaise and fatigue lasting for several weeks.

Hepatitis B Carriers

About 5–10% of HBV infections result in chronic carrier state. The latter may be defined as persistence of HBsAg in the circulation for more than six months. Carriers are of two types:

- *Super carriers*

  They have HBeAg, high titres of HBsAg and DNA polymerase in their blood. HBV may also be demonstrable in their blood. Very minute amount of serum or blood from such carriers can transmit the infection.

- *Simple carriers*

  These are more common types of carriers who have low level of HBsAg and no HBeAg, HBV and DNA polymerase in the blood. They transmit the infection only when large volumes of blood are transferred as in blood transfusion.

Laboratory Diagnosis

Laboratory diagnosis of HBV infections can be carried out by detection of HBsAg, anti-HBs, HBeAg, anti-HBe, IgM anti-HBc, IgG anti-HBc and HBV DNA in the serum (Table 39.2). These can be detected by sensitive and specific tests like ELISA and RIA.

Prophylaxis

Measures for the control of HBV infection are the same as those for HIV infection, i.e. screening of blood donors, use of sterile disposable syringes and needles by the healthcare workers (HCWs) and parenteral drug users, reduction of the number of sexual partners, the use of condoms, etc. HCWs should wear gloves, gowns, masks and eyeglasses to prevent exposure to blood and body fluids, avoidance of eating or smoking in the place of work and proper hand washing after work. Blood spills should be cleaned up with 2% glutaraldehyde or 0.5% sodium hypochlorite. Disposable equipment should be incinerated and other equipment should be properly sterilized.

Passive Immunization

Hepatitis B immune globulin (HBIG) is prepared from donors with high titres of anti-HBs. It can be given in the doses of 300–500 IU intramuscularly after accidental exposure, as may occur by needlestick injury or by splashing of blood from an HBsAg positive patient. HBIG should be administered as early as possible after exposure and preferably within 48 hours. A second dose is usually given 4 weeks after the first.

Active Immunization

Immunization against HBV is required for high risk individuals like:

TABLE 39.2: Serological markers of hepatitis B infection

Clinical condition	Serological marker						
	HBsAg	HBeAg	Anti-HBs	Anti-HBe	Anti-HBc		HBV DNA
					IgM	IgG	
Incubation period	+	+	–	–	–	–	+
Acute hepatitis	+	+	–	–	+	+	+
Chronic active hepatitis	+	+	–	–	+	+	+
Asymptomatic carrier state	+	–	–	+	–	+	–
Past infection	–	–	+	+	–	+	–
Immunization without infection	–	–	+	–	–	–	–

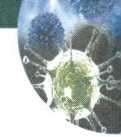

- HCWs, especially those in direct contact with blood and sharp instruments,
- Patients and HCWs of institutions for the mentally retarded,
- Patients requiring repeated transfusion of blood and blood products,
- Patients on maintenance dialysis,
- Patients receiving prolonged inpatient treatment,
- Patients who require frequent tissue penetration,
- Parenteral drug users,
- Sexually promiscuous individuals and prostitutes, and
- Spouses of those known to be infected with HBV.

Following vaccines are available for Hepatitis B:

- **Plasma-derived hepatitis B vaccine**

  It consists of purified 22 nm particles of HBsAg, prepared from the plasma of symptomless carriers.

- **Recombinant yeast hepatitis B vaccine**

  It is produced by cloning the *S* gene of HBV in yeast *Saccharomyces cerevisae* and the HBsAg particles produced are extracted and purified for use as vaccine. This vaccine is safe, antigenic, free from side effects and as immunogenic as plasma-derived vaccine.

- **Recombinant chinese hamster ovary (CHO) cell hepatitis vaccine**

  Expression system of CHO cells has been successfully used and the product is commercially available. This is the first vaccine using mammalian cell expression system.

- **Synthetic peptide vaccines**

  As the name indicates these are chemically synthesized polypeptide vaccines. These are safe and cheap. These are still under experimental stage.

Three doses at 0, 1 and 6 months are administered intramuscularly into the deltoid region.

HEPATITIS C VIRUS (HCV)

A virus of growing importance, hepatitis C virus, belongs to the genus *Hepacivirus* in the family Flaviviridae. The HCV viral particle is 50–60 nm in diameter and consists of an envelope derived from host cell membrane into which are inserted the virally encoded glycoproteins (E1 and E2) surrounding a nucleocapsid and a positive-sense, single-stranded RNA genome of about 9,500 nucleotides.

The virus shows extensive genome heterogeneily and has been classified into 6 genotypes (1–6) and more than 80 subtypes. Genotype 1 is the main HCV genotype prevalent worldwide and accounts for 40–80% of all isolates.

HCV transmission occurs by needlestick injuries or cuts with sharps, use of contaminated needles and syringes, transfusion of unscreened blood and sexual intercourse. HCV can be transmitted *in utero*, during parturition and by breast milk.

Incubation period of hepatitis C averages 6–8 weeks though it may range up to several months. As compared to hepatitis B, clinical infection with hepatitis C is generally less severe, has shorter preicteric period, milder symptoms, absent or less marked jaundice, somewhat lower serum alanine aminotransferase (ALT) levels and the case-fatality rate from fulminant hepatitis is 1% or less. However, 85% or more of the acute HCV infections become chronic. The affected individuals have persistence of the virus in their blood, elevated ALT levels for at least a year or two or more and they are at risk, just as in hepatitis B, of developing **cirrhosis and hepatocellular carcinoma**.

Diagnosis of HCV infection can be established by:
- Detection of anti-HCV by ELISA, viral genome by PCR, and by immunofluorescence, and
- *In situ* hybridization on biopsy and autopsy specimen.

Prophylaxis

HCV infection can be prevented by screening of blood donors, avoidance of use of unsterile needles for intravenous drug abuse, tattooing and for medical and dental procedures. Many of the public health measures adopted to prevent transmission of human immunodeficiency virus and HBV by parenteral routes will assist efforts at controlling HCV.

HEPATITIS D VIRUS (HDV)

The HDV, also known as the delta hepatitis virus, is a defective satellite virus requiring HBV as helper virus. It is the sole member of the genus *Deltavirus*. It is spherical, 36–38 nm in diameter with HBsAg coat and HDAg nucleoprotein (Fig. 39.2). The genome consists of a single small circular molecule of minus sense RNA of 1.7 kilobase pairs (Table 39.1).

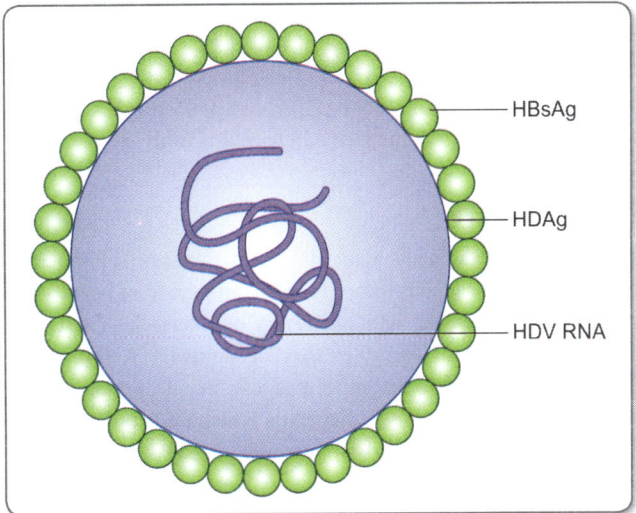

Fig. 39.2: Hepatitis D virus.

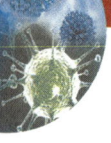

Pathogenesis

HDV is transmitted principally by blood and blood products, but also by sexual contact. Vertical transmission is also possible (Table 39.1).

Two types of HDV infections are possible:

- **Simultaneous coinfection with HBV and HDV in the same inoculum**.
- **Superinfection of an HBsAg carrier by HDV**. It is commoner and more serious because a large number of hepatocytes are already producing HBsAg, and HDV can replicate without delay with a relatively short incubation period. It leads to severe liver damage, fulminant HBsAg positive hepatitis and elevated mortality (up to 20%).

In simultaneous acute HBV and HDV infections, IgM anti-HBc will be detectable, while in acute HDV infection superimposed on chronic HBV infections, anti-HBc will be of IgG class.

Laboratory Diagnosis

In patients with HBV-HDV coinfection, shortly before the end of incubation period, HBsAg appears in the serum and towards the end of incubation period HDAg appears which can be detected by ELISA. In the later stages of acute disease, anti-HD IgM appears followed by anti-HD IgG. These can be detected by ELISA.

Prophylaxis

HDV infection can be prevented by prevention of coinfection with HBV or of superinfection of HBV carriers and hence requires all the measures that apply to the prevention of HBV infection, including vaccination against HBV. HBV vaccine is effective as HDV cannot infect persons immune to HBV.

HEPATITIS E VIRUS (HEV)

Morphology

Hepatitis E virus is small (32–34 nm), naked, single-stranded, RNA virus classified in the genus *Hepevirus*, family Hepeviridae.

Pathogenesis

Hepatitis E is primarily associated with ingestion of **faecally contaminated drinking water**. **Incubation period** of hepatitis E ranges from 2–9 weeks, with an average of 5–6 weeks. Clinically, the disease closely resembles that of hepatitis A. However, bilirubin levels tend to be higher and jaundice deeper and more prolonged. **Like hepatitis A, hepatitis E also does not progress to chronic hepatitis, cirrhosis, cancer or carrier state**.

Laboratory Diagnosis

- Exclusion of hepatitis A by IgM serology and hepatitis B by absence of HBsAg and IgM anti-HBc.
- Immunoelectron microscopic examination of patient faeces for aggregated hepatitis E virus particles using monoclonal antibodies.
- ELISA tests for IgM and IgG anti-HEV.
- A Western blot assay for IgM and/or IgG anti-HEV.

Prophylaxis

Hepatitis E can be prevented by improved standards of sanitation and provision of chlorinated water throughout the developing world. During the epidemic, take boiled water and only cooked food. No vaccine or effective antiviral drugs exist.

HEPATITIS G VIRUS (HGV)

Hepatitis G virus has been placed in family Flaviviridae genus *Hepacivirus*. The genome of HGV consists of 9.4 kb molecule of ssRNA of positive polarity (Table 39.1).

The virus is present worldwide. Majority of the individuals with HGV infection have no detectable evidence of liver disease. There have been, however, cases of acute, fulminant and chronic hepatitis where HGV is presently the only explanation for their liver disease.

HGV infection is mainly detected by reverse transcriptase polymerase chain reaction (RT-PCR).

SEN VIRUS (SEN-V)

SEN-V is named after the initials of the patient from whom the virus was isolated. It was discovered by an Italian research group led by Dr. Daniele Primi in 1999. It is a circular, single-stranded DNA virus with an average length of 3900 nucleotides. It is unenveloped virus. It has eight highly divergent genotypes—SEN-V A through H. Studies employing PCR DNA detection indicate that SEN-V exists in the blood and is transmitted parenterally.

SEN-V is associated with transfusion associated non-A, non-E (NANE) hepatitis.

TRANSFUSION-TRANSMITTED VIRUS (TTV)

TTV was first identified in the serum of a Japanese patient in 1997. It is a single-stranded DNA virus. The role of TTV in human disease is unknown but it may be associated with some cases of post-transfusion hepatitis.

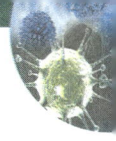

🎵 Key Points

- Hepatitis A infection does not produce extrahepatic manifestations, no carrier state and it is not associated with cirrhosis or hepatocellular carcinoma.
- Hepatitis B virus, SEN virus and transfusion-transmitted virus are DNA viruses while all other hepatitis viruses are RNA viruses.
- *Hepatitis A vaccine is safe and effective, and recommended for professionals working with institutionalized patients.*
- **HBV** is transmitted by parenteral, perinatal and sexual routes.
- *HBV vaccine is safe, effective and relatively long-lasting, and also protects against hepatitis D infection.*

❓ ASSESS YOURSELF

SHORT ANSWER QUESTION

Write short notes on:

(a) Hepatitis A virus

(b) Hepatitis B virus

(c) Hepatitis C virus

(d) Hepatitis D virus

(e) Hepatitis E virus

MULTIPLE CHOICE QUESTIONS

1. All of the following hepatitis viruses are RNA viruses except:
   (a) hepatitis A virus
   (b) hepatitis B virus
   (c) hepatitis E virus
   (d) hepatitis G virus

2. Hepatocellular carcinoma may be caused by:
   (a) hepatitis B virus
   (b) hepatitis C virus
   (c) Both of the above
   (d) None of the above

3. Which of the following viruses is/are transmitted by parenteral and sexual routes?
   (a) Hepatitis B virus
   (b) Hepatitis C virus
   (c) Hepatitis G virus
   (d) All of the above

4. Which of the following is a defective satellite virus?
   (a) Hepatitis B virus
   (b) Hepatitis C virus
   (c) Hepatitis D virus
   (d) Hepatitis E virus

5. Which of the following serological markers is/are positive in super carriers of hepatitis B?
   (a) HBeAg
   (b) HBsAg
   (c) DNA polymerase
   (d) All of the above

6. Which of the following hepatitis viruses is/are DNA virus/viruses?
   (a) Hepatitis B virus
   (b) SEN virus
   (c) Transfusion-transmitted virus
   (d) All of the above

7. Which of the following hepatitis viruses is not DNA virus?
   (a) Hepatitis A virus
   (b) Hepatitis B virus
   (c) SEN virus
   (d) Transfusion-transmitted virus

ANSWERS TO MCQS

1. b   **2.** c   **3.** d   **4.** c   **5.** d   **6.** d   **7.** a

NOTES

Section

VI

Pathogenic Organisms-III
Fungi

Chapter 40

Medical Mycology

Fungi are eukaryotic organisms which exist as saprophytes, parasites or commensals. They reproduce by means of spores or conidia. On or in the appropriate substrates, the spores germinate to form yeasts or molds or both. In yeasts (Fig. 40.1A) a spore forms round, oval or elongated single cell that reproduces by budding. In molds, spores germinate to form branching filaments called hyphae. They may be septate or non-septate (coenocytic).

MORPHOLOGICAL CLASSIFICATION OF FUNGI

On the basis of morphology, there are four groups of fungi (Fig. 40.1):

- **Yeasts:** Yeasts are round, oval or elongated unicellular fungi. Most of them reproduce by an asexual process called budding in which the cell develops a protuberance which enlarges and eventually separates from the parent cell (Fig. 40.1A).
- **Yeast-like:** In some yeasts like *Candida*, the bud remains attached to the mother cell and elongates, followed by repeated budding forming chains of elongated cells known as pseudohyphae (Fig. 40.1B). *C. albicans* and *C. stellatoidea* also produce germ tubes (Fig. 40.1C). Germ tubes are the begining of true hyphae and appear as filaments that are not constricted at their points of origin on the parent cells. If the filaments are constricted at their points of origin on the parent cell, they are pseudohyphae, not germ tubes.
- **Molds:** In molds, spores germinate to produce branching filaments called hyphae (singular hypha). They are 2–10 µm in diameter. They may be septate (Fig. 40.1D) or non-septate (coenocytic) (Fig. 40.1E). The hyphae continue to grow and branch to form tangled mass of growth called mycelium (pl., mycelia) (Fig. 40.1F).
- **Dimorphic fungi:** Many fungi pathogenic to man have a yeast form in the host tissue and *in vitro* at 37°C on enriched media, and hyphal (mycelial) form *in vitro* at 25°C. These are known as dimorphic fungi.

Dermatophytosis

Dermatophytosis, tinea or ringworm is the most common type of superficial mycosis seen in human beings. It infects keratinized tissues of the skin, hair and nails. Dermatophytosis is caused by 41 species of dermatophytes which belong to three genera (*Trichophyton*-24, *Microsporum*-16 and *Epidermophyton*-1).

Dermatophytes grow only on the keratinized layers of skin and its appendages and do not ordinarily penetrate the living tissues. Hypersensitivity to fungus antigens may lead to secondary eruptions occurring in sensitized patients because of circulation of allergenic products from the primary site of infection. It is known as **dermatophytid** or **id reaction**.

Clinically, ringworm can be classified depending on the site involved. Tinea corporis, tinea capitis, tinea barbae, tinea cruris, tinea manuum, tinea unguium and tinea pedis involve body, shaft of hair of scalp, beard and moustache, groin, hands, nail plates and feet, respectively. The lesions are circular which spread with an erythematous border with variable degree of scaling and inflammation.

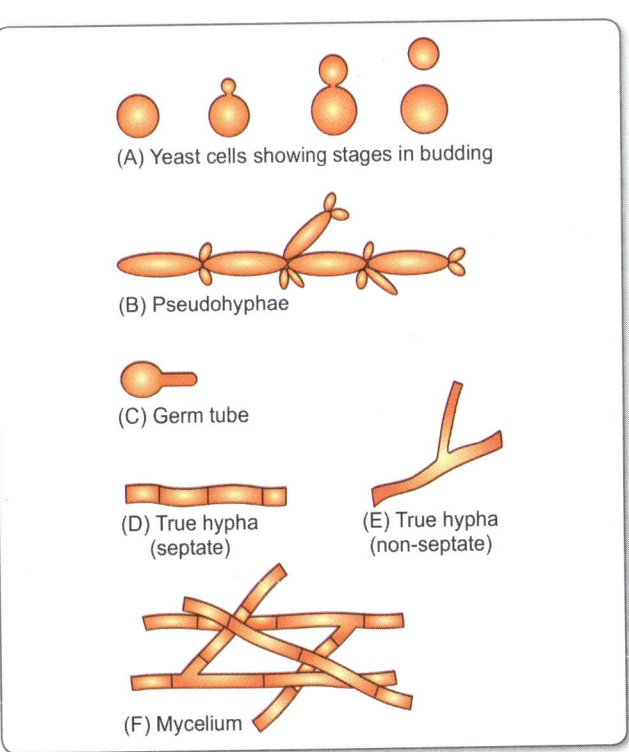

(A) Yeast cells showing stages in budding

(B) Pseudohyphae

(C) Germ tube

(D) True hypha (septate)

(E) True hypha (non-septate)

(F) Mycelium

Fig. 40.1: Basic fungal morphology.

In lesions, dermatophytes appear as hyphae and arthro-conidia. Three types of hair infection can be seen in 10% KOH wet mounts:

- **Ectothrix:** In this, the fungus is present on the surface of hair shaft. It is caused by *M. audouinii*, *M. canis* and *T. mentagrophytes* (Fig. 40.2A).
- **Endothrix:** In this, the arthroconidia formation occurs entirely within the hair completely filling the hair shaft without a conspicuous external sheath of arthroconidia. This is caused by *T. tonsurans* and *T. violaceum* (Fig. 40.2B).
- **Favus:** In this, there is sparse hyphal growth and formation of air spaces within the hair shaft. This is caused by *T. schoenleinii* (Fig. 40.2C).

In cultures on Sabouraud's dextrose agar, dermatophytes form characteristic colonies consisting of septate hyphae and two types of asexual spores, microconidia and macroconidia. Sexual spores of some species have also been identified. The differentiation of the three genera is based mainly on the nature of macroconidia (Table 40.1 and Fig. 40.3).

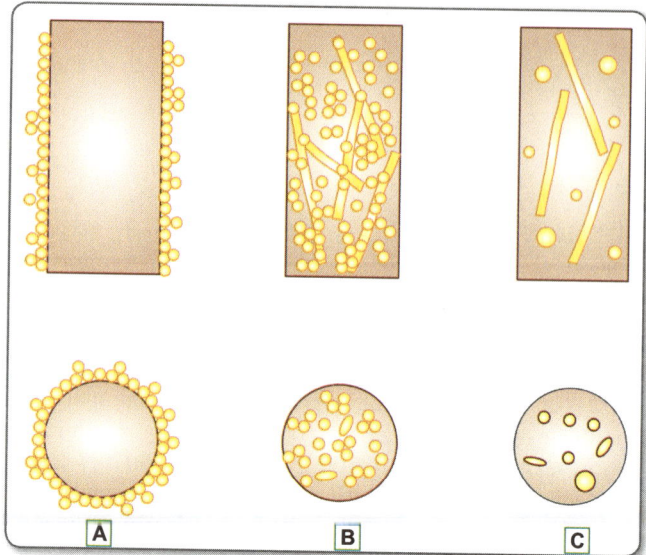

Fig. 40.2: Hair invasion of dermatophytes in longitudinal and transverse sections.

Trichophyton

Colonies may be powdery, velvety or waxy with pigmentation characteristic of different species. Macroconidia are usually rare but microconidia are abundant. The latter are arranged in clusters along the hyphae or borne on conidiophores. Some species possess special types of hyphae, i.e. spiral hyphae, racquet hyphae and favic chandeliers (Fig. 40.4). Fungi of this genus can infect skin, hair and nails. *T. rubrum* is the most common species infecting man.

Microsporum

Colonies of the fungi of this genus are cottony, velvety or powdery with white to brown pigmentation. Macroconidia are very numerous and microconidia are relatively scanty. They infect skin and hair but not the nails.

Epidermophyton

Colonies are powdery and greenish-yellow. Microconidia are absent and macroconidia are club-shaped and are arranged in groups of two or three. It infects skin and nails but not the hair.

Salient characteristics of common dermatophytes are given in Table 40.2.

Laboratory Diagnosis

The site should be cleaned with spirit and scrapings from the skin lesions should be collected by scraping outwards with a blunt scalpel from the edges of the lesions. Infected hair and nail clippings can also be collected. The specimen is mixed with a drop of 10% KOH on a slide, and after placing a coverslip, the preparation is gently heated to bring about clearing. Microscopy reveals branching septate hyphae or chains of arthroconidia. Three types of hair infection may be distinguished in wet mounts—**ectothrix, endothrix** and **favic-type hair invasion**. Demonstration of fungus in nails may be possible only after clearing with KOH for a day or two.

Species identification is possible only by culture examination. Keratinous material is inoculated on SDA with chloramphenicol and cycloheximide and incubated at 25–30°C for three weeks. Identification of dermatophytes is based on colonial morphology,

TABLE 40.1: Generic characteristics of dermatophyte macroconidia

Genus	Frequency	Size	Number of septations	Thickness of wall	Surface of wall	Manner of attachment
Microsporum	Very numerous (except *M. audouinii*)	5–100 × 3–8 µm	3–15	Thick (except *M. gypseum* and *M. nanum*)	Rough	Singly
Trichophyton	Usually rare	20–50 × 4–6 µm	2–8	Thin	Smooth	Singly
Epidermophyton	Numerous	20–40 × 6–8 µm	2–4	Both thin and slightly thick	Smooth	Singly or in clusters

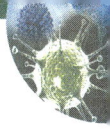

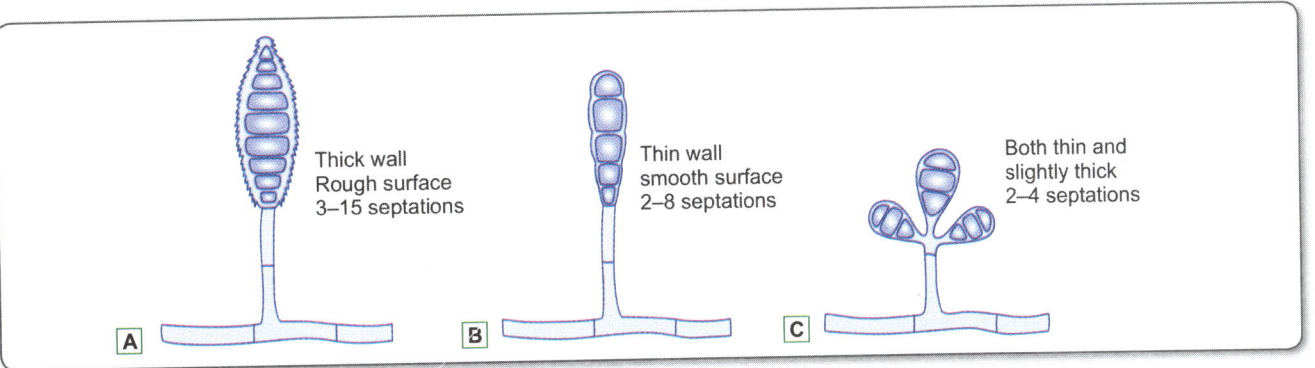

Fig. 40.3: Macroconidia in the three genera of dermatophytes: (A) Microsporum, (B) Trichophyton, and (C) Epidermophyton.

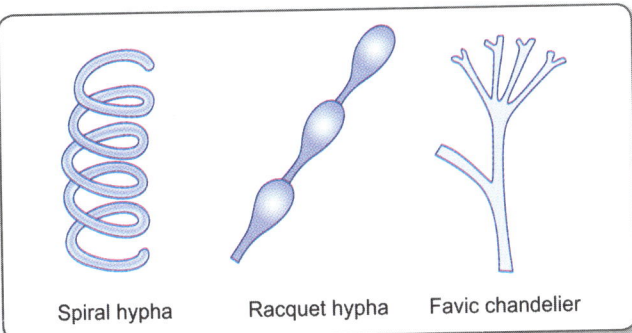

Spiral hypha   Racquet hypha   Favic chandelier

Fig. 40.4: Special types of hyphae in dermatophytes.

colour, pigment production and production of microconidia and macroconidia (Tables 40.1 and 40.2, and Figs 40.3 and 40.4).

Sporotrichosis

Sporotrichosis is a chronic pyogenic granulomatous infection of the skin and subcutaneous tissues, although it may become disseminated by lymphatic spread. It is caused by *Sporothrix schenckii*, a dimorphic fungus. The infection is due to the implantation of spores through injured skin. It is more common in farmers and gardeners.

TABLE 40.2: Salient characteristics of common dermatophytes

Species	Colony character	Morphology
T. rubrum	Cottony which later becomes velvety with a blood-red pigment on the reverse side.	Few, long, narrow, pencil-shaped macroconidia.
T. mentagrophytes	Flat with a cream to buff or tan powdery surface. The reverse side of colonies on SDA may be brown, yellow or dark-red. However, dark-red colour is not produced on potato dextrose agar with 1% glucose.	Numerous microconidia. Thin-walled, club-shaped, spindle-shaped or long pencil-shaped macroconidia.
T. tonsurans	White, tan, yellow or reddish brown with central furrows.	Abundant clavate to tear-shaped microconidia and few irregular thick-walled macroconidia.
T. schoenleinii	White to tan, glabrous, waxy, heaped and folded.	Microconidia very rare, macroconidia absent. Hyphae tend to become knobby and clubbed at ends (favic chandeliers).
T. violaceum	Heaped and verrucose, glabrous with a deep violet colour.	Irregularly branched hyphae. Microconidia usually not found. Macroconidia resembling those of T. rubrum may be formed.
M. audouinii	Slow growing, velvety, brownish.	Terminal chlamydoconidia, conidia rarely produced. Some isolates show large, irregular, spindle-shaped, thick-walled with smooth or echinulate surface macroconidia. Some isolates produce pectinate hyphae.
M. canis	White to bright yellowish colony with bright yellow to orange-brown on reverse.	Abundant, thick-walled, spindle-shaped macroconidia and a few clavate, sessile microconidia.
M. gypseum	Powdery, buff coloured.	Abundant, spindle-shaped macroconidia with thick and finely rough wall. Microconidia are clavate, sessile and rare.
E. floccosum	Powdery, greenish-yellow, radially folded.	Macroconidia are numerous, club-shaped and are arranged in groups of two or three. Microconidia absent.

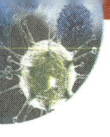

The initial lesion is a small ulcerated nodule commonly on the hand or the forearm. Nodules and abscesses occur along the draining lymphatics and the regional lymph nodes enlarge, suppurate and ulcerate. The primary lesion may remain localized or disseminate to involve the bones, joints, lungs and rarely CNS particularly in debilitated or immunosuppressed individuals.

In infected tissues, *S. schenckii* appears in the form of round, oval (2–3 μm) or elongated or cigar-shaped (1–5 μm) yeast-like cells with irregular budding. With ordinary stains, they are difficult to find. The use of PAS or methenamine silver stain and fluorescent antibody technique facilitates detection of these organisms. The abscesses may show the **asteroid body**. This consists of central basophilic budding yeast cell with eosinophilic material (antibody complex) radiating from it (Fig. 40.5).

The diagnosis is confirmed by isolation of the causative organism by culture of swabs from the ulcerated lesions or pus aspirated from subcutaneous nodules or biopsy material. *S. schenckii* grows well on routine agar media, and at room temperature (25°C). The young colonies are blackish and shiny, becoming wrinkled and fuzzy with age. Strains vary in pigmentation from shades of black and grey to whitish. Microscopic examination reveals thin, delicate hyphae bearing conidia developing in a 'rosette' pattern at the ends of delicate conidiophores (Fig. 40.6). Conidia are also produced along the sides of the hyphae. To induce mycelial to yeast conversion, the fungus is inoculated on blood agar tubes and incubated at 37°C.

Histoplasmosis

Histoplasmosis is an intracellular mycosis of reticuloendothelial system. It is caused by a dimorphic fungus, *Histoplasma capsulatum*. *H. capsulatum* grows in soil with high nitrogen content. The growth of the fungus appears to be most frequently associated with soil enriched by excreta of bats, chickens and other birds. From the soil, the conidia of *H. capsulatum* are airborne and these are inhaled leading to infection.

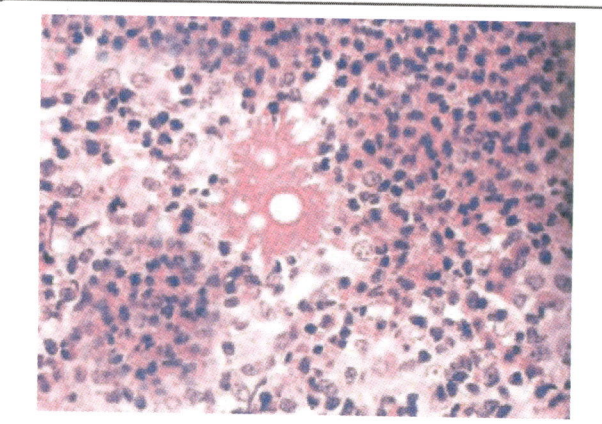

Fig. 40.5: Asteroid body in sporotrichosis. The yeast-like cells are surrounded by eosinophilic Splendore-Hoeppli material (haematoxylin and eosin stain, × 400).

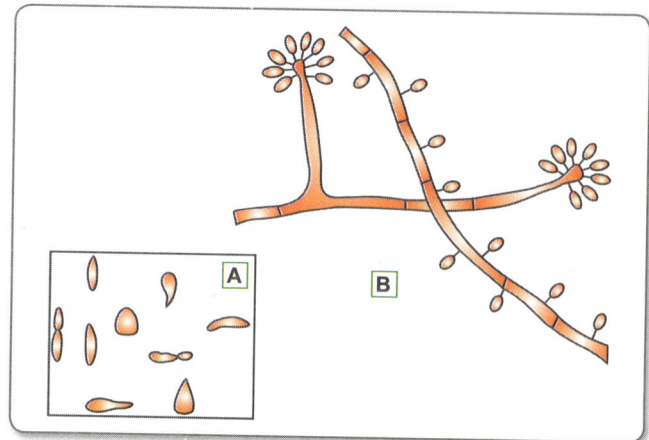

Fig. 40.6: *Sporothrix schenckii:* (A) yeast phase; and (B) mycelial phase.

Histoplasmosis is ordinarily an asymptomatic or relatively mild, self-limiting pulmonary infection, although chronic or acute disseminated disease with poor prognosis may occur. In addition, it may also involve lymph nodes, spleen, liver, adrenals, kidneys, skin, CNS and other organs of the body. Granulomatous and ulcerative lesions may develop on the skin and mucosa.

In tissues, *H. capsulatum* is present inside phagocytic cells in yeast phase. They are round or oval, yeast-like cells, 2–5 μm in diameter. They fill the cytoplasm of macrophages, monocytes and occasionally polymorphonuclear leucocytes. With Giemsa or Wright stain, the cell wall and the cell protoplasm stain light blue and dark blue, respectively. A clear space is usually seen between the protoplasmic mass and the cell wall.

With H & E staining, only a central protoplasmic mass surrounded by a halo is seen (Fig. 40.7). Only a dark staining can outline the cell wall. In the PAS stain, the wall is stained pink to purplish red with pallor coloured protoplasm filling the cell. In the Gomori methenamine silver stain the cell wall stains intense black (Fig. 40.8). The so called 'capsule' of *H. capsulatum* is considered to be an artifact resulting from the shrinkage of the protoplasm within the cell wall.

On SDA, at 25–30°C, it forms white to tan fluffy colony with septate branching hyphae with two types of unicellular, asexual spores:

- Large round, tuberculate macroconidia (8–14 μm) are most prominent and are diagnostic.
- Small spores or microconidia usually appear first. They are sessile or stalked, smooth-walled, round to pyriform, 2–5 μm in diameter (Fig. 40.9A). On blood agar or other enriched media containing cysteine, small, round or oval budding yeast cells are produced (Fig. 40.9B).

Diagnosis may be made by microscopic examination of stained smears of sputum, bone marrow, peripheral blood, scrapings from dermal or mucosal ulcers and biopsies of lymph nodes and other organs and by culture of the fungus from these materials. Serological tests like latex agglutination, precipitation and

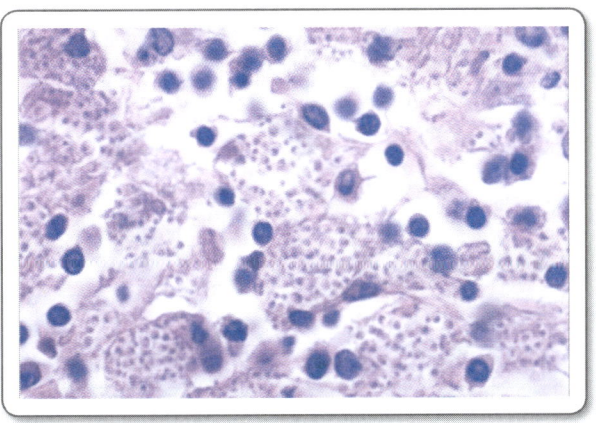

Fig. 40.7: Section of skin stained with haematoxylin and eosin showing *Histoplasma capsulatum*: surrounded by clear halo filling the cytoplasm of phagocytes (× 400).

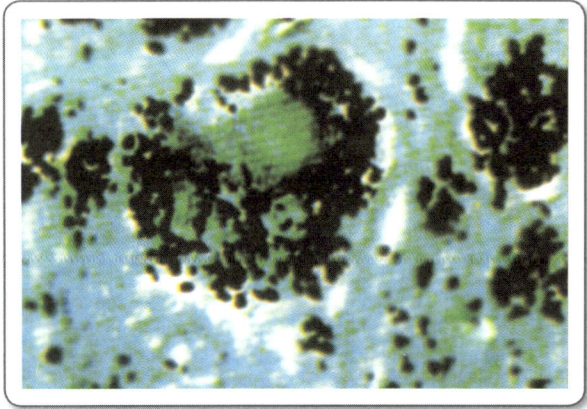

Fig. 40.8: Section of skin stained with Gomori methenamine silver staining. It shows black budding yeast cells (× 400).

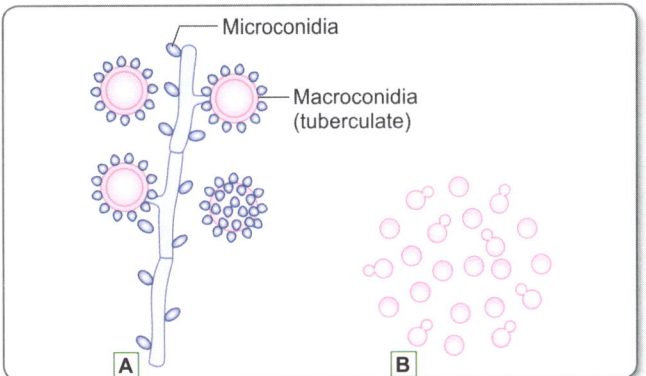

Fig. 40.9: *Histoplasma capsulatum*: (A) mycelial phase, and (B) yeast phase.

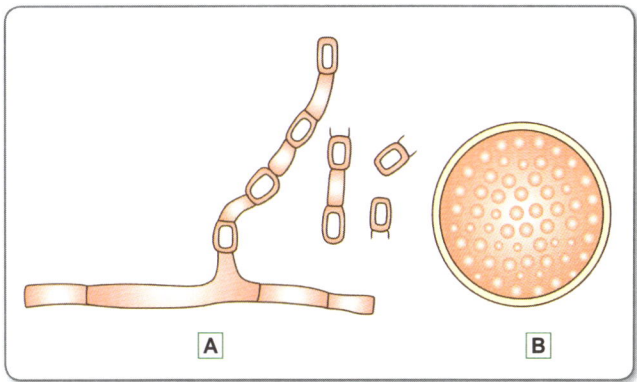

Fig. 40.10: Coccidioides immitis: (A) mycelial phase, and (B) tissue phase.

complement fixation become positive two weeks after infection. Delayed hypersensitivity to the fungus can be demonstrated by histoplasmin skin test.

Coccidioidomycosis

Coccidioidomycosis is primarily an infection of the lungs caused by *Coccidioides immitis*, a dimorphic fungus. It exists as a saprophyte in the soil. The arthroconidia of the saprophytic phase are carried by the wind and are inhaled by man and animals. Sixty per cent of the infections in man are asymptomatic. In 39.8% cases, various degrees of symptomatology result that range from self-limiting influenza like fever to pulmonary infection with cavities. Only 0.2% develop secondary coccidioidomycosis or coccidioidal granuloma which is the progressive and often fatal form of the disease.

In soil and in culture (both at room temperature and at 37°C), *C. immitis* grows as a mold. The hyphae develop barrel-shaped arthroconidia measuring 2.5–4 × 3–6 μm. They characteristically alternate with smaller intervening empty cells (Fig. 40.10A).

The hyphae fragment easily and release the arthroconidia. The latter are highly infectious and are readily airborne, therefore, the handling of a well developed culture is hazardous. *C. immitis* is probably the most virulent of all human mycotic agents. The inhalation of only a few arthroconidia produces primary coccidioidomycosis.

In the lungs, the arthroconidia form **spherules** (30–100 μm or more in diameter). These contain numerous **endospores**, 2–5 μm in diameter (Figs 40.10B and 40.11). The mature spherules have double wall measuring 2 μm in thickness. At maturity, the spherules rupture and their endospores are released which develop to form new spherules in adjacent tissue or following dissemination, in other organs of the body.

Diagnosis may be made by microscopic examination of sputum, pus and biopsy material, and culture on SDA incubated at 25–30°C. Since arthroconidia are highly infectious and readily airborne, therefore, Petri dish should not be used for isolation of *C. immitis* and all procedures should be carried out in a safety cabinet.

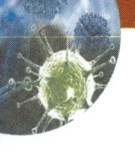

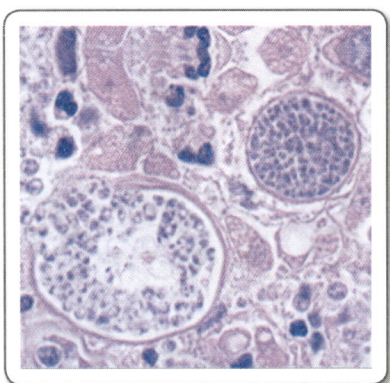

Fig. 40.11: Spherules of *Coccidiodes immitis* containing endospores (H & E stain, × 400).

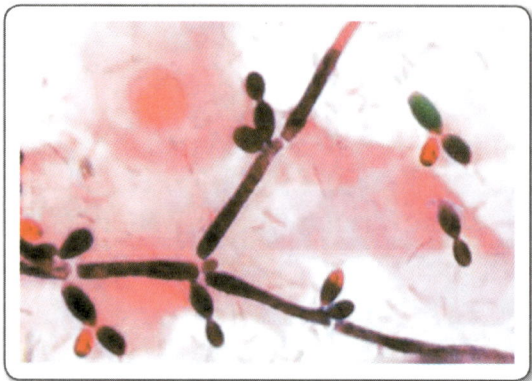

Fig. 40.12: Vaginal smear showing budding yeast cells, true hyphae and epithelial cells (PAS stain, × 400).

Candidiasis

Candidiasis is the commonest mycosis involving skin and its appendages, mucosa, and the internal organs. The infection may be acute or chronic and has a worldwide distribution. It is caused by a yeast-like fungus *Candida albicans* (80–90% of cases) and occasionally by other *Candida* species *C. tropicalis*, *C. parapsilosis*, *C. krusei*, *C. guilliermondii*, *C. glabrata*, *C. kefyr*, *C. lusitaniae*, *C. rugosa*, *C. viswanathii* and *C. stellatoidea* which is a variant of *C. albicans*.

They occur as normal flora of skin, mucous membranes and gastrointestinal tract. Candidiasis is an opportunistic endogenous infection. Predisposing factors for candidiasis are AIDS, diabetes, iatrogenic immunosuppression, intravenous catheters, prolonged administration of antimicrobial agents, neutropenia, haematologic malignant diseases, burns and intravenous drug use. It may cause:

- *Mucocutaneous lesions:* These include oral candidiasis (oral thrush), oesophageal candidiasis, vulvovaginitis, balanitis, balanoposthitis, conjunctivitis and keratitis.
- *Skin and nail infections:* These include infection of the skin at moist sites such as axillae, groins, perineum, submammary folds and occasionally in toe clefts. Persons who frequently immerse their hands in water may develop infection of the finger webs, nail folds and nails. In infants it may lead to napkin dermatitis.
- *Systemic candidiasis:* It may lead to urinary candidiasis, pulmonary candidiasis, hepatosplenic candidiasis, endocarditis, meningitis, endophthalmitis, arthritis, osteomyelitis and candidaemia.

C. albicans is an oval or spherical budding yeast cell 3–5 μm in diameter. It produces pseudohyphae when the buds continue to grow but fail to detach, producing chains of elongated cells that are pinched or constricted at the septations between cells (Figs. 40.1A and B). It also can produce true hyphae (Fig. 40.12). Diagnosis can be established by microscopy and culture.

Gram-stained smears and KOH wet mounts from lesions, exudates, patches from the mucous membrane of the mouth, oesophagus and vagina, and skin and nail scrapings show budding Gram-positive yeast cells and pseudohyphae.

Candida species grow well on SDA and on ordinary bacteriological culture media at 25–37°C. Cream-coloured, smooth, pasty colonies appear in 1–2 days. Lactophenol cotton blue preparation and Gram-stained smears show budding yeast cells and pseudohyphae. *C. albicans* can be differentiated from other species by sugar fermentation and sugar assimilation reactions.

Two simple morphologic tests distinguish *C. albicans*, the most common pathogen, from other species of *Candida*:

- After incubation in sheep, horse or normal human serum for about 90 minutes at 37°C, yeast cells of *C. albicans* will begin to form true hyphae or **germ tubes** (Fig. 40.1C).
- On Cornmeal-Tween 80 agar at 25°C for 72 hours, pseudohyphae (and some true hyphae) form with clusters of round blastoconidia at the septa. Large thick-walled, usually single terminal chlamydospores are characteristically formed (Fig. 40.13).

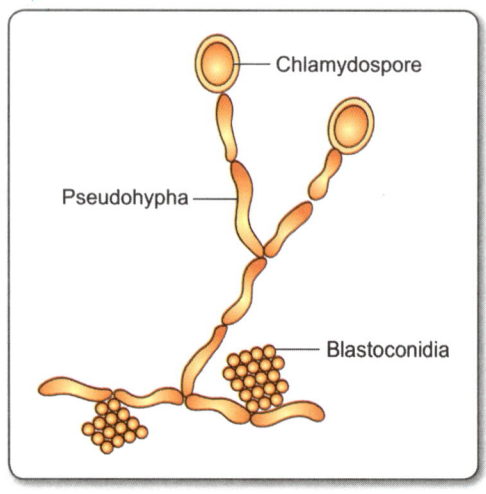

Fig. 40.13: Chlamydospores.

CRYPTOCOCCOSIS

Cryptococcosis is an infection caused by the encapsulated yeast, *Cryptococcus neoformans*. It is ubiquitous in the soil and in the avian faecal material, such as pigeon droppings which apparently provide a reservoir of the organisms. Infection follows airborne exposure and inhalation of yeast cells. In nature, yeast cells are minimally encapsulated, small, dry and easily aerosolized. From lungs, the yeast may metastasize to virtually any organ in the body. Cryptococcosis is basically an opportunistic infection. It occurs most frequently in patients with abnormalities of T lymphocyte function. The commonest form of the cryptococcosis is a mild, self-limiting pulmonary infection. Dissemination of infection may lead to the involvement of CNS, skin, mucosa, bone and other organs. Cryptococcosis is worldwide in distribution.

C. neoformans is by far the most life-threatening fungal pathogen that accounts for about 5–8% of all opportunistic infections in patients with advanced HIV disease. Clinical presentations in these patients include, meningitis, nerve palsies, seizures and cryptococcoma of the CNS. Other uncommon manifestations include pulmonary disease, myocarditis associated with acute heart failure and pleural effusion.

C. neoformans is a true yeast. Both in the tissues and culture at room temperature as well as at 37°C, only budding yeasts are seen. Diagnosis is established by demonstration of budding yeast cells in CSF, sputum, pus or brain tissue by direct microscopy, culture and serological tests for capsular antigen. The direct microscopy of CSF, mixed with a drop of India ink or nigrosin shows round budding yeast cells, 4–10 μm in diameter. The organisms are surrounded by a wide refractile gelatinous capsule that may be twice the size of the yeast cell. In India ink preparation, it appears as a clear halo around the yeast cells (Fig. 40.14). Sputum, pus and brain tissue should be examined after digestion in KOH. The histopathological examination of biopsy material can be done by staining with Mayer's mucicarmine, PAS, GMS and H & E staining. Tissue stained with Mayer's mucicarmine shows the capsule as bright carmine red (Fig. 40.15).

Sediment from a centrifuged CSF specimen is inoculated on SDA. It is incubated at 30–35°C. *C. neoformans* readily grows on this medium forming smooth, mucoid, cream-coloured colonies. Lactophenol cotton blue (LCB) mount shows budding yeast cells. Hyphae or pseudohyphae are not normally produced. *C. neoformans* possesses the enzyme phenol oxidase, and testing for its presence is another means of accurate identification. This can be done by culturing the suspected yeasts on special agars such as niger seed agar, bird seed agar and caffeic acid agar, and looking for the black colonies (phenol oxidase-positive).

Pathogenic *C. neoformans* can be differentiated from non-pathogenic species by its ability to:
- Grow at 37°C,
- Hydrolyze urea,
- Produce black colonies on niger seed agar, bird seed agar and caffeic acid agar, and

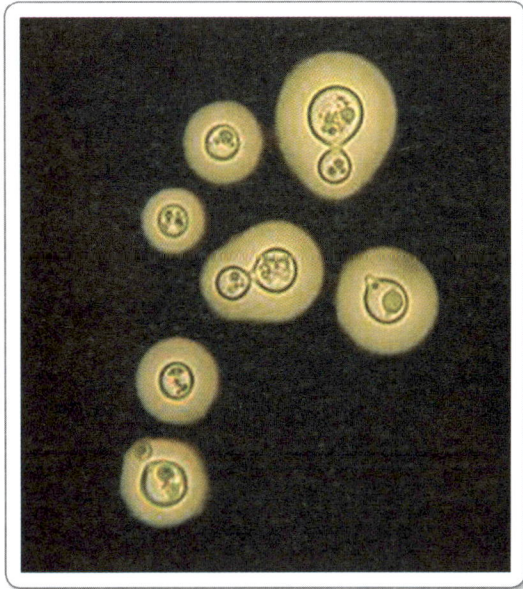

Fig. 40.14: An India ink wet mount of *Cryptococcus neoformans* showing encapsulated budding yeast cells (× 400).

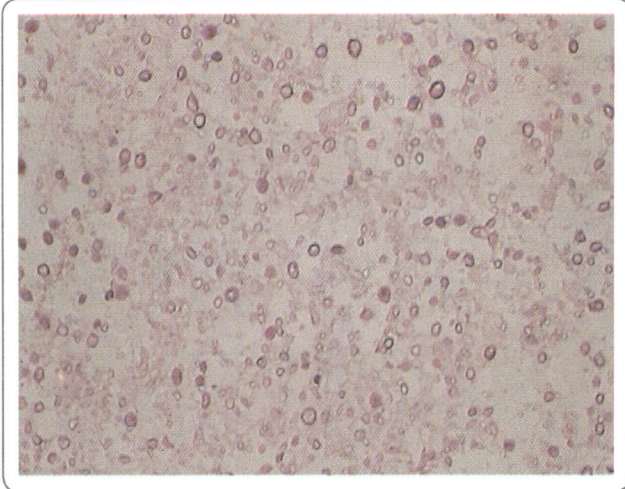

Fig. 40.15: Cryptococci stained with Mayer's mucicarmine stain. The capsule is stained red in colour (× 400).

- Produce disease in mice on intracerebral and intraperitoneal inoculation.

Cryptococcal capsular polysaccharide antigen can be detected in serum and CSF by latex agglutination and ELISA test.

ASPERGILLOSIS

There are 339 species of *Aspergillus*, however, approximately 20 species have been implicated in human disease (aspergillosis), which is worldwide in occurrence. Of these *A. fumigatus* is most important. Other important pathogens in this group are *A. niger*,

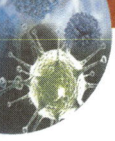

A. flavus, *A. terreus* and *A. nidulans*. Aspergilli are ubiquitous in nature. Aspergillosis is caused by inhalation of *Aspergillus* conidia or mycelial fragments which are present on vegetation (especially nuts and grains), decaying matter, soil and air. A high degree of natural resistance exists in healthy host, but when the host defence is compromised, as in AIDS and in patients on immunosuppressive therapy, aspergillosis may develop. It may cause:

- *Allergic bronchopulmonary aspergillosis*
- *Intracavitary aspergilloma (fungus ball)*
- *Invasive aspergillosis*
- *Endocarditis*
- *Paranasal granuloma.*

Diagnosis may be made by microscopic examination and by culture. Ten per cent KOH preparation of sputum, broncho-alveolar lavage, transbronchial biopsy and other biopsies reveal non-pigmented septate hyphae, 3–5 μm in diameter with characteristic dichotomous branching. The hyphae have a tendency to branch repeatedly. The branches arise at an angle of approximately 45 degrees (Fig. 40.16). In a majority of pulmonary and disseminated lesions, only hyphal forms are seen. Histological sections can be stained with H&E and GMS and examined for characteristic hyphae (Fig. 40.17).

For species identification, the clinical material is inoculated on SDA without cycloheximide and incubated at 25°C. Colonies appear after incubation for 1–2 days. The isolate is identified on the basis of growth characteristics and microscopic morphology. Lactophenol cotton blue mount shows branching and septate hyphae. From the latter arise conidiophores, the ends of which are expanded to form vesicles. The vesicle bears phialides which arise directly from the vesicle (uniseriate) or from sterile cells called metulae (biseriate).

Aspergillus Fumigatus

The colonies of *A. fumigatus* are granular to cottony and usually have some shades of green, green-grey or green-brown pigmentation. Microscopically, the conidiophores are short (usually less than 300 μm long) and 5–10 μm in diameter. Vesicles

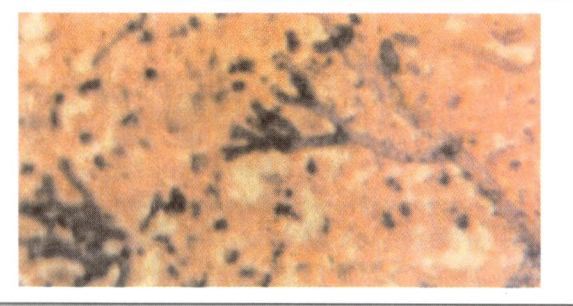

Fig. 40.16: *Aspergillus* showing septate hyphae with characteristic dichotomous branching (H & E stain, × 400).

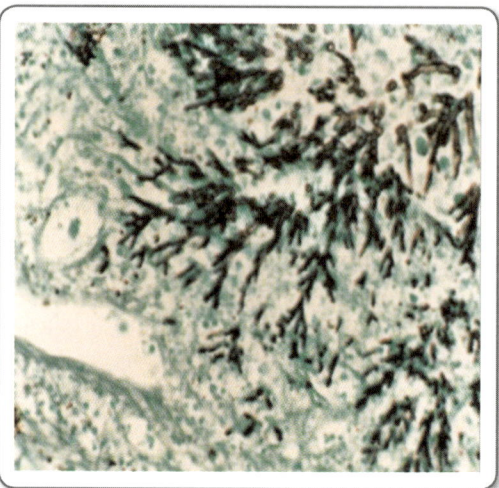

Fig. 40.17. Section stained by Gomori's methanamine silver stain. The hyphae of *Aspergillus* are stained black in colour (× 400).

are 20–30 μm in diameter. The phialides are uniseriate, compact, forming only on the upper two thirds of the vesicle, parallel to the axis of the conidiophore. Conidia are round, smooth, or slightly rough and 2–3.5 μm in diameter (Fig. 41.18A).

Aspergillus Flavus

The colonies of *A. flavus* are granular to woolly and have some shade of yellow or yellow-brown. Microscopically, the conidiophores are long (400–800 μm), the vesicles are 25–45 μm in diameter. The phialides may arise directly from three fourth or the entire circumference of the vesicle (uniseriate) or from sterile cells called metulae (biseriate). Conidia are spherical, smooth, or slightly roughened with maturity and form long chains (Fig. 40.18B).

Aspergillus Niger

The surface of the colonies of *A. niger* is covered by a dense aggregate of jet black conidia. The underside of the colony is buff or yellow-grey, distinguishing *A. niger* from the dematiaceous fungi. Microscopically, the conidiophores are long 400–3000 × 12–17 μm. The vesicles are globose and measure 30–75 μm in diameter. Phialides arise from metulae (biseriate) from the entire circumference of the vesicle. Conidiation is extremely profuse, to the extent that the vesicles are obscured by dense aggregates of 3–5 μm diameter, spherical, black conidia that become roughened with maturity (Fig. 40.18C).

Aspergillus Terreus

The colonies of *A. terreus* are cinnamon buff, brown or orange-brown. Radial folds emanating from the centre of the colony are often observed. Microscopically, the vesicles are relatively small (10–20 μm in diameter) flask-shaped or hemispherical. Phialides arise

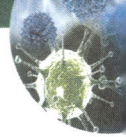

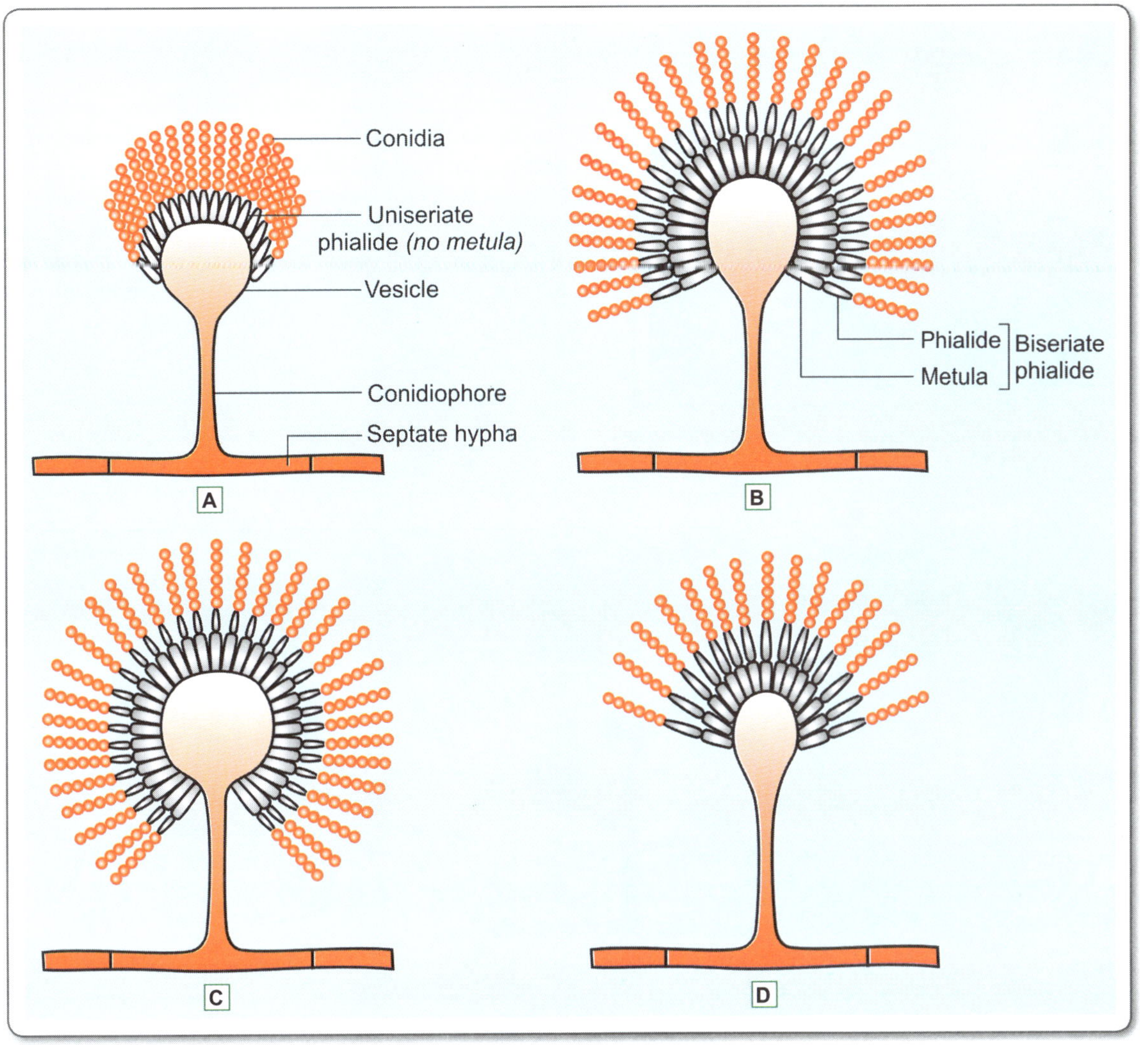

Fig. 40.18: *Aspergillus* spp.: (A) *A. fumigatus*, (B) *A. flavus*, (C) *A. niger*, and (D) *A. terreus*.

from metulae (biseriate) on the upper half only. Conidia are smooth, elliptical, measure 2–2.5 µm in diameter (Fig. 40.18D).

Aspergillus Nidulans

A. nidulans may rarely be recovered from cases of human infections. Phialides arise from metulae (biseriate) on their upper half surface. *A nidulans* may form sexually derived ascospores contained within sac-like structures called cleistothecia.

MUCORMYCOSIS

Mucormycosis is an opportunistic infection caused by saprophytic fungi, notably species of *Mucor*, *Rhizopus* and Lichtheimia (*Absidia*) of the family Mucoraceae, order Mucorales. These fungi are common saprophytes of soil, manure and decaying vegetables, and fruits. These are essentially opportunistic fungi.

The major predisposing factors to mucormycosis are acute diabetes mellitus, metabolic acidosis, debilitating diseases such as leukaemia or lymphoma, immunosuppression, starvation, and widespread use of broad spectrum antibiotics, steroids and antimetabolites. Mucormycosis may lead to:

- *Rhinocerebral mucormycosis*
- *Pulmonary mucormycosis*
- *Gastrointestinal mucormycosis*
- *Disseminated mucormycosis*
- *Dermal mucormycosis*
- *Subcutaneous mucormycosis*

The characteristic pathological changes in mucormycosis are suppuration and necrosis. Invasion of thrombosed blood vessels by the fungus is a conspicuous feature. In tissues (Fig. 40.19), the organisms appear as irregularly branched, non-septate, very broad hyphae (7–15 µm in diameter) which characteristically are deeply stained with routine H&E stain.

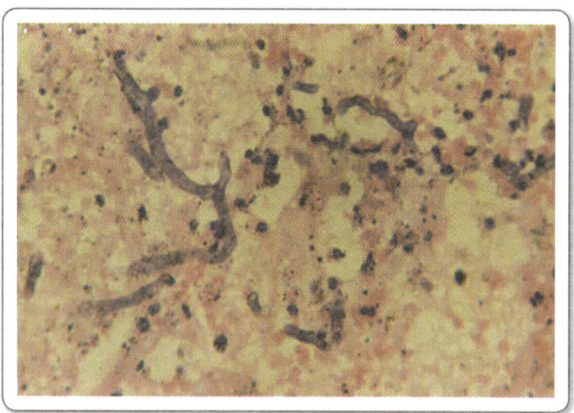

Fig. 40.19: Mucormycosis showing broad non-septate hyphae (H&E stain, × 400).

Diagnosis can be made by examination of KOH wet mounts of scrapings from the lesions, pus, sputum and nasal discharge. It shows characteristic hyphae. The fungi can be readily seen by histological sections stained with routine H&E stain. Fungi can be readily isolated on SDA at 37°C. *Rhizopus* has rhizoids and sporangiophores that arise in groups directly above the rhizoids. *Mucor* does not possess rhizoids and shows branched sporangiophores arising randomly along aerial mycelium. *Lichtheimia* has rhizoids and sporangiophores that arise from the aerial mycelium in between the rhizoids (Fig. 40.20).

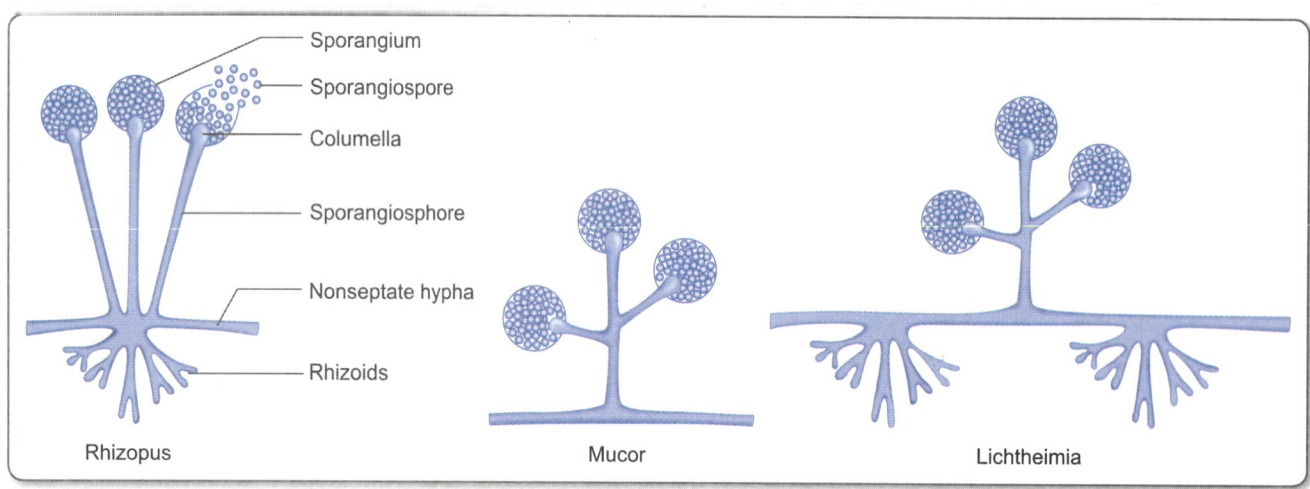

Fig. 40.20: Rhizopus, Mucor and Lichtheimia.

🔖 Key Points

- *Fungi* constitute a large, diverse group of heterotrophic organisms, most of which are found as **saprophytes in the soil and on decaying plant material**.
- *Fungi* can be classified into **yeasts, yeast-like, molds** and **dimorphic fungi**.
- *Mycoses* can be classified into **superficial, subcutaneous, systemic** and **opportunistic**.
- **Dermatophytosis** is caused by 41 species of dermatophytes which belong to three genera (*Trichophyton*-24, *Microsporum*-16 and *Epidermophyton*-1).
- **Sporotrichosis** is caused by *Sporothrix schenckii*, a saprophyte in nature.
- *Histoplasma capsulatum* is found in **soil enriched with the droppings of birds and bats**, and infection results from the **inhalation of infectious propagules**.
- *Candidiasis* is the commonest mycosis involving **skin and its appendages, mucosa**, and **internal organs**.
- *Cryptococcosis* is most frequently recognized as disease of the **CNS**, although the primary site of infection is the **lungs**.
- There are **339 species of** *Aspergillus* however, approximately 20 species have been implicated in human disease. The most important are *Aspergillus fumigatus, A. niger, A. flavus, A. terreus* and *A. nidulans*.
- **Mucormycosis** is an **opportunistic infection** caused by **saprophytic fungi** notably species of *Rhizopus, Mucor* and *Lichtheimia*.

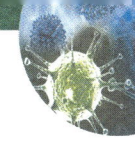

? ASSESS YOURSELF

LONG AND SHORT ANSWER QUESTIONS

1. Discuss the morphology, cultural characters and pathogenicity of dermatophytes.
2. Write short notes on:
   (a) Classification of fungi
   (b) Sporotrichosis
   (c) Histoplasmosis
   (d) Coccidioidomycosis
   (e) Candidiasis
   (f) Cryptococcosis
   (g) Mucormycosis

MULTIPLE CHOICE QUESTIONS

1. Which of the following fungi is not a mold?
   (a) *Aspergillus*
   (b) *Penicillium*
   (c) *Mucor*
   (d) *Candida*
2. Asteroid bodies may be seen in:
   (a) sporotrichosis
   (b) Rhinosporidiosis
   (c) Chromoblastomycosis
   (d) Mycetoma
3. Histoplasmosis is acquired from:
   (a) Soil
   (b) Animals
   (c) Man
   (d) Water
4. Which of the following fungi is/are responsible for mucormycosis?
   (a) Mucor
   (b) Rhizopus
   (c) Lichtheimia
   (d) All of the above

ANSWERS TO MCQs

1. d   2. a   3. a   4. d

NOTES

Pathogenic Organisms-IV
Parasites and Medically Important Arthropods

Chapter **41**

Commonly Seen Protozoans and Helminths

Parasitology is the area of biology concerned with the phenomenon of dependance of one living organism on another. Medical parasitology deals with the parasites which infect man, the diseases they produce, the response generated by him against them, and various methods of diagnosis, prevention and treatment.

- **Parasite:** It is defined as an animal or plant which lives in or upon another organism and derives its nutrient directly from it.
- **Host:** It is defined as an organism which harbours the parasite and provides the nourishment and shelter to the latter. It is of following types:
    - **Definitive host:** The host which harbours the adult parasite, the most highly developed form of a parasite or where the parasite replicates sexually. When the most highly developed form is not obvious, the definitive host is the mammalian host.
    - **Intermediate host:** This is the host which alternates with the definitive host and harbours the larval or asexual stages of a parasite. Some parasites require two intermediate hosts for completion of their life cycle.
    - **Reservoir host:** It is the host that harbours the parasite and serves as an important source of infection to other susceptible hosts.
    - **Vector:** It is the insect host which transmits parasites to man and animals.

Host-parasite relationships

Host-parasite relationship is of following types:
- **Symbiosis:** An association in which both host and parasite are so dependent upon each other that one cannot live without the help of the other. Neither of the partners suffers from any harm from this association.
- **Commensalism:** An association in which only parasite derives benefit without causing any injury to the host. A commensal lives on food residues or waste products of the body and is capable of leading an independent life.
- **Parasitism:** An association in which the parasite derives benefit and host gets nothing in return and always suffers from some injury. The parasite is so adapted to this association that it cannot live an independent life.

CLASSIFICATION OF PARASITES

Parasites are classified into protozoa (unicellular organisms) and helminths (multicellular organisms).

Protozoa

Principal protozoan pathogens of man are given in Table 41.1.

ENTAMOEBA HISTOLYTICA

This is the most important amoebic parasite of humans. It is worldwide but more common in tropical and subtropical countries. In India, the problem of amoebiasis is widespread and the disease is prevalent in all parts of the country. It resides in mucosa and submucosa of large intestine of man.

TABLE 41.1: Principal protozoan pathogens of man

Group	Species
Amoebae	*Entamoeba histolytica* *Acanthamoeba* spp.
Flagellates	*Naeglaria fowleri* *Giardia lamblia* *Trichomonas vaginalis* *Trypanosoma brucei gambiense* *T. brucei rhodesiense* *T. cruzi* *Leishmania* spp.
Sporozoa	*Plasmodium falciparum* *P. vivax* *P. malariae* *P. ovale* *P. knowlesi* *Toxoplasma gondii* *Cryptosporidium parvum* *Cytoisospora belli*
Others	*Balantidium coli* *Babesia microti* *B. divergens* *Pneumocystis jirovecii*

Morphology

The parasite exists in three morphological forms—trophozoite, precyst and cyst (Fig. 41.1).

Trophozoite

It measures 10–60 μm (average 20–30 μm) in diameter. The cytoplasm of the trophozoite can be divided into a clear outer ectoplasm and an inner finely granular endoplasm in which red blood cells, leucocytes and tissue debris are found within the food vacuoles. Trophozoites are motile with active, unidirectional and purposeful motility. Movement results from long finger-like pseudopodial extensions of ectoplasm into which endoplasm flows.

Nucleus

It is spherical in shape varying in size from 4–6 μm in diameter. In stained preparations it shows a central dot-like karyosome which is surrounded by a clear halo. The nuclear membrane is delicate and is lined by a single layer of fine chromatin granules. The space between the karyosome and the nuclear membrane is traversed by linin network (achromatic fibrils) having spoke-like radial arrangement.

Precyst

It is smaller in size, varying from 10–20 μm in diameter. It is oval with a blunt pseudopodium projecting from the periphery.

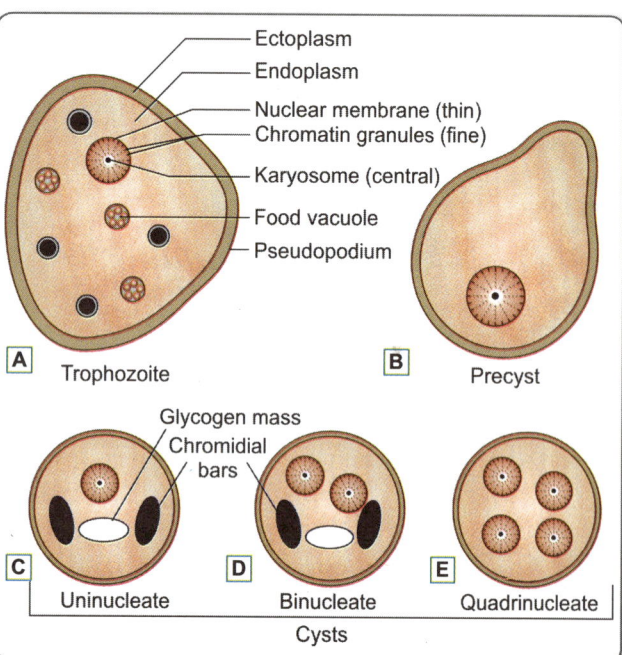

Fig. 41.1: Various morphological forms of *Entamoeba histolytica*. (A) Trophozoite, (B) Precystic stage, (C) Uninucleate cyst, (D) Binucleate cyst, E. Mature quadrinucleate cyst.

Food vacuoles disappear. There is no change in the nucleus which shows characteristics of that of the trophozoite.

Cyst

It is spherical, 10–15 μm in diameter. It is surrounded by a thick chitinous wall which makes it highly resistant to the gastric acid, adverse environmental conditions and the chlorine concentration found in potable water. It starts as a uninucleate body, but later the nucleus divides to form two and then four nuclei. Uninucleate and binucleate cysts in addition also possess a glycogen mass, which stains brown with iodine, and 1–4 chromidial or chromatoid bars. These do not stain with iodine but appear as refractile oblong bars with rounded ends in normal saline preparations. With iron-haematoxylin stain they stain black in colour.

Life Cycle

It passes its life cycle in only one host (Fig. 41.2). Man acquires the infection by ingestion of water or food contaminated with mature quadrinucleate cysts. In the small intestine the cyst wall is lysed by trypsin and a single tetranucleate amoeba (**metacyst**) is liberated. Each nucleus divides by binary fission giving rise to eight nuclei. Almost immediately the cytoplasm becomes separated into as many parts as there are nuclei, thus from each mature cyst eight small **metacystic trophozoites** are produced. This process is known as **excystation**. Metacystic trophozoites are carried in the faecal stream into the caecum. They invade the mucosa and ultimately lodge in the submucous tissue of large intestine. Here they grow and multiply by binary fission.

During growth, *E. histolytica* secretes a proteolytic enzyme of the nature of histolysin which brings about destruction and necrosis of tissue and produces flask-shaped ulcers (Fig. 41.3). The amoebae are mostly present at the periphery of the lesion. At this stage, a large number of trophozoites are excreted along with blood and mucus in the stool leading to amoebic dysentery. In a few cases, erosion of the large intestine may be so extensive that trophozoites gain entrance into the radicals of portal vein and are carried away to the liver where they multiply leading to amoebic hepatitis and amoebic liver abscess.

After some time, when the effect of the parasite on the host is toned down and patient has developed resistance, the lesions start healing and patient starts passing normal (formed) stools. The trophozoites, in the lumen of the large intestine, discharge undigested food particles and transform into precysts and then into mature quadrinucleate cysts. These are the infective stages of the parasite. This process is known as **encystation**. Cyst formation occurs only within the intestinal tract; once the stool has left the body, cyst formation does not occur.

Pathogenicity

E. histolytica causes intestinal and extraintestinal amoebiasis.

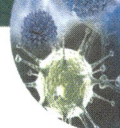

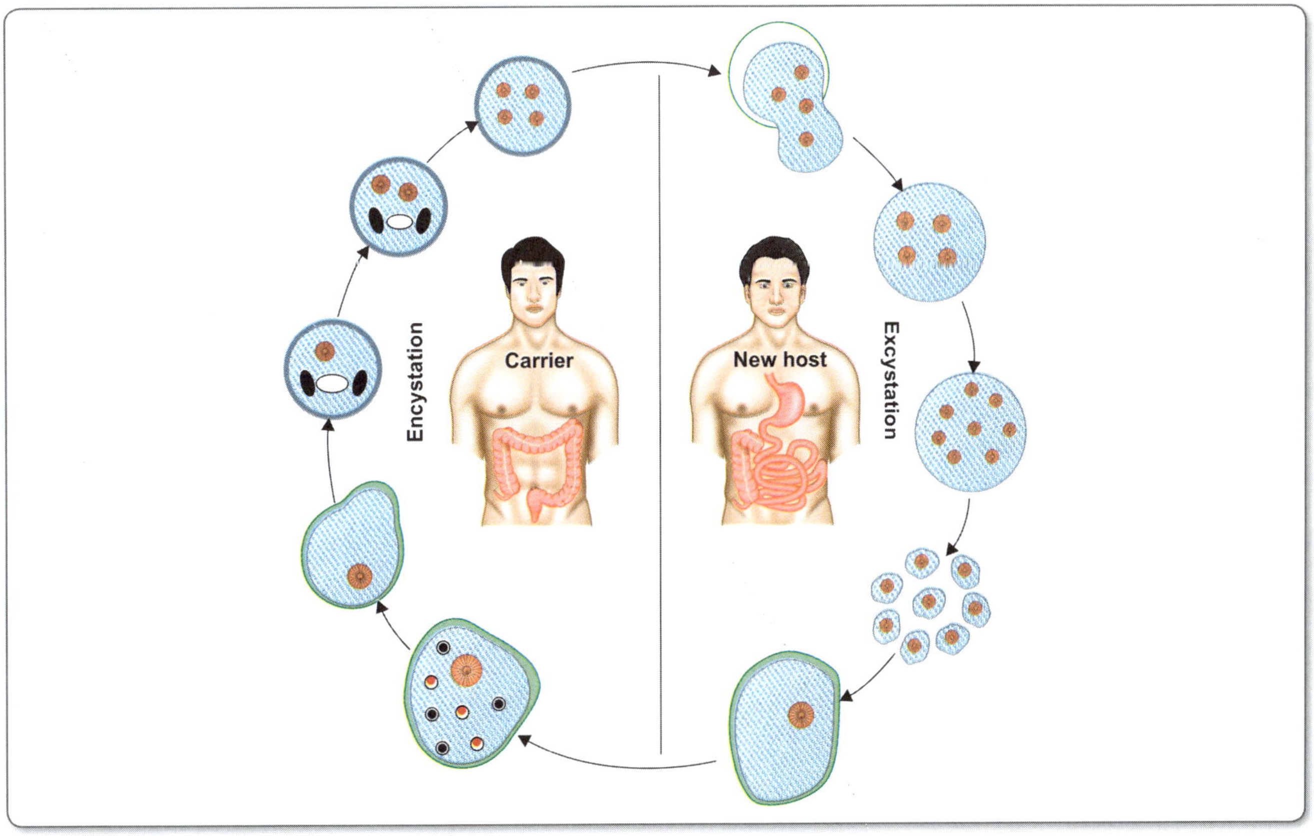

Fig. 41.2: Life cycle of *Entamoeba histolytica*.

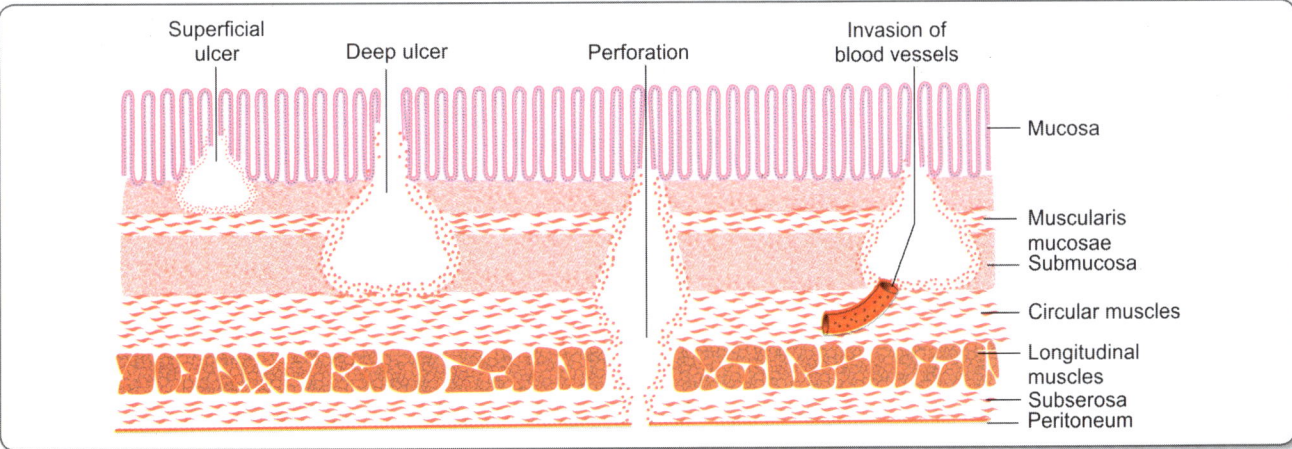

Fig. 41.3: Pathogenesis of intestinal amoebiasis.

Intestinal Amoebiasis

After an incubation period of 1–4 weeks, the amoebae invade the colonic mucosa, producing characteristic ulcerative lesions and a profuse bloody diarrhoea (amoebic dysentery). The ulcers may be generalized involving the whole length of the large intestine or they may be localized in the ileocaecal (caecum, ascending colon,

ileocaecal valve and appendix) or sigmoidorectal (sigmoid colon and rectum) region. Ulcers are discrete with intervening normal mucosa. They vary in size from pin-head size to more than 2.5 cm in diameter. They may be deep or superficial. Base of the deep ulcers is generally formed by muscular coat. However, superficial ulcers do not extend beyond muscularis mucosae (Fig. 41.3).

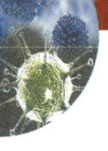

Extraintestinal Amoebiasis

About 5% individuals with intestinal amoebiasis, 1–3 months after the disappearance of the dysenteric attack, develop hepatic amoebiasis. Trophozoites of *E. histolytica* are carried as emboli by the radicles of the portal vein from the base of the amoebic ulcer in the large intestine (Fig. 41.3). The capillary system of the liver acts as an excellent filter and holds these parasites. They multiply in the liver and lead to cytolytic action. The amoebae cause obstruction of the portal venules resulting in anaemic necrosis of hepatic cells. The destruction starts here and continues in concentric layers. Necrosis is followed by cytolysis. Small miliary abscesses coalesce to form big liver abscess.

Amoebic liver abscess varies greatly in size. It has been reported in patients of all ages, but predominate in adults between 20–60 years. It has a marked preference for the right lobe of the liver and it is at least three times more frequent in males than in females. The wall of the abscess cavity is ragged with shreds of connective tissue running across the abscess cavity. A section through the margin of the liver abscess can be differentiated into three zones:

- A necrotic centre filled with thick pus with no amoebae.
- An intermediate zone consisting of degenerated liver cells, a few red blood cells, leucocytes and occasional trophozoites of *E. histolytica*.
- An outer zone of nearly normal hepatic tissue just being invaded by amoebae.

Pus of liver abscess: The centre of an amoebic liver abscess contains a viscous red-brown (anchovy sauce appearance) or grey-yellow fluid consisting of cytolysed liver cells, red blood cells and leucocytes. It is referred to as 'pus' but contains very few pus cells. Since the amoebae actively multiply in the walls of the abscess, the last few drops of pus obtained from the lesion are most likely to yield recognizable trophozoites of the parasite.

From the liver, *E. histolytica* may enter into general circulation involving other organs of the body like lungs, brain, spleen, skin, etc. Both faecal and sigmoidoscopic examinations for the parasite are negative in approximately half of the patients in extraintestinal disease.

Laboratory Diagnosis

Intestinal Amoebiasis

- **Stool examination:** In acute amoebiasis, stool or colonic scrapings from ulcerated areas are examined by macroscopic and microscopic examination. It should be carefully differentiated from bacillary dysentery (Table 41.2). For microscopic examination stool is picked up with a matchstick

TABLE 41.2: Differences between amoebic and bacillary dysentery

Character	Amoebic dysentery	Bacillary dysentery
Macroscopic		
Number	6–8 motions a day	Over 10 motions a day
Amount	Copious	Small
Odour	Offensive	Odourless
Colour	Dark red	Bright red
Reaction	Acidic	Alkaline
Consistency	Not adherent to the container	Adherent to the container
Microscopic		
RBCs	In clumps	Discrete, sometimes in clumps due to rouleaux formation
Pus cells	Few	Numerous
Macrophages	Few	Numerous, many of them contain RBCs hence may be mistaken for *E. histolytica*
Eosinophils	Present	Scarce
Charcot-Leyden crystals	Present	Absent
Pyknotic bodies	Present	Absent
Ghost cells	Absent	Present
Parasites	Trophozoites of *E. histolytica*	Absent
Bacteria	Many motile bacteria	Few or absent

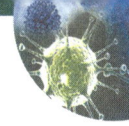

or a platinum loop and emulsified in a drop of normal saline on a clean glass slide. A clean coverslip is placed over it and examined under microscope first under low power and then under high power. This method is specially useful for the demonstration of the actively motile trophozoites of *E. histolytica*.

For the demonstration of cysts or dead trophozoites, stained preparation may be required for the study of the nuclear character. For this purpose iodine stained preparation is commonly employed. Stool is emulsified in a drop of five times diluted solution of Lugol's iodine, covered with a clean coverslip and examined under microscope. Both saline and iodine preparations may be prepared on the same slide. Since excretion of cysts in the stool is often intermittent, at least three consecutive specimens should be examined. **DNA probe** has been used recently to identify *E. histolytica* in the stool specimen and specific sequences can be amplified by **polymerase chain reaction** (PCR).

- **Blood examination:** It shows moderate leucocytosis.
- **Serological tests:** These are negative in early cases. However, in later stages of invasive intestinal amoebiasis antibodies appear and serological tests become positive. These tests include indirect haemagglutination (IHA), indirect fluorescent antibody test (IFA) and enzyme-linked immunosorbent assay (ELISA).

Hepatic Amoebiasis

- **Diagnostic aspiration:** Trophozoites of *E. histolytica* can be demonstrated by microscopy of the pus aspirated by exploratory puncture of amoebic liver abscess. Trophozoites can be demonstrated in the pus in less than 15% cases of amoebic liver abscess (Fig. 41.4).
- **Liver biopsy:** Trophozoites of *E. histolytica* can be demonstrated in the specimens of liver biopsy from cases of amoebic hepatitis or the wall of the liver abscess.
- **Blood examination:** It shows leucocytosis with total leucocyte count of 15,000–30,000/µl, of which 70–75% are polymorphonuclear leucocytes.

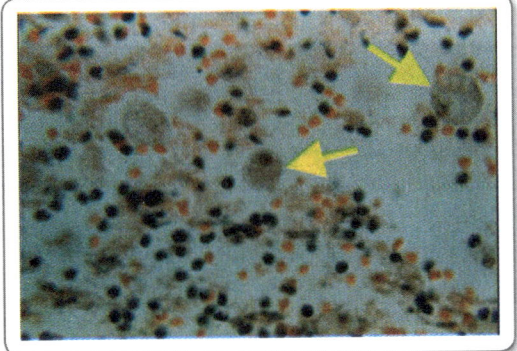

Fig. 41.4: Trophozoites of *Entamoeba histolytica* in liver aspirate.

- **Stool examination:** In about 15% cases of amoebic hepatitis cysts of *E. histolytica* can be demonstrated in the stool. This indicates persistence of intestinal infection.
- **Serological tests:** Serological tests like IHA, IFA and ELISA are of immense value in the diagnosis of hepatic amoebiasis. IHA and IFA tests have been reported positive with titres of ≥ 1 : 256 and ≥ 1 : 200, respectively in almost 100% cases of amoebic liver abscess.
- **Molecular methods:** DNA probes and PCR are molecular methods of promise for the detection of *E. histolytica* in stool and liver aspirates. The sensitivity is estimated at 87%.
- **Histology:** A histological diagnosis of amoebiasis can be made when the trophozoites within the tissue are identified.

ENTAMOEBA COLI

It is a worldwide parasite. It lives freely in the lumen of large intestine of man and is non-pathogenic. Like *E. histolytica* it exists in three stages – trophozoite, precyst and cyst (Table 41.3). Life cycle of *E. coli* is similar to that of *E. histolytica*.

GIARDIA LAMBLIA

Giardia lamblia is worldwide. This lives attached to the mucosal surface of the small intestine, notably in duodenum and upper part of jejunum of man. It exists in two stages – trophozoite and cyst.

Morphology

Trophozoite

It is pear-shaped with rounded anterior and pointed posterior end (Fig. 41.5A and B). It measures 14 µm in length and 7 µm in maximum width. The dorsal surface is convex while on the ventral surface it has a shallow posteriorly notched concavity (sucking disc) that embraces anterior half of the organism. It acts as an organ of attachment. It is bilaterally symmetrical and has one pair of nuclei, one on each side of the midline, one pair of axostyles, one pair of parabasal bodies present on the axostyles and four pairs of flagella and probably four pairs of blepharoblasts from which the flagella arise.

The cytoplasm is finely granular. The nuclei are rounded and possess a central karyosome. The nuclear membrane is delicate and is not lined by chromatin material. By rapid movement of flagella, the trophozoites move from place to place.

Cyst

Mature cyst is oval in shape and measures 12 × 7 µm in size. It has two pairs of nuclei which may remain clustered at one end or lie in pairs at opposite ends. The remains of the flagella and margins of the sucking disc may be seen inside the cytoplasm of the cyst (Figs 41.5C and 41.6).

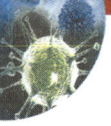

TABLE 41.3: Trophozoites, precysts and cysts of *E. histolytica* and *E. coli*

	E. histolytica	E. coli
Trophozoite		
Size	20–30 μm	20–50 μm
Motility	Active	Sluggish
Cytoplasm	Clearly defined into ectoplasm and endoplasm.	Not defined.
Cytoplasmic inclusions	Red blood cells, leucocytes and tissue debris but no bacteria.	Bacteria and cellular debris but never red blood cells.
Nucleus	Central karyosome, the nuclear membrane is delicate and is lined by fine chromatin granules. It is not visible in unstained preparations.	Eccentric karyosome, the nuclear membrane is thick and is lined by coarse chromatin granules. It is visible in unstained preparations.
Precyst	Oval with a blunt pseudopodium, 10–20 μm in diameter. Nucleus shows characteristics of that of its trophozoite.	20 μm in diameter, resembles in shape with that of *E. histolytica*. Nucleus shows characteristics of that of its trophozoite.
Cyst		
Size	Spherical, 10–15 μm in diameter.	Spherical, 15–20 μm in diameter.
Number of nuclei	1–4	1–8
Chromatoid bars	Rounded	Filamentous

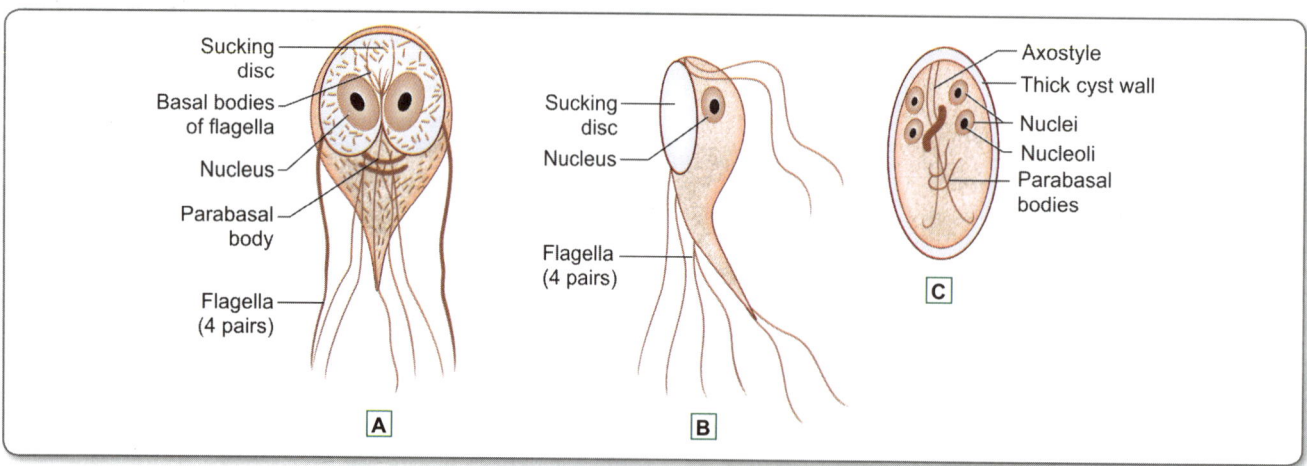

Fig. 41.5: Morphological forms of *Giardia lamblia*. (A) Trophozoite, (B) Lateral view of trophozoite, (C) Cyst.

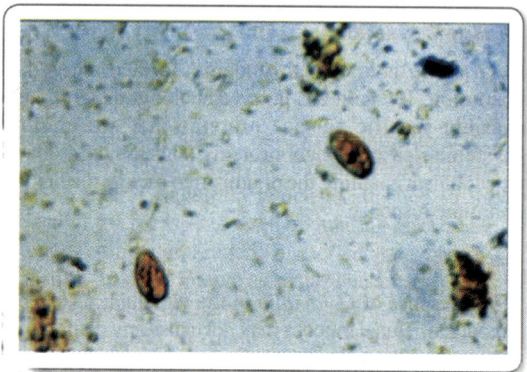

Fig. 41.6: Cysts of *Giardia lamblia* in stool (iodine preparation).

Life Cycle

It passes its life cycle in one host. Mature cyst is the infective form of the parasite. Man acquires infection by ingestion of water and food contaminated with the cysts. Within 30 minutes of ingestion **excystation** occurs in the duodenum. The cyst hatches out two trophozoites, which then multiply to form enormous numbers and colonize in the duodenum and upper part of jejunum. To avoid acidity of duodenum, it may localize in biliary tract.

By means of the concavity on its ventral surface the trophozoite attaches to the mucosal surface of the duodenum and jejunum. In frankly diarrhoeic stools, it is usual to find only the trophozoites. **Encystation** occurs commonly in transit down the colon where the intestinal contents lose moisture and patient starts passing formed stools. The trophozoites retract their flagella and secrete a thin, tough and hyaline cyst wall. As cyst matures, the internal structures are doubled, so that when excystation occurs, the cytoplasm divides, thus producing two trophozoites.

Pathogenicity

The presence of *G. lamblia* in the glandular crypts of duodenal-jejunal mucosa ordinarily causes no irritation. These flagellates do not invade the tissues, but feed on mucous secretions. With the help of sucking disc the parasite attaches itself to the surface of the epithelial cells in the duodenum and jejunum and may cause duodenal and jejunal irritation leading to duodenitis and jejunitis. Patient may complain of dull epigastric pain, flatulence and chronic diarrhoea of steatorrhoea type. The stool is voluminous, foul smelling and contains large amount of mucus and fat but no blood. This is due to malabsorption since the parasites are coated on the mucosa, thus absorption suffers. Patient loses weight. When *Giardia* localizes in the biliary tract, it may lead to chronic cholecystitis and jaundice.

Laboratory Diagnosis

Giardiasis can be diagnosed by identification of cysts of *G. lamblia* (Fig. 41.6) in the formed stools, the trophozoites of the parasite in diarrhoeal stools and bile aspirated from duodenum by intubation by normal saline and iodine preparation as in case of *E. histolytica*.

TRICHOMONAS

Genus *Trichomonas* contains three species which occur in humans – *T. tenax*, *T. hominis* and *T. vaginalis*. These flagellates exist only in trophozoite stage. Cystic stage is absent. They have four anterior flagella and one lateral flagellum which is attached to the surface of the parasite to form undulating membrane. The undulating membrane is supported at the base by a rod-like structure known as costa. The axostyle runs down the middle of the body and ends in the pointed tail-like extremity. A round nucleus is located in the anterior portion.

Trichomonas tenax

It is a pyriform flagellate. It measures 5–12 µm in length and 5–10 µm in width (Fig. 41.7). **It is a harmless commensal of the human mouth**, living in the tartar around the teeth, in cavities of carious teeth, in necrotic mucosal cells in the gingival margins of gums and in pus pockets in tonsillar follicles. It is transmitted by kissing, salivary droplets and fomites.

Diagnosis can be made by demonstration of *T. tenax* in the tartar by microscopy. Better oral hygiene will rapidly eliminate the infection.

Trichomonas hominis

It is pyriform, measuring 5–14 µm in length and 7–10 µm in width (Fig. 41.7). **It inhabits the caecum of man and several other primate species** and feeds on enteric bacteria. It does not invade the intestinal mucosa. Though it has been occasionally found in the diarrhoeic stools, its pathogenicity is yet to be established.

Trichomonas vaginalis

Morphologically, it resembles *T. tenax* but it is larger than this. It measures 7–23 µm in length and 5–15 µm in width (Figs 41.7 and 41.8). In a wet mount the trophozoite has a characteristic jerky motility. **The normal habitat of the parasite is the vagina and urethra of women and the urethra, seminal vesicles and prostate of man**. It may also be found in the Bartholin's glands and urinary bladder in female.

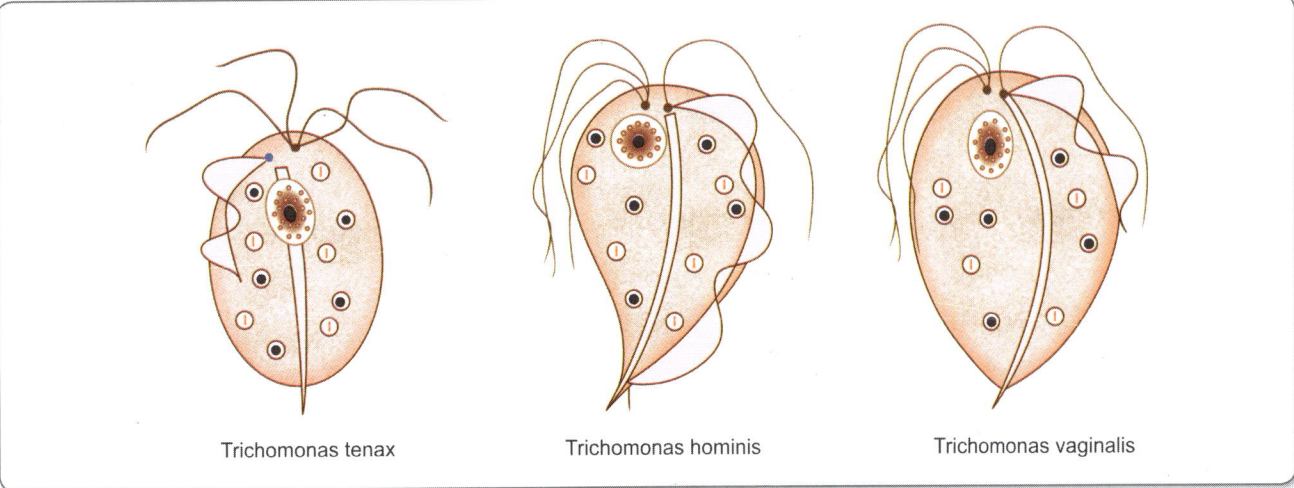

Trichomonas tenax   Trichomonas hominis   Trichomonas vaginalis

Fig. 41.7: Trophozoites of *Trichomonas* spp.

SECTION VII • PATHOGENIC ORGANISMS-IV PARASITES AND MEDICALLY IMPORTANT ARTHROPODS

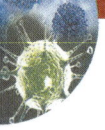
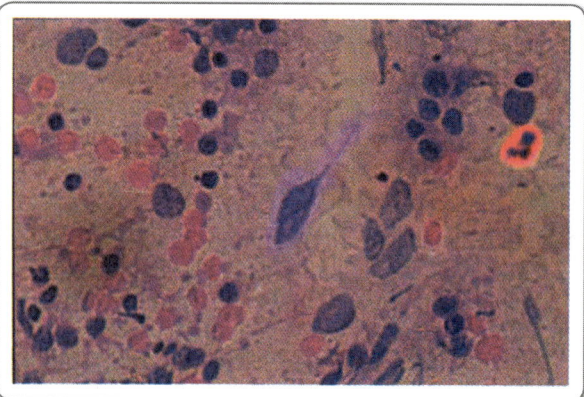

Fig. 41.8: Trophozoites of *Trichomonas vaginalis* in vaginal smear (Papanicolaou stain × 400).

Pathogenicity

The parasite lives on the mucosa feeding on bacteria and leucocytes. *T. vaginalis* is an **obligate parasite**. It cannot live without close association with the vaginal, urethral or prostatic tissues.

The organism is responsible for a **mild vaginitis** with discharge. Vaginal discharge contains a large number of parasites and leucocytes and is liquid, greenish or yellow. It covers the mucosa down to the urethral orifice, vestibular glands and clitoris. Male patients usually have mild or asymptomatic infections. They may develop itching and discomfort inside penile urethra, especially during urination. The parasite is transmitted by sexual intercourse.

Laboratory Diagnosis

The diagnosis can be made by demonstration of trophozoites of *T. vaginalis* in wet mounts of the sedimented urine, vaginal secretions or vaginal scrapings. In males it may be found in urine or prostatic secretions. Fixed smears may be stained with Papanicolaou stain and seen under microscope (Fig. 41.8).

PLASMODIUM

Genus *Plasmodium* has five species – *P. vivax*, *P. falciparum*, *P. malariae*, *P. ovale*, and *P. knowlesi*, a species of monkeys can also infect humans. They cause the most important life-threatening protozoan disease called malaria.

Life Cycle

Malaria parasites exhibit a complex life cycle (Figs 41.9 and 41.10) involving alternating cycles of asexual division (schizogony) occurring in man (intermediate host) and sexual development (sporogony) occurring in female *Anopheles* mosquito (definitive host). Therefore, **malaria parasites exhibit alternation of generations and alternation of hosts**.

Human Cycle

The sporozoites are the infective form of the parasite. They are present in the salivary glands of female *Anopheles* mosquito. It usually bites at night. Man gets infection by the bite of infected mosquito. During the act of biting, the proboscis of the mosquito pierces the skin and saliva containing sporozoites is injected directly into the blood stream. The cycle in man comprises of following stages:

- Pre-erythrocytic schizogony
- Erythrocytic schizogony
- Gametogony
- Exo-erythrocytic or dormant schizogony

Pre-erythrocytic schizogony

Within one hour all the **sporozoites** leave the blood stream and enter into liver parenchyma cells. The sporozoites which are elongated, spindle-shaped bodies become rounded inside the liver cells. They undergo a process of multiple nuclear division, followed by cytoplasmic division and develop into **schizont**. In different species it varies in size from 24–60 μm in diameter and contains 2,000–50,000 merozoites. Primary exoerythrocytic schizogony consists of only one generation. The duration of this cycle of *P. falciparum*, *P. vivax*, *P. ovale* and *P. malariae* is 6, 8, 9 and 13–16 days, respectively. When primary exoerythrocytic schizogony is complete, the liver cell ruptures and releases merozoites into blood stream.

Erythrocytic schizogony

The **merozoites** liberated from pre-erythrocytic schizogony penetrate red blood cells where they multiply at the expense of the host cells. Here they pass through the stages of trophozoites, schizonts and merozoites (Table 41.4 and Figs 41.9 to 41.12). Depending on the species about 6–24 nuclei are produced before cytoplasmic division occurs, and the red cell ruptures to release the individual merozoites, which then infect fresh red blood cells.

The parasitic multiplication during the erythrocytic phase is responsible for bringing on a clinical attack of malaria. Erythrocytic schizogony may be continued for a considerable period, but in the course of time the infection tends to die out. *P. falciparum* differs from the other forms of malaria parasites in that developing erythrocytic schizonts aggregate in the capillaries of the brain and other internal organs, so that only young ring forms are found in peripheral blood.

Gametogony

After malaria parasites have undergone erythrocytic schizogony for certain period, some merozoites develop within red cells into male and female gametocytes known as **microgametocytes** and **macrogametocytes**, respectively (Figs 41.9, 41.10 and 41.12). They develop in the red blood cells of the capillaries of internal organs like spleen and bone marrow. Only mature gametocytes

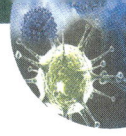

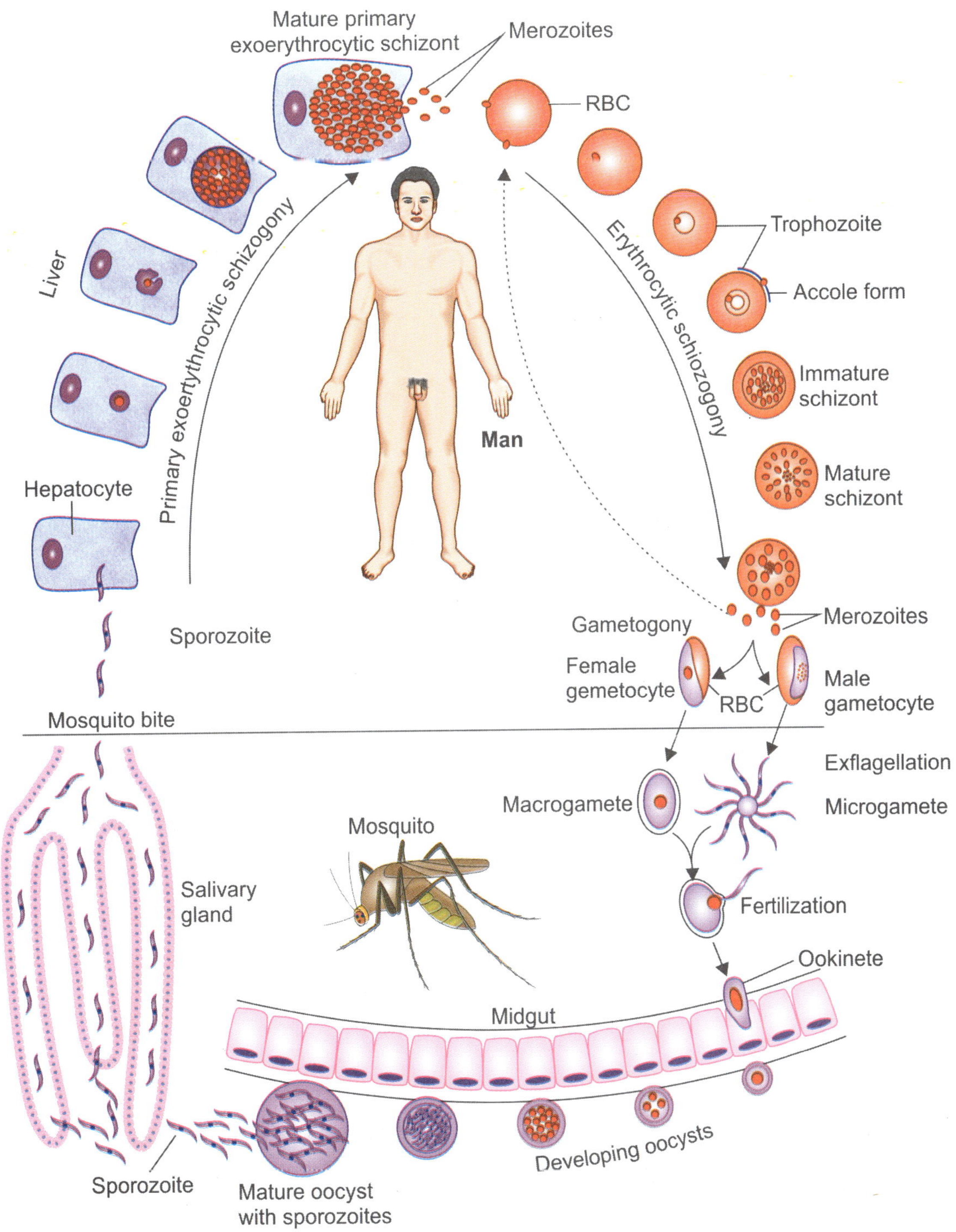

Mature primary exoerythrocytic schizont

Merozoites

RBC

Liver

Trophozoite

Accole form

Immature schizont

Mature schizont

Primary exoerythrocytic schizogony

Erythrocytic schiozogony

Hepatocyte

Man

Sporozoite

Merozoites

Gametogony

Female gametocyte

RBC

Male gametocyte

Mosquito bite

Exflagellation

Microgamete

Salivary gland

Mosquito

Macrogamete

Fertilization

Ookinete

Midgut

Developing oocysts

Sporozoite

Mature oocyst with sporozoites

Fig. 41.9: Life cycle of malaria parasite.

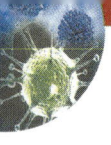

Plasmodium vivax

Early trophozoite
(Ring stage)

Late trophozoite with
Schüffner's dots

Amoeboid form with
Schüffner's dots

Early schizont

Maturing schizont

Mature schizont

Male gametocyte

Female gametocyte

Plasmodium falciparum

Early trophozoite
(Ring stage)

Multiple infections
with accolé form

Ring with Maurer's dots

Early schizont

Maturing schizont

Mature schizont

Male gametocyte

Female gametocyte

Plasmodium malariae

Early trophozoite
(Ring stage)

Band form

Band form

Early schizont

Maturing schizont

Mature schizont

Male gametocyte

Female gametocyte

Plasmodium ovale

Early trophozoite (Ring stage)
with James's dots

Early trophozoite
(enlarged RBC)

Slightly amoeboid

Early schizont

Maturing schizont

Mature schizont

Male gametocyte

Female gametocyte

Fig. 41.10: Morphological forms of malaria parasites.

TABLE 41.4: Differential characters of erythrocytic phase of plasmodia of man

	P. vivax	*P. falciparum*	*P. malariae*	*P. ovale*
1. Forms in peripheral blood	Trophozoites, schizonts and gametocytes.	Rings and crescents (gametocytes).	Trophozoites, schizonts and gametocytes.	Trophozoites, schizonts and gametocytes.
2. Early trophozoite or ring stage	Large, 2.5 μm in diameter, usually one prominent chromatin dot, sometimes two, cytoplasm opposite the chromatin dot thicker, usually one and occasionally two rings in one red blood cell.	Small, delicate, 1.25– 1.5 μm in diameter, often with two chromatin dots, two rings in one red blood cell common. Some parasites lie along the red cell membrane. These are known as accolé forms.	Similar to that of *P. vivax.*	Similar to that of *P. vivax.*
3. Late trophozoite	Large, markedly amoeboid, prominent vacuole.	Medium-sized, compact and rounded.	Small, compact, band-shaped, slightly amoeboid, vacuole disappears early.	Slightly amoeboid.
4. Schizont	Large, 9–10 μm in diameter, almost fills an enlarged red cell.	Small, 4.5–5.0 μm in diameter, fills two-thirds of normal-sized red blood cell which is not enlarged.	Small, 6.5–7.0 μm in diameter, almost fills a normal-sized red blood cell.	Small 6.2 μm in diameter, fills about three quarters of slightly enlarged red blood cell.
5. Number of merozoites	12–24	14–32	6–12	8–12
6. Microgametocytes	Spherical, 9–10 μm in diameter, compact, no vacuole, diffuse chromatin, cytoplasm stains light blue or reddish.	Crescent-shaped (banana-shaped), 8–10 μm × 2–3 μm, chromatin diffuse.	Similar to that of *P. vivax* but smaller.	Similar to that of *P. vivax* but smaller.
7. Macrogametocytes	Spherical, 10–12 μm in diameter, compact, larger than microgametocyte, compact chromatin, cytoplasm stains dark blue.	Crescent-shaped, longer and more slender, 10–12 μm × 2–3 μm, chromatin compact, cytoplasm stains dark blue.	Similar to that of *P. vivax* but smaller.	Similar to that of *P. vivax* but smaller.
8. Malaria pigment	Yellowish-brown; fine granules	Dark-brown; one or two solid blocks	Dark-brown coarse granules	Dark yellowish-brown, coarser than those of *P. vivax*
9. Age of red blood cells invaded	Young	All ages (young and old)	Old	Young
10. Alterations in infected red cell	Enlarged, pale and the portion of the cytoplasm not occupied by the parasite shows a dotted or stippled appearance, called Schüffner's dots. With Leishman stain they appear as fine pink granules.	Normal size and possesses 6–12 Maurer's dots which stain brick-red with Leishman stain.	Normal size and occasionally show fine stippling (Ziemann's dots) on prolonged staining.	Enlarged, pale James's dots resembling Schüffner's dots appear early and infected cell may be oval.
11. Duration of erythrocytic schizogony	48 hours	36–48 hours	72 hours	48 hours
10. Presence of secondary exoerythrocytic cycle	Yes	No	No	Yes

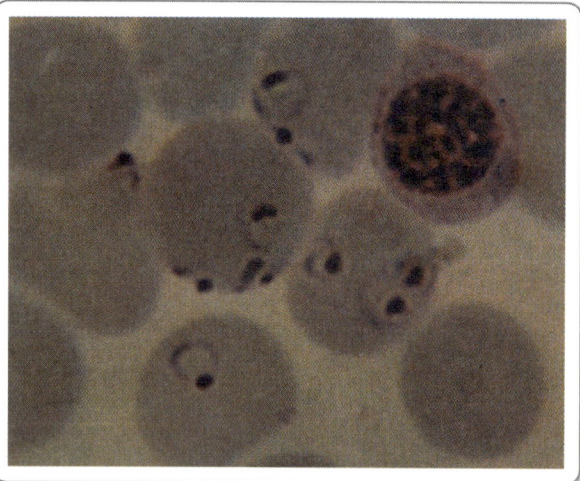

Fig. 41.11: Early trophozoites (ring forms) of *Plasmodium vivax* (Giemsa strain × 1000).

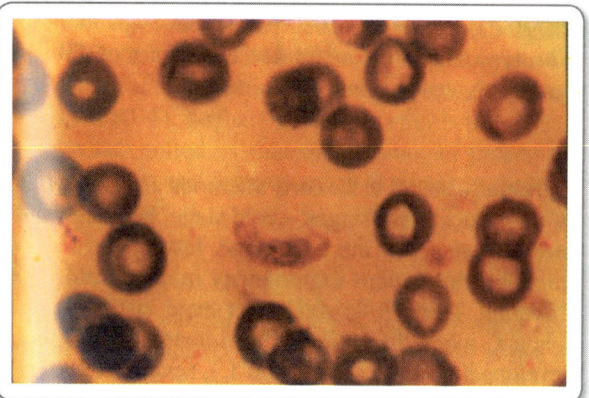

Fig. 41.12: Gametocytes (crescents) of *Plasmodium falciparum* in peripheral blood (Giemsa stain × 1000).

are found in the peripheral blood. They do not cause any febrile condition in human host. These are produced for the propagation and continuance of the species. The host carrying gametocytes is known as **carrier**. The microgametocytes of all the species of *Plasmodium* are smaller in size, cytoplasm stains light blue and the nucleus (chromatin) is diffuse and large. On the other hand the macrogametocytes are larger, the cytoplasm stains deep blue and the nucleus is compact and small.

Exo-erythrocytic or Dormant Schizogony

In case of *P. vivax* and *P. ovale*, some sporozoites on entering into hepatocytes enter into a resting (dormant) stage before undergoing asexual multiplication while others undergo multiplication without delay. The resting stage of the parasite is rounded, 4–6 μm in diameter, uninucleate and is known as **hypnozoite or sleeping form**. After a period of weeks, months or years (usually up to 2 years) hypnozoites are reactivated to

become schizonts and release merozoites which infect red blood cells producing **relapse** of malaria. Hypnozoites are not formed in case of *P. falciparum* and *P. malariae*, therefore, relapses do not occur in disease caused by these species.

Mosquito (Sexual) Cycle

Sexual cycle actually starts in the human host itself by the formation of gametocytes which are present in the peripheral blood. Both asexual and sexual forms of the parasite are ingested by female *Anopheles* mosquito during its blood meal from the patient. In the mosquito, only the mature sexual forms are capable of further development and rest die.

In the stomach of the mosquito (Fig. 41.9) from one microgametocyte 5–8 thread-like filamentous structures called **microgametes** are formed by the process of exflagellation. The macrogametocyte does not show any exflagellation. It develops into a **macrogamete**, its nucleus shifts to the surface, where a projection is formed. **Fertilization** occurs when a microgamete penetrates this projection. The fertilized macrogamete is known as **zygote**. This occurs in 20 minutes to 2 hours. In next 24 hours, the zygote lengthens and matures into **ookinete**, a motile vermiculate stage. It penetrates the epithelial lining of the stomach of the mosquito and comes to lie between the external border of the epithelial cell and peritrophic membrane.

Here it develops into **oocyst**. It is rounded, 6–12 μm in diameter with a single vesicular nucleus. It increases in size from 6 μm to 60 μm in diameter. Inside this develop sporozoites. The number of sporozoites in each oocyst varies from a few hundreds to a few thousands and number of oocysts in the stomach wall varies from a few to more than a hundred. On about 10th day the oocyst is fully mature, ruptures and releases sporozoites in the body cavity of the mosquito. Through the body fluid the sporozoites are distributed to various organs of the body except the ovaries. They have special predilection for salivary glands and ultimately reach in maximum numbers in the salivary ducts. At this stage the mosquito is capable of transmitting infection to man.

Pathogenicity

Man develops infection by the bite of infected female *Anopheles* mosquito. However, infection may also be transmitted by:

- Transfusion of blood from a patient of malaria. This is known as **transfusion malaria**. Plasmodia can remain viable in refrigerated blood for up to 10 days.
- Transmission of infection to foetus *in utero* through some placental defect. This is known as **congenital malaria**.
- By the use of contaminated syringes particularly in drug addicts.

The above conditions are also known as **trophozoite-induced malaria**. In this condition there is no pre-erythrocytic and exo-erythrocytic schizogony, incubation period is short and there is no relapse.

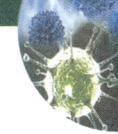

After an incubation period of 12 days for *P. falciparum*, 13–17 days for *P. vivax* and *P. ovale*, and 28–30 days for *P. malariae* patient develops malaria. The typical picture of malaria consists of febrile paroxysm, anaemia and splenomegaly.

The periodicity of the febrile attack varies with the species of the infecting parasite. The periodicity is 48 hours in *P. vivax* (**benign tertian**) and *P. ovale* (**ovale tertian**), and 72 hour in *P. malariae* (**quartan**). However, with *P. falciparum*, the cycles of different broods of parasite do not become synchronized as they do in other species. Therefore, typical tertian fever is not usual in falciparum (**malignant tertian**) malaria. **Quotidian periodicity** with the fever occurring at 24-hour intervals may be due to two broods of tertian parasites maturing on successive days or due to mixed infection.

Pernicious Malaria

Pernicious malaria is a complex of **life-threatening complications** that sometimes supervene in acute falciparum malaria. It is due to heavy parasitization and is of three types:

- *Cerebral malaria:* Cerebral malaria is a severe complication of falciparum malaria and frequently leads to death, even when appropriate therapy has been given. It is characterized by hyperpyrexia, coma and paralysis. Brain is congested. Capillaries of the brain are plugged with parasitized red blood cells, each cell containing malaria pigment.
- *Algid malaria:* It resembles surgical shock with cold clammy skin, peripheral circulatory failure and profound shock. Patient may also develop vomiting and diarrhoea or dysentery.
- *Septicaemic malaria:* It is characterized by a high degree of prostration, there is high continuous fever with involvement of various organs.

Blackwater Fever

It is a manifestation of repeated infections with *P. falciparum* which were inadequately treated with quinine. Sometimes resumption of quinine therapy for new attack is followed by massive destruction of RBCs, fever and haemoglobinuria and renal failure.

The exact mechanism of haemolysis in blackwater fever is not known. An **autoimmune mechanism** has been suggested. Parasitized and quininized red blood cells, during previous infection, act as antigen against which antibodies are formed. With subsequent infection and treatment with quinine, there is massive destruction of both infected and uninfected red blood cells. As other antimalarials have replaced quinine, blackwater fever has now become rare.

Laboratory Diagnosis

Malaria is one of the few parasitic infections considered to be **immediately life-threatening**, and a patient with diagnosis of *P. falciparum* malaria should be considered a medical emergency because the disease can be rapidly fatal.

Microscopy

Diagnosis of malaria can be established by demonstration of malaria parasites in the blood. Thick and thin smears of the blood are prepared on the same or different slides. Blood is taken by pricking a finger or ear lobule before starting treatment with antimalarials. For preparation of thick smear take a large drop of blood on the slide. Spread it in an area of 1 cm square. Dehaemoglobinization of thick smear is done by keeping the slide in distilled water in Koplin's jar in vertical position for 5–10 minutes till the slide becomes white and then it is dried in air. Both thick and thin smears are stained with Leishman stain. The smears are then examined under oil-immersion lens.

The parasites are most abundant in peripheral blood late in the febrile paroxysm (a few hours after the height of paroxysm). Therefore, blood for smear should be collected at this period. All asexual erythrocytic stages, as well as gametocytes can be seen in peripheral blood in infection with *P. vivax*, *P. malariae* and *P. ovale*, but in *P. falciparum* infection, only the ring forms and crescent-shaped gametocytes can be seen. Late trophozoite and schizont stages of *P. falciparum* are usually confined to the internal organs and appear in peripheral blood only in severe or pernicious malaria.

The occurrence of **multiple rings** in an individual red blood cell with **accolé forms** is diagnostic of *P. falciparum* infection. Malaria pigments may be demonstrated inside the monocytes and polymorphonuclear leucocytes. The presence of malaria pigments only, in the absence of malaria parasites, suggests *P. falciparum* infection. Schüner's, Maurer's, Ziemann's and James's dots can be seen in red blood cells infected with *P. vivax, P. falciparum, P. malariae* and *P. ovale* respectively. Red blood cells are enlarged in *P. vivax* infection.

Thin film is examined first and if parasites are found, there is no need for examining the thick film. If parasites are not seen in thin film in a few minutes the thick film should be examined. If parasites are seen in thick film but identity is not clear, the thin film is re-examined more thoroughly to determine the identity of the species. **The parasites are more along the upper and lower margins of the "tail" of the film.** Examination of thin film usually takes 15–20 minutes ($\geq$300 oil-immersion fields), and examination of thick film usually requires 5–10 minutes (at least 100 oil-immersion fields).

Immunodiagnosis

Serological tests which can be carried out for the diagnosis of malaria include indirect immunofluorescence test, indirect haemagglutination and enzyme-linked immunosorbent assay.

DNA probes

These provide rapid, sensitive and specific diagnostic tools for the diagnosis of malaria.

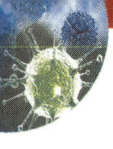

Treatment

Chloroquine was the standard treatment for acute malaria for many years. However, **resistance to this drug in *P. falciparum* is widespread**. Less commonly *P. vivax* may also be chloroquine-resistant. **Quinine is the most reliable alternative to chloroquine** for the treatment of malaria caused by chloroquine-resistant strains. Tetracycline and clindamycin exhibit some antimalarial activity and are used as an adjunct to quinine therapy. **Mefloquine and halofantrine** are also active against chloroquine-resistant strains, but resistance to these drugs has also been reported.

Chloroquine and quinine do not eliminate exoerythrocytic parasites in the liver. For this primaquine (8-aminoquinoline drug) should be used. However, this drug may precipitate haemolysis in individuals who are deficient in the enzyme glucose-6-phosphate dehydrogenase.

PLASMODIUM KNOWLESI

A fifth species, *P. knowlesi*, which normally infects long-tailed macaques (*Macaca fascicularis*) and pig-tailed macaques (*Macaca nemestrina*), is a significant cause of human malaria in Southeast Asia. It is transmitted by *Anopheles leucosphyrus* group of mosquitoes that reside in the upper canopy of the forests and has infrequent contact with humans. Similar to *P. falciparum*, the erythrocyte invasion by *P. knowlesi* is not restricted to young or old RBCs which allows the development of high levels of parasitemia. It has a short life cycle of 24 hours (quotidian), and the development of the parasite in RBCs is not synchronous. *P. knowlesi* infection is usually misidentified as *P. falciparum* or *P. malariae* because its early trophozoites resemble the ring forms of *P. falciparum* and the later stages mimic those of *P. malariae*. In contrast to *P. falciparum*, *P. knowlesi* does not appear to sequester in the microvasculature, and the neurologic complications seen with *P. falciparum* infection have not been described.

RBCs infected with *P. knowlesi* exhibit a normal morphology, and all developmental stages may be seen in peripheral blood.

P. knowlesi, similar to *P. falciparum* and *P. malariae*, does not appear to produce hypnozoites in the liver. Relapses from the liver are not known to occur.

Helminths

Medical helminthology deals with the study of helminths (parasitic worms). Most helminths are truly parasitic because they have no independent existence outside the host. Pathogenic manifestations of helminthic disease are due to the location of the worms, their size and life style. Helminths are divided into two major groups – nematodes or round worms and platyhelminths or flat worms. The latter are further divided into trematodes (flukes) and cestodes (tapeworms). Common helminths of man are given in Table 41.5.

TABLE 41.5: Common helminths of man

Species	Common name
Nematodes	
Enterobius vermicularis	Threadworm
Ascaris lumbricoides	Common roundworm
Ancylostoma duodenale	Old world hookworm
Necator americanus	New world hookworm
Wuchereria bancrofti	Bancroft's filaria
Cestodes	
Enchinococcus granulosus	Dog tapeworm
Taenia solium	Pork tapeworm
Taenia saginata	Beef tapeworm

ENTEROBIUS VERMICULARIS

Enterobius vermicularis (threadworm, pinworm, seatworm) infects children throughout the world. The adult worms live in caecum, vermiform appendix and adjacent portions of ascending colon.

Morphology

Adult Worms

These are small, white, spindle-shaped and resemble short pieces of thread. At the anterior end, both male and female worms possess a pair of wing-like expansions, known as cervical alae. The male measures 2–4 mm in length and 0.1–0.2 mm in breadth. The posterior one-third of the body is curved. The female is longer, 8–12 mm in length and 0.3–0.5 mm in width. Its posterior extremity is straight and drawn out into a thin pointed pin-like tail (Fig. 41.13).

Eggs

The eggs are colourless, non-bile stained and flattened on one side (planoconvex). They measure 60 µm in length and 30 µm in width. They are surrounded by a transparent shell and usually contain fully developed larvae (Figs 41.13 and 41.14). **They float in saturated solution of common salt.**

Life Cycle

Of all the intestinal worms, it has the simplest life cycle (Fig. 41.13). It is completed in a **single host**. The adult worms live in caecum, appendix and adjacent portions of ascending colon. Male fertilizes female and dies, and is excreted in faeces. The gravid female migrates down the colon to the rectum. At night, when the host is in bed, it comes out of the anus. It then crawls on the perianal skin and deposits the eggs. Crawling of the gravid female worm leads to intense pruritis and the patient scratches the affected part.

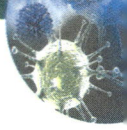

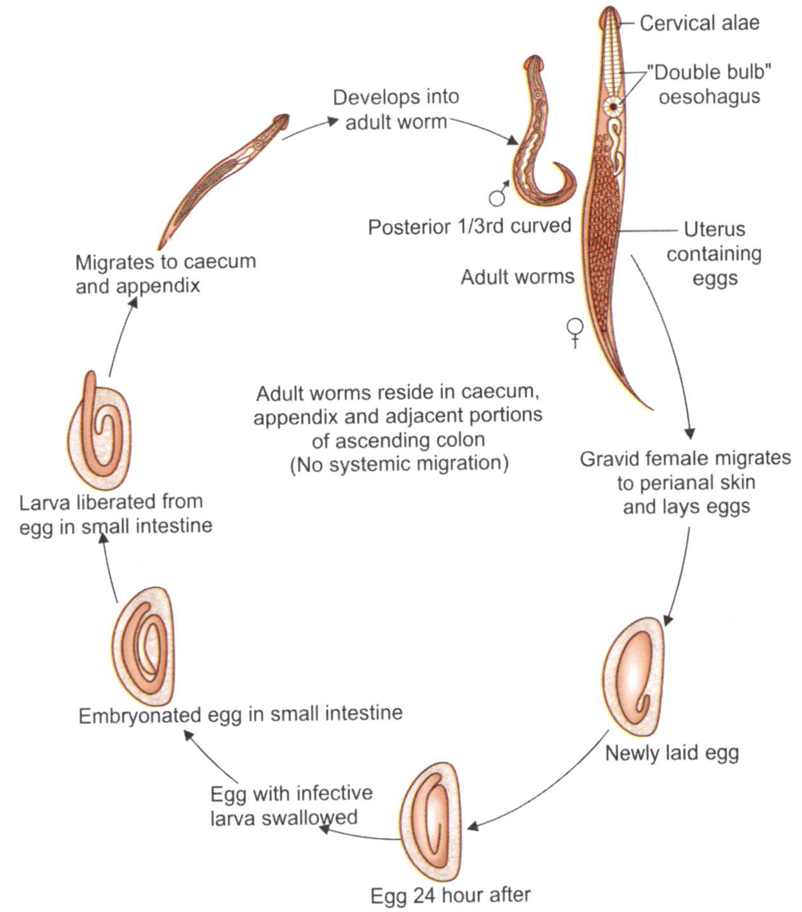

Cervical alae

"Double bulb"
oesophagus

Develops into
adult worm

Uterus
containing
eggs

Posterior 1/3rd curved

Adult worms

Migrates to caecum
and appendix

Adult worms reside in caecum,
appendix and adjacent portions
of ascending colon
(No systemic migration)

Gravid female migrates
to perianal skin
and lays eggs

Larva liberated from
egg in small intestine

Embryonated egg in small intestine

Newly laid egg

Egg with infective
larva swallowed

Egg 24 hour after

Fig. 41.13: Life cycle of *Enterobius vermicularis*.

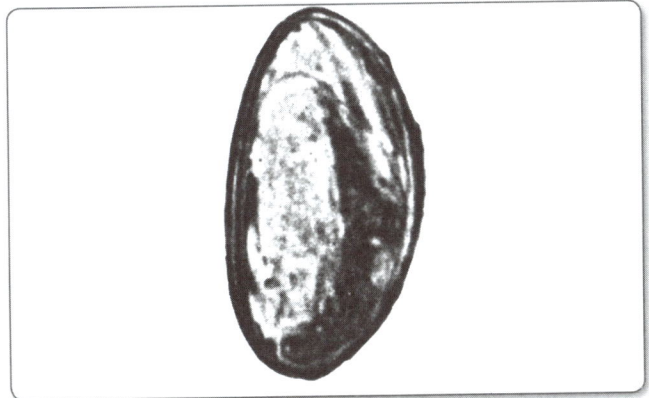

Fig. 41.14: Egg of *Enterobius vermicularis*.

also contract infection. Infection may also be acquired from contaminated objects like door knobs, table tops, etc. Airborne eggs that are dislodged from bed linens and clothes may get into mouth and swallowed.

The larvae, from embryonated eggs, hatch out in the small intestine. They then migrate to the caecum and vermiform appendix and develop into adult worms. Eggs laid on perianal skin may immediately hatch into infective-stage larvae and may ascend through anus to develop into adolescent worms in the caecum and vermiform appendix.

After laying eggs on the perianal skin the worm may retreat into the anal canal and come out again to lay more eggs. The worm may also wander into the vulva, vagina, uterus, fallopian tubes and peritoneum.

Pathogenicity

It causes nocturnal perianal pruritis. It may also lead to appendicitis, vulvovaginitis and salpingitis.

Such patients have eggs of *E. vermicularis* on the fingers and under the nails. These individuals may develop autoinfection by direct anus-to-mouth transfer by finger contamination. Persons handling night clothes and bed linen of infected patients can

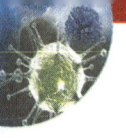

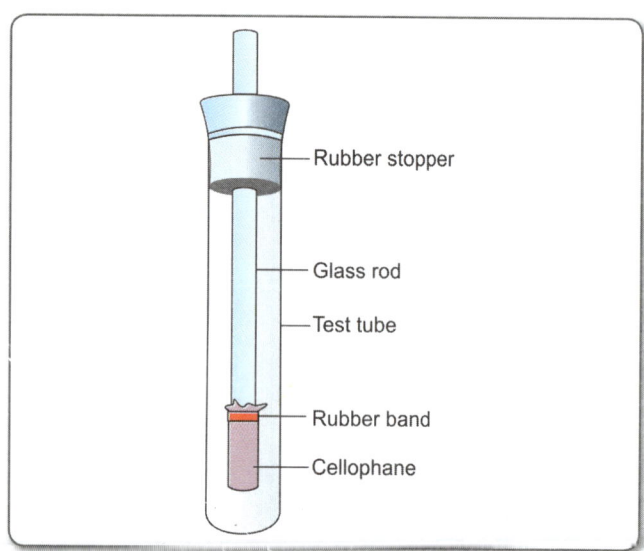

Fig. 41.15: NIH swab.

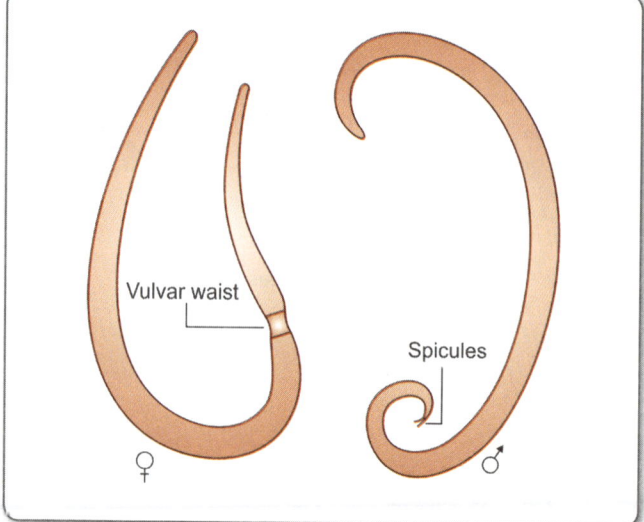

Fig. 41.16: Adult worms of *Ascaris lumbricoides*.

Laboratory Diagnosis

Detection of Adult Worms

The adult worms may be noticed by the patient or by the parents of the patient at the time of commencement of pruritis. They may be recovered in the stools after administration of a purgative or in the vermiform appendix during appendicetomy.

Demonstration of Eggs

Since eggs are not discharged by the worm into faeces, therefore, faecal examination is not useful in the laboratory diagnosis of threadworm infection. However, in a small proportion of patients stool examination may show the presence of eggs of *E. vermicularis*.

Eggs which are deposited in large numbers on the perianal skin at night can be demonstrated by scraping these areas with NIH (National Institute of Health) swab (Fig. 41.15) in the morning before the child goes to toilet and takes bath. NIH swab consists of a glass rod at one end of which a piece of transparent cellophane (with sticky surface out) is wrapped and held in place with a rubber band. The other end of the glass rod is fixed in a rubber stopper and kept in a test tube. The cellophane part is used for swabbing by rolling over the perianal skin. Then the cellophane is detached, spread over glass slide and examined microscopically. This procedure should be repeated on three successive days. Eggs may also be recovered from under the fingernails and the washings from garments.

ASCARIS LUMBRICOIDES

Ascaris lumbricoides, the common roundworm, has worldwide distribution. Adult worm resides in the small intestine, particularly the jejunum of man. It resembles an ordinary earthworm and is **the largest intestinal nematode parasitizing man**.

Morphology

Adult Worm

It is elongated and cylindrical in shape with both ends tapering. The mouth opens at the anterior end. It possesses three finely toothed lips – one dorsal and two ventral. The digestive and respiratory organs of the worm float inside the body cavity possessing a **toxic fluid known as ascaron**. Allergic reactions seen in infected individuals are due to this toxin.

Male Worm

It measures 15–30 cm in length and 3–4 mm in diameter. The posterior end is curved ventrally to form a hook. The ejaculatory duct along with the anus open into the cloaca from which arise a pair of copulatory spicules of equal size (Fig. 41.16).

Female Worm

It is longer and stouter than the male worm and measure 25–40 cm in length and 5 mm in diameter. The tail is straight and conical. The anus is subterminal and opens on the ventral surface in the form of a transverse slit. The vulva opens at the junction of anterior and middle-third of the body on the midventral part of the worm. This part of the worm is narrow and is known as vulvar waist (Fig. 41.16). A mature female *A. lumbricoides* lays enormous number of eggs (nearly 200,000 eggs daily) which are passed in the faeces. Eggs are of two types:

• **Fertilized eggs**
  The fertilized eggs are round or oval in shape and measure 60–75 µm in length and 40–50 µm in breadth (Figs 41.17 and 41.18A). They are bile-stained and brown in colour. They are surrounded by a thick, transparent shell, consisting

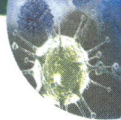

of a relatively nonpermeable innermost lipoidal vitelline membrane, a thick transparent middle layer and an outermost coarsely mammillated albuminoid layer. Outer mammillated coat is sometimes lost. Such eggs are called **decorticated eggs**. They contain a large conspicuous unsegmented ovum with **a clear crescentic area at each pole. Fertilized eggs float in saturated solution of common salt**.

- **Unfertilized eggs**

In the absence of a male worm, the female produces unfertilized (infertile) eggs. These are narrower and longer and measure 90 µm in length and 55 µm in breadth (Figs 41.17 and 41.18B). They are bile-stained and brown in colour. They have a small atrophied ovum and a thin shell within an irregular coating of albumin. The innermost lipoidal vitelline membrane of the shell is absent. The unfertilized eggs

are heaviest of all the helminthic eggs, therefore, they **do not float in saturated solution of common salt**.

Life Cycle

The life cycle of *A. lumbricoides* (Fig. 41.17) is passed in only **one host, man**. No intermediate host is required. Adult worms reside in the small intestine, particularly the jejunum of man. Fertilized eggs containing unsegmented ovum are passed in the faeces. However, they are not immediately infective to man. They have to undergo a period of incubation in soil before acquiring infectivity. Depending on the temperature and humidity, a **rhabditiform larva** develops from the unsegmented ovum and undergoes first moulting within the egg shell in 10–40 days. The optimum temperature and humidity for the development

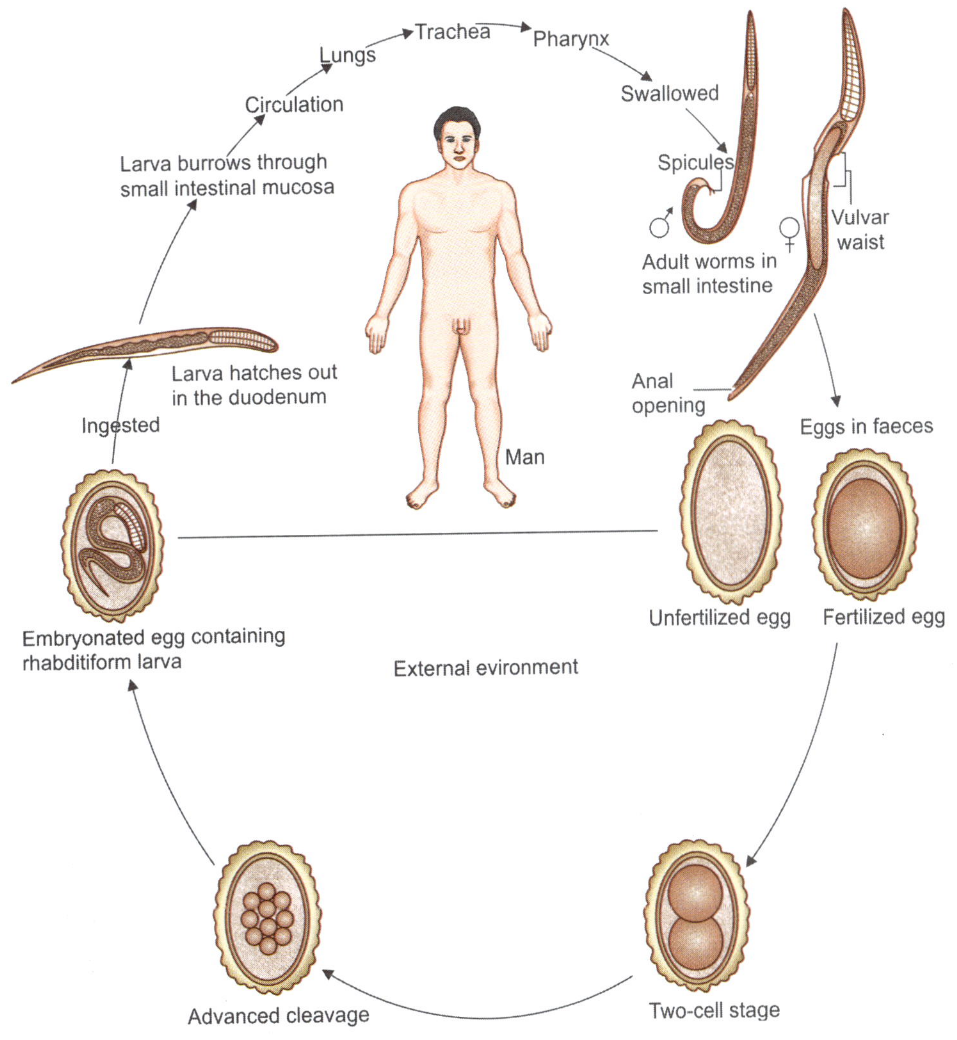

Trachea → Pharynx

Lungs

Swallowed

Circulation

Spicules

Larva burrows through small intestinal mucosa

♂   ♀ Vulvar waist

Adult worms in small intestine

Larva hatches out in the duodenum

Anal opening

Eggs in faeces

Ingested

Man

Embryonated egg containing rhabditiform larva

Unfertilized egg   Fertilized egg

External evironment

Advanced cleavage   Two-cell stage

Fig. 41.17: Life cycle of *Ascaris lumbricoides.*

SECTION VII • PATHOGENIC ORGANISMS-IV PARASITES AND MEDICALLY IMPORTANT ARTHROPODS

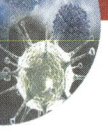
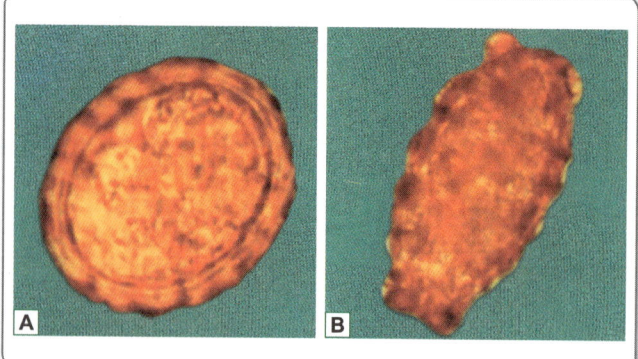

Fig. 41.18: Fertilized (A) and unfertilized (B) eggs of *Ascaris lumbricoides* (saline wet mount, × 400).

of the larva within the egg shell is 20–40°C and more than 40%, respectively. **The embryonated eggs containing rhabditiform larvae are pathogenic to man**.

Man acquires infection by ingestion of food, water or raw vegetable contaminated with embryonated eggs. In the small intestine (duodenum) rhabditiform larvae are hatched out of the ingested eggs. These larvae then burrow their way through the mucous membrane of the small intestine and are carried by the portal circulation to the liver, where they reside for 3–4 days. They then pass via hepatic vein, inferior vena cava, right heart and pulmonary artery and reach the lungs. Here they grow in size and moult twice (first on 5th day and second on 10th day). The larvae then break through the capillary wall and reach the lung alveoli.

From the alveoli, the larvae migrate up the bronchi, trachea and larynx, crawl over the epiglottis to the pharynx and are swallowed. They pass down the oesophagus and stomach and localize in the upper part of the small intestine, their normal abode. On twenty-fifth to twenty-ninth day of infection, the larvae undergo another moulting and transform into adult worms. In about 6–10 weeks they become sexually mature and by 12 weeks the gravid females begin to discharge eggs in the stool and the cycle is repeated.

Pathogenicity

Disease produced by *A. lumbricoides* is known as **ascariasis** and is caused by both adult worms and migrating larvae.

Pathogenicity of Adult Worms

- By robbing the host of its nutrition, the adult worms affect the nutritional status of the host leading to **malnutrition and night blindness** due to vitamin A deficiency. The long-term effect of the malnutrition caused by ascariasis is **retardation of growth**.
- The presence of adult worms in the intestine may also lead to intermittent colicky cramps and loss of appetite. In

heavy infection, adult worms may cause **obstruction of the intestinal tract**.

- **The worms are restless wanders**. They tend to probe and insinuate themselves into any aperture they find on the way. They may crawl out of mouth or may enter the nasal meatus via nasopharynx and pass out of a naris. From the oropharynx, the worm may enter a eustachian tube and penetrate to the middle ear and through the tympanic membrane to external auditory meatus. The worm may also enter into the trachea leading to **respiratory obstruction**. The worms may migrate downwards and lodge in appendix, bile duct and pancreatic duct leading to appendicitis, obstructive jaundice and acute haemorrhagic pancreatitis, respectively. They may perforate the intestinal wall weakened by ulcers or gangrene (Fig. 41.19).
- Release of toxic body fluid (ascaron) of the adult worm in the body of the patient may lead to various **allergic manifestations** such as fever, urticaria, angioneurotic oedema, wheezing and conjunctivitis.

Pathogenicity of Migrating Larvae

In persons repeatedly infected with *Ascaris* and sensitized to the parasite antigens, the migrating larvae may lead to inflammatory and hypersensitivity reactions in the lungs. There is formation of granuloma and eosinophilic infiltrates. It leads to fever, cough, dyspnoea, urticarial rash and eosinophilia. The sputum may be blood-tinged and may contain *Ascaris* larvae and Charcot-Leyden crystals. This condition is known as **Loeffler's syndrome**.

Laboratory Diagnosis

Parasitic Diagnosis

Diagnosis of *A. lumbricoides* infection can be made by:
- *Demonstration of adult worms:*

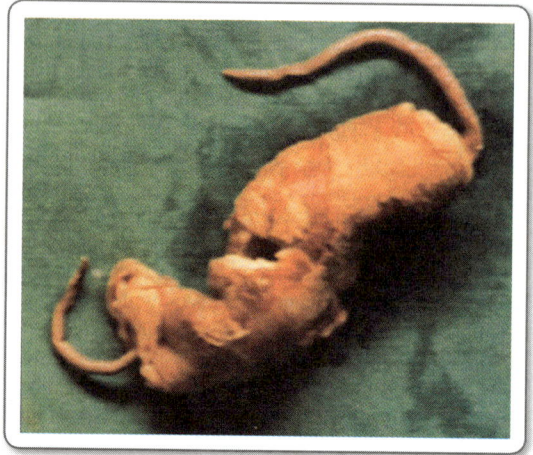

Fig. 41.19: *Ascaris lumbricoides* perforating the wall of small intestine.

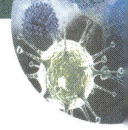

Worm may be passed through anus, mouth, nose and rarely through ear. Barium meal may occasionally reveal the presence of adult worms in the small intestine.

- *Demonstration of larvae:*
  Ascaris larvae may be detected in the sputum during the stage of migration.
- *Demonstration of both fertilized and unfertilized eggs:*
  These may be detected by direct microscopy or concentration of the faeces by salt floatation or formalin-ether sedimentation method. However, eggs may not be seen if only male worms are present.

Serodiagnosis

Ascaris antibody can be detected by indirect haemagglutination (IHA) and immunofluorescence antibody (IFA) test. These tests are useful for the diagnosis of extra-intestinal ascariasis like Loeffler's syndrome.

Visceral larva migrans

Visceral larva migrans (VLM) is a syndrome caused by ingestion of embryonated eggs of nematodes of animals like *Toxocara canis* (dog roundworm) and *T. cati* (cat roundworm). These eggs are usually found in soil contaminated by dog or cat faeces. Larvae hatch in the small intestine and immediately penetrate the intestinal wall and migrate to liver. They may move onto the lungs or to other parts of the body or remain in the liver. Occasionally, the larvae reach the eye and cause serious retinal lesions. Several other roundworms, including *Angiostrongylus*, *Gnathostoma* and *Anisakis* species are occasionally implicated in visceral larva migrans.

Wherever the larvae settle, they are attacked by phagocytic cells, consisting mainly of eosinophils, histiocytes and occasionally giant cells leading to the formation of a granulomatous lesion and their progress is arrested. From lungs, like *A. lumbricoides*, they may even migrate through trachea and oesophagus and reach small intestine but, in the human body, they do not convert into adult worms.

Visceral larva migrans is characterized by hyper-eosinophilia (15–80%) together with hepatomegaly or pneumonitis or both, hypergammaglobulinaemia and fever. The larvae may invade the eye producing an **eosinophilic granulomatous reaction**, usually in the retina, and lead to **endophthalmitis**. Visceral larva migrans can be diagnosed by IHA and IFA test.

HUMAN HOOKWORMS

Human hookworms, *Ancylostoma duodenale* and *Necator americanus*, are common throughout the tropics and subtropics. Adult worms reside in small intestine mostly in jejunum, sometimes in duodenum and rarely in ileum.

ANCYLOSTOMA DUODENALE

Morphology

Adult Worms

They are small, pinkish and fusiform in shape (Fig. 41.20). The anterior end is curved dorsally, hence the name hookworm. This curve is in the same direction as the general body curvature. The oral cavity is provided with four hook-like teeth on ventral surface and two knob-like teeth on dorsal surface (Fig. 41.21). The differences between male and female *A. duodenale* are given in Table 41.6. Owing to the position of genital openings of male and female worms they assume a Y-shaped figure during copulation.

Copulatory Bursa

Copulatory bursa is present in the male worm for attachment with the female during copulation. This consists of three lobes. These lobes are supported by 13 chitinous rays, five each in lateral lobes and three in dorsal lobe (Figs. 41.21).

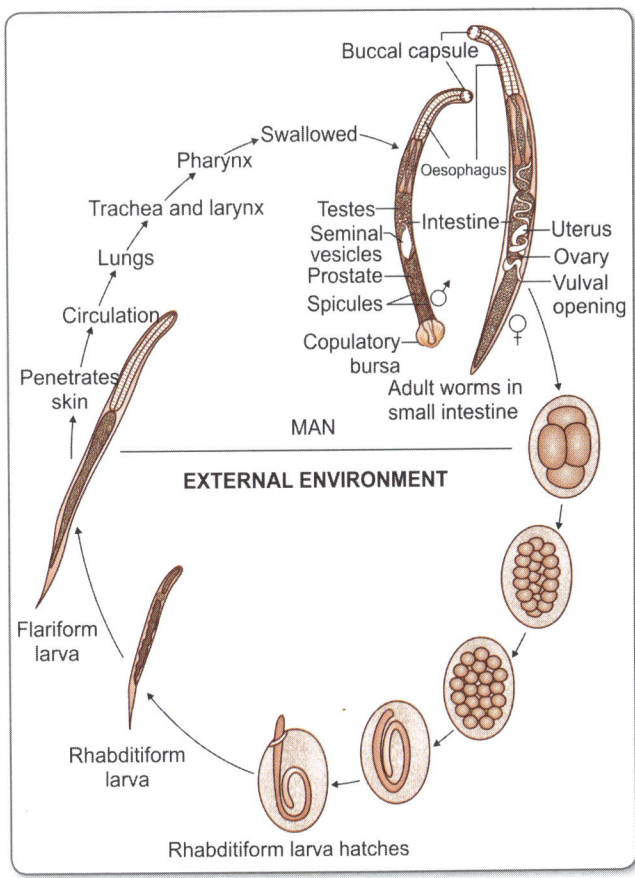

Fig. 41.20: Life cycle of *Ancyclostoma duodenale*.

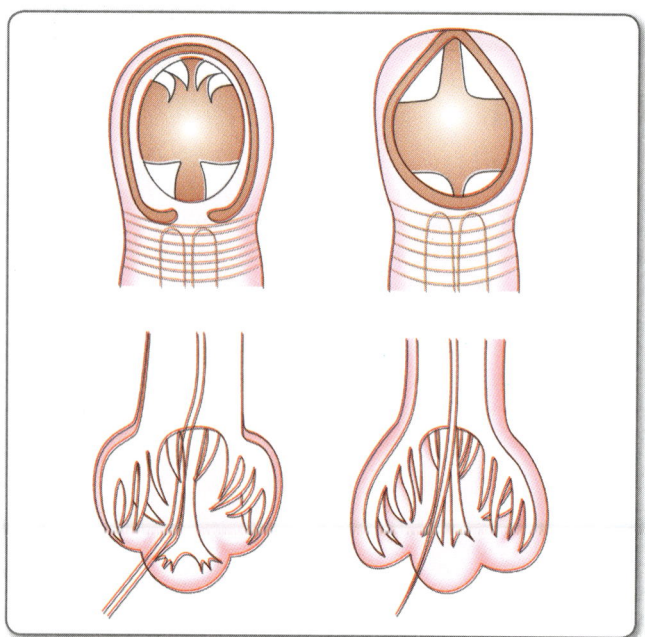

Fig. 41.21: Buccal capsule and copulatory bursa of (A) *Ancylostoma duodenale*, and (B) *Necator americanus*.

TABLE 41.6: Differences between male and female *A. duodenale*

	Male	**Female**
Size	8 mm	12.5 mm
Posterior end	Expanded in an umbrella-like fashion. This is known as copulatory bursa	Tapering
Genital opening	Opens posteriorly with cloaca	Opens at the junction of posterior and middle third of the body

Eggs

Eggs are oval measuring 60 μm in length and 40 μm in width. They are colourless (not bile-stained) and are surrounded by a thin transparent hyaline shell. They possess a segmented ovum with usually four blastomeres. **There is a clear space between the segmented ovum and the egg shell** (Figs 41.20 and 41.22). The eggs float in saturated salt solution.

Life Cycle

Man is the only host (Fig. 41.20). No intermediate host is required. Adult worms inhabit the small intestine of man attaching themselves to the mucous membrane by means of their mouthparts. The eggs containing segmented ova are passed out in the faeces of infected person. In the warm and moist soil,

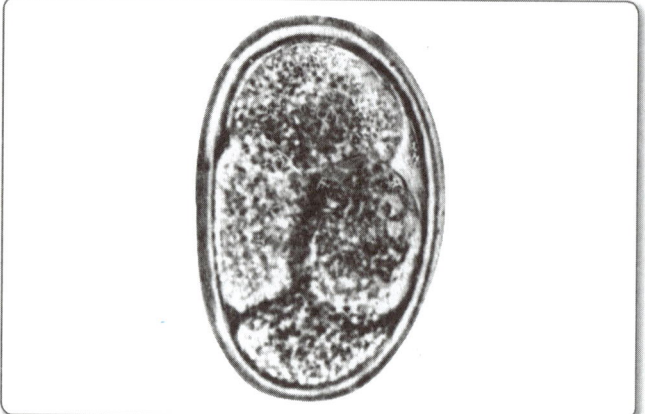

Fig. 41.22: Egg of *Ancylostoma duodenale* (saline wet mount, × 400).

rhabditiform larva hatches out from the egg in 24–48 hours. The rhabditiform larva moults twice on the third and fifth day and develops into a **filariform larva**. This is capable of penetrating unbroken skin and is the **infective stage of the parasite**.

When a person walks barefooted on soil containing the filariform larvae they penetrate the skin, particularly the skin between the toes, the dorsum of the foot and the medial aspect of the sole. In farm workers the larvae may penetrate the skin of the hands. On reaching the subcutaneous tissue the larvae enter into the lymphatics or small venules and begin a migratory phase similar to that of *Ascaris*. Through lymph-vascular system they enter into venous circulation and are carried via the right heart into the pulmonary capillaries. Here they break through the capillary walls and enter into the alveolar spaces. From alveoli, the larvae migrate up the bronchi, trachea and larynx, crawl over the epiglottis to the pharynx and are swallowed.

During migration or on reaching oesophagus they undergo third moulting. Thereafter they reach small intestine, undergo fourth moulting and develop into **adult worms**. They attach themselves to the mucous membrane of small intestine by means of their mouthparts. In about six weeks, from the time of infection, adult worms become sexually mature. Male fertilizes female and the latter lays eggs which are passed in faeces and the cycle is repeated.

Pathogenicity

Clinical disease in *A. duodenale* infection may be caused by the migrating larvae or adult worms.

Pathogenicity of Migrating Larvae

Migrating larvae of *A. duodenale* may cause three types of lesions:
- **Ancylostoma dermatitis or ground itch**
  When filariform larvae enter the skin they may lead to dermatitis. This causes intense itching and burning followed by erythema and oedema of the area which soon develops into papular and vesicular eruptions. This condition is

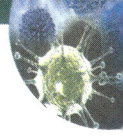

more common with *N. americanus* than with *A. duodenale* infection. It disappears in 1–2 weeks.

- **Creeping eruption or cutaneous larva migrans**
  It is a cutaneous lesion commonly resulting from exposure of human skin to filariform larvae of animal (canine or feline) hookworms, which are not adapted to man, e.g. *A. brasiliensis, A. ceylanicum* and *A. caninum*. Occasionally it may be caused by the larvae of *A. duodenale* and *N. americanus*.

  The filariform larvae of animal hookworms are not able to penetrate below the level of stratum germinativum of human skin. They are, therefore, unable to negotiate their way into blood vessels and proceed to small intestine. They migrate in tortuous tunnels between the stratum germinativum and stratum corneum of the skin, causing a serpiginous vesicular lesion. This leads to intense pruritis with subsequent pyogenic infection. As the larvae move onwards, the abandoned portion of the tunnel becomes dry and crusty. The migration persists for many months before the larva dies. Biopsy shows larvae with round cells, particularly eosinophil, infiltration.

- **Pulmonary lesions**
  When the filariform larvae break through the pulmonary capillaries and enter the alveoli, they may lead to bronchitis and bronchopneumonia. A marked eosinophilia occurs at this stage.

Pathogenicity of Adult Worms

The disease caused by adult worms is responsible for the syndrome commonly referred to as hookworm disease. The maturing and adult worms attach themselves to the mucosa of small intestine by means of their mouthparts. Hookworms ingest blood. One adult worm of *A. duodenale* and *N. americanus* sucks 0.2 ml and 0.03 ml of blood daily, respectively. In addition, the worms frequently leave one site and attach themselves to another site leaving behind small bleeding lesions.

This leads to microcytic, hypochromic type of iron deficiency anaemia. The degree of anaemia depends on the number of worms, body iron store and dietary iron. Patient develops epigastric pain, dyspepsia, vomiting and diarrhoea, the stool being reddish or black. Tongue, conjunctiva and skin become pale. Skin, in addition, becomes cold and dry. Hair become dry and lusterless and there is oedema of feet and ankles.

Laboratory Diagnosis

Diagnosis of hookworm infection can be established by:

Direct Methods

- Demonstration of characteristic eggs in the faeces by direct microscopy or by concentration method.
- Adult worms may also be detected in the stool.
- Aspiration of duodenal contents by Ryle's tube may reveal eggs or the adult worms.

Indirect Methods

- Blood examination may reveal microcytic, hypochromic anaemia and eosinophilia.
- In many cases of hookworm disease stool examination may show occult blood and Charcot-Leyden crystals.

NECATOR AMERICANUS

Necator americanus adult worms are slightly smaller and thinner than those of *A. duodenale*. Differences between the adult worms of these two human hookworms are given in Table 41.7. The eggs of *N. americanus* are indistinguishable from those of *A. duodenale*, and the life cycle, pathogenicity and diagnosis of the former are also similar to those of the latter.

WUCHERERIA BANCROFTI

Wuchereria bancrofti occurs in tropical and subtropical countries. In India, it is distributed along the sea coast and along the banks of big rivers. Adult worms inhabit lymph nodes and lymphatic vessels of man (Fig. 41.23). The microfilariae (embryonic forms) are found in peripheral blood.

TABLE 41.7: Differences between the adult worms of *A. duodenale* and *N. americanus*

	A. duodenale	N. americanus
Size	Larger and thicker	Smaller and thinner
Anterior end	Bends in the same direction as the body curvature	Bends in the opposite direction of the body curvature
Buccal capsule	Six teeth, four hook-like on ventral surface and two knob-like on dorsal surface	Four chitinous plates, two each on ventral and dorsal surface
Number of rays in copulatory bursa	Thirteen	Fourteen
Posterior end of female	A posterior spine is present	No posterior spine is present
Vulval opening	Situated behind the middle of the body	Situated in front of the middle of the body
Pathogenicity	More pathogenic	Less pathogenic

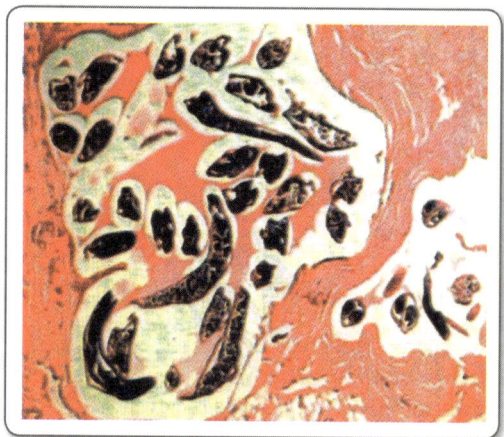

Fig. 41.23: *Wuchereria bancrofti* in lymph node (haematoxylin and eosin stain).

Morphology

Adult Worms

Adult worms (Fig. 41.24) are transparent, creamy white, long, hair-like structures. They are filiform in shape with both ends

tapering. The male and female worms measure 2.5–4 cm × 0.1 mm and 8–10 cm × 0.2–0.3 mm, respectively. The posterior end of the female worm is straight, while that of the male is curved ventrally and contains two spicules of unequal length. Both male and female worms remain coiled together and it is difficult to separate them. The female is viviparous and liberates sheathed embryos (microfilariae) into lymph from where they find their way into blood.

Microfilaria

It is transparent and colourless with blunt head and pointed tail. It measures 290 × 6–7 μm in size and is covered by a hyaline sheath which is much longer (359 μm) than the microfilaria. It can move forwards and backwards within the sheath. The somatic cells appear as granules in the central axis of the microfilaria. At places, these granules are absent. These form the landmarks for recognition of various microfilariae. The tail-tip is free from nuclei (Figs 41.25 and 41.26).

Life Cycle

W. bancrofti passes its life cycle in two hosts. Man is the definitive host and the female mosquitoes belonging to the genera *Culex*,

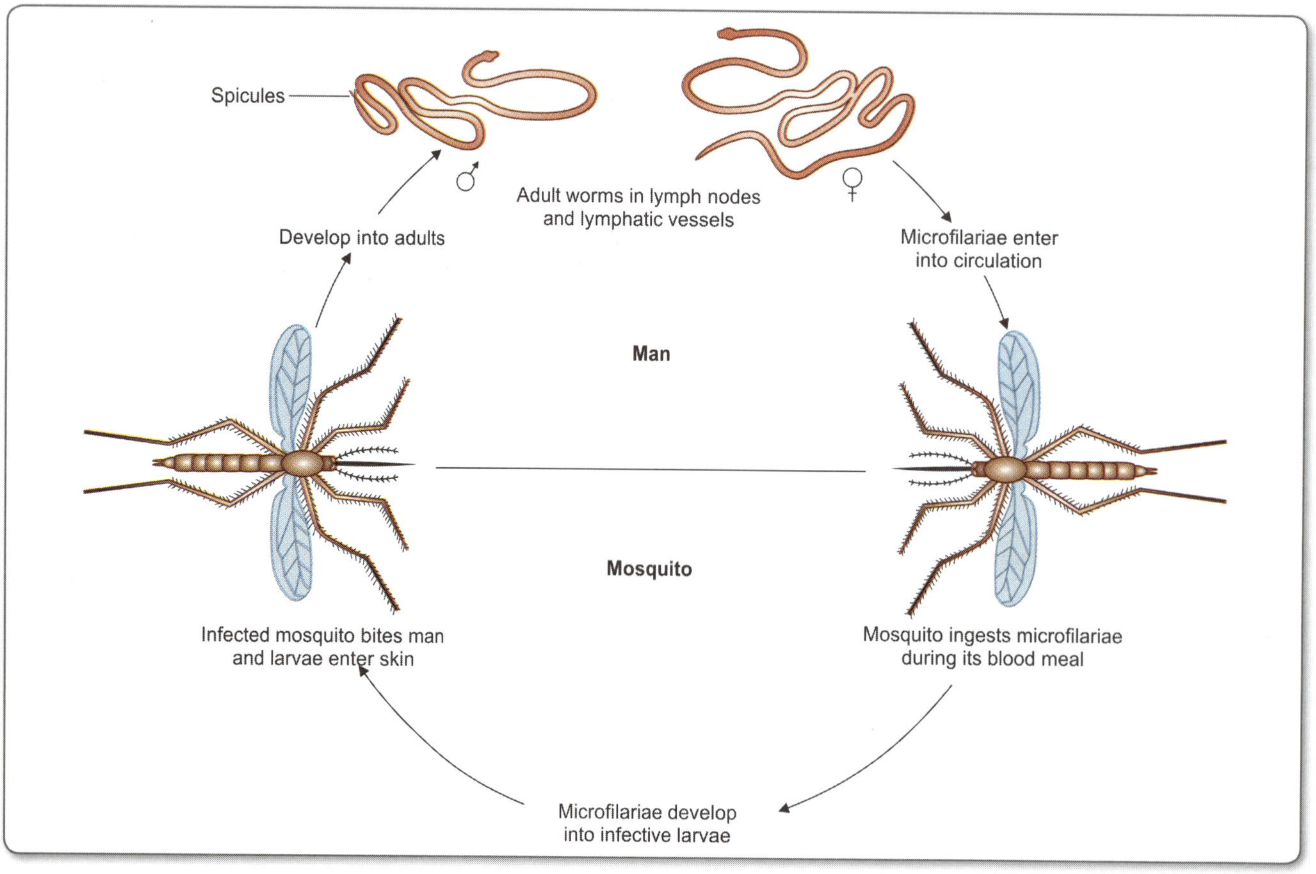

Fig. 41.24: Life cycle of *Wuchereria bancrofti*.

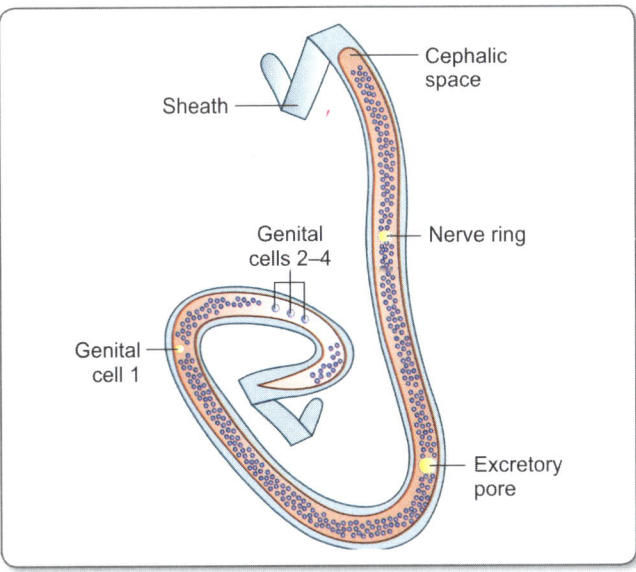

Fig. 41.25: *Microfilaria bancrofti.*

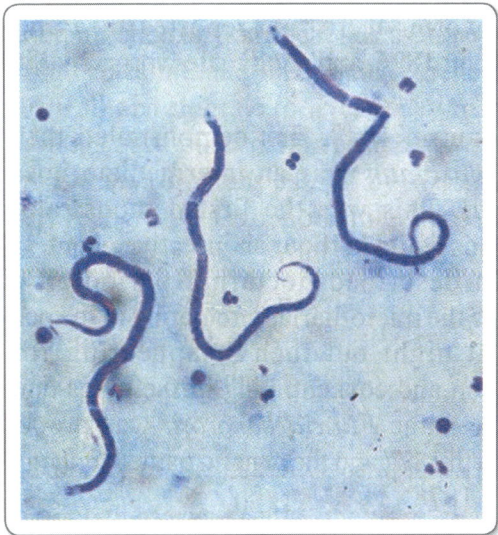

Fig. 41.26: Microfilaria bancrofti in peripheral blood (Giemsa stain × 400).

Aedes and *Anopheles* act as intermediate host. Adult worms reside in lymph nodes and lymphatics (usually inguinal, scrotal and abdominal) of man. The lymph provides nutrition to the adult worms. The male fertilizes female and the gravid female gives birth to microfilariae. Through lymphatics, they find their way into general circulation. The microfilariae appear in large numbers in peripheral blood at night, between 10 pm and 2 am. This correlates with the nocturnal biting habit of the insect vector. The periodicity may also be related to the sleeping habits of the hosts. It has been reported that if the sleeping habits of the hosts are reversed, over a period of time, the microfilariae change their periodicity from night to day.

Sheathed microfilariae are ingested by the mosquito during its blood-meal and reach the stomach of the mosquito. They cast off their sheaths, penetrate the stomach wall and reach thoracic muscles. Here they develop into infective stage of the larvae. These larvae then migrate from thoracic muscles to the proboscis sheath of the mosquito. When the infected mosquito bites a human being, the larvae, in its proboscis, are deposited on the skin near the site of puncture. They then either enter through the puncture wound or penetrate through the skin on their own. Thereafter, they enter into lymphatics and settle down usually in inguinal, scrotal and abdominal lymph nodes, where they develop into adult worms. They become sexually mature. Male fertilizes female, the gravid female gives birth to microfilariae and the cycle is repeated.

Pathogenesis

Infection caused by *W. bancrofti* is known as **wuchereriasis** or **filariasis**. The disease is mainly caused by adult worms (classical filariasis) and sometimes by larvae (occult filariasis).

Classical Filariasis

Presence of the adult worms leads to lymphangitis, lymphadenitis, lymphangiovarix, gross lymphoedema with hypertrophy of the affected part (elephantiasis) (Figs 41.27 and 41.28), hydrocele and chyluria.

Occult Filariasis

This is a hypersensitivity reaction to microfilarial antigens. Patient develops massive eosinophilia (30–80%; absolute count >3000/µl), generalized lymph node enlargement, hepatosplenomegaly and pulmonary symptoms. Microfilariae are not found in the peripheral blood and classical features of lymphatic filariasis are absent.

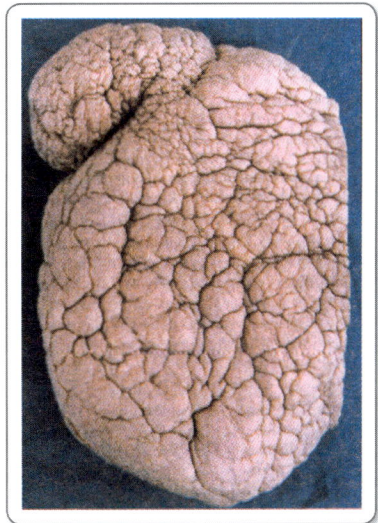

Fig. 41.27: Elephantiasis penis and scrotium.

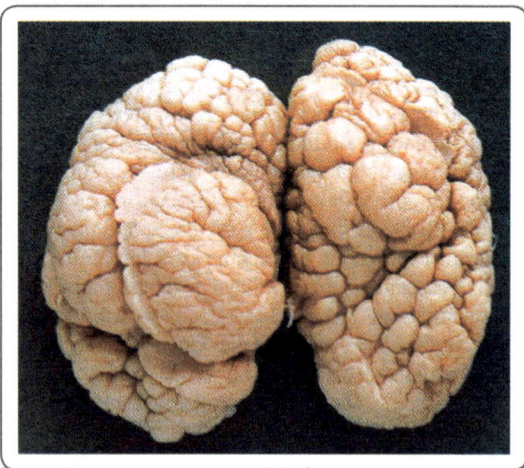

Fig. 41.28: Elephantiasis vulva.

Laboratory Diagnosis

Direct Evidence

- Demonstration of microfilariae in peripheral blood film, chylous urine and hydrocele fluid.
- Demonstration of adult worm in biopsied lymph nodes (Fig. 41.23) and calcified worm can be seen on X-ray.

Indirect Evidence

Filarial antigen may be detected in the patient serum by enzyme immunoassay using monoclonal antibodies against microfilarial surface antigens.

TAENIA SAGINATA AND TAENIA SOLIUM

T. saginata (beef tapeworm) and *T. solium* (pork tapeworm) are worldwide, however the former is much more prevalent than the latter.

Adult Worms

The adult worms live in small intestine (upper jejunum) of man. The adult worms consist of scolex (head), neck, and strobila which is made up of a large number of proglottids (segments). The differentiating features of *T. saginata* and *T. solium* are given in Table 41.8.

Eggs

Eggs (Figs 41.29 and 41.30) of both species are indistinguishable. They are spherical, brown in colour (bile-stained) and measure 31–43 μm in diameter. They are surrounded by embryophore which is brown, thick-walled and radially striated. Outside this may be present thin transparent shell which represents the remnant of yolk mass. Inside the embryophore is present hexacanth embryo (oncosphere) with three pairs of hooklets. **It does not float in saturated solution of common salt. The eggs of *T. solium* are infective to pig and also to man, while those of *T. saginata* are infective only to cattle**.

Life Cycle of T. saginata

It is passed in two hosts (Fig. 41.29). Definitive host is man and intermediate host is cattle (cow and buffalo). The adult worm

TABLE 41.8: Differentiating features of *T. saginata* and *T. solium*

	T. saginata	*T. solium*
Length	5-10 metres	2-3 metres
Scolex	Large, quadrate without rostellum and hooklets. Possesses four suckers which may be pigmented.	Small, globular, armed with a double row of alternating large and small hooklets. Possesses four suckers which are not pigmented.
Neck	Long	Short
Proglottids		
Number	1000-2000	800-1000
Expulsion	Expelled singly	Expelled in chains of 5 or 6
Number of lateral branches of uterus	15-30	5-10
Vaginal sphincter	Present	Absent
Ovaries	Two without any accessory lobe	Two with an accessory lobe
Testes	300-400 follicles	150-200 follicles
Measurement of gravid segment	20 mm in length and 5 mm in breadth	12 mm in length and 4 mm in breadth
Larva	Cysticercus bovis, present in cow and not in man	Cysticercus cellulosae, present in pig and may also develop in man

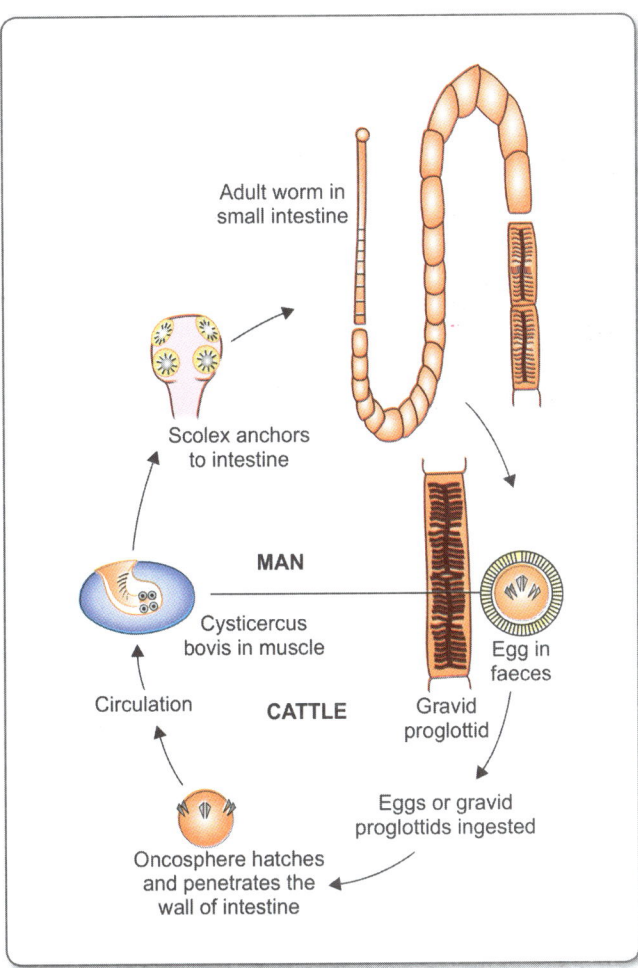

Fig. 41.29: Life cycle of *Taenia saginata*.

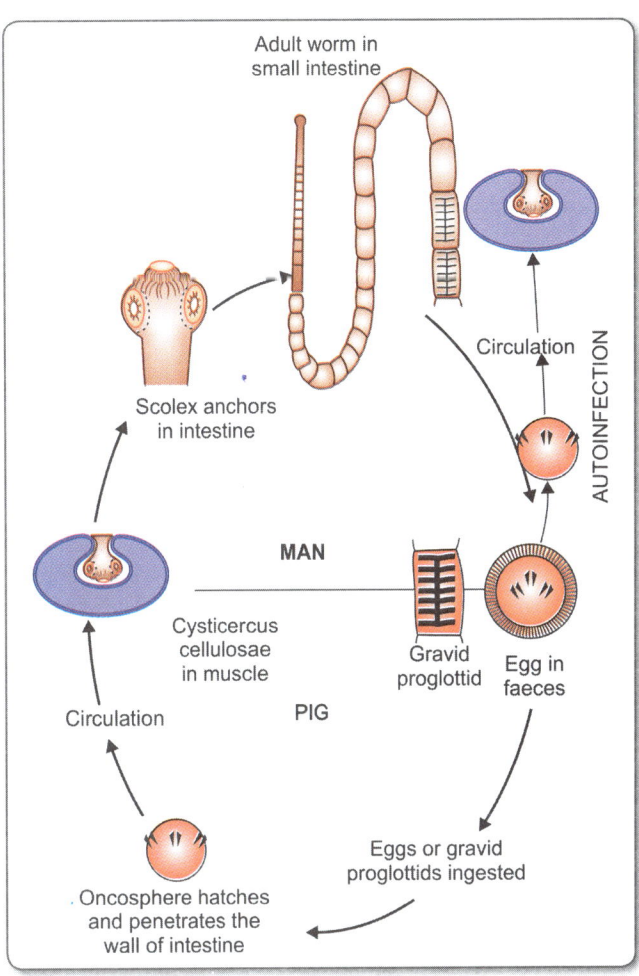

Fig. 41.30: Life cycle of *Taenia solium*.

lives in the small intestine (upper jejunum) of man. Eggs or gravid segments are passed out with the faeces on the ground. These are ingested by cows or buffaloes while grazing in the field. When they reach the duodenum, the embryophore of the eggs ruptures and liberates **oncospheres**. With the help of their hooklets they penetrate the wall of the intestine and enter into portal vessels or mesenteric lymphatics. Then they reach general circulation via liver, right side of the heart, lungs and left side of the heart. From general circulation, they are filtered out in striated muscles where in 60–75 days, they develop into bladder worm – **cysticercus bovis**.

The mature cysticerci are ovoid in shape, milky-white, opalescent and measure 7.5–10 mm in breadth and 4–6 mm in length. They have unarmed scolices (scolices without hooklets) invaginated in them. These can live in flesh of cattle for about 8 months, but can develop further only when ingested by man, its definitive host. **Cysticercus bovis is unknown in humans**.

Man acquires infection by eating raw or undercooked beef containing encysted larval stage (cysticercus bovis). The larvae hatch out in the small intestine, the scolices exvaginate and anchor to the mucosal surface by means of their suckers and develop into adult worms. They grow to sexual maturity in 2–3 months, lay eggs which are passed out in faeces along with the gravid segments and the cycle is repeated.

Life Cycle of T. solium

It is similar to that of *T. saginata* (Fig. 41.30). However, the intermediate host for *T. solium* is pig and its larval form is known as **cysticercus cellulosae**. Man acquires infection by eating raw or undercooked pork containing the encysted larval stage. Mature cysticercus cellulosae is an opalescent, ellipsoidal body and measures 8–10 mm in breadth and 5 mm in length. Its long axis lies parallel to the muscle fibres. It has an invaginated scolex with its four suckers and a rostellum with a double row of alternating large and small hooklets.

Cysticercus bovis and cysticercus cellulosae occur in cattle and pig (intermediate hosts), respectively. However, the latter can also develop in man as follows:

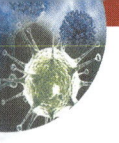

- By ingesting the eggs with contaminated water and food.
- A man harbouring adult worms may autoinfect oneself either by unhygienic personal habits or by reverse peristaltic movements of the intestine whereby the gravid segments are thrown into the stomach, equivalent to the swallowing of thousands of eggs. Further development to cysticercus cellulosae in man is similar to that in pig.

Pathogenicity

Adult worms in the small intestine usually produce no symptoms. But at times, they may cause vague abdominal discomfort, indigestion, persistent diarrhoea or diarrhoea alternating with constipation and loss of appetite.

Cysticerosis is a disease caused by larval stage of *T. solium* an important public health problem of the tropical countries including India. Cysticercus cellulosae (larval form of *T. solium*) may develop in any organ and the effects produced depend on the location of cysticerci. They usually occur in large numbers (Fig. 41.31), sometimes they may occur singly. They usually develop in the subcutaneous tissues and muscles forming visible nodules. It may also develop in brain leading to epileptic attacks and in anterior and vitreous chamber of the eye. *In India, it is regarded as second most important cause of intracranial space-occupying lesions following tuberculosis and the most common cause of epilepsy. It is estimated that 5–20% of all cases with epilepsy in India have neurocysticercosis.*

Laboratory Diagnosis

- The diagnosis of *T. saginata* and *T. solium* adult worm infection can be carried out by:
  - **Demonstration of characteristic eggs** in the stool by direct and concentration method by sedimentation technique (formalin-ether sedimentation technique). **They do not float in saturated solution of common salt.**
  - Since eggs of both *T. saginata* and *T. solium* are similar, therefore for the species diagnosis, the **demonstration of gravid proglottids and scolices is essential** (Table 41.8).

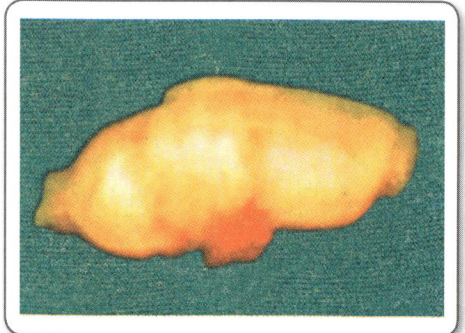

Fig. 41.31: Cysticerci (three in number) in the abdominal muscle.

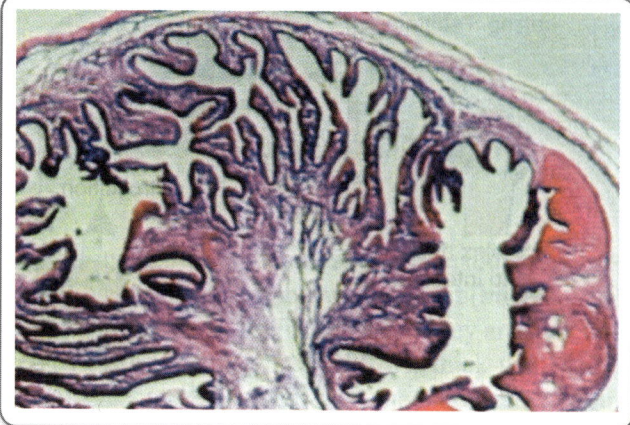

Fig. 41.32: Cysticercus cellulosae in tongue muscle.

- The diagnosis of cysticercosis can be carried out by:
  - **Biopsy of nodule:**
    It may reveal cysticerci (Fig. 41.32).
  - **X-ray of skull and soft tissue:**
    It may reveal calcified cysticerci.
  - **CT scan of the brain:**
    It can accurately locate the lesion in the brain.
  - **Differential leucocyte count:**
    It reveals eosinophilia.
  - **Serological tests:**
    Serological tests such as indirect haemagglutination (IHA), indirect fluorescent antibody (IFA) and enzyme-linked immunosorbent assay (ELISA) can be used for demonstration of specific antibodies in the serum.

ECHINOCOCCUS GRANULOSUS

Echinococcus granulosus or dog tapeworm is worldwide, but it is more common in sheep and cattle-raising countries. Adult worm resides in the small intestine of dog and other canine animals (wolf, fox and jackal). Larval form is seen in man and other intermediate hosts (sheep, goat, cattle, pig and horse). **The dog and sheep are the optimum definitive and intermediate hosts, respectively** and the cycle of transmission is maintained between them.

Morphology

It is a very small tapeworm measuring 3–6 mm in length. It consists of a scolex, neck and strobila (Fig. 41.33).

Scolex

It is piriform in shape and measures about 300 μm in diameter. It possesses four suckers and a protrusible rostellum with two circular rows of hooklets.

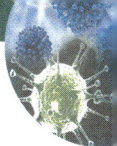

Neck

It is short and thick.

Strobila

It consists of three segments (occasionally four). The first segment is immature, the second is mature and the third (and the fourth when present) is gravid.

Eggs

These are indistinguishable from those of other *Taenia* species. These measure 32–36 µm in length and 25–32 µm in breadth and contain hexacanth embryos with three pairs of hooklets.

Larval Form

This is found within the hydatid cyst which develops in the intermediate host (see pathogenicity).

Life Cycle

E. granulosus passes its life cycle in two hosts (Fig. 41.33). The adult worm lives attached to the mucosa of small intestine of dog and other canine animals. The eggs are discharged in the faeces.

These are swallowed by the intermediate hosts while grazing in the fields. Man acquires infection by a direct contact with infected dog or by ingesting water or food contaminated with dog's faeces containing eggs of *E. granulosus*.

In the duodenum the hexacanth embryos hatch out. These penetrate the intestinal wall and enter into the radicals of portal vein and are carried to the liver. The liver acts as the first filter where about 70% of human infections are located. Some embryos may pass through the hepatic capillaries and enter the pulmonary circulation. Lungs act as the second filter. A few of these embryos may pass pulmonary circulation too and enter general circulation and may lodge in various organs.

Wherever the embryos settle an active cellular reaction consisting of monocytes, giant cells and eosinophils takes place around the parasite. A large number of the parasites may thus be destroyed by host defence mechanism. Some of the embryos, however, escape destruction and develop into hydatid cysts (Figs 41.34 to 41.41). The cellular reaction in these cases gradually disappears, followed by appearance of fibroblasts and the formation of new blood vessels. Fibroblasts lay fibrous tissue, which envelops the growing embryo. This is known as **pericyst**. This merges with surrounding normal tissue. The parasite derives its nutrition through this layer. In old cysts the pericyst may become sclerosed or calcified and parasite within it may die.

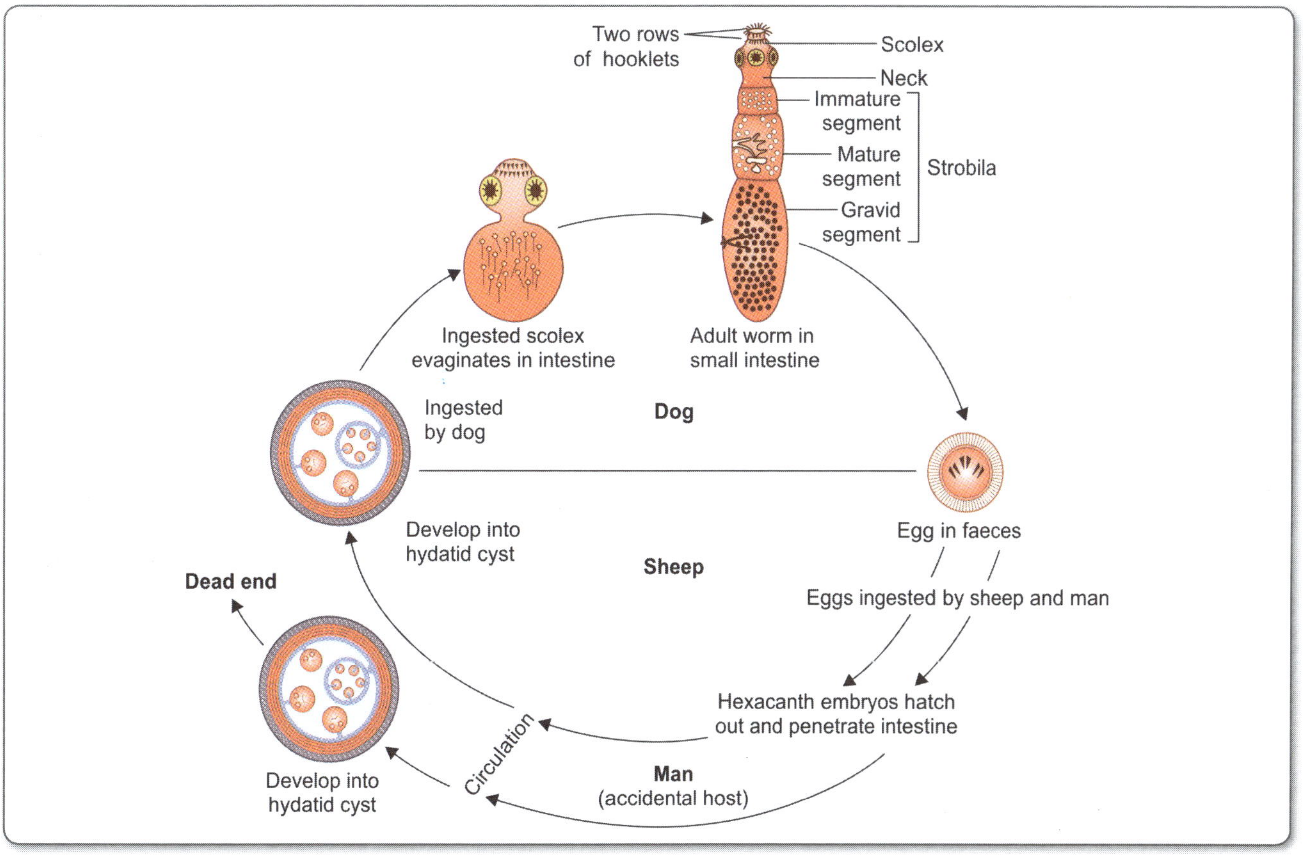

Fig. 41.33: Life cycle of *Echinococcus granulosus*.

SECTION VII • PATHOGENIC ORGANISMS-IV PARASITES AND MEDICALLY IMPORTANT ARTHROPODS

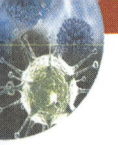

Inside the pericyst, the embryo develops into a fluid-filled bladder known as hydatid cyst. From inner side of the cyst, brood capsules with a number of scolices are developed. The mature hydatid cyst when ingested by dog and other canine animals develop into a number of adult worms. These lay eggs which are passed in the faeces of infected animals and the cycle is repeated. Since dog has no access to the hydatid cysts developed in viscera of man, therefore, the life cycle of the parasite comes to a dead end.

Pathogenicity

E. granulosus causes **echinococcosis** or hydatid disease or **hydatid cyst** in man. It represents larval form of the parasite. The cyst wall secreted by the embryo consists of two layers (Figs 41.33, 41.39 to 41.41).

- **Ectocyst:**

 It is outer layer. It is laminated hyaline membrane about 1 mm in thickness. It resembles white of a hard-boiled egg. It is elastic, therefore, when excised or ruptured, it curls on itself thus exposing the inner layer containing brood capsules, scolices and daughter cysts.

- **Endocyst:**

 It is inner or germinal layer. It consists of a number of nuclei embedded in a protoplasmic mass. It measures 22–25 μm

in thickness. It gives rise to ectocyst on outside and brood capsules and scolices on inside. It also secretes hydatid fluid.

- **Hydatid fluid:**

 It is clear, colourless or pale yellow. It has specific gravity of 1.005–1.010. It is slightly acidic (pH 6.7) and contains sodium chloride, sodium sulphate, sodium phosphate and sodium and calcium salts of succinic acid. It is antigenic, therefore, it is used for **Casoni's test** and when absorbed it leads to anaphylactic shock. Centrifuged deposit of the hydatid fluid shows **hydatid sand** which consists of brood capsules, free scolices and hooklets.

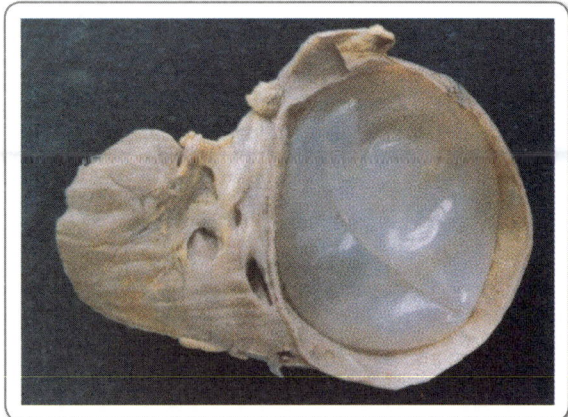

Fig. 41.36: Hydatid cysts of the kidney.

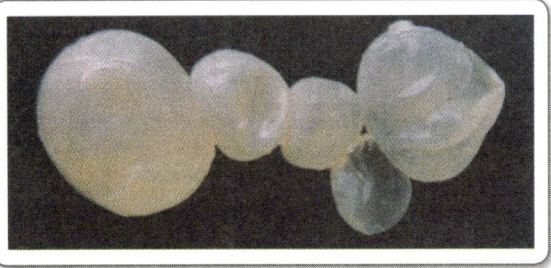

Fig. 41.34: Hydatid cyst.

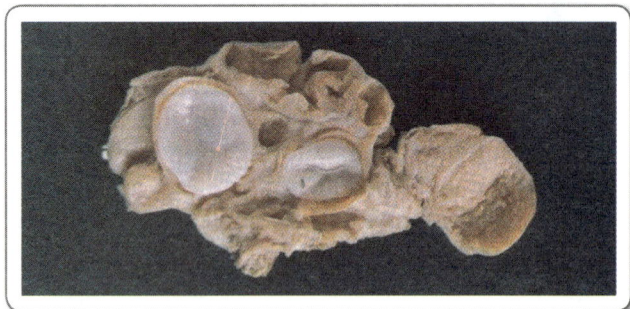

Fig. 41.37: Hydatid cysts of the spermatic cord.

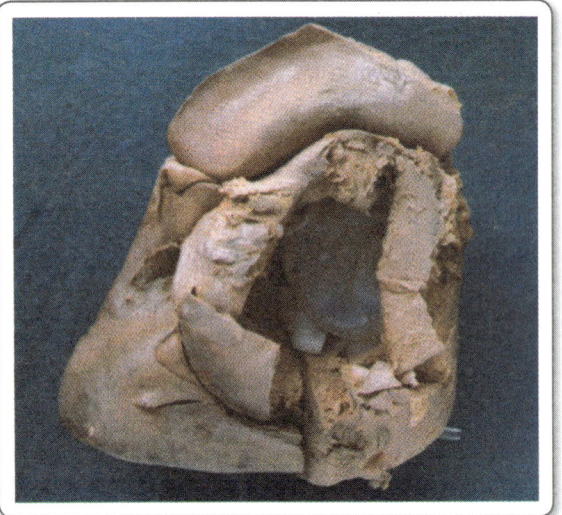

Fig. 41.35: Hydatid cysts of the liver.

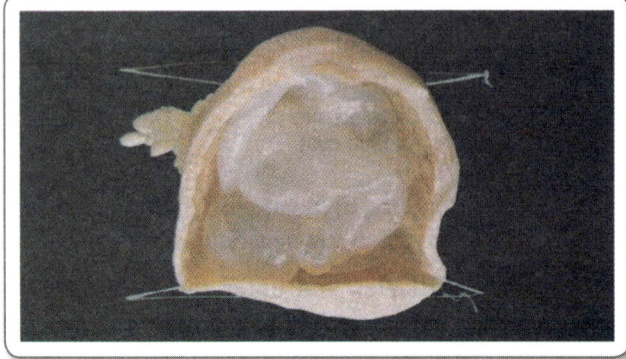

Fig. 41.38: Hydatid cysts ovary.

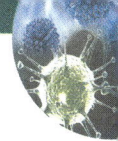

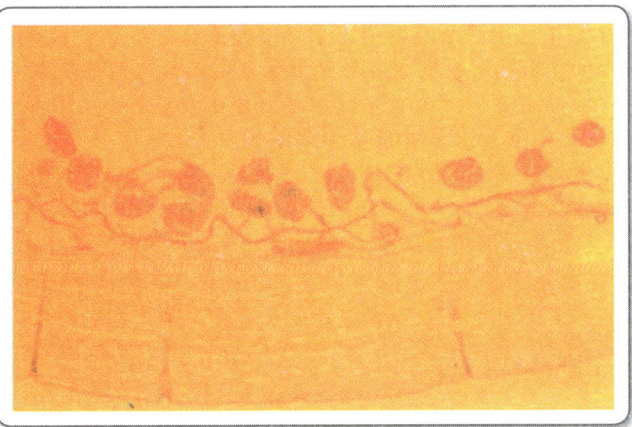

Fig. 41.39: Hydatid cysts armed scolices and free hooklets (haematoxylin and eosin stain × 400).

- **Acephalocysts:**
  Sometimes brood capsules and/or scolices are not formed. These types of hydatid cysts are known as acephalocysts. These are sterile and if ingested by definitive host do not lead to infection.
- **Endogenous daughter cyst:**
  Sometimes a fragment of the germinal layer may detach and develop daughter cyst inside the mother cyst. This is known as endogenous daughter cyst (Fig. 41.40). It also has both ectocyst and endocyst with brood capsules and scolices. Granddaughter cysts may also be formed.
- **Exogenous cyst:**
  In case of hydatid disease of bone, because of high intracystic pressure, herniation or rupture of germinal and laminated layer may occur through some weaker part of the bone resulting in formation of exogenous cyst.

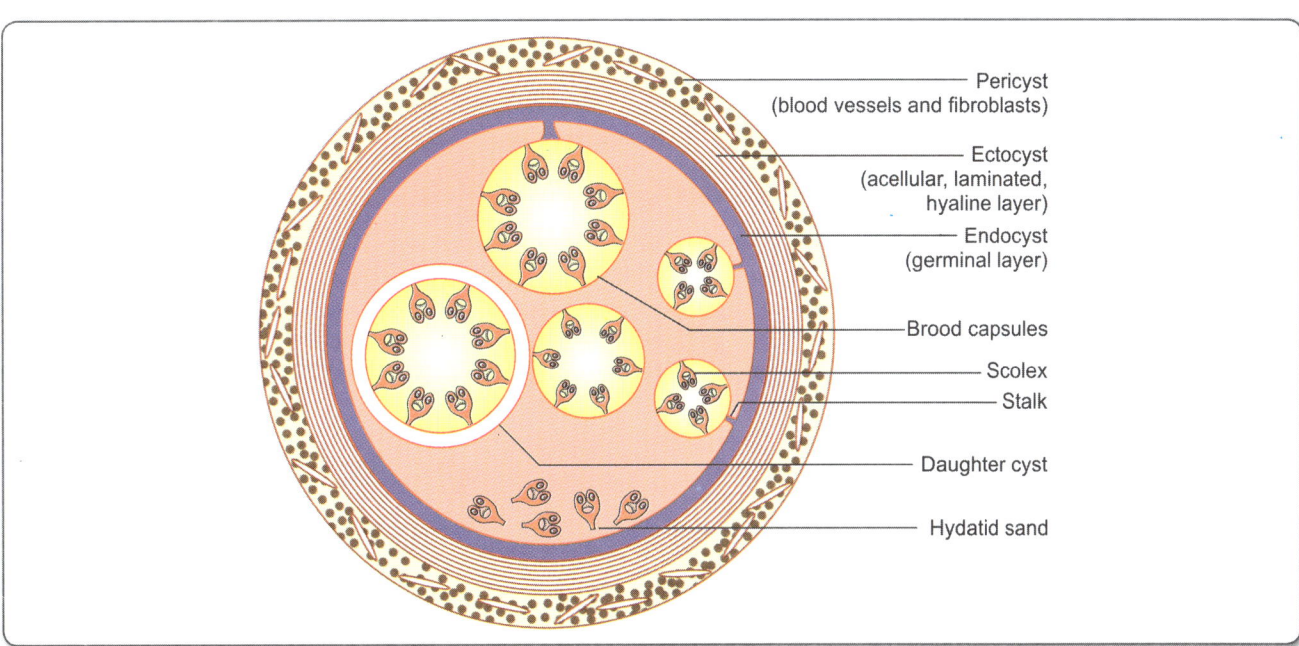

Fig. 41.40: Hydatid cyst.

- **Organs involved:**
  Hydatid cyst may involve liver, lung, central nervous system, heart, spleen, kidneys, bone, muscles, female genital tract, eye, etc. It may lead to visible swelling and pressure effects.

Laboratory Diagnosis

It can be carried out by the following tests:

Casoni's Test

It is an immediate hypersensitivity skin test which was introduced by Casoni in 1911. Antigen for the Casoni test is sterile hydatid

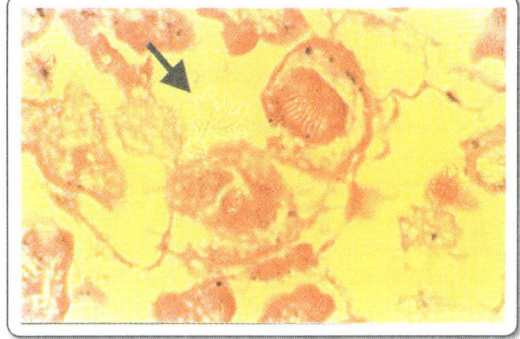

Fig. 41.41: Hydatid cyst showing armed scolices and free hooklets (haematoxylin and eosin stain × 400).

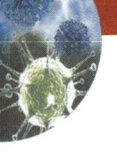

fluid drawn from **unilocular hydatid cysts** from sheep, pigs, cattle or man. The fluid is filtered, tested for sterility and stored in sealed ampoules under refrigeration. For the test, 0.2 ml of the antigen is injected intradermally in one arm. For control, an equal amount of sterile normal saline is injected intradermally on the other arm. The control fades almost immediately, while the tested site in positive cases develops a large wheal measuring 5 cm or more in diameter with multiple pseudopodia. This test has a low sensitivity (55–70%) and gives false positive reactions in patients suffering from other cestode infections.

Differential Leucocyte Count

Differential leucocyte count may reveal eosinophilia (20–25%).

Serological Tests

Serodiagnosis of hydatid cyst may be carried out by enzyme-linked immunosorbent assay (ELISA), radioimmunoassay (RIA),

complement fixation, indirect haemagglutination (IHA) and latex agglutination tests.

Examination of Cyst Fluid

Examination of cyst fluid reveals the typical invaginated scolices, brood capsules and hooklets. Because leakage of fluid in the adjoining tissue may lead to anaphylactic shock, therefore, the fluid aspirated from surgically removed cyst should be examined and diagnostic puncture of cyst is not recommended.

Histological Examination

Histological examination of surgically removed cyst reveals different layers of the hydatid cyst, i.e. pericyst, ectocyst and endocyst (Figs 41.39 and 41.41).

Radiodiagnosis

X-ray, ultrasound and CT scan are also helpful in the diagnosis of hydatid cyst.

Key Points

- **Host parasite relationship is of 3 types:** Symbiosis, commensalism and parasitism.
- *Entamoeba histolytica* causes intestinal and extraintestinal amoebiasis.
- *Giardia lamblia* is responsible for duodenitis and jejunitis and may also cause chronic cholecystitis and jaundice.
- The normal habitat of *Trichomonas vaginalis* is vagina and urethra of women, and urethra, seminal vesicles and prostate of man.
- *Plasmodium vivax* and *P. falciparum* are most common in India.
- *Enterobius vermicularis* causes nocturnal perianal pruritis.
- *Ascaris lumbricoides* is the largest intestinal nematode parasitizing man and causes ascariasis.
- *Ancylostoma duodenale* may cause ground itch, cutaneous larva migrans, and bronchitis and bronchopneumonia.
- *Wuchereria bancrofti* leads to filariasis.
- *Taenia solium* leads to cysticercosis which is caused by larval stage and is an important public health problem of tropical countries including India.
- *Echinococcus granulosus* leads to hydatid cyst in man.

Assess Yourself

Long and Short Answer Questions

1. Discuss geographical distribution, morphology, cultivation, life cycle, pathogenicity and laboratory diagnosis of *Entamoeba histolytica*.
2. Discuss geographical distribution, morphology, life cycle, pathogenicity, laboratory diagnosis and treatment of *Giardia lamblia*.
3. Discuss morphology, life cycle, pathogenicity and laboratory diagnosis of Malaria parasites.
4. Tabulate differences between Human malaria parasites.
5. Describe morphology, life cycle, pathogenicity and laboratory diagnois of:
   (a) *Taenia saginata*
   (b) *Echinococcus granulosus*

Contd...

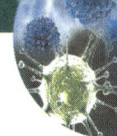

? ASSESS YOURSELF

6. Discuss geographical distribution, habitat, morphology, life cycle, pathogenicity and laboratory diagnosis of:
   (a) *Ascaris lumbricoides* (b) *Wuchereria bancrofti*

7. Write short note on cutaneous larva migrans.

MULTIPLE CHOICE QUESTIONS

1. Mature cyst of *Entamoeba histolytica* is:
   (a) Uninucleate (b) Binucleate
   (c) Quadrinucleate (d) Octanucleate

2. Cysts of *Entamoeba histolytica* are formed in
   (a) The lumen of the intestine (b) The tissues
   (c) The soil (d) All of the above

3. Infective stage of *Entamoeba histolytica* is
   (a) Trophozoite (b) Binucleate cyste
   (c) Quadrinucleate cyst (d) None of the above

4. How many pairs of flagella are present in the trophozoite of *Giardia lamblia* ?
   (a) One pair (b) Two pairs
   (c) Three pairs (d) Four pairs

5. *Trichomonas tenax* resides in:
   (a) Vagina (b) Mouth
   (c) Duodenum (d) Caecum

6. Which is the infecive form of the malaria parasite?
   (a) Oocyst (b) Sporozoite
   (c) Bardyzoite (d) Tachyzoite

7. Relapse of malaria is **not** seen in infection with:
   (a) *Plasmodium vivax* (b) *Plasmodium ovale*
   (c) *Plasmodium falciparum* (d) All of the above

8. Crescent-shaped or banana-shaped gametocytes are seen in infection with:
   (a) *Plasmodium vivax* (b) *Plasmodium falciparum*
   (c) *Plasmodium ovale* (d) *Plasmodium malariae*

9. In which of the following cestodes man can act as both definitive and intermediate host?
   (a) *Taenia saginata* (b) *Taenia slium*
   (c) *Diphyllobothrium latum* (d) *Hymenolepis nana*

10. Which is the intermediate host for Taenia saginata?
    (a) Man (b) Cattle
    (c) Pig (d) Sheep

11. Larval form of *Taenia solium* is seen in:
    (a) Pig (b) Cattle
    (c) Dog (d) Cat

ANSWERS TO MCQs

1. c **2.** a **3.** c **4.** d **5.** b **6.** b **7.** c **8.** b **9.** b **10.** b **11.** a

42 Chapter

Medically Important Arthropods

Arthropods belong to the phylum Arthropoda. They are animals with jointed legs, segmented bodies and chitinous exoskeletons. There are over one million species in the phylum Arthropoda (insects and their allies). *Arthron* in Greek means jointed and *poda* means feet. Arthropods are one of the most important sources, other than man himself, of human pathogens. Scientific study of insects is known as *entomology*. *Entom* in Greek means insect and *logas* means scientific study.

Medical entomology is the branch of this science that deals with the arthropods, which are involved with the spread of disease in human beings. Medical significance of arthropods is attributed mainly due to their blood sucking habits, and their role as vectors of the agents of bacterial, viral or parasitic infection. They can transmit infection in the following ways:

- **Mechanical transmission**, in which the arthropod vector merely transports the organisms from one host to another or from the environment to a host and is not a part of the life cycle of the organism.

- **Biological transmission**, requiring a period of incubation or development in this host. For example, malaria parasites undergo multiplication in the female anopheles mosquito before becoming infective for man.

There are five main classes in the phylum Arthropoda (Table 42.1). Class Insecta, class Arachnida and class Crustacea are of medical importance. Other classes include primarily parasites of the animals. Class Insecta includes mosquitoes, flies, fleas, bugs and lice; and class Arachnida includes ticks, mites, spiders and scorpions. Class Crustacea includes cyclops, crabs and crayfish.

Arthropods of medical interest ingest the pathogenic organisms and convey these to man by following methods:

- Arthropods may obtain the parasitic organisms in a blood meal from an infected person and deposit them in a vomit-drop in the puncture wound (plague) or in faecal pellets near the puncture wound (epidemic and endemic typhus, trench fever, and Chagas' disease) made in the skin of an uninfected person.
- Contamination from infected hemolymph may occur when the arthropod is crushed on the skin (epidemic typhus and epidemic relapsing fever).

TABLE 42.1: Classification of medically important arthropods

Class	Order	Common names
Insecta	Diptera	Mosquitoes, sandflies, tsetse flies, blackflies, deerflies, botflies, warble flies, house flies, flesh flies, blowflies and kads
	Hemiptera	Bed bugs and assassin bug
	Coleoptera	Beetles
	Siphonaptera	Fleas
	Anoplura	Sucking lice
	Mallophaga	Biting lice
	Hymenoptera	Wasps, honeybees and ants
	Dictyoptera	Cockroaches
Arachnida	Acari	Hard ticks, soft ticks, chiggers, itch mites and follicle mites
	Araneae	Spider
	Scorpiones	Scorpions
Crustacea	Copepoda	Cyclops
	Decapoda	Crabs and crayfish
Pentastomida		Tongue worm
Myriapoda	Diplopoda	Millipedes
	Chilopoda	Centipedes

TABLE 42.2: **Common arthropods and diseases transmitted by them**

Arthropod	Diseases transmitted
Mosquitoes	
• Anopheles	Malaria, filariasis (not in India)
• Culex	Filariasis, Japanese encephalitis, West Nile fever
• Aedes	Yellow fever, dengue, chikungunya haemorrhagic fever, Rift Valley fever, filariasis
• Mansonia	Brugian filariasis
Flies	
• House fly	Typhoid and paratyphoid fever, diarrhoea, dysentery, cholera, gastroenteritis, amoebiasis
• Sand fly	Kala-azar, oriental sore, espundia, oroya fever
• Tsetse fly	African trypanosomiasis
Louse	Epidemic typhus, relapsing fever, trench fever
Rat flea	Bubonic plague, endemic typhus, *Hymenolepis diminuta* infection
Black fly	Onchocerciasis
Reduviid bug	Chagas' disease
Ticks	
• Hard ticks	Spotted fever group, viral encephalitis, Colorado tick typhus, tularaemia, human babesiosis
• Soft ticks	Q fever, relapsing fever, Kyasanur Forest disease
Mites	
• Trombiculid mite	Scrub typhus
• Gamasid mite	Rickettsial pox
• Itch mite	Scabies
Cyclops	Dracunculosis, diphyllobothriasis
Cockroaches	Same as in case of house fly

- Some arthropods discharge the pathogens (malaria sporozoites and virus particles) through the hypopharynx in minute droplets of salivary secretion at the time they procure a blood meal. Filarial larvae from the proboscis (labium and mouth area) of the mosquito are deposited on the skin near the site of the puncture. They then enter through puncture wound or penetrate through the skin on their own.

In many arthropod-associated diseases, the etiologic agents were undoubtedly parasites of their invertebrate hosts long before man came into the life cycle. In some cases the parasite has been so long and so well adjusted to the arthropod that it produces no obvious injury, namely, *Rickettsia rickettsii* and *Borrelia duttoni* in ticks, and *R. tsutsugamushi* in trombiculid mites. In the tick and in the mite the respective parasites are even transmitted vertically (congenitally) and require no vertebrate host for at least several generations. On the other hand, *R. prowazekii* in the body louse can cause extensive and often fatal damage to this ectoparasite, suggesting that the vector-pathogen relationship is an imperfect one. Vector-borne human infections are given in Table 42.2, and biting characteristics of medically important arthropods are given in Table 42.3.

TABLE 42.3: **Biting characteristics of medically important arthropods**

Only females bite
- Mosquitoes of genera *Anopheles* and *Culex*
- Sandflies of genera *Phlebotomus* and *Lutzomyia*
- Blackflies (*Simulium* spp.)
- Deerflies or mango flies (*Crysops* spp.)
- Biting midges (*Culicoides* spp.)

Both males and females bite
- Tsetse flies (*Glossina* spp.)

Usually bite at night
- *Anopheles* mosquitoes
- Sandflies of the genera *Phlebotomus* and *Lutzomyia*
- Triatomine bugs

Usually bite during the day time
- *Aedes* mosquitoes
- Blackflies (*Simulium* spp.)
- Biting midges (*Culicoides* spp.)
- Deerflies or mango flies (*Chryosops* spp.)

Insects those are able to pass through ordinary mosquito net
- Sandflies of the genera *Phlebotomus* and *Lutzomyia*

INSECTS

Mosquitoes

Mosquitoes are readily recognised by a long needle-like proboscis. Adult males and females both feed on plant juices, but the female needs blood for the development of her eggs, and is also a voracious predator on a wide variety of vertebrate animals throughout the world. Mosquitoes of importance in human medicine are divided into two broad types:

- **Anopheline mosquitoes**, numerous species of which transmit malaria.
- **Culicine mosquitoes**, which are the vectors of many arbovirus infections.

Both anopheline and culicine mosquitoes also act as the intermediate hosts of certain filarial worms. Female mosquitoes lay their eggs on water; larvae and pupae are both aquatic. Most anopheline mosquitoes prefer relatively large expanses of water that do not dry up, but many culicine mosquitoes, particularly *Aedes* spp. will breed in small pockets of water, such as tree holes, water butts, etc. Adults have wide flight range and may be found several kilometres from their breeding ground.

Sandflies

Sandflies are tiny flies that are well able to penetrate ordinary mosquito net. They have a restricted flight range, so that the diseases they transmit – notably kala-azar and other forms of leishmaniasis, bartonellosis and sandfly fever – tend to be localized in distribution. Female flies suck blood, usually at night, and breed in dark, moist areas, often in or around human dwellings. Species associated with disease transmission in Africa, the Middle East, Asia and the Mediterranean littoral belong to the genus *Phlebotomous*. In Central and South America, *Lutzomyia* spp. act as vectors of leishmaniasis and Oroya fever.

Beetles

Some beetles act as intermediate host of the dwarf tapeworm *Hymenolepis diminuta*, an uncommon human parasite of minor importance.

Reduviid bugs

Reduviid bugs transmit *Trypanosoma cruzi*, causative agent of Chagas' disease, in South America. They are about 2.5 cm in length – much larger than bed bugs – and unlike them, they have wings. They are usually active at night, settling on the face of an unsuspecting sleeper to take a blood meal and to defecate. The infective trypanosomes are in the hindgut and the bitten person becomes infected by rubbing the bug's faeces into the irritating bite wound.

Fleas

Fleas are small blood-sucking parasites. They have laterally flattened bodies and lack wings. Well developed hind legs enable them to jump from host to host. Many fleas feed on man if given the opportunity. However, the species that is adapted for life on man is the human flea, *Pulex irritans*. It is common throughout the world. Female fleas of another species, *Tunga penetrans*, attack man once they have been fertilized. The fleas burrow into the skin, or under the toe-nails, of human host and are known as *jiggers*. The abdomen of the gravid female becomes grossly distended *with eggs*, causing pain, irritation and, sometimes secondary infection. Jigger fleas are common in dry, sandy soil, mainly in Africa and parts of Central and South America.

Human fleas are seldom implicated in the transmission of disease, but some other species are important disease vectors. Most notorious is the rat flea, *Xenopsylla cheopis*, which is the most important, but not the sole vector of plague. Some forms of typhus are also transmitted by *X. cheopis* and other fleas.

Lice

Lice are wingless insects that undergo incomplete metamorphosis during their development. The ones that parasitize man are blood-sucking species with flattened bodies and short legs that are adapted to cling to hair. Body lice and head lice are considered to be variants of the same species, *Pediculus humanus*. Body louse, *P. humanus corporis* is somewhat larger than the head louse, *P. humanus capitis*, and there are other minor differences. A third species *Phthirus pubis* is quite distinct morphologically and is known as 'crab' louse.

Head lice are usually confined to the hair of the scalp, but body lice live in clothing covering the body, rather than on the skin. *Phthirus pubis* is usually found on pubic hair, but may also infest other hairy parts including eyelashes. All types attach their characteristic eggs (*nits*) to body hair and effective treatment involves removal of the *nits* as well as dealing with the adults.

Crab lice are not known to be involved in disease transmission, but body and head lice are classic vectors of epidemic typhus and relapsing fever. Treatment with insecticides such as permethrin, malathion and carbaryl may be effective, but resistance occurs.

Other Biting Flies

The tsetse flies, *Glossina* spp., are found in the so called 'fly belts' of sub-Saharan Africa, where they are responsible for transmission of trypanosomiasis in man as well as in cattle and other animals. Usually both male and female feed on blood. Other biting flies responsible for transmission of disease in Africa include species of *Chrysops* (deerflies or mango flies) which act as vectors of *Loa loa* and *Simulium* (blackflies) which act as vectors of onchocerciasis.

Midges

Biting midges are tiny flies. The females attack in swarms, usually in the evening, and may give rise to painful reactions. Like mosquitoes, they are mostly aquatic. One genus *Culicoides* spp. transmits filarial worms of *Mansonella* spp.

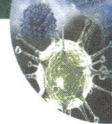

ARACHNIDS

This group includes spiders, scorpions, ticks and mites. They have four pairs of legs. They do not have wings, nor do they have antennae.

Ticks

Ticks are important vectors of human disease. They are of two types: **hard (ixodid) ticks**, which have a chitinous shield on the back and **soft (argasid) ticks**, which lack this feature. Ticks are obligate blood-feeders. They parasitize a wide variety of animals.

Ixodid ticks transmit many rickettsiae of the spotted fever group as well as agents of Q fever, Lyme disease, tularaemia, babesiosis and some arboviruses.

Other Arthropods

Crustaceans (crabs and crayfish) are of interest in human medicine mainly as intermediate hosts of *Paragonimus westermani*, the lung fluke. Copepods (water fleas) are similarly important only as hosts of guinea worm, *Dracunculus medinensis* and the fish tapeworm, *Diphyllobothrium latum*.

🖊 Key Points

- Arthropods transmit infections by mechanical or biological transmission.
- Anopheline mosquitoes and culicine mosquitoes are of importance to human medicine.
- *Phlebotomus* species of sandfly is associated with widespread transmission in most of the parts of the world.
- Ticks are very important vectors of human disease.

❓ ASSESS YOURSELF

MULTIPLE CHOICE QUESTIONS

1. Which type of vector is *Culex quinquefasciatus* for the transmission of *Wuchereria bancrofti*?
   - (a) Propagative
   - (b) Cyclopropagative
   - (c) Cyclodevelopmental
   - (d) Transovarian

2. Sandflies belong to which of the following classes?
   - (a) Insecta
   - (b) Arachnida
   - (c) Pentastomida
   - (d) Crustacea

3. Both males and females of which of the following genera of arthropods bite?
   - (a) *Phlebotomus*
   - (b) *Glossina*
   - (c) *Crysops*
   - (d) *Anopheles*

4. Which of the following arthropods bite during daytime?
   - (a) *Anopheles*
   - (b) Reduviid bugs
   - (c) *Phlebotomus*
   - (d) *Aedes*

5. Which of the following genera of arthropods can pass through ordinary mosquito net?
   - (a) *Phlebotomus*
   - (b) *Culicoides*
   - (c) *Anopheles*
   - (d) *Aedes*

6. In which of the following arthropods transovarial transmission of pathogens occurs?
   - (a) Sandflies
   - (b) Ticks
   - (c) Head lice
   - (d) Reduviid bugs

ANSWERS TO MCQs

1. c   2. a   3. b   4. d   5. a   6. b

Section
VIII

Immunity

Immunity

Immunity refers to resistance of a host to pathogens and their toxic products. It is of two types:

- **Innate immunity**
  - ▪ Non-specific ⎫ Species
  - ▪ Specific ⎬ Racial
  - Individual
- **Acquired immunity**
  - ▪ *Active*
    - ♦ Natural
    - ♦ Artificial
  - ▪ *Passive*
    - ♦ Natural
    - ♦ Artificial

INNATE IMMUNITY

It is due to genetic and constitutional make-up of an individual. Prior contact with microorganisms or their products is not essential. It may be specific against a particular organism or non-specific. Innate immunity may be further divided into species, racial or individual immunity.

Species Immunity

It is total or relative resistance to a pathogen shown by all the members of a species. For example, all human beings are resistant to plant pathogens and many animal pathogens. Rat is strikingly resistant to diphtheria whilst guinea pig and man are highly susceptible. This is due to physical and biochemical differences between the tissues of different host species which determine if a pathogen can multiply in them.

Racial Immunity

Within a species, there may be marked racial differences in resistance to infection, e.g. in the USA, Negroes are more susceptible to tuberculosis than whites. Racial differences in immunity are known to be genetic in origin. A hereditary (genetic) abnormality of red blood cells (sickling) confers immunity to infection by *Plasmodium falciparum* because such RBCs cannot be parasitized by these parasites. This may provide survival advantage to such individuals in malaria-infested areas.

Individual Immunity

Different individuals in a race differ in their resistance to microbial infections. The genetic basis of individual immunity is apparent from the observation that if one homozygous twin develops tuberculosis, there is a 75% chance that the other twin will develop overt tuberculosis. In contrast, for heterozygous twins, there is only 33% chance that the second twin will contract overt disease.

Factors Influencing Innate Immunity

Age

In general, very young and very old are more susceptible to infectious diseases than persons in other age groups. This appears to be due to the immaturity of immune system in very young and gradual waning of immune response in very old.

Hormonal Influences and Sex

There is an increased susceptibility to infection in endocrine disorders such as diabetes mellitus, hypothyroidism and adrenal dysfunction. Pregnant women are more susceptible to microbial infections due to increased steroid levels during pregnancy.

Nutritional Factors

Both antibody-mediated and cell-mediated immunity are lowered in malnutrition.

Mechanism of Innate Immunity

Mechanical Barriers and Surface Secretions

The intact skin and the mucous membranes provide a high degree of protection against pathogens. If skin is damaged, as in case of injury or burns, infections may be a serious problem. Fatty acids secreted by the sebaceous glands, propionic acid produced by the normal flora of the skin and high salt concentration in drying sweat contribute to bactericidal action. Secretions from sebaceous glands contain both saturated and unsaturated fatty acids that kill many bacteria and fungi.

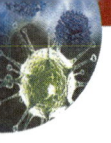

SECTION VIII • IMMUNITY

We have a specialized epithelial lining in our respiratory and gastrointestinal tract to minimize infection. **Mucous membrane** is composed of specialized epithelial cells which secrete a sticky substance called mucus. This traps dust. In respiratory tract there are also ciliated cells, which move the dust-laden mucus up and out of respiratory tract (**mucociliary escalator**) enabling it to be swallowed or coughed out. When swallowed they are destroyed in the stomach's highly acidic environment and digestive juices.

Gastrointestinal Tract

Following factors protect gastrointestinal tract from infection:
- The mouth is constantly bathed in saliva which has an inhibitory effect on many microorganisms.
- **Physical barrier** produced by mucus-secreting epithelial cells.
- **Secretory IgA antibodies** produced here.
- **Highly acidic environment of stomach** may hydrolyse microbial invaders.
- Already established **normal flora** such as *Escherichia coli* serves to inhibit invasion and repopulation by pathogenic microparasites.

Urogenital Tract

Kidneys produce sterile urine which travels down the ureter to the bladder and passes out through the urethral opening. Although, urethra has normal flora, invading microorganisms usually do not gain access to the bladder. It is mainly due to frequent flushing of urethra by sterile urine. However, if organisms have mechanism to attach to epithelial cells lining the tract even frequent flushing might not evacuate them. Because of short urethra, bladder infection is more common in females than in males.

Conjunctiva

Conjunctiva is continually being assaulted by microbe-laden dust. Whenever the dust hits the conjunctiva we blink and tears are produced. Tears mechanically wash away the particles and a hydrolytic enzyme, lysozyme, destroys most viruses and bacteria.

Humoral Defence Mechanisms

Many microbicidal substances are present in the tissues and body fluids. They are responsible for innate immunity. Following are the bactericidal substances present in the tissues and body fluids:

Lysozyme

This is a basic protein of low molecular weight (approximately 20,000 daltons) found in high concentrations in polymorphonuclear leucocytes as well as in most tissue fluids except CSF, sweat and urine. It has bactericidal action by splitting of certain polysaccharide components of cell walls of susceptible bacteria.

Basic Polypeptides

Several basic proteins, derived from tissues and blood cells, possess antibacterial activity. These include spermine and spermidine which can kill tubercle bacilli and some staphylococci.

Complement

The term **complement** (C) is applied to a system of components present in the serum of man and animals. It consists of nine different proteins denoted C1–C9. The fraction C1 occurs in serum as calcium ion dependent complex, which on chelation with EDTA yields three protein subunits called C1q, C1r and C1s. Thus C is made up of 11 different proteins. Though some of its components are stable, C as a whole is heat-labile undergoing spontaneous denaturation slowly at room temperature and in 30 minutes at 56°C. Serum deprived of C activity by heating it at 56°C for 30 minutes is said to be inactivated.

C is normally present in the body in an inactive form but can be activated to form an enzyme cascade. The cascade is a series of reactions in which the preceding components act as enzymes on the succeeding components cleaving them into dissimilar fragments. The larger fragments join the cascade and the smaller fragments are released which often possess biological effects which contribute to defence mechanism by:
- Initiating an inflammatory response,
- Causing the destruction of parasites, bacteria, virus-infected cells or red blood cells,
- Clearing dead cells and immune complexes,
- Detoxifying endotoxins, and
- Effecting release of histamine from mast cells.

There are two activation mechanisms through which complement system executes its role. These are known as classical pathway and alternative or properdin pathway. The former requires the presence of antibody for activation. In contrast, the alternative pathway does not need antibody and can be triggered by the mere presence of bacterial or viral components. For example, the lipopolysaccharide layer of Gram-negative bacterial cell wall is enough to activate alternative pathway. However, both these pathways lead to the same physiological consequences i.e. opsonization, cellular activation and lysis.

Biological Effects of Complement

- Complement mediates immunological membrane damage. This results in bacteriolysis and cytolysis. Different cells vary in their susceptibility to complement-mediated lysis. Gram-negative bacteria are generally sensitive to lysis, while Gram-positive are killed without lysis. Neutralization of certain viruses requires the participation of C, e.g. neutralization of herpes virus by IgM antibody requires the binding of C1, C4 and possibly C3 too.
- C fragments released during cascade reaction help in amplifying the inflammatory response. Proteolytic cleavage of C3 and C5, in either the classical or alternative pathway,

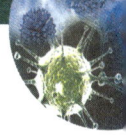

generates two potent mediators of inflammation, C3a and C5a. Mast cells and basophils possess receptors for C3a and C5a. Binding of C3a or C5a to these receptors causes these cells to release histamine. This may lead to contraction of the uterus, trachea, arteries, atrium of the heart and intestines, and increased vascular permeability leading to oedema. C5a, in addition exerts a series of unique effects on white blood cells. These include:

- Degranulation and lysosomal enzyme release.
- Promotes adherence of granulocytes to the endothelium.
- Induces chemotactic migration of granulocytes.

- Phagocytes such as macrophages, monocytes and neutrophils possess surface receptors for C3b. If immune complexes have activated the complement system, the C3b bound to them facilitates their recognition and ingestion by these phagocytes. This facilitated phagocytosis is referred to as **opsonization**.

- Complement participates in **type II** (cytotoxic) and **type III** (immune complex) hypersensitivity reactions. The destruction of erythrocytes, following incompatible blood transfusion is an example of type II hypersensitivity. Participation of C is required for the production of immune complex diseases such as serum sickness and Arthus reaction (type III hypersensitivity).

- Several serum C components are lowered in many autoimmune diseases such as systemic lupus erythematosus and rheumatoid arthritis. They may, therefore, be involved in the pathogenesis of autoimmune diseases. C plays a major role in the pathogenesis of autoimmune haemolytic anaemia, paroxysmal nocturnal haemoglobinuria and hereditary angioneurotic oedema.

- C3 and C6 participate in coagulation process.

- C bound to antigen-antibody complexes adheres to erythrocytes. This is known as **immune adherence**. It contributes to defence against pathogenic microorganisms as such adherent particles are rapidly phagocytosed. C3 and C4 are necessary for immune adherence.

Interferons

These are a family of antiviral agents produced by cells stimulated by live or killed viruses and certain other inducers. A number of molecules have been described. α and β interferons are part of innate immunity and γ interferon is produced by T cells as part of acquired immunity.

Cellular Defence Mechanisms

Microparasites (viruses, bacteria, fungi and protozoa) that penetrate the physical barriers are confronted, in addition to humoral defence mechanism, by non-specific cellular defences. Cellular defence against microparasites is provided by **phagocytes** and a subpopulation of lymphocytes known as **natural killer (NK) cells**. Phagocytes are classified into microphages and macrophages. **Microphages** are polymorphonuclear leucocytes and **macrophages** consist of histiocytes which are the wandering amoeboid cells seen in tissues, fixed reticuloendothelial cells and monocytes of blood.

Phagocytic cells reach the site of inflammation in large numbers. They engulf, kill and digest bacteria. On the other hand, viral invasion is countered by NK cells. Residing in the peripheral lymphoid organs, NK cells recognize virus-infected cells, bind to them and subsequently lyse them. NK cells have also been implicated in host defence against cancers. They are thought to recognize the changes in the cell membranes of transformed cells in a mechanism similar to that used to combat virus infection. Fungi are confronted by polymorphonuclear leucocytes, macrophages and NK cells.

Phagocytic cell engulfs microparasite by extending pseudopodia around it. These fuse and microorganism is internalized into a vacuole (**phagosome**) which fuses with lysosomes found in the cell to form **phagolysosome** (Fig. 43.1). Microparasites are subjected to the lytic enzymes in the phagolysosome and are destroyed.

Eosinophils are polymorphonuclear leucocytes with cytoplasmic granules and bilobed nucleus. Their number in the blood of normal individuals is 3–5%. But in patients with parasitic infections and allergies their number increases. They are not efficient phagocytic cells. However, their granules possess molecules that are toxic to parasites. Large parasites such as helminths cannot be internalized. Therefore, they must be killed extracellularly.

Fever

A rise in temperature following infection is a natural defence mechanism. It inhibits or kills the infecting organisms.

Inflammation

It is the cellular and vascular response to injury such as invasion by an infectious agent, exposure to a noxious chemical or physical trauma. The signs of inflammation are redness, swelling,

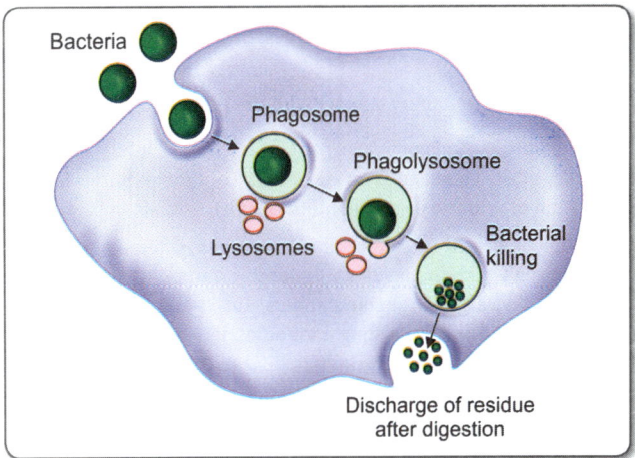

Fig. 43.1: Events of phagocytosis.

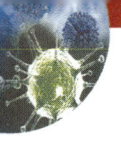

SECTION VIII • IMMUNITY

heat, pain and disturbed or altered functions. Inflammation leads to vasodilation, increased vascular permeability and cellular infiltration. **Polymorphonuclear leucocytes** escape into the tissues by diapedesis and accumulate in large numbers attracted by the chemotactic substances released at the site of injury. They then phagocytose microorganisms and their products. Because of increased vascular permeability, there is an **outpouring of plasma** which helps to dilute the toxic products present. In addition, plasma contains a number of non-specific (complement, properdin, beta lysin, leukins and plakins) and specific (antibodies) inhibitors.

ACQUIRED IMMUNITY

Most potential pathogens are checked by innate immunity before they establish an overt infection. If these defences are breached the acquired immune system is called into play. The resistance that an individual acquires during his life-time is known as acquired immunity. It is antigen-specific and may be antibody-mediated or cell-mediated. It is of two types—active immunity and passive immunity (Table 43.1 and Flowchart 43.1).

Both active and passive immunity may be further divided into natural and artificial.

Active Immunity

This involves the active involvement of the person's own immune apparatus leading to the synthesis of antibodies and/or the production of immunocompetent cells (ICCs). It appears only after a **lag (latent) period**, i.e. the time required for generation of antibodies and ICCs. During development of active immunity there is often a negative phase during which the level of measurable immunity may actually be lower than before antigenic stimulus. This is due to antigen combining with pre-existing antibodies and lowering its level.

If an individual who has been actively immunized against an antigen, experiences the same antigen subsequently, the immune response occurs more quickly and more abundantly than during the first encounter. This is known as **secondary response**.

Immune system is able to retain the memory of a prior antigenic exposure for long periods and produces a secondary type response when encountered with the same antigen. This is known as **immunological memory**. Active immunity may be natural or artificial.

Natural Active Immunity

Natural active immunity results either from a subclinical or clinical infection. A large majority of adults in the developing countries possess natural active immunity to poliomyelitis due to repeated subclinical infections with poliovirus during childhood. Some infections like diphtheria, whooping cough, measles and mumps induce long-lasting immunity. Others such as common cold and influenza confer immunity which lasts for a short time.

Artificial Active Immunity

This is the resistance induced by vaccines which are preparations of live or killed microorganisms or their products:

- **Bacterial vaccines**
  - *Live*
    - B.C.G. for tuberculosis
    - Ty 21a for typhoid
  - *Killed*
    - TAB for enteric fever
    - Cholera
    - Pertussis
  - *Bacterial products*
    - Tetanus toxoid
    - Diphtheria toxoid

TABLE 43.1: Differences between active and passive immunity

Active immunity	Passive immunity
Produced actively by host's immune system as a result of antigenic stimulation.	Received passively by the host. No participation of host's immune system.
Induced by infection or by contact with antigens.	Conferred by administration of antibodies.
Long-lasting.	Transient.
Immunity effective only after a lag period, i.e. time required for generation of antibodies and immunocompetent cells.	Immunity effective immediately.
During development of active immunity there is often a negative phase during which the level of measurable immunity may actually be lower than before antigenic stimulus. This is due to antigen combining with the pre-existing antibodies and lowering its level.	No negative phase.
Immunological memory present, therefore, subsequent challenge (secondary response) is more effective.	No immunological memory. Subsequent administration of antibodies is less effective due to immune elimination.
More effective and confers better protection.	Less effective and provides inferior immunity.
Not applicable in immunodeficient individuals.	Applicable in immunodeficient individuals

Flowchart 43.1: Types of immunity.

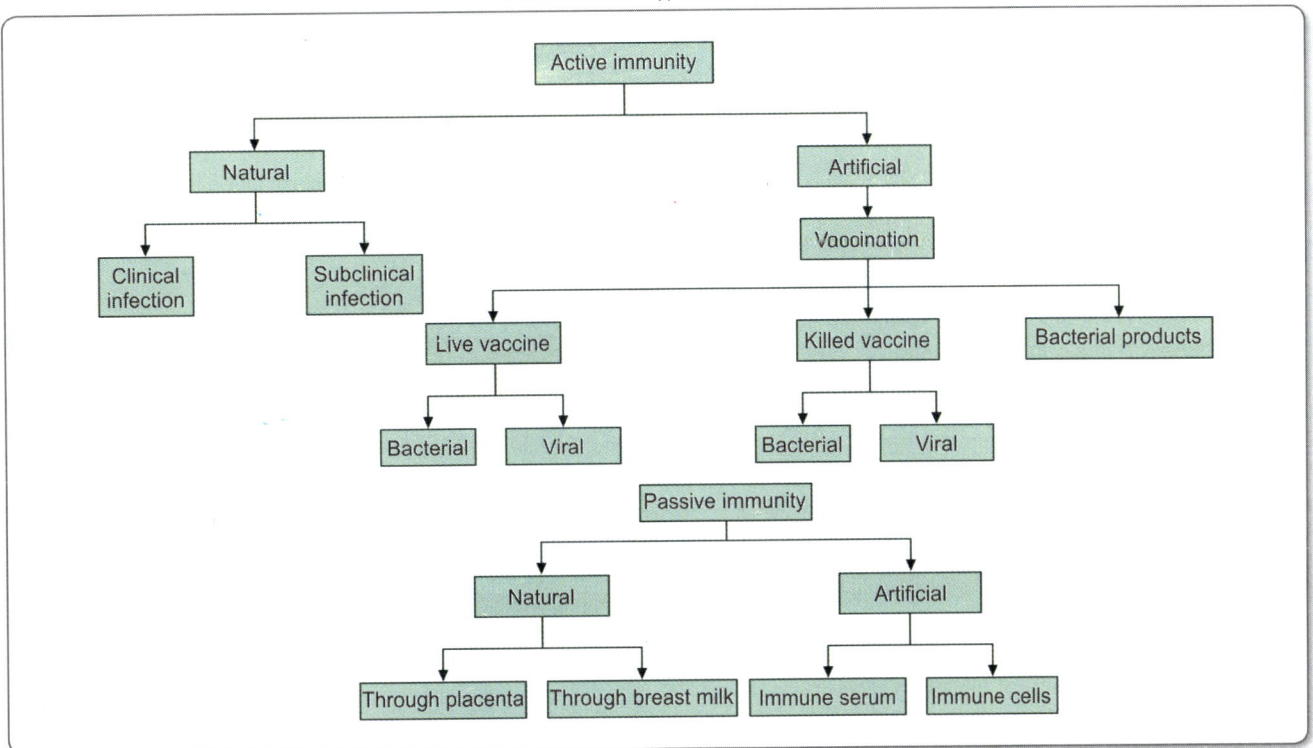

- ◆ Capsular polysaccharide of meningococci
- ◆ Capsular polysaccharide of *Haemophilus influenzae* type b
- **Viral vaccines**
  - ■ *Live*
    - ◆ Sabin vaccine for poliomyelitis or oral polio vaccine (OPV)
    - ◆ 17D vaccine for yellow fever
    - ◆ MMR vaccine for measles, mumps, rubella
    - ◆ Varicella-zoster
  - ■ *Killed*
    - ◆ Salk vaccine for poliomyelitis or inactivated polio vaccine (IPV)
    - ◆ Neural and non-neural vaccines for rabies
    - ◆ Influenza
    - ◆ Hepatitis A
    - ◆ Hepatitis B
    - ◆ Japanese encephalitis

Live vaccines initiate a sort of mini infection without causing disease. The immunity following vaccination, therefore, parallels that following natural infection. However, it is of lower order than that induced by infection. Since live vaccines undergo limited multiplication in the body, therefore, number of organisms required in a dose is less; single doses may be sufficient and they are relatively cheaper. Live vaccines may be administered orally. However, since they are live, therefore, strict conditions of storage are required.

Killed vaccines are generally less immunogenic than live vaccines and protection lasts only for a short period. Therefore, they have to be administered repeatedly. At least two doses are required. First dose is known as **primary** and subsequent doses as **booster doses**. In killed vaccines since the organisms are killed, therefore, larger number of these are required in each dose. Oral route for killed vaccines is generally not effective. Antibody response to killed vaccines is improved by addition of adjuvants, for example, aluminium phosphate adjuvant vaccine for cholera.

Passive Immunity

The immunity that is transferred to a recipient in a ready-made form is known as passive immunity. Here the recipient's immune system plays no active role. There is no lag or latent period, the immunity is effective immediately after passive immunization. There is no negative phase. It confers only transient immunity lasting usually for days or weeks till the antibodies are metabolized and eliminated. There is no secondary type response. Rather subsequent administration of antibodies is less effective due to **immune elimination**.

Natural Passive Immunity

This is the resistance transferred from mother to foetus through placenta. IgG antibodies can cross placental barrier to reach the foetus. After birth, immunoglobulins are passed to the newborn through the breast milk. Human colostrum is rich in IgA

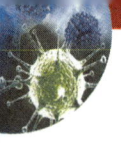

antibodies which are resistant to digestion in stomach and small intestine, hence confers immunity on the neonate up to three months of age.

Artificial Passive Immunity

This is the immunity transferred passively to the recipient by administration of antibodies. This is done by administration of hyperimmune sera of man or animals. For example, tetanus antitoxin is prepared in horses by active immunization of horses with tetanus toxoid, bleeding them and separating the serum. Similarly, diphtheria antitoxin and gas gangrene antitoxin are also prepared. However, since these antitoxins are foreign proteins and are liable to cause serious or even fatal hypersensitivity reactions, these should be administered only after testing for hypersensitivity. After first administration, it is removed by metabolism and following subsequent injections by metabolism and immune elimination. Therefore, immunity conferred is short-lived.

Sera collected from patients convalescing from infectious diseases contain high levels of specific antibodies. Convalescent sera have, therefore, been employed for passive immunization against viral infections such as measles and rubella. Sera of healthy adults contain antibodies against infectious agents prevalent in a community. Therefore, sera from a large number of individuals can be collected and used for passive immunization. Placenta provides a convenient source of human immunoglobulins. Human immune serum does not lead to any hypersensitivity reaction, there is no immune elimination and its half-life is more than that of animal sera. However, with human serum there is a grave risk of transmission of human immunodeficiency virus and hepatitis B, C and D viruses.

Indications of Passive Immunization

- To provide immediate protection to a non-immune individual exposed to an infection, when there is insufficient time for active immunization, e.g. administration of tetanus antitoxin and gas gangrene antitoxin to a non-immune individual with crushing road-side injury, and administration of diphtheria antitoxin to a non-immune child exposed to diphtheria.
- Administration of anti-Rh(D) IgG to Rh-negative mother, bearing Rh-positive baby at the time of delivery to prevent Rh isoimmunization.

- For suppression of active immunity, when it is injurious, for example, administration of antilymphocytic serum for suppression of lymphocytes in transplantation surgery to suppress the immune response towards the transplant.

Combination of active and passive immunization may also be employed. For example, a person exposed to tetanus may be injected tetanus antitoxin on one arm and tetanus toxoid on the other with separate syringes followed by full course of tetanus toxoid. Diphtheria antitoxin and diphtheria toxoid can also be practised similarly.

ADOPTIVE IMMUNITY

Injection of immunologically competent lymphocytes is known as adoptive immunity. Instead of whole lymphocytes, an extract of immunologically competent lymphocytes known as **transfer factor** can be used. This has been attempted in the treatment of lepromatous leprosy.

LOCAL IMMUNITY

This means immunity at a particular site, generally the site of invasion and multiplication of pathogen. For example, in case of poliomyelitis, parenteral vaccine provides systemic immunity. The antibodies neutralize virus only after blood invasion. It does not prevent multiplication of the virus at the site of entry, the gut mucosa, and its faecal excretion. However, when live oral vaccine is given it leads to local immunity. Similarly, live influenza vaccine administered intranasally provides local immunity while killed influenza vaccine evokes humoral antibody response. Local immunity is conferred by **secretory IgA antibodies** produced locally by plasma cells present on mucosal surfaces or in secretory glands.

HERD IMMUNITY

Overall level of immunity in a community is known as herd immunity. When a large number of individuals in a community (herd) are immune to a pathogen the herd immunity to a pathogen is said to be satisfactory. When herd immunity is low, epidemics are likely to occur on the introduction of the pathogen. This is due to the fact that a larger number of individuals are susceptible.

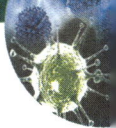

🌱 Key Points

- The *innate system* of immune defence consists of a formidable *barrier to entry* and *second-line phagocytes and circulatory soluble factors*.
- *The cells which mediate immunity include lymphocytes and phagocytes.* Lymphocytes recognize antigens on pathogens. Phagocytes internalize pathogens and degrade them.
- The main phagocytic cells are *polymorphonuclear neutrophils* and *macrophages*.
- *Specificity and memory* are two essential features of acquired Immunity. The immune system mounts a more effective immune response on second and subsequent encounters with a particular antigen.
- Injection of immunologically competent lymphocytes is known as *adoptive immunity*.
- Immunity at the site of invasion and multiplication of a pathogen is known as *local immunity*.
- Overall level of immunity in a community is known as *herd immunity*.
- Components of innate immune system include *phagocytes, natural killer cells*, the *alternative complement pathway* and *inflammation*.

❓ ASSESS YOURSELF

LONG ANSWER QUESTIONS

1. Discuss mechanisms of innate immunity.
2. What is the role of mechanical barriers and surface secretions in providing immunity against infections?
3. What is artificial active immunity? Describe it giving suitable examples.

MULTIPLE CHOICE QUESTIONS

1. Passive immunization is indicated in:
   - (a) Tuberculosis
   - (b) Enteric fever
   - (c) Diphtheria
   - (d) Rubella

2. Lysozyme is present in:
   - (a) Tears
   - (b) CSF
   - (c) Sweat
   - (d) Urine

3. Large parasites such as helminths may be killed extracellularly by the action of:
   - (a) Neutrophils
   - (b) Eosinophils
   - (c) Basophils
   - (d) Monocytes

4. Inflammation is influenced by histamine, which is released by:
   - (a) Basophils
   - (b) Eosinophils
   - (c) Erythrocytes
   - (d) Platelets

5. The cells responsible for killing intracellular viruses are:
   - (a) Natural killer cells
   - (b) Eosinophils
   - (c) Basophils
   - (d) Platelets

6. Which of the following leads to longest-lasting immunity to an infectious agent?
   - (a) Naturally acquired passive immunity
   - (b) Artificially acquired passive immunity
   - (c) Naturally acquired active immunity
   - (d) None of the above

ANSWERS TO MCQsv

1. c   2. a   3. b   4. a   5. a   6. c

Antigen and Antibody

ANTIGEN

Antigens (*antibody* generator) are substances that can stimulate an immune response and, given the opportunity, react specifically by binding with the effector molecules (antibodies) and effector cells (lymphocytes) produced. Most antigens are proteins, but some are carbohydrates, lipids or nucleic acids. Some antigens such as proteins may possess a number of small chemical groups that are called antigenic determinants or **epitopes** which can bind specifically to antigen binding site (**paratope**) of the antibody molecule (Fig. 44.1) and T cell receptors. Each determinant can stimulate the formation of a particular kind of antibody or effector cell. Thus, a pure protein antigen may give rise to many distinct antibodies and effector cells.

Incomplete Antigen or Hapten

This is a chemical substance of low molecular weight that cannot induce an immune response by itself. Nevertheless, haptens can induce a response if combined with larger molecules (normally proteins) which serve as carriers. In contrast to complete antigens, haptens contain a single epitope. In response to hapten carried on carrier particle, antibodies are produced not only against the hapten but also against the carrier particle. The antihapten antibodies produced then bind to the hapten even when it is not linked to the carrier protein. Virtually, any chemical substance can serve as an antigenic determinant or epitope.

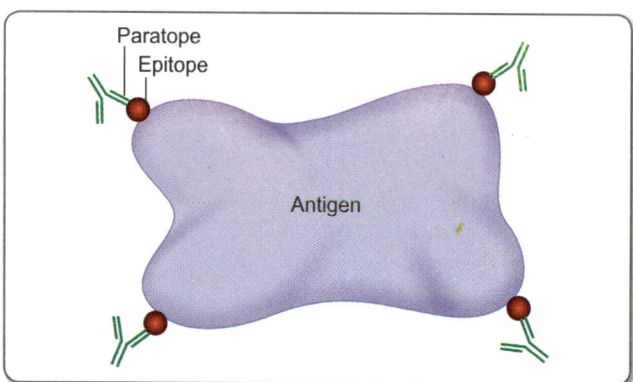

Fig. 44.1: Epitopes of antigen and paratopes of antibody.

Immunogenicity

This refers to the ability of an antigen to stimulate an immune response.

Determinants of Antigenicity

- **Size**
  Antigenicity depends upon the molecular weight. Very large molecules such as haemocyanins are highly antigenic and particles with low molecular weight (less than 5,000) are non-antigenic or feebly so.
- **Foreignness**
  Only antigens which are foreign to the individual (non-self) induce an immune response because host distinguishes self from non-self and normally does not respond to self.
- **Chemical nature**
  Proteins and polysaccharides are most antigenic. Lipids and nucleic acids are less antigenic.
- **Susceptibility to tissue enzymes**
  Only those substances which can be metabolized and are susceptible to the action of tissue enzymes behave as antigens. Antigens introduced into the body are degraded by the host into the fragments of appropriate size containing antigenic determinants. Phagocytosis and intracellular enzymes appear to play an essential role in breaking down antigens into immunogenic fragments.

Antigenic Specificity

It is determined by chemical grouping and acid radicals. Antigenic specificity varies with the position of antigenic determinant, i.e. whether it is in *ortho*, *meta* or *para* positions. However, antigenic specificity is not absolute. Cross reactions can occur between antigens which bear stereochemical similarities.

Species Specificity

Tissues of all individuals in a species contain species-specific antigens. However, some degree of cross reactivity is seen between antigens from related species. **Species-specific antigens possess forensic applications in the identification of species of blood and seminal stains.**

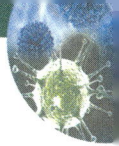

Isospecificity

Isoantigens are antigens found in some but not all members of a species. On the basis of isoantigens a species may be divided into different groups. The best example of isoantigens is human blood group antigens on the basis of which all humans can be divided into different groups—A, B, AB and O. Each of these groups may be further divided into Rh-positive or Rh-negative. **This carries clinical importance in blood transfusion and isoimmunization during pregnancy.**

Histocompatibility Antigens

These are the antigens present on the cells of each individual of a species. Histocompatibility typing is essential in organ/tissue transplantation from one individual to another within a species. These antigens are associated with plasma membrane of tissue cells and are responsible for evoking immunological response against graft unless it is antigenically identical to that of the recipient. These antigens are encoded by genes known as histocompatibility genes which collectively constitute **major histocompatibility complex** (MHC). These are located on short arm of chromosome 6. MHC products present on the surface of leucocytes are known as **human leucocyte-associated (HLA) antigens**. These have been studied extensively in organ transplantation. Major histocompatibility antigens in man and mouse are known as HLA and H2 respectively.

Autospecificity

Autologous or self antigens are ordinarily non-antigenic. However, hidden or sequestrated antigens that are not normally found free in circulation or tissue fluids are not recognized as self antigens. For example, **lens protein** which is normally confined within the capsule of the lens, and antigens that are absent during the embryonic life and develop later, such as **spermatozoa**, are also not recognized as self antigens. But if these antigens are released into the tissues, as for instance following injury to lens or damage to the testis, antibodies are produced against them. This is one of the mechanisms of pathogenesis of autoimmune diseases. Cells or tissues may undergo **antigenic alteration** as a result of infection or irradiation and may thus become immunogenic leading to **autoimmunity**.

Organ Specificity

Some organs such as brain, kidney and lens protein of different species share the same antigens. These are known as organ specific antigens. The neuroparalytic complications following antirabic vaccination are a consequence of brain specific antigens shared by sheep and man.

Heterogenetic (Heterophile) Specificity

Same or closely related antigens occurring in different biological species, classes and kingdoms are known as heterogenetic or heterophile antigens. The best example of such heterophile antigens is the **Forssman antigen** which is a lipid carbohydrate complex widely distributed in man, animals, birds, plants and bacteria. It is absent in rabbits, therefore, anti-forssman antibody can be prepared in these animals. Examples of tests based on the principle of heterophile antigens used in diagnostic serology are as under:

Weil-Felix Reaction

It is an agglutination test in which patient sera are tested for agglutinins to O antigens of non-motile strains of *Proteus* OX2, OX19 and OXK. Cross reaction between O antigen of these strains of *Proteus* and certain rickettsial antigens is the basis of this test.

Paul-Bunnell Test

In patients with infectious mononucleosis heterophile antibodies appear in the serum of the patient. These antibodies agglutinate sheep erythrocytes. This test is known as Paul-Bunnell test.

Cold Agglutinin Test

Agglutination of human O group erythrocytes at 4°C by the sera of patients suffering from primary atypical pneumonia.

Agglutination of Streptococcus MG

Agglutination of *Streptococcus* MG by the sera of the patients of primary atypical pneumonia.

ANTIBODY

Antibodies or immunoglobulins (Igs) are γ globulins which are produced in response to antigenic stimulation. These react specifically with the antigens which stimulated their production. Igs are produced by plasma cells and to some extent by lymphocytes also. On the basis of physicochemical and antigenic structure Igs can be divided into five distinct classes or isotypes namely IgG, IgA, IgM, IgD and IgE.

Antibody Structure

IgG has been studied extensively and serves as a model of basic structural unit of all Igs. It is a Y-shaped four polypeptide chain molecule. Of the four chains, two each are light (L) and heavy (H). These are held together by disulphide bonds (Fig. 44.2). L chain has a molecular weight of 25,000 daltons and H chain 50,000 daltons. H chains are structurally and antigenically distinct for each class and are designated with Greek letters α (alpha), δ (delta), ε (epsilon), γ (gamma) and μ (mu) in IgA, IgD, IgE, IgG and IgM respectively. L chains are of two types—κ (kappa) and

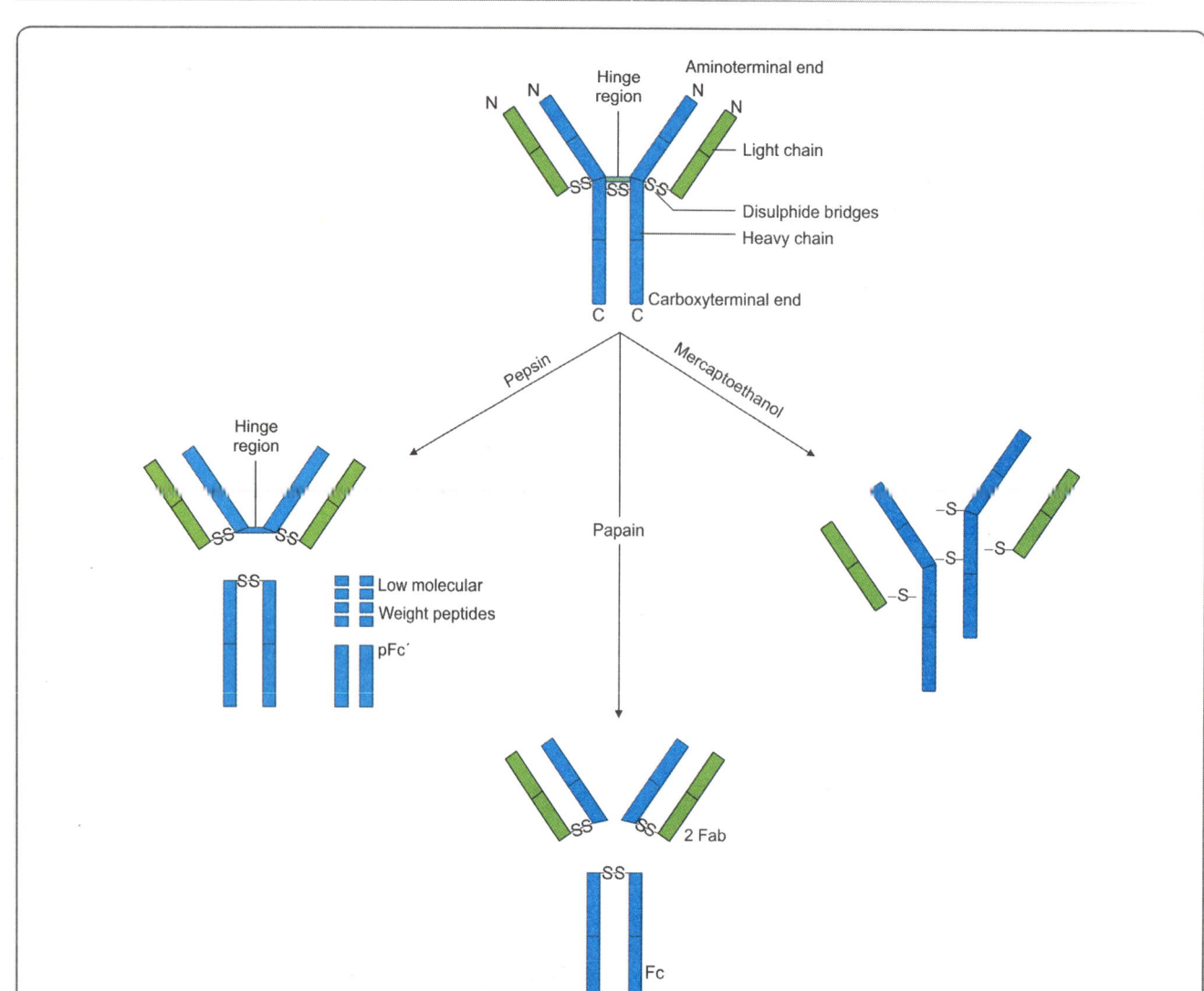

Fig. 44.2: Basic immunoglobulin structure.

λ (lambda). A molecule of Ig may have either κ or λ chains but never both together. κ and λ chains occur in a ratio of about 2 : 1 in human serum.

IgG when treated with proteolytic enzyme papain in the presence of cysteine cleaves it into three fragments. Two identical fragments (45,000 daltons each) still possess the antigen-binding sites and are thus named **fragment antigen binding** or **Fab**. These two fragments represent bivalency of IgG molecule. The third fragment (50,000 daltons) which lacks the ability to bind to antigen can be crystallized. It is, therefore, known as **fragment crystallizable (Fc)**.

Functions of Fc

● Binds complement leading to complement fixation.

● Binds to cell receptors (FcRs).
● Determines passage of IgG across the placental barrier.
● Determines skin fixation and catabolic rate.
● Antigenic determinants that distinguish one class of antibody from another are also located on Fc fragment.

Treatment of the IgG antibody molecule with proteolytic enzyme pepsin cleaves H chains on the carboxy-terminal side of the interchain disulphide bonds of the hinge region. Therefore, 2 Fab fragments remain united. This fragment is designated as $F(ab')_2$ with two antigen-binding sites. Pepsin also degrades part of the Fc portion to small peptides and leaves a dimer of the carboxy-terminal quarter of the chain, termed **pFc′**.

When IgG is treated with reducing agent, such as mercapto-ethanol in the presence of urea, the disulphide bonds are reduced releasing four peptide chains – two heavy and two light.

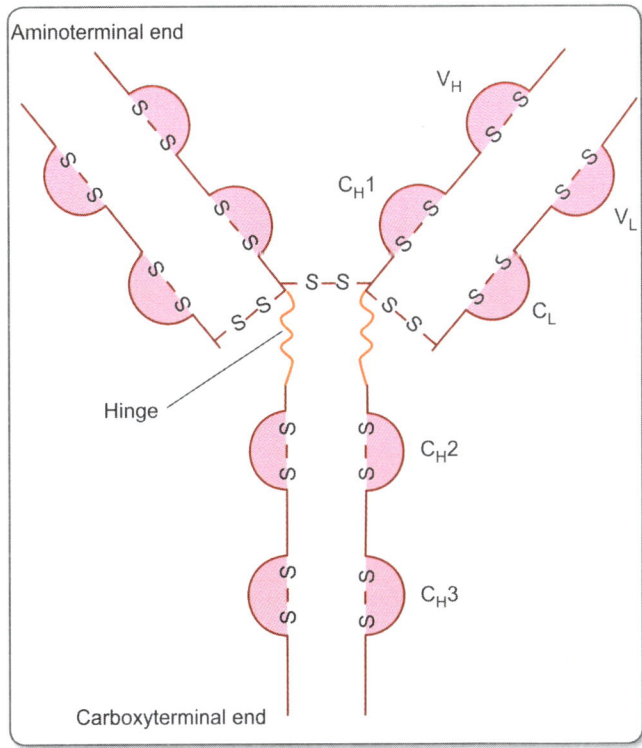

Aminoterminal end

V_H

C_H1

V_L

C_L

S–S

Hinge

C_H2

C_H3

Carboxyterminal end

Fig. 44.3: Variable and constant domains of immunoglobulin molecule.

Structural Basis of Antibody Diversity

Two H chains are always identical in a given molecule and the same is true of L chains. Each H chain of IgG contains 440 amino acids while each L chain contains 220 amino acids. H chain has four domains of 110 amino acids each, while L chain has two domains of 110 amino acids each (Fig. 44.3). The antigen combining sites of the molecule are at its aminoterminal end. These are composed of both H and L chains. Of the 220 amino acids, those that constitute carboxyterminal half of L chain occur in a constant sequence. This part of the chain is called **constant region** (C_L). Only two sequence patterns are seen in constant region of κ and λ chains. On the other hand, amino acid sequence in aminoterminal half of the L chain is highly variable; the variability determines the immunological specificity of the antibody molecule. It is, therefore, called **variable region** (V_L).

A similar pattern is seen in H chains. The variable region of H chain, however, is only 25% as long as constant region. The variable region of H chain like that of L chain has highly variable sequence of amino acids and is known as V_H. The constant region of H chain is divided into three portions C_H1, C_H2 and C_H3. The infinite range of specificity of Igs depends upon the variability of amino acid sequences at the variable regions of H and L chains which form antigen combining sites.

Fd piece

It is the portion of H chains present in Fab fragment. H chains carry a carbohydrate moiety which is distinct for each class of immunoglobulins.

Each Ig peptide chain has internal disulphide links in addition to interchain disulphide bonds which bridge H and L chains. These intrachain disulphide bonds form loops in the peptide chain and each of the loops is completely folded to form a globular domain and each domain has its separate function. Variable region domains V_L and V_H are responsible for the formation of a specific antigen-binding site. C_H2 region in IgG binds C1q in the classical complement sequence and C_H3 domain mediates adherence to monocyte surface. The area of H chain in the C region between C_H1 and C_H2 is the **hinge region**. It is more flexible and is more exposed to enzymes and chemicals.

Immunoglobulin Classes

Human serum contains five classes of immunoglobulins: IgG, IgA, IgM, IgD and IgE. Table 44.1 shows their differentiating features.

Immunoglobulin G

This is the most abundant class of Ig in the body constituting approximately 75% of the total Igs. This is distributed equally within the intravascular and extravascular pools. Very little IgG is produced during the early stages of the primary response to antigen, but it is the major form of antibody produced during the secondary response. It is not synthesized by the foetus in any significant amounts. IgG is also most commonly seen **myeloma protein**. It has a half-life of 21 days. The normal serum concentration of IgG is about 12 mg/ml. It is a glycoprotein with a molecular weight of 150,000 daltons.

There are **four subclasses** of human IgG (IgG1, IgG2, IgG3 and IgG4). Each subclass possesses a distinct type of γ chain which can be identified with specific antiserum. They constitute about 59%, 30%, 8% and 3% respectively of the total human IgG. All normal humans possess all four subclasses of IgG, just as they possess all classes of Igs. IgG binds complement in classical pathway. IgG3 is most effective in binding complement followed by IgG1 and IgG2. It can bind to protein A (from *Staphylococcus aureus*) and protein G (from group G streptococci). IgG is the only class of Igs that can cross the placenta and is responsible for the protection of the infant during first few months of life. However, subclass IgG2 does not cross the placenta. IgG is also found, along with IgA, in milk during the first few weeks after birth, providing additional protection if the infant is breast-fed.

Macrophages and monocytes bear Fc receptors (FcRs) which bind to the Fc portion of IgG1 and IgG3 in C_H3 domain. Such binding permits these cells to exhibit antibody-dependent cellular toxicity. IgG usually exhibits high affinity for antigens leading to efficient neutralization of toxins. Among null cells, a distinct subpopulation of cytotoxic cells has been recognized which also possesses FcRs for Fc part of IgG. They are capable of lysing or killing target cells sensitized with IgG. They are known as **killer cells**. They are responsible for **antibody-dependent cell-mediated cytotoxicity (ADCC)**. Platelets also possess FcRs for Fc portion of IgG leading to aggregation, degranulation and release of histamine. IgG is the only Ig which has the property of fixing to guinea pig skin.

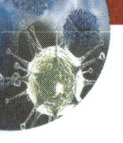

TABLE 44.1: Properties of various immunoglobulin classes

	IgG	IgA	IgM	IgD	IgE
Molecular weight in kDa	150	160,385	900	180	190
Sedimentation coefficient (s)	7	7, 11	19	7	8
Carbohydrate content (%)	3	8	12	13	12
Heavy chain	$\gamma_1, \gamma_2, \gamma_3, \gamma_4$	α_1, α_2	μ	δ	ϵ
Light chain	κ or λ	κ or λ	κ or λ	κ or λ	κ or λ
Serum concentration (mg/ml)	12	2	1.2	0.03	0.00004
Half-life (days)	21	6	5	3	2
Complement binding	Classical pathway	Alternative pathway	Classical pathway	None	None
Binding to tissue	Heterologous	None	None	None	Homologous
Secretion from serous membranes	No	Yes*	No	No	Yes
Placental passage	Yes	No	No	No	No
Heat stability (56°C)	Yes	Yes	Yes	Yes	No

Secretory IgA.

Catabolism of IgG is unique in that it varies with its serum concentration. When its level is raised, as in chronic malaria, kala-azar or myeloma, the IgG synthesized against a particular antigen will be catabolised rapidly and may result in the particular antibody deficiency. Conversely, in hypogammaglobulinaemia, the IgG given for treatment will be catabolised slowly.

IgG participates in most immunological reactions such as complement fixation, precipitation and neutralization of toxins and viruses. Passively administered IgG suppresses the homologous antibody synthesis by a feedback process. This property is utilized for prevention of isoimmunization of Rh-negative mother bearing Rh-positive baby by administration of anti-Rh (D) IgG at the time of delivery.

Immunoglobulin M

It is so named because it is a macroglobulin at least five times larger than IgG. It is a glycoprotein with molecular weight of about 900,000–1,000,000 daltons (millionaire molecule). It is present on the surface of virtually all uncommitted B cells. About 10% of normal serum Igs consist of this class. The normal serum level of IgM is 1.2 mg/ml. It has a half-life of about 5 days. IgM normally exists as a pentamer, consisting of 5 Ig subunits (Fig. 44.4).

In contrast to IgG, IgM remains almost exclusively in the serum and is not usually found extravascularly in body cavities or secretions. Therefore, IgM is believed to be responsible for protection against blood invasion by microorganisms. Pentameric IgM is apparently too large to cross the placenta. The H μ chain has four C_H domains rather than three as seen in H chains of IgG. H chains are held together by disulphide bonds between C_H3 domains. There is an additional peptide chain called the

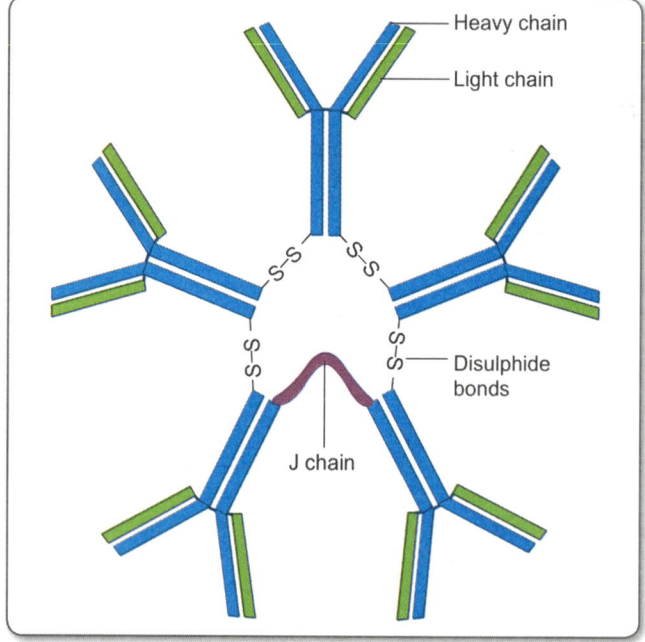

Fig. 44.4: IgM immunoglobulin.

joining (J) chain. The J chain may be largely responsible for the polymerization process, which occurs shortly before the molecule is secreted by plasma cell.

IgM contains 10 Fab fragments, and thus 10 antigen-binding sites. Therefore, theoretically it can bind to 10 antigen molecules. However, it appears that many antigens are so large that when bound to one site, they physically prevent the binding of another antigen molecule to an adjacent binding site. Thus, generally, IgM is capable of binding as few as five molecules of antigen.

Phylogenetically IgM is the oldest Ig class. It is usually the first antibody to appear following stimulation by an antigen. However, IgM synthesis is usually not prolonged, and IgG antibodies soon become the most prevalent class. IgM is also the earliest to be synthesized by foetus beginning by about **20 weeks of gestation**. As it cannot cross the placental barrier, the presence of IgM in the foetus or newborn indicates intrauterine infection. Its detection is, therefore, useful for the diagnosis of congenital syphilis, rubella, HIV infection, and toxoplasmosis. IgM antibodies are relatively short-lived, hence their demonstration in the serum indicates recent infection. Treatment of serum with 0.12 M 2-mercaptoethanol selectively destroys IgM without affecting IgG antibodies. This provides a simple method for differential estimation of IgG and IgM antibodies.

IgM is much more efficient than IgG in its ability to fix complement, promoting lysis and death of most Gram-negative bacteria. This greater efficacy is due to the fact that complement may bind to several Fc regions of pentameric IgM simultaneously thus initiating complement cascade and target cell lysis with a single molecule. IgM is also more effective than IgG in opsonization, bactericidal action and in bacterial agglutination. However, in neutralization of toxins and viruses, it is less active than IgG.

Isohaemagglutinins (anti-A and anti-B) and antibodies to *Salmonella* serotype Typhi O antigen and Wassermann reaction antibodies in syphilis are usually IgM. In certain disease states such as lupus erythematosus and rheumatoid arthritis, IgM may occur in monomeric form in high concentration. Monomeric IgM has lower avidity for antigen than does the pentameric form.

Immunoglobulin A

The basic structure of IgA is similar to that of IgG. It contains two identical light chains (either κ or λ) and two heavy α chains. It is the second most abundant class, constituting about 15% of human serum Igs where it exists as a monomeric Ig. More important form is the dimeric form, known as **secretory IgA (sIgA)**. It is the predominant class of Igs in secretions such as milk, tears, nasal secretions, saliva, perspiration, genitourinary secretions and seromucous secretions.

On mucus surfaces sIgA antibodies form an antibody paste and is believed to play an important role in local immunity against respiratory and intestinal pathogens. sIgA is relatively resistant to digestive enzymes and reducing agents. Many infectious organisms cause disease by attaching to glycoproteins on the surface of epithelial cells of secretory gland. If this adhesion is sufficiently strong, the organism will divide, establish a colony and cause disease by any of a number of mechanisms, e.g. secretion of toxins that cause local and systemic injury. Secretory IgA when present in the secretions prevents attachment of organisms to epithelial cells thus preventing adhesion, colonization and infection.

Serum IgA is principally a 7S molecule with a molecular weight of 160,000 daltons. Secretory IgA is synthesized by

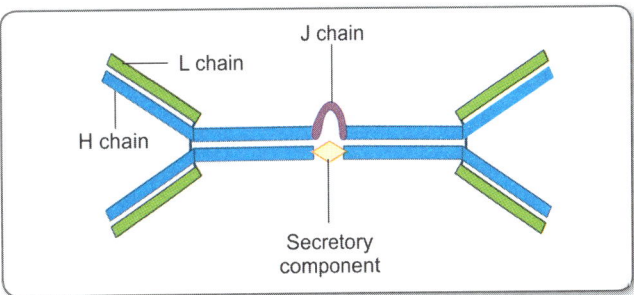

Fig. 44.5: Secretory IgA.

plasma cells in the subepithelial tissue and secreted as a dimer containing four heavy chains, four light chains and one **J chain** which is similar to J chain found in pentameric IgM (Fig. 44.5). sIgA also possesses an additional structural unit called secretory component (SC). It is synthesized not in lymphoid cells but in epithelial cells of glands of intestine, and the respiratory tract and is attached to IgA molecules at their Fc portions producing 11S dimer with a molecular weight of 385,000 daltons. sIgA is relatively resistant to digestive enzymes, which may be due to the secretory component. IgA does not fix complement in classical pathway but can activate the alternative complement pathway. It promotes phagocytosis and intracellular killing of microorganisms.

There are two subclasses of IgA in humans—IgA1 and IgA2. In serum, IgA1 constitutes 80%–90% of IgA while sIgA consists of about equal amounts of the two subclasses.

Certain streptococci and pathogenic *Neisseria* produce proteases that specifically cleave the heavy chain of IgA1. IgA2 is resistant to such cleavage because it has a shorter hinge region and lacks the proline-rich site cleaved by the proteases.

Immunoglobulin D

Like other monomeric antibodies IgD is composed of two light and two heavy chains. The latter are designated as δ chains. It contains about 13% carbohydrate. Its molecular weight is 180,000 daltons. It does not bind complement. It does not cross placenta and does not bind to cells via Fc region. IgD is present on the surface of B lymphocytes which are destined to differentiate into antibody-producing plasma cells and its serum concentration is very low (0.03 mg/ml). Reaction of antigen with surface immunoglobulin may lead to cell differentiation and antibody synthesis.

Immunoglobulin E

It resembles IgG structurally. Its molecular weight is 190,000 daltons. Its half-life is about two days. It does not fix complement or cross placental barrier. In contrast to other Igs it is heat-labile and gets inactivated by heating it at 56°C for 30 minutes. It is susceptible to 2-mercaptoethanol. It is chiefly produced in the linings of the respiratory and intestinal tracts.

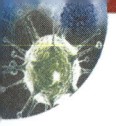

It is present in extremely low concentrations (0.00004 mg/ml) in the serum. But raised serum levels are seen in atopic (type I hypersensitivity) conditions like asthma and hay fever.

Most of a person's IgE is fixed to the surface of mast cells and basophils and when a specific antigen binds with IgE bound to mast cell or basophil membrane, the reaction results in the release of pharmacologically active substances such as histamine and serotonin which dilate capillaries, increase vascular permeability and cause bronchial constriction. Fc portion of IgE binds to the Fc receptors present on the surface of mast cells and basophils leaving antigen-binding sites free to react with specific antigen.

So far, no beneficial effect of IgE has been identified. It has been observed that IgE levels may rise following infections with parasites especially helminths. It has been suggested that mast cell-bound IgE reacts with antigens on the parasite followed by release of histamine. This results in increased vascular permeability followed by influx of plasma and cells (particularly eosinophils) and destruction of parasite. IgE mediates **Prausnitz-Kustner reaction**.

From available information it appears that:

IgG : Protects the body fluids
IgA : Protects the body surfaces
IgM : Protects the blood stream
IgE : Mediates type I hypersensitivity
IgD : Present on the surface of B lymphocytes

which are destined to differentiate into antibody producing plasma cells.

Key Points

- **Antigens** are substances that can stimulate an immune response and, given the opportunity, react specifically by binding with the effector molecules (antibodies) and effector cells (lymphocytes).
- A substance capable of eliciting immune response is known as **immunogen**.
- **Antibodies** or immunoglobulins are γ globulins which are produced in response to antigenic stimulation. These react specifically with the antigens which stimulated their production.
- **The immunoglobulins have a basic unit of two light chains and two heavy chains in a light-heavy-light arrangement.**
- **There are five classes of antibody – IgG, IgA, IgM, IgD and IgE.**
- IgG is the **most abundant** class of immunoglobulins in the body constituting approximately 75% of total immunoglobulins.
- **Joining (J) chain** is present in **IgM** and **secretory IgA**.
- **Secretory IgA** is relatively **resistant to digestive enzymes**, which may be due to the **secretory component** of this immunoglobulin.
- In contrast to other immunoglobulins, **IgE** is **heat-labile** and gets inactivated by heating at 56°C for 30 minutes.

? Assess Yourself

Long Answer Questions

1. What is an antigen? Discuss briefly various determinants of antigenicity.
2. What are heterophile antigens? Name various serological tests which are based on the principle of heterophile antigens. Discuss briefly their principles and uses.
3. What is an antibody? Draw labelled diagram of IgG, IgA and IgM.
4. Name various classes of immunoglobulins and describe structure and functions of IgG, IgA and IgM.

Multiple Choice Questions

1. The chemical nature of an antigen may be:
   (a) Protein
   (b) Polysaccharide
   (c) Lipid
   (d) All of the above

Contd...

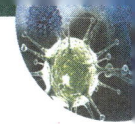

? ASSESS YOURSELF

2. The determinants of antigenicity is/are:
   (a) Size of the antigen
   (b) Foreignness
   (c) Chemical nature
   (d) All of the above

3. Isoantigens are:
   (a) Antigens found in all members of a species
   (b) Antigens found in some members of a species
   (c) Antigens found in all members of different species
   (d) Antigens found in some members of different species

4. The function/s of Fc fragment of IgG is/are:
   (a) It binds complement
   (b) It is related to passage of IgG across the placental barrier
   (c) It determines catabolic rate
   (d) All of the above

5. Which immunoglobulin class is heat-labile?
   (a) IgG
   (b) IgM
   (c) IgA
   (d) IgE

6. IgG participates in which of the following reactions?
   (a) Complement fixation
   (b) Precipitation
   (c) Neutralization of toxins and viruses
   (d) All of the above

7. J chain is present in:
   (a) IgG
   (b) IgM
   (c) IgD
   (d) IgE

8. IgM is the earliest class of immunoglobulin to be synthesized by foetus beginning by about:
   (a) 15 weeks of gestation
   (b) 20 weeks of gestation
   (c) 25 weeks of gestation
   (d) 30 weeks of gestation

ANSWERS TO MCQs

1. d   **2.** d   **3.** b   **4.** d   **5.** d   **6.** d   **7.** b   **8.** b

45 Chapter

Antigen-Antibody Reactions

When an antigen is mixed with its specific antibody, in the presence of electrolytes at a suitable temperature and pH, they combine with each other in an observable manner. **In the body** they form the basis of:

- Antibody-mediated immunity in infectious diseases.
- Tissue injury in some types of hypersensitivity and autoimmune diseases.

In the laboratory, they help in the diagnosis of:
- Infectious diseases.
- Noninfectious agents such as enzymes.

These reactions can be used for the detection and quantitation of either antigen or antibody. Antigen-antibody reactions *in vitro* are known as serological reactions.

CHARACTERISTICS OF ANTIGEN-ANTIBODY REACTIONS

- Antigen-antibody reaction is specific but cross reactions may occur.
- Antigen-antibody combination is firm but reversible.
- Binding takes place on the surface. Therefore, surface antigens are more relevant.
- Entire molecules react. Therefore, when an antigenic determinant present on a large molecule or a carrier particle reacts with antibody, whole molecules or particles are agglutinated.

For better understanding of antigen-antibody reactions a few terms are defined below:

Affinity: Intensity of the attraction between an antibody-combining site and an antigenic determinant.

Avidity: Strength of the bond after the formation of antigen-antibody complexes.

Sensitivity: Ability of a test to identify correctly all those who have the disease i.e. true positives. A 90% sensitivity means that 90% of the diseased persons screened by the test will give a true positive and 10% a false negative result.

Contd...

Specificity: Ability of a test to identify correctly all those who do not have the disease i.e. true negatives. A 90% specificity means that 90% of non-diseased persons screened by the test will give a true negative and 10% a false positive result. In other words, 10% of non-diseased persons will be wrongly classified as diseased when they are not.

TYPES OF ANTIGEN ANTIBODY REACTIONS

Precipitation Reactions

Precipitation

When a soluble antigen is mixed with its specific antibody in the presence of electrolytes at a suitable temperature and pH, the antigen-antibody complex forms an insoluble precipitate. This precipitate usually settles down at the bottom of the tube. Precipitation can take place in liquid media and in gels such as agar, agarose and polyacrylamide. The process of precipitation can be hastened by electrically driving the antigen and antibody.

Flocculation

When instead of sedimenting the precipitate remains suspended as floccules, the reaction is called flocculation.

Zone Phenomenon

If a series (10–12) of tubes is set up (Fig. 45.1), each containing a constant amount of antiserum, and increasing amounts of antigen are added to the tubes in the row, precipitation will be found to occur most rapidly and abundantly in one of the middle tubes, in which antigen and antibody are in optimal or equivalent proportion. In the preceding tubes, in which the antibody is in excess, and in the later tubes, in which the antigen is in excess, the precipitation will be weak or absent. Therefore, the amount of precipitation will be seen to increase along the row, reaching a maximum and then falling off with higher antigen concentration.

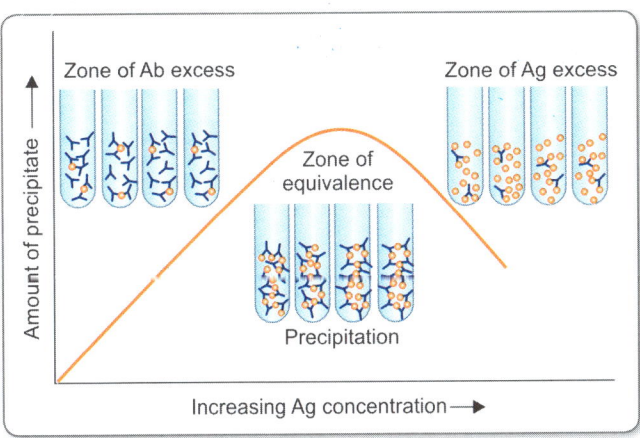

Fig. 45.1: Zone phenomenon.

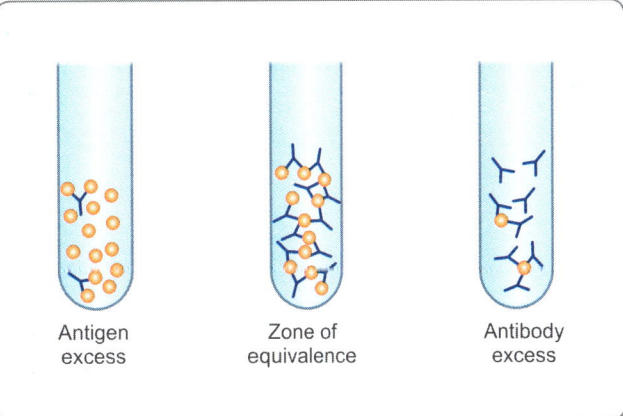

Fig. 45.2: Lattice formation.

If the amounts of precipitate in different tubes are plotted on a graph, the resulting curve will have **three phases**—an ascending part (**prozone** or zone of antibody excess), a peak (**zone** of equivalence), and a descending part (**postzone** or zone of antigen excess). This is called **zone phenomenon**. Assay of supernatant solution will show that those tubes containing too little antigen still contain free antibody and in the tubes with antigen excess, little precipitate forms, although soluble immune complexes and free antigens are present in the supernatant fluid. Only in tubes of maximum precipitation is all antibody removed from solution. *The prozone is of importance in clinical serology as sera rich in antibody may sometimes give false negative results, unless several dilutions are tested.*

Mechanism of Precipitation

To explain the mechanism of precipitation, Marrack, 1934 proposed a lattice hypothesis. Multivalent antigens combine with bivalent antibodies in varying proportions, depending upon the antigens and antibodies in the reacting mixture. When the antigens and antibodies are in optimal proportion a large lattice is formed consisting of alternating antigen and antibody molecules. Therefore, most abundant precipitation occurs when both antigens and antibodies are in optimal proportion. In antibody excess each antigen or two combine with an independent molecule of antibody. Therefore, the lattice does not enlarge. Similarly, in antigen excess the lattice does not enlarge (Fig. 45.2).

Applications of Precipitation Reactions

Some of the precipitation and flocculation tests which have application in diagnostic bacteriology are as under:

Ring Test

This test is done by layering antigen solution over a column of antiserum in a capillary tube. After a short while a ring of precipitate forms at the interface. Typing of streptococci and pneumococci, C-reactive protein test and Ascoli's thermo-precipitin test for the diagnosis of anthrax, are some of the uses of ring test.

Slide Test

This is an example of flocculation test. When a drop each of antigen and antiserum are placed on a slide and mixed by shaking, floccules appear. VDRL, a most widely used test for the diagnosis of syphilis, is an example of slide flocculation test.

Tube Test

Flocculation test can be carried out in the tubes also. Kahn test for syphilis and standardization of toxins and toxoids are examples of tube flocculation.

Immunodiffusion (Precipitation in Gel)

When an antibody and its antigen are placed in an agar gel they diffuse towards each other and form an opaque band of precipitation at the junction of their diffusion front.

Types of Immunodiffusion Tests

Single diffusion in one dimension (Oudin procedure)

Antibody is incorporated in agar gel in a test tube. Antigen solution is then layered over it. The antigen diffuses downwards and wherever it reaches in optimum concentration with antibody a line of precipitation is formed (Fig. 45.3A). As more antigen diffuses, the line of precipitation moves downwards. Number of lines of precipitation indicates the number of antigens and antibodies present.

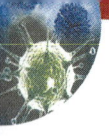

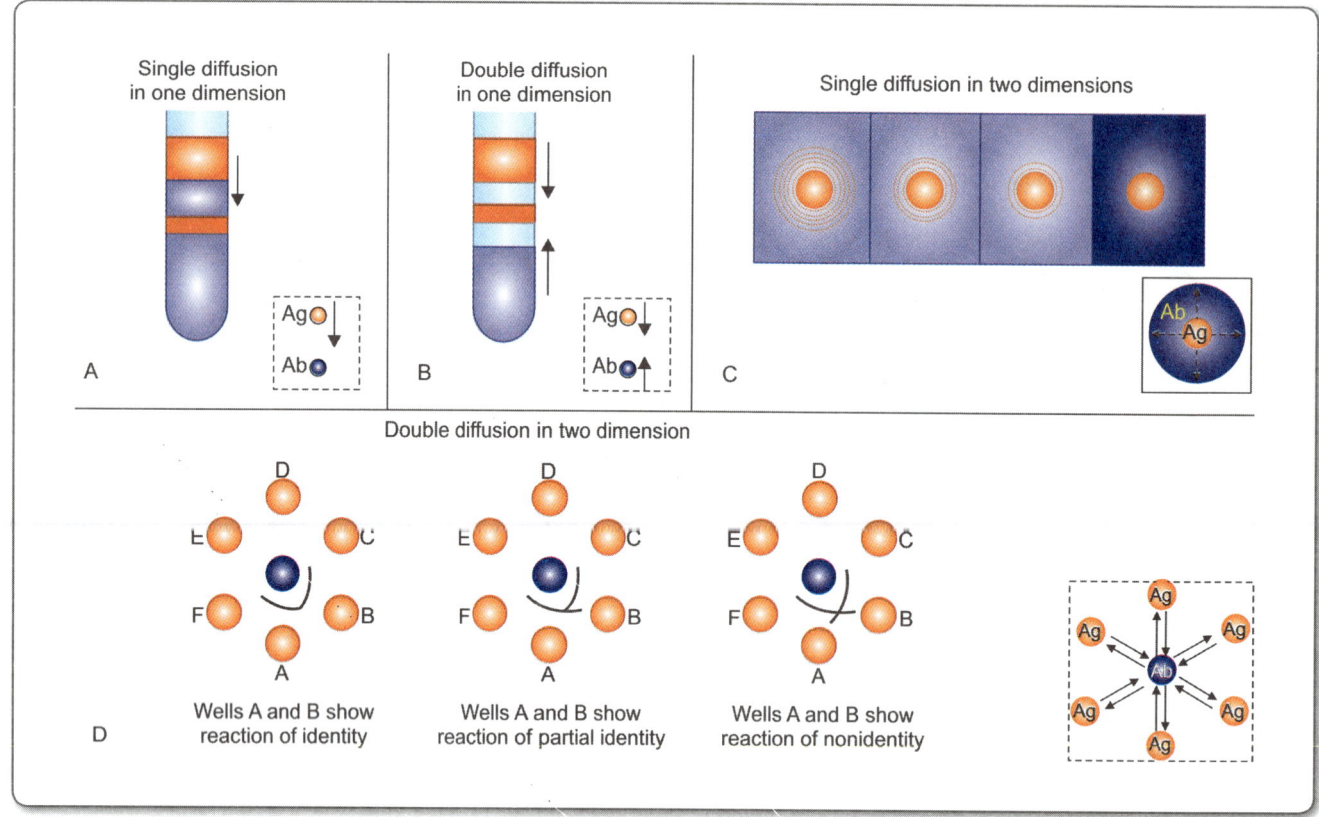

Fig. 45.3: Immunodiffusion.

Double diffusion in one dimension (Oakley-Fulthorpe)

Antibody is incorporated in agar gel in a test tube. Above this is placed a column of plain agar which in turn is overlaid with antigen, either as liquid or incorporated into agar (Fig. 45.3B). Antigen and antibody diffuse (double diffusion) towards each other (in one dimension) through the intervening column of plain agar and form a band of precipitation where they meet in optimum concentration.

Single diffusion in two dimensions (Radial immunodiffusion)

Here monospecific antiserum (antiserum containing only antibody against the antigen which is to be assayed) is incorporated in agar gel. It is poured on a glass slide or a petri dish and a number of wells are punched into it, and different dilutions of the antigen are placed into various wells. As the antigen diffuses from the well, a ring of precipitate forms at that position where antigen and antibody are in optimal proportions. Larger the concentration of antigen, the farther it diffuses to be in optimal proportions with the antibody incorporated in the gel. Therefore, the diameter of the ring gives the estimate of the concentration of the antigen (Fig. 45.3C).

Double diffusion in two dimensions (Ouchterlony procedure)

Agar is poured on the slide and wells, usually seven, are punched in it using a template. The known antiserum is placed in the central well and different antigens in surrounding wells. One of these contains known positive antigen. It acts as a positive control. This technique is also useful for comparing different antigens for the presence of identical or cross reacting components. The samples are placed in adjacent wells, and the corresponding antibody is placed in the central well.

Reaction of Identity

If two precipitin bands fuse completely (Fig. 45.3D), the pattern is termed reaction of identity. It indicates that the antigens in the adjoining wells are identical.

Reaction of Nonidentity

If unrelated antigens are placed in adjacent wells, they diffuse towards central well containing antibodies for both, the two precipitin bands form independently and cross each other. This is known as reaction of nonidentity.

Reaction of Partial Identity

If the antigens in the two adjacent wells are cross reacting (partial identity), the precipitation bands fuse but form a spurlike projection. This is known as reaction of partial identity.

A special variety of double diffusion in two dimensions is the **Elek's test** for toxigenicity of diphtheria bacilli.

Immunoelectrophoresis

Immunoelectrophoresis combines electrophoresis and immuno-diffusion (immune precipitation in gel). This method can be used for analyzing complex antigens in biological fluids. A glass slide is covered with molten agar or agarose. A well for antigen and a trough for antiserum is cut on it (Fig. 45.4). Antigen well is filled with antigen mixture (human serum). The slide is then placed in an electric field for about an hour to allow for the electrophoretic migration of various antigens. Different antigens will migrate at different rates or even in different directions, depending upon their size and charge and the conditions of electrophoresis.

After the completion of electrophoresis, antiserum trough is filled with appropriate antiserum (antiserum to whole human serum). Antigens and antibodies diffuse towards each other, resulting in the formation of precipitin bands, for individual antigens and antibodies, where they are both in zones of optimal proportions, in 18–24 hours. Because immunoelectrophoresis uses electric charge in addition to diffusion, it is more likely to separate antigen than is simple diffusion alone. By this method, over 30 different antigens can be identified in human serum. This technique is useful for detection of normal and abnormal serum proteins.

Electroimmunodiffusion

Immunodiffusion is a slow process. The development of precipitin lines can be speeded up by electrically driving antigens and antibodies in a gel, rather than simply allowing them to come in contact by diffusion. Of these, one dimensional double electroimmunodiffusion and one dimensional single electroimmunodiffusion are used frequently in the clinical laboratory.

- *One-dimensional double electroimmunodiffusion (counterimmunoelectrophoresis or CIE):* This method can be used for those antigens and antibodies that migrate in opposite directions in electric field. The wells are punched about 1 cm apart in an agar slab on a glass plate. Antigen and antibody solutions are placed in wells towards cathode and anode sides respectively. Electric field is then applied electrophoresing both antigens and antibodies from separate wells. The antigen migrates towards antibody and antibody migrates towards antigen. A precipitin band is formed, in between the two wells, where they meet in optimum proportions (Fig. 45.5). This method has several advantages over simple diffusion in agar.
  - The electrophoresis forces the reactants into a small area allowing the detection of small quantities of antigens and antibodies. Therefore, **it is 10 times more sensitive than simple diffusion in agar**.
  - It is a rapid assay. Precipitin bands may form in just 30 minutes.

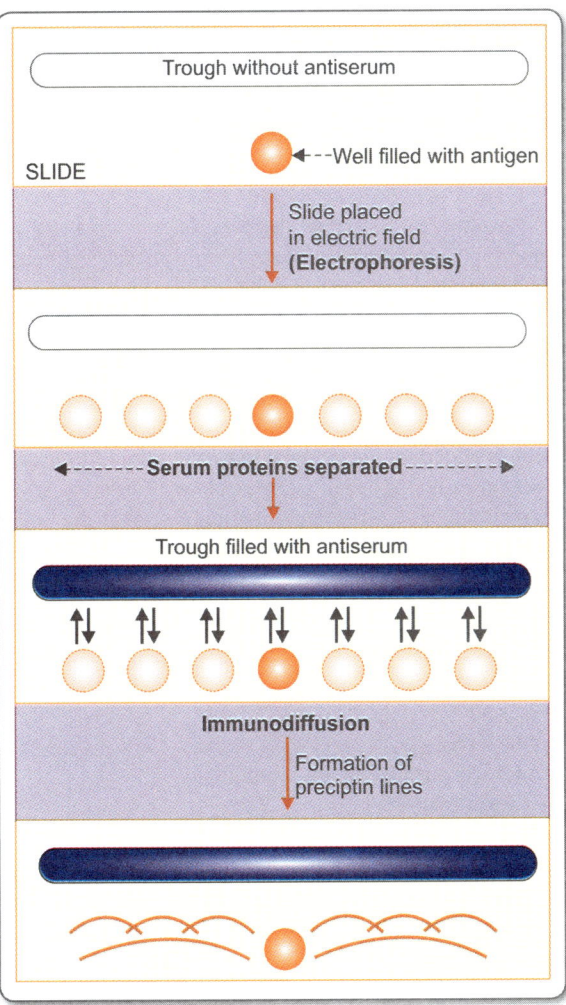

Fig. 45.4: Immunoelectrophoresis.

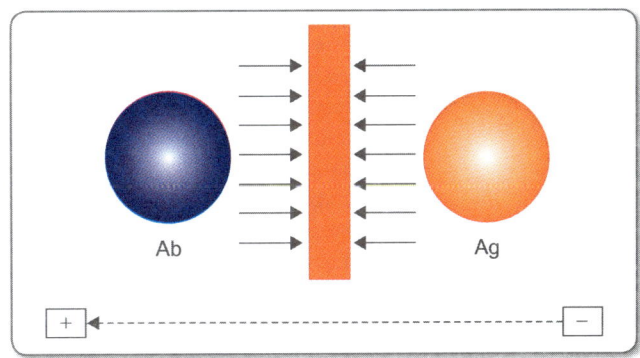

Fig. 45.5: Counterimmunoelectrophoresis.

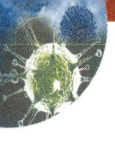

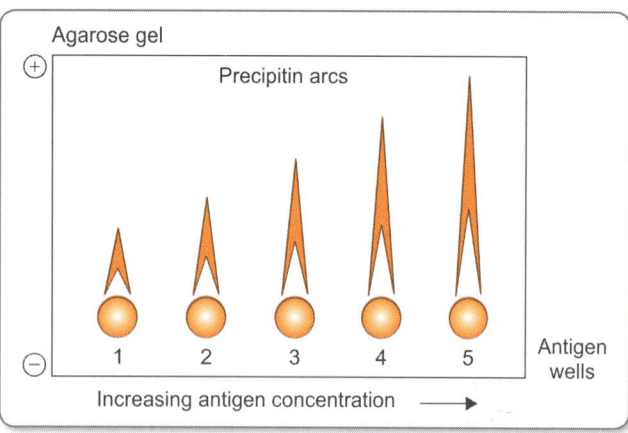

Fig. 45.6: Rocket electrophoresis.

This method is used for detection of various antigens such as:

- hepatitis B surface antigen (HBsAg) and alpha-fetoprotein in serum;
- meningococcal and cryptococcal antigens in CSF; and
- detection of anti-DNA antibody in the serum of patients with several autoimmune disorders.

- *One-dimensional single electroimmunodiffusion (rocket electrophoresis):* As in case of radial immunodiffusion, wells are cut in an agarose gel slab on a glass plate. Agarose contains the antiserum to the antigen of interest. The antigen, in increasing concentrations, is placed in wells. The antigen is then electrophoresed into the agarose containing antibody that does not migrate. The pattern of immunoprecipitation resembles a rocket (hence the name), since precipitation occurs along the moving boundary of antigen, as it migrates into the agarose (Fig. 45.6). The height (distance from the antigen well to the top of the precipitin band) is proportional to the antigen concentration. The main application of this technique, therefore, is for quantitative estimation of antigen.

Agglutination Reactions

When a particulate antigen or an antigen present on the surface of a cell (red cell or bacterium) or an inorganic particle (e.g. polystyrene latex coated with antigen) is mixed with its antibody in the presence of electrolytes at a suitable temperature and pH, the particles are clumped or agglutinated. This reaction is analogous to precipitation reaction, in that antibody merely acts as a bridge to form a lattice network of antibody and cells or inorganic particles coated with antigen. Because cells or particles are much larger than soluble antigen, therefore, they aggregate into clumps. Agglutination reaction is more sensitive than precipitation for detection of antibodies.

- **Prozone phenomenon:**
  False negative agglutination reactions can occur with some antisera in antibody excess (first few dilutions). This is known as prozone phenomenon. Unagglutinated cells in prozone actually have antibody molecules adsorbed on their surface, with both sites of bivalent antibody attached to the same cell resulting into poor or no lattice formation.

- **Blocking antibodies:**
  Occasionally, antibodies (e.g. anti-Rh and anti-*Brucella*) are formed that react with the antigenic determinants on a cell but do not cause agglutination. Such antibodies are called blocking antibodies, because they inhibit agglutination by complete antibody added subsequently.

Applications of Agglutination Reactions

Slide Agglutination

A drop of saline is placed on a clean glass slide and a small amount of culture from a solid medium is emulsified in it by means of inoculating loop. It is then examined through a hand lens or low-power microscope that the suspension is even and bacteria are not autoagglutinable. Then with a platinum loop a drop of specific antiserum is placed on the slide near the bacterial suspension. The serum and the bacterial suspension are then mixed and examined with naked eye or with hand lens or under low-power microscope for the evidence of agglutination within a minute. Slide agglutination test is rapid and convenient, but in order to obtain rapid agglutination serum is used undiluted or in low dilutions.

Uses

- Identification of bacterial isolates (e.g. *Salmonella* spp. *Shigella* spp. and *Vibrio cholerae*) from clinical specimens.
- Blood grouping and cross matching.

Tube Agglutination

This is done in round-bottomed test tubes or perspex plates with round-bottomed wells. A fixed volume of a particulate antigen suspension is added to an equal volume of serial dilutions of the patient serum in test tubes or perspex plates. Following several hours of incubation at 37°C, agglutination is seen at the bottom of the tubes. The titre of the serum is given as the reciprocal of the highest dilution that causes agglutination.

Uses

Serological diagnosis of:

- Enteric fever.
- Brucellosis.
- Typhus fever.
- Streptotococcus MG agglutination.
- Cold agglutination.
- Paul-Bunnel test.

In the **Widal test** used for the diagnosis of enteric fever, two types of antigens are used—the flagellar (H) antigen and somatic (O) antigen. H antigen is a formolised suspension of the organisms which on combination with antibody, forms large, loose and fluffy clumps resembling wisps of cotton-wool. For H agglutination conical (Dreyer's) tubes are used. O antigen is prepared by

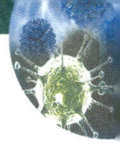

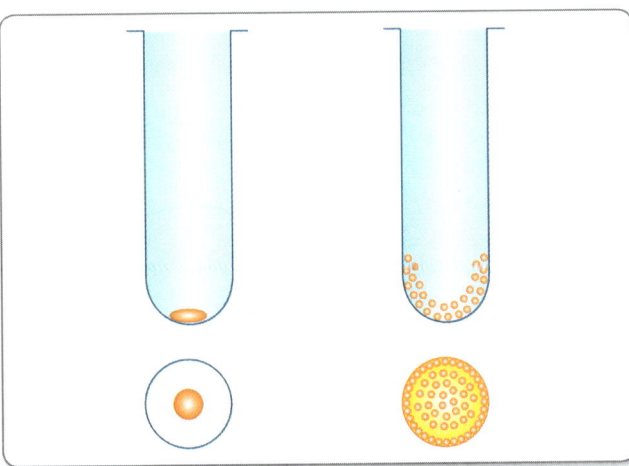

Fig. 45.7: Tube agglutination test.

treating the bacterial suspension with alcohol. On combination with antibody it forms fine granular deposit resembling chalk powder at the base of round-bottomed (Felix) tubes, whereas, negative reaction shows a compact button-like deposit (Fig. 45.7).

Tube agglutination test for brucellosis may be complicated by prozone phenomenon and the presence of blocking antibodies. To avoid false negative results due to prozone, several dilutions of the serum should be tested. *Blocking antibodies may be detected by doing the test in hypertonic (5%) saline, albumin saline or more reliably by the antiglobulin (Coombs') test.* Rh antibodies are also blocking antibodies.

Heterophile Agglutination

Weil-Felix reaction for serodiagnosis of typhus fever and *Streptococcus* **MG agglutination** for the diagnosis of primary atypical pneumonia are the examples of heterophile agglutination test.

Antiglobulin (Coombs') Test

Anti-Rh antibodies are of IgG type, but they normally do not agglutinate Rh-positive RBCs (blocking antibodies). The inability of these antibodies to agglutinate is perhaps due to the presence of insufficient antigenic determinants on the RBCs to permit the antibody to overcome the normal electrostatic repulsion that exists among RBCs. When sera containing blocking anti-Rh antibodies are mixed with Rh-positive red cells, the antibody coats the surface of erythrocytes but they are not agglutinated. When such antibody-coated erythrocytes are washed to free all unattached protein and are treated with anti-human gammaglobulin (**antiglobulin or Coombs' serum**), the cells are agglutinated.

Coombs' test is of two types—direct and indirect.
1. **Direct Coombs' test:** The sensitization of erythrocytes with incomplete antibodies takes place *in vivo* as in case of haemolytic disease of newborn due to Rh incompatibility.

Therefore, when washed RBCs from such patient are mixed with antiglobulin, agglutination takes place.
2. **Indirect Coombs' test:** The sensitization of RBCs with incomplete antibodies is performed *in vitro*. Rh-positive RBCs are mixed with the serum to be tested for Rh-antibodies and then after a short incubation and washing, antiglobulin or Coombs' serum is added. If the test serum contained anti-Rh antibodies, agglutination will take place.

Passive (Indirect) Agglutination

A precipitation reaction can be converted into agglutination reaction by coating soluble antigen onto the surface of carrier particles such as RBCs, latex, bentonite and gelatin particles. Such test is more convenient and more sensitive for detection of antibodies. Some of the examples of passive agglutination are given below:

- In rheumatoid arthritis, **RA factor** (an antigammaglobulin autoantibody) appears in the serum of the patient. It acts as an antibody to human IgG. Latex polystyrene beads coated with denatured human IgG when mixed with patient serum leads to agglutination of latex polystyrene beads.
- Latex particles coated with antibodies to meningococci, *Haemophilus influenzae* type b and pneumococci can be used to detect corresponding antigens in cases of **pyogenic meningitis**.
- Latex agglutination tests are also widely used for detection of hepatitis B, antistreptolysin O, C-reactive protein, human chorionic gonadotropin hormone and many other antigens.
- One of the most widely used passive agglutination test employing erythrocytes is **Treponema pallidum haemagglutination (TPHA)** for serological diagnosis of treponemal infection.
- For the detection of **anti-HIV antibodies**, gelatin particles can be sensitized (coated) with inactivated HIV antigen. When these sensitized particles are mixed with the patient serum or plasma these particles are agglutinated if the anti-HIV antibodies are present in the sample. The test procedure is extremely simple using a microtitre technique and is particularly suitable for mass screening of specimens. The test is time-saving and results are readable by the naked eye after about two hours.

When, instead of antigen, antibody is adsorbed on the carrier particles in tests for estimation of antigens, the technique is known as **reversed passive agglutination**.

Coagglutination

This is based upon the principle that most strains of *Staphylococcus aureus* (especially Cowan strain I) possess protein A on their surface. Protein A binds IgG molecules, non-specifically, through Fc region leaving specific Fab sites free to combine with specific antigen. When suspension of such sensitized staphylococcal cells is treated with homologous (test) antigen, the antigen combines

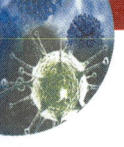

with free Fab sites of IgG attached to staphylococcal cells leading to visible clumping of staphylococci within two minutes. This is known as coagglutination (COA).

COA test can be used for detecting the presence of bacterial antigens in serum, urine and CSF. For example, typhoid bacillus antigen is consistently present in the blood in the early phase of disease, and also in the urine of the patients. This antigen can be detected by COA test. Similarly, meningococcal, pneumococcal and *Haemophilus* antigens can be detected by COA test in the CSF. Identification of *Neisseria gonorrhoeae* and serogrouping of β-haemolytic streptococci A, B, C, D and G can also be carried out by COA test.

Complement Fixation Test (CFT)

The ability of antigen-antibody complexes to fix complement is made use of in complement fixation test (CFT). This is a very versatile and sensitive test for antibody and antigen detection. This can detect as little as 0.04 µg of antibody nitrogen and 0.1 µg of antigen. CFTs include **Wassermann reaction** and **Reiter protein complement fixation test** (RPCFT) for the serodiagnosis of syphilis. Similarly, CFTs for the identification of various viral antigens are also available.

In most of the cases fixation of complement with antigen-antibody complex causes in itself no visible effect. Therefore, it is necessary to use an **indicator system** consisting of sheep red cells coated with anti-sheep red cell antibody. Complement lyses antibody coated red cells. CFT, therefore, is performed in two stages.

- **Stage 1:** Test serum (for the detection of antibody) and the antigen are mixed in the presence of carefully measured amount of complement and then incubated at 37°C for 1 hour. If the patient serum had specific antibody to the test-antigen, complement would be unavailable to lyse the erythrocytes.
- **Stage 2:** Indicator system, antibody-coated sheep red cells, is added to determine whether the complement has been fixed in stage 1 reaction or not. If the patient serum did not have specific antibody, to the antigen, complement would be fixed by the indicator system, resulting in erythrocyte lysis. Therefore, a positive CFT is indicated by absence of lysis of red cells whilst a negative test, with unused complement, is shown by lysis of the red cells (Fig. 45.8).

Other Tests Employing Complement

Immune Adherence

Some bacteria, like *Vibrio cholerae* and *Treponema pallidum*, react with specific antibody in the presence of complement and particulate material such as erythrocytes or platelets; the bacteria are aggregated and adhere to the cells. This is known as immune adherence. Adherence occurs through the activated C3b component of complement.

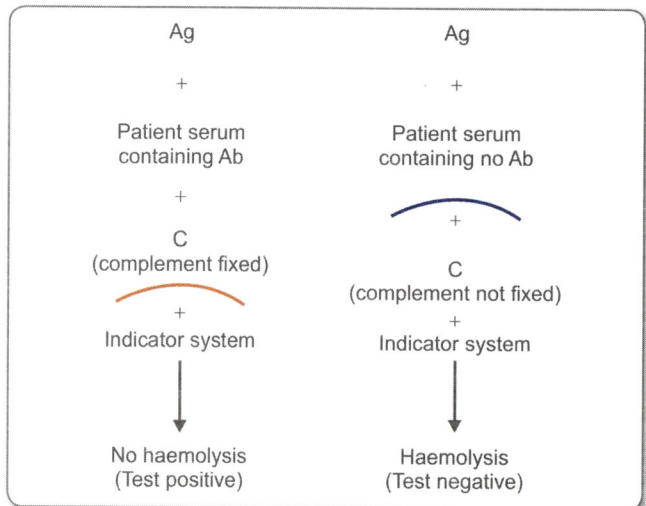

Fig. 45.8: Complement fixation test.

Treponema Pallidum Immobilization Test

The test serum is incubated anaerobically with a suspension of live treponemes and complement. If antibodies are present, the treponemes will be found to be immobilized.

Cytolytic or Cytocidal Tests

When *V. cholerae* is mixed with its antibody in the presence of complement, the bacterium is killed and lysed.

Neutralization Tests

These are of two types—virus neutralization tests and toxin neutralization tests.

Virus Neutralization Tests

Neutralization of viruses by their antibodies in a patient serum may be quantitated by their ability to reduce the infectivity of a stock virus preparation. The test serum is diluted serially, incubated with a known amount of virus and the mixture is then added to indicator systems—animals, embryonated hen's egg and tissue culture. The highest dilution of serum ablating infectivity in 50% of virus-serum mixtures tested is taken as the titre. **Neutralization of bacteriophages can be demonstrated by plaque inhibition test**. When bacteriophages are seeded in appropriate dilution on lawn cultures, plaques of lysis are produced. Specific antiphage serum inhibits plaque formation.

Toxin Neutralization

Bacterial exotoxins are highly antigenic and their activity may be completely neutralized by appropriate concentrations of

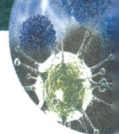

specific antibody. Antibody to bacterial exotoxin is usually referred to as antitoxin. Bacterial endotoxins are poorly antigenic and their toxicity is not neutralized by antisera.

The neutralizing capacity of an antitoxin can be assayed by neutralization test in which mixture of toxin and antitoxin is injected into a susceptible animal and the least amount of antitoxin that prevents death or disease in the animal is estimated. In case of diphtheria toxin, which in small doses causes cutaneous reaction, neutralization test can be carried out on the human skin. The **Schick test** is based on the ability of circulating antitoxin to neutralize the diphtheria toxin given intradermally. Neutralization (no reaction) indicates immunity, and erythema and induration indicates susceptibility to diphtheria.

If a toxin has a demonstrable *in vitro* effect, this effect can be neutralized by specific antitoxin. For example, antistreptolysin O, present in the serum of the patient suffering from *Streptococcus pyogenes* infection, neutralizes the haemolytic activity of the streptococcal O haemolysin. Another example of *in vitro* toxin-antitoxin neutralization is **Nagler's reaction**. *Clostridium perfringens* produces α-toxin which is a phospholipase (lecithinase-C). This produces opalescence in serum or egg yolk media. This reaction is specifically neutralized by the antitoxin.

Opsonization

A substance, such as complement or antibody, that can bind to the surface of a cell or a particle, making it more readily phagocytosed is known as opsonin. Enhanced complement-mediated phagocytosis can occur either in the presence or absence of antibody. Phagocytes such as macrophages, monocytes and neutrophils possess surface receptors (CR1) for C3b and Fc receptors for antibody. If immune complexes have activated the complement system then Fc and CR1 receptors, present on the phagocyte, bind Fc region of antibody and C3b bound on immune complexes respectively, thus facilitating their phagocytosis. This facilitated phagocytosis by antibody and complement is known as **immune opsonization**.

In contrast, **nonimmune opsonization** requires only C3b (opsonin) for opsonization. Bacteria in the blood stream can activate the alternative pathway and generate C3b, which coats the bacteria. C3b binds to CR1 receptors present on the phagocytes, thus facilitating their phagocytosis. Viruses, soluble immune complexes and tumour cells are also opsonized and removed by the same mechanism (Fig. 45.9).

Immunofluorescence

Fluorescent dyes absorb invisible UV light between 290 and 495 nm and emit visible longer wavelength (525 nm) green light. Therefore, if microorganisms or tissue cells are stained with a fluorescent dye and examined under the microscope with UV light instead of visible light they are seen as bright objects against a dark background. This principle is used in fluorescence microscopy. Coons and his colleagues (1942) showed that

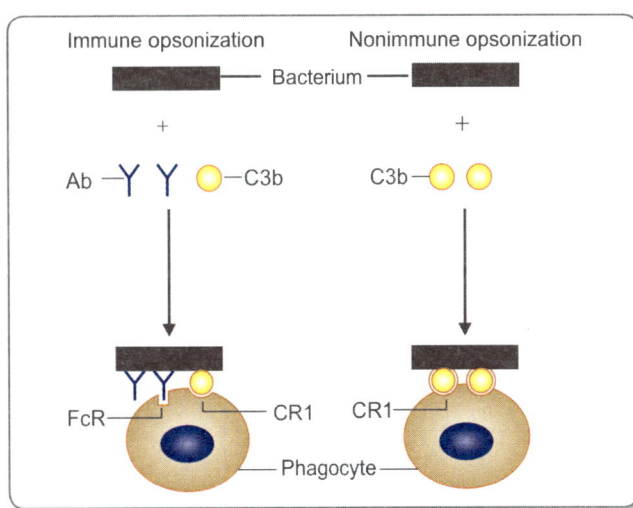

Fig. 45.9: Opsonization.

fluorescent dyes, such as fluorescein isothiocyanate (FITC), can be conjugated to antibodies (without affecting their specificity) permitting their ready detection, when attached to an antigen associated with a cell. Immunofluorescence (IF) is now used extensively to detect:

- Tissue antigens.
- Antibodies to tissues including autoantibodies.
- The antigens of infecting organisms in the body.
- Antigen-antibody complexes.

It is more sensitive than precipitation and complement fixation test. Fluorescence can be observed under a fluorescence microscope (FM), which contains a high intensity UV light source (mercury lamp) instead of visible light. Two types of filters are fitted in the FM:

- *Primary filter:* It is fitted close to the lamp. This ensures the maximum emission of radiation (UV light) of the required wavelengths.
- *Secondary filter:* It is placed in the eyepiece to cut out UV rays which might damage the observer's eye.

Fluorescence-staining techniques are of two types—direct and indirect (Fig. 45.10).

Direct IF

This consists of bringing fluorescein-tagged antibodies in contact with antigens (bacteria, viruses and other antigens) fixed on a slide (e.g. in the form of a tissue section or a smear of an organism), allowing them to react, washing off excess antibody and examining under FM. The site of union of the labelled antibody with its antigen can be seen by the apple-green fluorescent areas on the slide. **Direct IF is routinely used as a sensitive method of diagnosing rabies, by detection of rabies virus antigens in brain smears**. A disadvantage of this method is that separate fluorescent conjugates have to be prepared against each antigen to be tested.

SECTION VIII • IMMUNITY

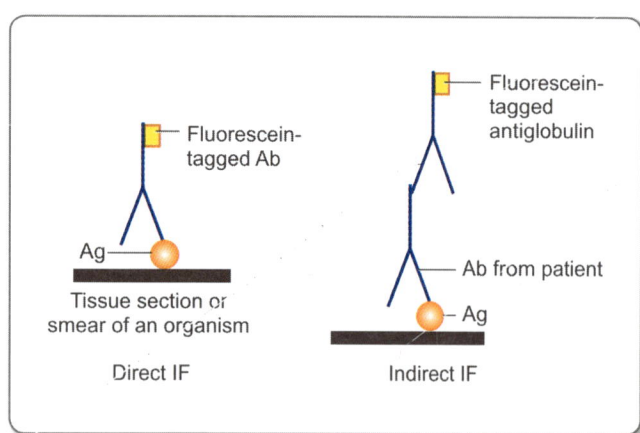

Fig. 45.10: Immunofluorescence.

Indirect IF

This method can be used for detection of specific antibodies in sera or other body fluids and also for identifying antigens. The disadvantage of direct IF, mentioned above, is overcome by this method. An example of this method is the **fluorescent treponemal antibody test for the diagnosis of syphilis**. Here a drop of the patient serum is placed on a smear of *T. pallidum* on a slide and after incubation, the slide is washed well to remove all free serum, leaving behind only antibody, if present, coated on the surface of the treponemes. Whether or not the patient serum contains antibodies to *T. pallidum* is shown by means of a fluorescein-tagged antihuman gammaglobulin (antiglobulin).

If patient serum contains anti-treponemal antibodies fluorescein-tagged antiglobulin will react with it. After washing away all the unbound fluorescent conjugate, when the slide is examined under FM the treponemes will be seen as bright objects against a dark background. If the patient serum is negative for anti-treponemal antibodies, there will be no antibody coating on the treponemes and, therefore, they will not take up the fluorescent conjugate. Therefore, they will not fluoresce. The advantage of this technique is that a single antihuman gammaglobulin fluorescent conjugate can be employed for detecting human antibody to any antigen. Indirect IF is also a convenient method for detecting auto-antibodies that have bound to membrane antigens, *in vivo*.

The direct method is simple and rapid to perform with fewer nonspecific reactions, however, it is less sensitive. The indirect method is more sensitive and gives brighter fluorescence, however, due to increased cross reactivity it is less specific.

Radioimmunoassay (RIA)

RIA is a very sensitive and specific method. It involves the use of either antiserum or more usually antigen labelled with ^{125}I. The amount of radioactive label bound to antigen-antibody complex can be measured, and hence the concentration of antigen or antibody in a specimen can be determined.

Enzyme Immunoassay (EIA)

Enzyme immunoassay is an important immunological method for detecting and measuring antigens or antibodies. It is based on the same principle as that of radioimmunoassay. The key difference is that for enzyme immunoassays the antigen or antibody is conjugated to an enzyme rather than a radioactive isotope. The enzyme is then detected by its ability to convert a colourless substance to a coloured one. Obviously the method requires that, in the enzyme immunoglobulin conjugate, the enzyme retains its enzymatic activity and the antigen or antibody its immunological activity.

Enzyme immunoassays have become very popular in view of their high sensitivity, safety, economy and the simple instrumentation requirements. Solid-phase immunoassays are more widely used. Such systems are called enzyme-linked immunosorbent assays (ELISAs). The ELISA can be used to detect and determine concentrations of antigen or antibody. The test may be done in polystyrene well (microtitre plate) or tube. Different types of ELISA have been developed (Fig. 45.11).

Indirect ELISA

The principle of this test can be illustrated by outlining its application for detection of anti-HIV-1 and anti-HIV-2 antibodies in the patient serum. The wells of the polystyrene microtitre plate are coated with purified HIV-1 and HIV-2 antigens or synthetic peptides representing immunodominant epitopes of HIV-1 and HIV-2, which constitutes the solid-phase antigen. Diluted test serum or plasma sample is added to such a well and incubated. If antibodies specific for HIV-1 and/or HIV-2 are present in the test sample they will form stable complexes

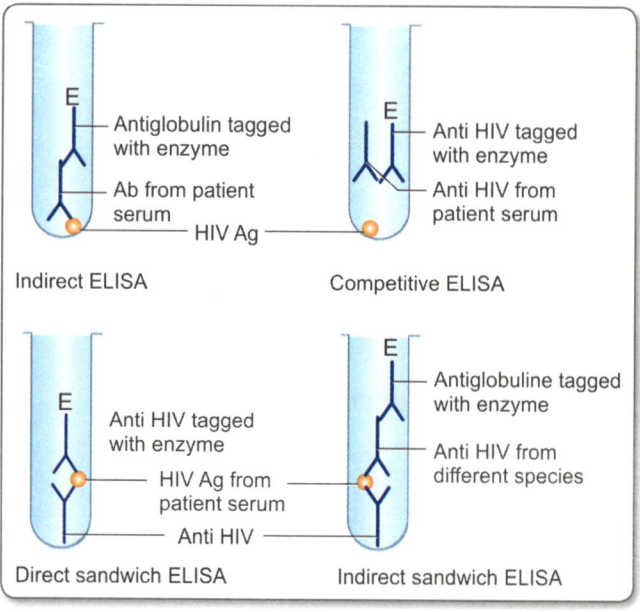

Fig. 45.11: ELISA.

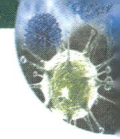

with antigens coated on the well. Well is then washed and a conjugate of goat antihuman immunoglobulin, which has been labelled with the enzyme horseradish peroxidase, is added. If the antigen-antibody complex is present, the peroxidase conjugate will bind to the complex and remains in the well. The conjugate fraction remaining free in the well is removed by washing and the presence of enzyme immobilized on the complexes is shown by incubation in the presence of a colourless enzyme substrate (H_2O_2) and chromogen (orthophenylene-diamine dihydrochloride solution). Incubation with enzyme substrate produces a yellow-orange colour in the test well. If the sample contains no anti-HIV-1 and/or anti-HIV-2, then the labelled antibody cannot be found and no colour develops. The absorbance value of each well is read by an ELISA plate reader at wavelength of 492 ± 2 nm.

Competitive ELISA

The principle of this test too can be illustrated by outlining its application for detection of anti-HIV antibodies in the patient serum. The wells of the polystyrene microtitre plate are coated with HIV antigens which constitutes the solid-phase antigen. The test sample and human anti-HIV, which has been labelled with the enzyme horseradish peroxidase, are incubated in such a well. When the sample contains no anti-HIV, solid-phase antigen-labelled antibody complex will be formed. The incubation with enzyme substrate produces a yellow-orange colour in the test well. If anti-HIV is present in the test sample, it competes with the labelled antibody for the available solid-phase antigen and no colour or reduced colour develops.

Sandwich ELISA

The most frequently used ELISA for detecting microbial antigen is the sandwich solid-phase ELISA. It is of two types:

Single-antibody or Direct Sandwich ELISA

Antibody is attached to the solid-phase. The test sample is then exposed to the solid-phase antibody, to which the antigen, if present, will bind. The solid-phase antibody-antigen complex is then rinsed free of unbound test sample and exposed again to antibodies reactive against the test antigen and conjugated with the enzyme. The conjugated antibody will react with the antigen held to the solid-phase by the first antibody, forming an antibody-antigen-antibody sandwich on the solid-phase. The solid-phase sandwich is again separated from unreacted test sample by rinsing. The second antibody (conjugated to an enzyme) can be detected with an appropriate substrate. This is a single antibody or direct sandwich ELISA.

Double Antibody or Indirect Sandwich ELISA

In the double-antibody ELISA the second antibody as above is not conjugated with the enzyme. The second antibody can be detected by treating it with an antiimmunoglobulin-enzyme conjugate. In the double antibody ELISA, the second antibody of the sandwich must be from a different species than the solid-phase antibody, otherwise, the antiimmunoglobulin conjugate reacts with the solid-phase antibody, producing high background activity.

ELISA is a simple and versatile technique. It needs only microlitre quantities of reactants. ELISA kits are commercially available for the detection of anti-HIV, hepatitis B surface antigen, rotavirus and antigens of a number of other organisms.

Western Blotting

Western blotting is analogous to Southern blotting, for isolated DNA, and Northern blotting, for isolated RNA. In Western blotting, protein antigens are separated according to their electrophoretic mobility and molecular weight by polyacrylamide gel electrophoresis, then blotted onto nitrocellulose paper by standard blotting procedure. The patient serum is allowed to react with the blot. Antibodies attached to separated viral antigens on the nitrocellulose paper are detected by enzyme tagged-anti-human gammaglobulin. Enzyme substrate is subsequently added which indicates positive test. The substrate changes colour in the presence of enzyme and permanently stains the nitrocellulose paper. The position of the band on the paper indicates the antigen with which the antibody has reacted.

Chemiluminescence Immunoassay (CLIA)

Chemiluminescence refers to a chemical reaction emitting energy in the form of light. As radioactive conjugates are employed in RIA, fluorescent conjugates in fluorescence microscopy and enzymes in ELISA, chemiluminescent compounds such as luminol or acridinium esters are used in CLIA as label to provide the signal during the antigen-antibody reaction. The signal (light) can be amplified, measured and the concentration of analyte calculated. This method has been fully automated.

Immunoelectron Microscopy

When the virus particles, for example, rotavirus and hepatitis A virus in stool, are scanty in the specimen they can be treated with specific antisera. It leads to clumping of virus particles which can be seen under electron microscope. This is known as immunoelectron microscopy and it finds application in detection of some viruses causing diarrhoea.

Capsule Swelling or Quellung Reaction

Mixing capsulated bacteria, such as *S. pneumoniae* and *Klebsiella pneumoniae*, with homologous antibody makes possible the direct microscopic visualization of capsules. Binding of the homologous type specific antibody increases the refractility and apparent thickness of the capsule thus making direct microscopic visualization of the capsule possible.

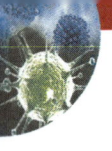

Immunoenzyme Test

Some stable enzymes, such as peroxidases, can be conjugated with antibodies. Antigens in tissue sections can be detected by treating them with peroxidase conjugated specific antibody. If the tissue section possesses specific antigen then antigen-enzyme conjugated antibody complexes will be formed which can be detected by treatment with enzyme substrate.

🔑 Key Points

- *Antigen-antibody reactions are specific* but cross reactions may occur.
- When a *soluble antigen* is mixed with its *specific antibody* in the presence of *electrolytes* at a *suitable temperature* and *pH*, the antigen-antibody complex forms an *insoluble precipitate*.
- The ability of *antigen-antibody complexes* to *fix complement* is made use of in *complement fixation test*.
- A substance, such as complement or antibody, that can bind to the surface of a cell or a particle, making it more readily phagocytosed is known as *opsonin*.
- Radioactive conjugates are employed in radioimmunoassay, fluorescent conjugates in fluorescence microscopy, enzymes in enzyme-linked immunosorbent assay and chemiluminescent compounds are used in chemiluminescence immunoassay.

❓ ASSESS YOURSELF

LONG ANSWER QUESTIONS

1. Define antigen-antibody reaction. Name various antigen-antibody reactions and describe the principle and applications of precipitation reaction giving suitable examples.
2. Define agglutination reaction and discuss the principle and applications of agglutination reactions giving suitable examples.
3. Describe the principle of complement fixation test and discuss in brief the various complement dependent serological tests.
4. Discuss the principle, various types and clinical applications of ELISA technique.

MULTIPLE CHOICE QUESTIONS

1. A large lattice is formed when:
   (a) Antigen is in excess
   (b) Antibody is in excess
   (c) Antigens and antibodies are in optimal proportion
   (d) All of the above

2. Ring test is used for:
   (a) Typing of streptococci and pneumococci
   (b) C-reactive protein test
   (c) Ascoli's thermoprecipitation test
   (d) All of the above

3. VDRL test is an example of:
   (a) Ring test
   (b) Slide flocculation test
   (c) Tube test
   (d) None of the above

4. Anti-Rh antibodies are:
   (a) IgG type
   (b) IgD type
   (c) IgA type
   (d) IgE type

5. Test employing complement is:
   (a) Widal test
   (b) VDRL test
   (c) *Treponema pallidum* immobilization test
   (d) Coagglutination test

Contd...

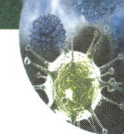

? ASSESS YOURSELF

6. ELISA kits are commercially available for detection of:
    (a) Anti-HIV antibodies
    (b) Hepatitis B surface antigen
    (c) Rotavirus
    (d) All of the above

7. Widal test is an example of:
    (a) Agglutination test
    (b) Precipitation test
    (c) Flocculation test
    (d) Complement-fixation test

8. Coombs' test is:
    (a) Complement fixation test
    (b) Antiglobulin test
    (c) Agglutination test
    (d) Precipitation test

ANSWERS TO MCQS

1. c   **2.** d   **3.** b   **4.** a   **5.** c   **6.** d   **7.** a   **8.** b

Hypersensitivity and Autoimmunity

HYPERSENSITIVITY

Hypersensitivity is an abnormal immune response which produces physiological or histopathological damage in the host. It may be divided into five types:

- Type I   :   Anaphylactic
- Type II   :   Cytotoxic
- Type III :   Immune complex
- Type IV   :   Cell-mediated or delayed
- Type V   :   Stimulatory or antireceptor

Type I, II, III and V hypersensitivity depend on the interaction of antigen with humoral antibodies and are known as immediate type reactions, although some are more immediate than others. Immediate hypersensitivity reactions develop in less than 24 hours after reexposure to an antigen. Type IV hypersensitivity or delayed hypersensitivity is mediated by T lymphocytes. Delayed hypersensitivity reactions develop in 24–48 hours.

Type I Hypersensitivity: Anaphylactic

It is **mediated by IgE antibody** and is due to the powerful effects of histamine and other vasoactive amines. Generally, small amount of antigen administered to mucous membrane or skin will induce local anaphylaxis, whereas larger amounts may induce a generalized reaction and antigen administered systemically may cause generalized anaphylaxis. Local anaphylaxis is exemplified by such conditions as hay fever and asthma. Systemic anaphylaxis is a shocklike condition that can occur in individuals who are intensely allergic to such things as bee venom, penicillin and horse serum.

An antigenic substance that can trigger the allergic state is known as **allergen**. It may be a protein or chemically complex low molecular weight substance. Most allergens are considered weakly immunogenic and most people do not respond to them adversely. However, an allergic person is often sensitive to several different allergens.

Mechanism of Type I Hypersensitivity

In order to produce type I hypersensitivity an individual must first come in contact with an antigen and produce IgE antibodies. These antibodies bind to mast cells and basophils (Fig. 46.1).

Basophils are found in the circulation while mast cells (or fixed basophils) are located in lymphoid regions of respiratory tract, gastrointestinal tract, reproductive tract, skin and lining of blood vessels including capillaries.

Thus, **after first exposure** allergen-specific IgE is fixed to the mast cells and basophils, thereby sensitizing them. The part of the IgE molecule that binds to the surface of mast cells and basophils is the Fc portion. These cells possess high affinity receptors specific for Fc portion of IgE antibodies. Thus, Fab portion of IgE remains exposed. IgE antibodies can remain attached on these cells for up to six weeks. Such an individual is said to be **sensitized**.

After a second exposure the allergen travels to the mast cells and basophils, where it binds to antigen-binding site on IgE molecule. Antigen-antibody binding triggers the process of degranulation through which the mast cell explosively discharges its pharmacologically active agents. These include histamine, serotonin, bradykinin, slow-reacting substance of anaphylaxis (SRS-A), platelet-activating factors, eosinophil chemotactic factor of anaphylaxis and prostaglandins.

Of these, histamine is the most abundant and fastest acting. It induces smooth muscle contraction, release of mucus, vasodilation and increased capillary permeability. All these reactions can have profound effects. For example, excessive smooth muscle contraction and release of mucus in respiratory tract can close the air passages of trachea and bronchi, causing asphyxiation and death by suffocation.

Another target area is the uterus. Pregnant women who are severely allergic may abort the foetus during an attack of histamine release and subsequent smooth muscle contractions in the uterus. Histamine also induces increased capillary permeability leading to oedema. Thus, there is extensive loss of blood fluids into the tissues. This may lead to circulatory shock and death.

Cutaneous Anaphylaxis

If a person is suspected to be allergic to a particular substance, a **skin test** can be done. In this test a small dose of allergen is injected intradermally. In less than 30 minutes results can be read. If the individual is allergic there will be a **wheal and flare response** at the site of injection. Wheal is a pale central area of puffiness due to oedema (caused by increased capillary permeability)

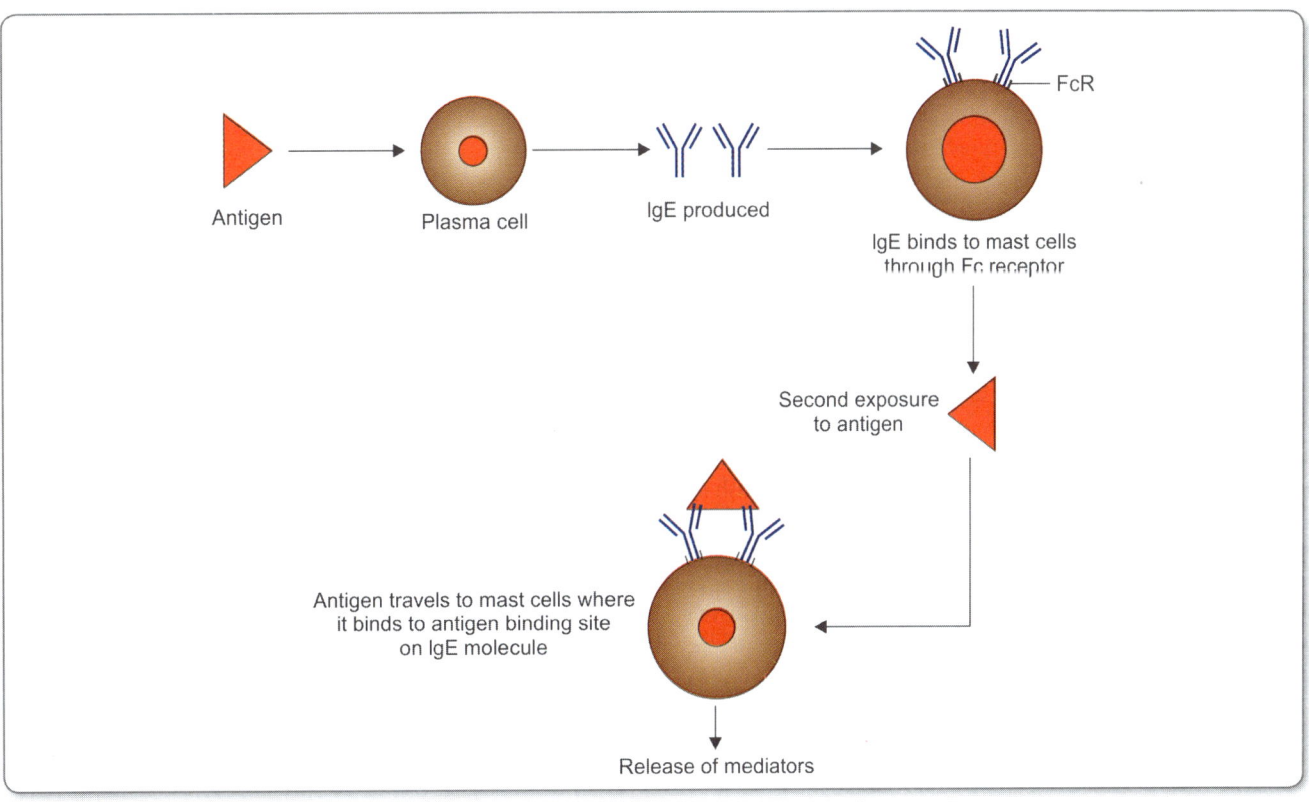

Fig. 46.1: Antigen-induced mediator release from mast cell.

which is surrounded by flare (caused by hyperaemia due to vasodilation). Since the injection site is small, it is possible to test for hypersensitivity to hundreds of substances on a person's back. The wheal and flare response can be used to determine the specific substance to which the atopic person is sensitive.

Prausnitz-Küstner (PK) Reaction

Prausnitz and Küstner in 1921 demonstrated transmission of IgE-mediated type I hypersensitivity by injecting serum containing IgE antibodies from allergic person into the skin of a normal or non-allergic person. Serum from Küstner, who was hypersensitive to certain species of cooked fish, was injected intracutaneously in Prausnitz (normal) followed 24 hours later by an intracutaneous injection of cooked fish, to which Küstner was sensitive, into the same site in Prausnitz. This led to wheal and flare reaction within 20 minutes. As IgE antibody is homocytotropic, the test has to be carried out on human skin, therefore, there is risk of transmission of hepatitis B and C viruses, and human immunodeficiency virus.

Anaphylaxis in vitro (Schultz-Dale Phenomenon)

In 1910, Schultz and Dale demonstrated that sensitized strips of smooth muscle contract, *in vitro*, following exposure to antigen.

Thus intestinal and uterine muscle strips from a sensitized animal (guinea pig) held in Ringer's solution bath contract vigorously on addition of specific antigen. Smooth muscle strips can be passively sensitized by bathing them in serum from a hypersensitive animal. The actual test is done by adding the antigen and observing subsequent contractions.

Atopy

The term atopy refers to chronic human allergic states. These include **hay fever**, **allergic asthma** and **food allergies**. The antigens commonly involved in atopy are inhalants (pollen, house dust, animal dander or other types of fine particles suspended in air) or ingestants (milk, milk products, eggs, meat, fish or cereal). Some of them are contact allergens, to which the skin and conjunctiva may be exposed. The mechanism of development of atopy is essentially the same as that of systemic anaphylaxis. Atopy is likely to develop when allergen is localized or absorbed slowly, on the other hand systemic anaphylaxis is likely to develop if large quantities of allergen are quickly distributed throughout the body.

Hay Fever (Allergic Rhinitis)

It is an IgE-mediated allergic reaction that affects the mucosal surfaces of upper respiratory tract. It leads to nasal congestion,

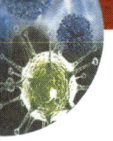

headache, running nose, watery eyes, itching and sneezing. The specific stimuli that cause allergic rhinitis include antigenic components of grass, weed and tree pollens, dust, mites, animal dander, organic dusts, components of tobacco smoke, and non-infectious components of fungal and bacterial allergens. If the allergen cannot be removed, then antihistaminics are the pharmacological agents of choice for the treatment of allergic rhinitis since histamine seems to be the major mediator of this allergy.

Allergic Asthma

It is a severe form of respiratory allergy. It leads to contraction of the trachea and bronchi. The specific stimuli that cause allergic asthma include airborne allergens. In addition, asthma-producing foods such as milk, milk products, eggs, meat, fish or cereal may also precipitate allergic asthma. Some patients may even be sensitive to normal microbial flora leading to endogenous asthma. The main mediators of this allergy are serotonin and SRS-A. Therefore, antihistaminics are not able to reverse the smooth muscle contraction. The drug of choice for the treatment of this allergy is adrenaline (epinephrine). It is dispensed as atomizers for quick delivery. In addition, corticosteroids and cromolyn sodium have proved beneficial in treating attacks of allergic asthma.

Food Allergies

Food allergy occurs in infants and children, but is uncommon in adults. Certain foods such as eggs, milk, peanuts, seafoods, citrus fruits and chocolate are frequent causes of food allergy. Consumption of the food in a patient with food allergy leads to nausea, vomiting, diarrhoea and cramps with typical urticaria and wheezing or upper airways congestion. Best cure for food allergy is to avoid that food unless it is a common ingredient of prepared foods such as flour.

Type II Hypersensitivity: Cytotoxic Reaction

This involves the combination of IgG and IgM serum antibodies with foreign antigenic components on a cell surface. Alternatively, a free foreign antigen or hapten such as a drug or microbial product may be adsorbed onto a cell membrane, which subsequently combines with antibody.

Clinically, antibody-mediated reactions occur in following situations:

Drug-induced Immune Haemolytic Anaemia

A type II hypersensitivity reaction involving haemolytic anaemia may be induced by administration of certain drugs. Drugs such as antibiotic penicillin, and alpha methyldopa for the treatment of hypertension can bind to the surface of red blood cell and form an antigenic complex with the surface of these cells. This can bring about the production of complement-fixing antibody to the drug. Reaction of this antibody with the RBC-bound drug activates the complement system, resulting in RBC lysis and anaemia.

Transfusion Reactions

When a person receives incompatible blood transfusion, the antibodies normally present in recipient's serum agglutinate and lyse donor RBCs with the liberation of free haemoglobin into the plasma. This leads to jaundice, fever and failure of kidney function. Serum of the donor may also agglutinate and lyse recipient's RBCs. For example, transfusion of group O whole blood or plasma to group A or group B or group AB recipients may lead to haemolysis. But this reaction is mild since the donor's serum gets considerably diluted in the circulation of the recipient.

Rh Incompatibility

Rh antibodies are major cause of **haemolytic disease of newborn (HDN)**. When an Rh-negative woman carries an Rh-positive foetus, she may be immunized against Rh antigen by passage of foetal red cells into maternal circulation. Minor transplacental leaks may occur any time during pregnancy, but it is during delivery that foetal cells enter the maternal circulation in large numbers. Therefore, the mother is usually immunized only at first delivery, and consequently, the first child escapes damage (except where the woman has been sensitized already by prior Rh incompatible blood transfusion). During subsequent pregnancy, Rh antibodies of IgG class pass from the mother to the foetus and damage its erythrocytes. The clinical features of HDN may vary from a mere accentuation of the physiological jaundice in the newborn to erythroblastosis fetalis or intrauterine death due to **hydrops fetalis**.

Type III Hypersensitivity: Immune Complex

If an antigen is not cell-bound but is rather small and soluble, the body can encounter severe difficulties if it is repeatedly exposed to that antigen. Antigen-antibody complexes formed under these conditions may lead to type III or immune complex-mediated hypersensitivity. Monocytes and macrophages are very efficient at binding and removing large precipitating antigen-antibody complexes. They can also eliminate the smaller complexes made in antibody excess but are relatively inefficient at removing those formed in antigen excess. The formation of antigen-antibody complexes in serum, with subsequent deposition of the complexes in tissues, is the key event in type III hypersensitivity. Antigen-antibody complexes can then activate serum complement, platelets and phagocytes, all of which lead to tissue damage.

Arthus Reaction (Local Immune Complex Disease)

Arthus (1903) observed that when rabbits were repeatedly injected subcutaneously with normal horse serum, the initial injections

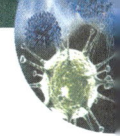

were without any local effect, but with later injections, there occurred intense local reaction consisting of oedema, induration and haemorrhagic necrosis. This is known as Arthus reaction. The tissue damage is due to formation of local precipitating immune complexes which are deposited on the endothelial lining of the blood vessels. Antigen-antibody complexes can then trigger and activate complement leading to inflammation and tissue damage.

Serum Sickness (Systemic Immune Complex Disease)

This is a systemic form of type III hypersensitivity. This develops in persons who receive a single injection of a high concentration of horse antitoxin against tetanus, gas gangrene, diphtheria, etc. for prophylactic and therapeutic purposes. Seven to 12 days after the injection, patient may develop fever, lymphadenopathy, splenomegaly, arthritis, glomerulonephritis, endocarditis, vasculitis, urticarial rash, abdominal pain, nausea and vomiting. It is due to the immune response to horse antigens and it has also been encountered in allergic reactions to certain drugs. After 7–12 days, antibodies to horse antigens appear while horse antigens are still persisting because a large dose was administered. Initially they form antigen-antibody complexes in antigen excess. These soluble complexes can circulate and get deposited in various sites throughout the body particularly in skin, joints, kidneys and heart.

Antigen-antibody aggregates can fix complement leading to inflammation and tissue damage. The plasma level of complement falls due to massive complement activation and fixation by antigen-antibody complexes. Initially, the circulating immune complexes are in antigen excess and produce inflammatory lesions, but as antibody production rises, the immune complexes increase in size as zone of equivalence is reached. These larger immune complexes are more easily phagocytosed and cleared by the cells of reticuloendothelial system of liver and spleen. Once all immune complexes are removed from the circulation, symptoms are usually resolved within a week.

Type IV Hypersensitivity: Cell-mediated or Delayed

Type IV hypersensitivity or delayed hypersensitivity (DH) is the clinically observable outcome of cell-mediated immune reaction in the tissues of a sensitized individual. The reaction is not brought about by circulating antibodies and B lymphocytes but by sensitized T lymphocytes and macrophages. It is named delayed hypersensitivity because it appears in 24–48 hours after the presensitized host encounters the antigen, while immediate hypersensitivity reactions develop in ½–12 hours (Table 46.1). Two types of DH are recognized: tuberculin (infection) type and contact dermatitis type.

Tuberculin (Infection) Type

The immune response to the tubercle bacillus, observed by Robert Koch in 1880, has served a general model for DH. When a small dose (1–3 units) of tuberculin or purified protein derivative (PPD) is injected intradermally in an individual sensitized to tuberculoprotein by prior infection or immunization, an indurated inflammatory reaction, 10 mm or more in diameter, develops at the site of injection within 48–72 hours. It is characterized by erythema due to increased blood flow to the damaged area and induration due to infiltration with a large number of mononuclear cells, mainly T lymphocytes and about 10–20% macrophages.

Contact Dermatitis Type

Contact dermatitis is cell-mediated allergic reaction that occurs when certain substances like metals (nickel and chromium), dyes (picryl chloride and dinitrochlorobenzene), drugs such as penicillin, and toiletries come in contact with skin. Sensitization is particularly liable to occur when contact is with an inflamed area and when chemical is applied in an oily base. Application of antibiotic ointments frequently provokes sensitization.

TABLE 46.1: Comparison of Type I–IV hypersensitivity reactions

Characteristic	Type I	Type II	Type III	Type IV
Approximate time to develop clinical signs	1/2–8 hours	5–12 hours	3–8 hours	24–48 hours
Reaction mediators	IgE, histamine, serotonin, SRS-A, etc.	IgG, IgM and complement	IgG, IgM, complement, neutrophils, eosinophils and lysosomal enzymes	T cells, macrophages and lymphokines
Response to intradermal injection of antigen	Wheal and flare	—	Erythema and oedema	Erythema and induration
Passive transfer with	Serum	Serum	Serum	T cells
Examples	Anaphylaxis, asthma, hay fever and, food and insect allergies	Transfusion reaction, HDN and drug-induced allergy	Arthus reaction and serum sickness	Tuberculin test, contact dermatitis, graft rejection and tumour immunity.

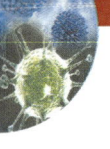

The substances involved are not antigenic by themselves but may acquire antigenicity on combination with skin proteins. Subsequent contact with allergen in a sensitized individual leads to contact dermatitis. The lesions vary from macules and papules to vesicles which break down leaving behind raw weeping areas typical of acute eczematous dermatitis.

This hypersensitivity can be detected by **patch test**. The allergen is applied to the skin under an adherent dressing. Sensitivity is indicated by itching, appearing in 4–5 hours and local reaction which may vary from erythema to vesicle or blister formation in 24 hours.

Type V Hypersensitivity: Stimulatory or Antireceptor

This is an antibody-mediated hypersensitivity. Here antibody reacts with a key surface component such as a hormone receptor and switches on or stimulates the cell. An example of this type of hypersensitivity is the thyroid hyperactivity in Graves' disease due to thyroid stimulating autoantibody.

Normally, thyroid stimulating hormone (TSH) from pituitary gland binds to thyroid cell receptors. This activates adenyl cyclase in the membrane which converts ATP to AMP. The latter stimulates activity of thyroid cells, thus secreting thyroxine. The thyroid stimulating antibody present in the sera of thyrotoxic patients is an autoantibody directed against receptors for TSH. This antibody, therefore, binds to these receptors and brings about the same effect as that of TSH.

AUTOIMMUNITY

Normally, we do not form potentially destructive antibodies and T cells against our own cells because our body has developed tolerance to self-antigens. However, sometimes we can produce antibodies and T cells against our own cell or tissue components leading to autoimmune diseases. **Autoimmunity may, therefore, be defined as immune response to self-antigens, which can generate autoantibodies and autocytotoxic T cells.**

Mechanism of Autoimmunity

There are several possible mechanisms involved in the development of autoimmunity:

Forbidden Clones

According to clonal selection theory, antibody-forming lymphocytes capable of reacting with different antigens are formed. Clones of cells that have immunological reactivity with self-antigens are eliminated during embryonic life. Such clones are called forbidden clones. Their persistence or development in later life by somatic mutations can lead to autoimmunity.

Hidden or Sequestrated Antigen

Certain self-antigens are present in closed systems and are not accessible to immune system. An example is the **lens antigen of the eye**. The lens protein is enclosed in its capsule and does not circulate in the blood. Therefore, immunological tolerance against this antigen does not develop during foetal life. When the lens protein antigen leaks out, following cataract surgery or injury to the eye, it leads to immune response and damage to the other eye.

Another example of hidden antigen is seen in case of **sperm antigens**. Since sperms develop only at puberty, therefore, the sperm antigens cannot induce tolerance during foetal life. Sperms may enter into blood stream following injury of the testes and mumps orchitis. Virus probably damages the basement membrane of seminiferous tubules leading to the leakage of sperms and initiation of an immune response resulting in orchitis.

Neoantigens or Altered Antigens

Cells or tissues may undergo antigenic alteration by physical agents such as irradiation. Several chemical agents including drugs can combine with cells and tissues and alter their antigenic structure. Skin contact with a variety of chemicals may lead to contact dermatitis. Drug-induced anaemia, leucopenia and thrombocytopenia often have autoimmune basis. Viruses and other intracellular pathogens may induce alterations of cell antigens leading to autoimmunity.

Cross Reacting Antigens

Immunological damage may result from immune response induced by cross reacting foreign antigens. For example, **Semple rabies vaccine** consists of infected sheep brain tissue inactivated with phenol. Its injection elicits an immune response against sheep brain antigens. This may lead to damage to patient's nervous tissue due to cross reaction between human and sheep brain leading to encephalitis.

Immunological injury may be due to cross reacting antigens present on microorganisms causing infection. An important example of this is the non-suppurative sequelae of *Streptococcus pyogenes* infection which include **acute rheumatic fever and acute glomerulonephritis**. M protein of *S. pyogenes* and heart of man share antigenic characteristics. The immune response induced by repeated streptococcal infections can, therefore, damage the heart. Nephritogenic strains of *S. pyogenes* share antigens with renal glomeruli. Therefore, immune response following infection with such strains may lead to acute glomerulonephritis.

Mutation

Immunocompetent cells may acquire an unnatural responsiveness to self-antigens by mutation.

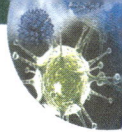

Activity of Helper and Suppressor T Cells

Helper T (Th) cells facilitate B cell response to many antigens. Suppressor T (Ts) cells inhibit antibody production by B cells. Optimal antibody response depends on the balanced activity of Th and Ts cells. *Overactivity of Th cells or decreased activity of Ts cells may lead to autoimmunity.*

AUTOIMMUNE DISEASES

These include systemic lupus erythematosus, rheumatoid arthritis, systemic sclerosis (scleroderma), dermatomyositis, and polyarteritis nodosa. Rheumatic fever is also sometimes classified as autoimmune disorder.

Key Points

- **Type I hypersensitivity** is mediated by **IgE antibodies**.
- **Type I hypersensitivity leads to anaphylaxis, hay fever, atopic dermatitis and allergic asthma.**
- **Type II hypersensitivity** is mediated by IgG or IgM antibodies against cell surface or extracellular matrix antigens.
- **Haemolytic disease of newborn** occurs when maternal antibodies to foetal blood group antigen cross the placenta and destroy the foetal erythrocytes.
- **Two types of type IV hypersensitivity** are recognized – tuberculin (infection) type and contact dermatitis type.
- **Autoimmunity** may be defined as *immune response to self antigens*.
- **Autoimmunity** may be due to *forbidden clones, sequestrated antigens, altered antigens, cross reacting antigens, mutation, and overactivity of Th cells or decreased activity of Ts cells*.

? ASSESS YOURSELF

LONG AND SHORT ANSWER QUESTIONS

1. What is hypersensitivity? Classify hypersensitivity reactions? Describe type I reactions.
2. Describe type II hypersensitivity reactions.
3. Write short notes on:
   - (a) Arthus reaction
   - (b) Serum sickness
   - (c) Type IV hypersensitivity
   - (d) Mechanism of autoimmunity

MULTIPLE CHOICE QUESTIONS

1. Anaphylactic reactions are mediated by which class of immunoglobulin?
   - (a) IgE
   - (b) IgM
   - (c) IgA
   - (d) IgD
2. Wheal and flare response is characteristic of:
   - (a) Type I hypersensitivity reaction
   - (b) Type II hypersensitivity reaction
   - (c) Type III hypersensitivity reaction
   - (d) Type IV hypersensitivity reaction
3. Which of the following is/are example/s of autoimmune disease/s?
   - (a) Rheumatoid arthritis
   - (b) Systemic lupus erythematosus
   - (c) Polyarteritis nodosa
   - (d) All of the above
4. Pathogenesis of rheumatic fever is due to immunological injury caused by:
   - (a) Cross reacting antigens
   - (b) Neoantigens
   - (c) Forbidden clones
   - (d) Hidden antigens

ANSWERS TO MCQs

1. a   **2.** a   **3.** d   **4.** a

47 Chapter

Prophylactic Immunization

Immunization against infectious diseases is one of the greatest successes of modern medicine. During the last 200 years, since the time of Edward Jenner, vaccination has controlled nine major diseases, namely, smallpox, diphtheria, pertussis, tetanus, poliomyelitis, mumps, measles, rubella and yellow fever. Major headway has been made against influenza, hepatitis B, pneumococci and *Haemophilus influenzae* type b infections, at least in some parts of the world. Of the major scourges of mankind, malaria, leprosy, helminthic diseases and human immunodeficiency virus infections have remained without useful vaccines. Immunization is of three types – active immunization, passive immunization and combined passive and active immunization.

ACTIVE IMMUNIZATION

Active immunization is done by use of vaccines which are preparation of live or killed microorganisms or their products.

Immunization Schedule

- **National immunization schedule:**
  The national immunization schedule is given in Table 47.1.
- **WHO EPI immunization schedule:**
  In May 1974, the WHO officially launched a global immunization programme known as *Expanded Programme of Immunization* (EPI) to protect all children of the world against six vaccine-preventable diseases, namely diphtheria, whooping cough, tetanus, poliomyelitis, tuberculosis and measles by the year 2000. EPI was launched in India in January 1978. WHO EPI immunization schedule is given in Table 47.2. This programme is now called Universal Child Immunization, 1990.

  The immunization schedule may be altered to suit the local needs of individuals and groups. Interruption of the schedule with a delay between doses does not interfere with the final immunity achieved.

  In addition, hepatitis B vaccine may be given at birth, 1 month and 6 months of age and booster dose at the age of 10 years. Children of the age of 15 months may be given MMR vaccine, followed by a booster at the age of 4–6 years.

TABLE 47.1: National Immunization schedule

Age	Vaccine
For infants	
• At birth (for institutional deliveries)	BCG and OPV-0 dose
• 6 weeks	BCG (if not given at birth) DPT-1 and OPV-1 and hepatitis B-1
• 10 weeks	DPT-2 and OPV-2 and hepatitis B-2
• 14 weeks	DPT-3 and OPV-3 and hepatitis B-3
• 9 months	Measles
16–24 months	DPT and OPV
5–6 years	DT*
10 years	TT**
16 years	TT**
For pregnant women	
• Early in pregnancy	TT-1 or booster
• One month after TT-1	TT-2

*   The second dose of DT should be given at an interval of one month if there is no clear history or documented evidence of previous immunization with DPT.

** The second dose of TT should be given at an interval of one month if there is no clear history or documented evidence of previous immunization with DPT, DT or TT.

TABLE 47.2: WHO EPI immunization schedule

Age	Vaccine
Birth	BCG, OPV
6 weeks	DPT, OPV
10 weeks	DPT, OPV
14 weeks	DPT, OPV
9 months	Measles

PASSIVE IMMUNIZATION

Passive immunization is used when it is considered necessary to protect a patient at short notice and for a limited period.

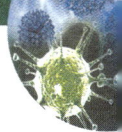

Three types of preparations are available for passive immunization – homologous and heterologous sera, pooled immunoglobulins and specific immunoglobulins.

Homologous and Heterologous Sera

Antitoxic, antibacterial or antiviral antibodies in human (homologous) or animal (heterologous) serum are injected to give temporary protection. Homologous sera confer protection for 3–6 months, whereas protection afforded by a heterologous serum is likely to last for only a few weeks.

Pooled Immunoglobulins

Pooled normal human serum contains protective levels of antibodies to a range of diseases. It may be used for short-term prophylaxis of hepatitis A in contacts or travellers who intend to visit countries where hepatitis A is common. It also protects an immunocompromised child temporarily against measles if given promptly after contact with a case.

For the prevention of nutritional blindness massive doses of vitamin A are given to the children up to the age of 5 years. First dose of 100,000 IU of vitamin A is given with measles vaccination at nine months of age. Subsequent doses of 200,000 IU each are given every six months up to the age of 5 years.

Specific Immunoglobulins

Specific immunoglobulins are available for passive immunization against tetanus (human tetanus immunoglobulin, HTIG), hepatitis B (HBIG), rabies (HRIG) and varicella-zoster (ZIG).

COMBINED PASSIVE AND ACTIVE IMMUNIZATION

In some diseases (e.g. tetanus, diphtheria, rabies) passive immunization is often undertaken in conjunction with inactivated vaccine products, to provide both immediate (but temporary) passive immunity and slowly developing active immunity. Both injections should be given at separate sites.

Key Points

- In May 1974, the WHO officially launched a *global immunization programme* known as **Expanded Programme of Immunization (EPI)** to protect all children of the world.
- **Passive immunization** is used when it is considered necessary to protect a patient at short notice and for a limited period.

? ASSESS YOURSELF

SHORT ANSWER QUESTION

1. Write short notes on:
   (a) Vaccines
   (b) National immunization schedule
   (c) WHO EPI immunization schedule
   (d) Passive immunization

MULTIPLE CHOICE QUESTIONS

1. Which of the following vaccines is/are killed vaccine/s?
   (a) Pertussis vaccine
   (b) Cholera vaccine
   (c) Japanese encephalitis vaccine
   (d) All of the above

2. Which of the following vaccines is/are prepared from live microbes manipulated and attenuated?
   (a) BCG vaccine
   (b) Oral polio vaccine
   (c) Measles vaccine
   (d) All of the above

3. Which of the following vaccines is/are prepared from microbial toxin/s?
   (a) Diphtheria vaccine
   (b) Tetanus toxoid vaccine
   (c) Both of the above
   (d) None of the above

Contd...

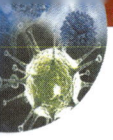

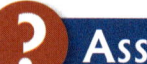

SECTION VIII ● IMMUNITY

? ASSESS YOURSELF

4. Which of the following vaccines should be administered at the birth of a child?

    (a) BCG   (b) DPT

    (c) Measles   (d) All of the above

5. Specific immunoglobulins are available for passive immunization against:

    (a) Tetanus   (b) Rabies

    (c) Hepatitis B   (d) All of the above

6. Which of the following diseases has/have remained without useful vaccine/s?

    (a) Malaria   (b) Leprosy

    (c) AIDS   (d) All of the above

ANSWERS TO MCQS

1. d   **2.** d   **3.** c   **4.** a   **5.** d   **6.** d

Section

IX

Miscellaneous

Chapter 48

Antimicrobial Stewardship

ANTIMICROBIAL RESISTANCE

Antibiotic resistance in bacteria may either be intrinsic or acquired. **Intrinsic resistance** means that the bacteria were resistant to the antibiotic even before the antibiotic was introduced. **Acquired resistance** means that a bacterium that was previously sensitive to an antibiotic has now turned resistant. It is the acquired resistance that is of great importance because it would result in treatment failure as well as potential dissemination of resistance to other bacteria.

The physiological mechanisms of antibiotic resistance include:

- Inactivation of the antibiotic by enzymes produced by the bacteria.
- Alteration of target proteins such that the antibiotic does not bind or binds with decreased affinity.
- Alteration of the membrane which decreases the permeability of the antibiotic.
- Active efflux of the antibiotic.
- Development of alternate metabolic pathway to bypass the action of antibiotic.

With antibiotics, as previously with sulphonamides, resistance began to arise. At first, organisms were encountered with low-level resistance to penicillin, and infections caused by these could be treated with larger doses of the antibiotics, because the low-level resistance was due to mutation which decreases the cell permeability to the antimicrobial agent and if larger doses are given then effective concentration of the drug can enter the bacterial cell. In time, however, highly resistant strains emerged which could not be therapeutically controlled.

Genetic Basis of Resistance

The initial low-level resistant microbial strains carried genes for resistance on the **chromosome**. These were soon replaced by higher-level resistant types, principally harbouring **plasmids**. Plasmid-mediated drug resistance is seen in various pathogenic and commensal bacteria of man and animals, e.g. *E. coli, Klebsiella pneumoniae, Proteus, Salmonella, Shigella* and *Pseudomonas*. Transfer of drug resistance occurs readily *in vitro*. It also occurs *in vivo* but in normal intestines it is inhibited by several factors like anaerobic conditions, bile salts, alkaline pH and abundance of anaerobic Gram-positive bacteria minimising the chances of

contact between donor cells and suitable recipient cells. But in intestines of persons on oral antibiotic therapy, transfer occurs readily due to the destruction of the sensitive normal flora and the selection pressure provided by the drug.

Transferable drug resistance involves all antibiotics in common use. Bacteria containing R plasmid can spread from animal to man. Therefore, indiscriminate use of antibiotics in man and animals or in animal feed can increase the spread of plasmid-mediated drug resistance in the community. Because of the misuse and overuse of antibiotics in the hospitals it is said *'hospital is the heaven for drug resistant bacteria'*.

Some chromosomal-mediated resistances remain a therapeutic problem, namely, those responsible for resistance to methicillin, rifampicin, nalidixic acid and isoniazid. However, most resistances of concern are associated with R plasmids. While plasmids may be the vectors of the resistance genes, the genes may themselves be located on discrete movable DNA elements called **transposons**. These are very often on plasmids, but have the ability to 'hop' from plasmid to plasmid or from plasmid to chromosome. In many bacteria, such as staphylococci, bacteriophages may also be important vectors for transposon spread.

Transposons may carry single or multiple resistance. The transposon can enter and remain stable in different species even if its entry vector (e.g. plasmid or phage) is lost, since the resistance transposon can be incorporated in a stable resident plasmid or the chromosome of the new host. The discovery of transposable resistance provided the basis for understanding the rapid spread of resistance markers throughout the bacterial kingdom and helped to explain why different genera seemed to have 'evolved' similar genes of resistance.

Bacteria resist antimicrobial agents by various mechanisms. **Chromosomal resistance**, except when resulting from transposon insertions, is generally mediated by a single low-level, non-enzymatic mechanism. In many organisms, these resistances seem related to decreased permeability, e.g. resistance in meningococci, mycobacteria, pneumococci and methicillin resistance in *S. aureus*. Exceptions are the chromosomally located degradative enzymes for the β-lactam antibiotics and the chromosomal-mediated resistance to rifampicin (via resistant RNA polymerases) and nalidixic acid (via resistant DNA gyrases).

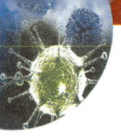
In general, **the plasmid- or transposon-mediated** resistances are of higher level and involve more active processes. Some plasmid-mediated resistance to penicillin and to chloramphenicol seems to involve decreased permeability, but the exact mechanism is not yet defined. Many plasmid-mediated resistances involve extracellular inactivation of the drug by enzymatic modification on degradation of its active element. In this category are the enzymes (β-lactamases) which destroy the β-lactam ring of the penicillins and cephalosporins, and those which inactivate chloramphenicol.

In clinical practice, resistance acquired by mutation is very important in tuberculosis. If a patient is put on streptomycin alone then initially organisms die in large numbers but soon resistant mutants appear which multiply in number while sensitive parents may be eliminated. If two or more drugs are used and if a mutant appears which is resistant to one of the drugs then it will be killed by other drug/s. **The chance of a mutant developing resistance to more than one drug at one time is remote**. This is the rationale of combined therapy in tuberculosis.

R plasmid-mediated resistance is usually to multiple drugs, therefore, there is no use of combined therapy. Acquisition of resistance by transduction is common in staphylococci. The penicillinase plasmids, which are transmitted by transduction, may also carry determinants of resistance to mercuric chloride and erythromycin.

Transposable Genetic Elements

Lederberg, in 1960, described an unusual class of *Gal*-mutants in *E. coli* caused by insertion of extra pieces of DNA called **insertion sequences** or **IS elements** at the point of mutation. Since then a large number of IS elements have been described in a wide variety of bacteria. They are common in bacterial plasmids and are common components of many if not all, bacterial chromosomes. They are also **cryptic** in the sense that they do not confer on the host bacterium a predictable phenotype. Their presence is usually indicated by mutation. IS elements possess ability to transpose, i.e. they can insert into different sites on the same or on different DNA molecules.

In 1974, the discovery of a new type of transposable element that encoded a recognizable gene product (β-lactam antibiotic resistance) was reported. It was termed a **transposon (tn)**. Since then many others carrying a variety of resistance and other genes have been identified. Because of the ability of transposable elements to move from one plasmid to another or to a phage or to the bacterial chromosome they have assumed the popular name of **jumping genes**. **Unlike plasmids, transposons do not contain genetic information necessary for their own replication**, and their replication, therefore, depends on their physical integration with a bacterial replicon.

Transposons are large (4–25 kb) transposable genetic elements. They encode at least one function that alters cell phenotype. Therefore, **transposon may be defined as a segment of DNA with one or more genes in the centre and the two ends**

carrying inverted repeat sequences of nucleotides—nucleotide sequences complementary to each other but in the reverse order. Because of this feature each strand of the transposon can form a single-stranded loop carrying the gene/genes and a double-stranded stem formed by hydrogen bonding between the inverted repeat sequences (Fig. 48.1).

The transfer of genetic material from one DNA molecule to another is known as **transposition**. It does not need genetic homology between transposable element and its site of insertion. It is, therefore, different from recombination. Insertion of a transposon leads to the acquisition of new characteristics by the recipient DNA molecule. **It has been suggested that R plasmids may have evolved as collections of transposons each carrying a gene that confers resistance to one or more antibiotics.**

Genetic Engineering (Recombinant DNA Technology)

Insertion of a foreign DNA molecule into DNA of a vector, which can replicate autonomously in a suitable host, is known as recombinant DNA (rDNA) technology or genetic engineering. This technique makes it possible to isolate any gene coding for any desired protein from microorganisms or from cells of higher forms of life including human beings, and their introduction into suitable microorganisms in which genes would be functional, directing the production of specific protein. Such cloning of

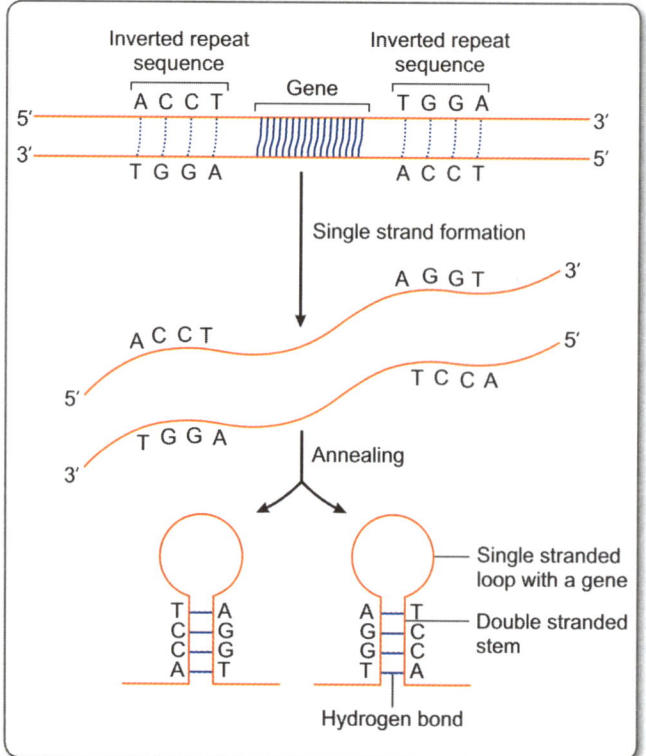

Fig. 48.1: Structure of transposon.

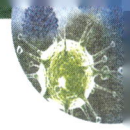

genes in microorganisms enables the preparation of the desired protein in pure form, in large quantities and at a reasonable cost. It has been made possible by the discovery of DNA endonucleases or restriction endonucleases which are enzymes able to cut DNA molecules at specific sequences. These enzymes are present in many prokaryotic organisms, e.g. restriction endonucleases *Eco*RI, *Hind*III, *Bam*HI, *Pst*I and *Sma*I are obtained from *E. coil*, *H. influenzae, Bacillus amyloliquefaciens, Providencia stuartii* and *Serratia marcescens* respectively.

Restriction enzymes are produced by bacterial cells as part of their defence against the incursion of foreign DNA particularly bacteriophages. The target sites for these enzymes normally comprise four to six base pairs of specific sequence and are palindromic meaning that the sequence is the same on both strands of double helix. These enzymes cut double-stranded DNA in two different ways. Some cut at positions on the DNA strands opposite to each other giving blunt ends. Other enzymes cut off-centre but at same relative location in each strand generating complementary or cohesive or sticky ends that can overlap for two to four bases.

Methicillin-resistant Staphylococci (MRSA)

MRSA is any strain of *S. aureus* that has developed, through the process of natural selection, resistance to beta-lactam antibiotics, which include the penicillins (methicillin, oxacillin, dicloxacillin, nafcillin, etc.) and the cephalosporins. It is also called oxacillin-resistant *Staphylococcus aureus* (ORSA). Strains unable to resist these antibiotics are classified as methicillin-sensitive *Staphylococcus aureus* or MSSA. The evolution of such resistance does not cause the organism to be more intrinsically virulent than strains of *S. aureus* that have no antibiotic resistance, but resistance does make MRSA infection more difficult to treat with standard types of antibiotics and thus more dangerous.

MRSA is responsible for several difficult-to-treat infections in humans. It is especially troublesome in hospitals, where patients with open wounds, invasive devices, and weakened immune systems are at a greater risk of infection than general public. The main cause of concern now is the emergence of community-acquired MRSA (CA MRSA) which were earlier restricted to the hospital setting, hospital-associated MRSA (HA-MRSA).

Importance of Antimicrobial Stewardship

Antimicrobial resistance is increasing; however, antimicrobial drug development is slowing. Therefore, antimicrobial stewardship is of utmost importance as a way to optimize the use of antimicrobials to prevent the development of resistance and improve patient outcomes. Antimicrobial surveillance programme has shown substantial increase in the rate of *Klebsiella* resistance to third-generation cephalosporins, extended-spectrum β-lactamase-producing *Klebsiella pneumoniae* and *Escherichia coli*, and *Pseudomonas* resistance to fluoroquinolones. During the past 30 years, antibiotic development has slowed considerably, and our options for treating increasingly resistant infections are becoming more and more limited.

Antimicrobial stewardship has been defined as "the optimal selection, dosage, and duration of antimicrobial treatment or prevention of infection, with minimal toxicity to the patient and minimal impact on subsequent resistance". There are three goals of antimicrobial stewardship:

1. Each patient should receive most appropriate antimicrobial with correct dose and duration.
2. Prevent antimicrobial overuse, misure and abuse. Antibiotics should not be given to patients with viral infection; noninfectious processes and bacterial infections that do not require antibiotics (such as small skin abscesses that will resolve with incision and drainage).
3. The third goal is to minimize the development of resistance. Patients exposed to antibiotics are at higher risk of becoming colonized or infected by resistant organisms. The most common cause of the development of *Clostridium difficile* infection is exposure to antibiotics. Gram-negative organisms, resistance to carbapenems and cephalosporins has been shown to increase 10- to 20-fold with exposure to these broad-spectrum antimicrobials.

Prevention of development of methicillin resistant staphylococci and multiple drug resistant organisms can be achieved by practising antimicrobial stewardship programme.

Blood and Blood Transfusion Policy

Life saving property of transfused blood became clear during the second world war, and thereafter blood transfusion became a suitable hospital function. There are a number of blood groups. ABO and Rh are the major blood groups. Forty percent individuals in India have O group followed by B (33%), A (22%) and AB (5%).

Rh isoimmunization can be prevented by adminstration of 100–300 μg of anti-Rh IgG prepared from human volunteers, at the time when the antigenic stimulation is expected to take place, i.e. immediately after delivery. To be effective, this should be employed from first delivery onwards.

COMPLICATIONS OF BLOOD TRANSFUSION

The complications of blood transfusion may be divided into immunological and non-immunological.

Immunological Complications

Immunological complications may be caused by red blood cell, leucocyte or platelet incompatibility or allergic reaction to plasma components.

Red blood cell incompatibility leads to acute intravascular haemolysis or the red blood cells may be coated by antibodies and engulfed by phagocytes, removed from the circulation and subjected to extravascular lysis. Haemolysis may also be due to transfusion of group O whole blood or plasma to group A or group B or group AB recipients.

Leucocyte incompatibility may cause fever, pulmonary infiltrates, dyspnoea, non-productive cough and chest pain. The risk of these reactions can be reduced by using leucocyte-poor red blood cells. Leucoagglutinins are probably the commonest cause of fever. Platelet incompatibility, allergy and infection may also lead to fever.

Allergic reactions may be caused by interaction of patient's preformed reagins with transfused allergens. When allergic reactions develop administer antihistaminics during transfusion.

Non-immunological Complications

Non-immunological complications of blood transfusion include transmission of infectious agents and circulatory overload. Infectious agents which may be transmitted during blood transfusion may be viruses, bacteria and protozoa (Table 49.1). Circulatory overload may be due to massive transfusion.

Transfusion-transmitted Infectious Agents

Infectious agents which may be transmitted during blood transfusion may be viruses, bacteria and protozoa. Therefore, before transfusion, blood should be screened for hepatitis B virus, hepatitis C virus, human immunodeficiency virus 1 and 2, *Treponema pallidum* and *Plasmodium* spp.

TABLE 49.1: Non-immunological complications of blood transfusion

I. Transmission of infectious agents
• Viruses
▪ Hepatitis B virus*
▪ Hepatitis C virus*
▪ Human immunodeficiency virus 1 and 2*
▪ Human T cell lymphotrophic virus 1 and 2
▪ Cytomegalovirus
• Bacteria
▪ *Treponema pallidum* *
▪ *Leptospira interrogans*
▪ *Borrelia burgdorferi*
• Protozoa
▪ *Plasmodium* spp.*
▪ *Babesia* spp.
▪ *Trypanosoma cruzi*
▪ *Leishmania donovani*
▪ *Toxoplasma gondii*
II. Circulatory overload

*Mandatory tests in India.

Chapter 50

Healthcare Worker Immunization Programme, Needle Stick Injuries and Prevention, and Post-exposure Prophylaxis

Healthcare staff should be vaccinated against vaccine-preventable diseases, e.g. hepatitis B, and BCG in tuberculin negative individuals, etc.

NEEDLE STICK INJURY, AND PREVENTION AND POST-EXPOSURE PROPHYLAXIS OF AIDS

Post-exposure Prophylaxis

Occupational Exposure

Occupational exposure refers to exposure to potential blood-borne infections (HIV, hepatitis B virus and hepatitis C virus) that may occur in healthcare settings during performance of job duties. Post-exposure prophylaxis (PEP) refers to comprehensive medical management to minimise the risk of infection among healthcare personnel following potential exposure to blood-borne pathogens. This includes counselling, risk assessment, relevant laboratory investigations based on informed consent of the source and exposed person, first-aid and depending on the risk assessment, the provision of short-term (4 weeks) of antiretroviral drugs, with follow-up and support.

Healthcare workers (HCW) are normally at very low risk of acquiring HIV infection during management of the infected patient. However, the absence of a vaccine or effective curative treatment makes the HCW apprehensive. Most exposures do not result in infection. The risk of infection varies with:

(a) amount of blood, body fluid and other potentially infectious material involved in exposure,

(b) number of viruses in patient blood at the time of exposure, and

(c) whether post-exposure prophylaxis (PEP) was taken within recommended time.

Exposure may be due to percutaneous injury (needle-stick exposure or cut with a sharp instrument) or contact of the mucous membrane of the eye, nose or mouth or non-intact skin (abraded and afflicted with dermatitis), contact with intact skin when the duration of contact is prolonged (e.g. several minutes) with blood or other potentially infectious body fluids. Body fluids that are potentially infectious include blood, semen, vaginal secretions, cerebrospinal fluid, synovial, pleural, peritoneal, pericardial and amniotic fluid or other body fluids contaminated with visible blood. Exposure to tears, sweat, urine, faeces and saliva of an infected person is normally not considered as an 'exposure' unless these secretions contain visible blood. **Risk of transmission of blood-borne viruses of HCW by percutaneous exposure is 0.3%, 9–30% and 1–10% for HIV, HBV and HCV, respectively.** Following exposure:

- Wash needle-stick exposures and cuts with soap and water.
- Flush with water splashes to the nose, mouth or skin. Irrigate eyes with clean water.
- Do not put pricked finger into mouth.
- Do not squeeze blood from wound, this causes trauma and inflammation, increasing risk of transmission.
- Do not use spirit, betadine or iodine. These may also cause trauma.
- After a splash of blood or body fluids in the eye, irrigate exposed eye immediately with water or normal saline. Sit in a chair, tilt head back and ask a colleague to gently pour water or normal saline over the eye. If wearing contact lens, leave it in place while irrigating, as it forms a barrier over the eye and will help protect it. Once the eye is cleaned, remove the contact lens and clean it in the normal manner. This will make it safe to wear again.

Administration of PEP to HCW depends upon the nature of exposure of the HCW and HIV status of exposure source. Two main factors determine the risk of infection—the nature of exposure and the status of the source patient.

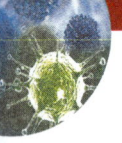

TABLE 50.1: Categories of exposure

Category	Definition and example
Mild exposure	Mucous membrane/non-intact skin with small volumes, e.g. a superficial wound (erosion of the epidermis) with a plain or low calibre needle, or contact with eyes or mucous membranes, subcutaneous injections following small-bore needles
Moderate exposure	Mucous membrane/non-intact skin with large volume or percutaneous superficial exposure with solid needle, e.g. a cut or needle-stick injury penetrating gloves
Severe exposure	Percutaneous with large volume, e.g. • an accident with a high calibre needle (≥18G) visible contaminated with blood; • a deep wound (haemorrhagic wound and/or very painful); • transmission of a significant amount of blood; • an accident with material that has previously been used intravenously or intra-arterially

Assessing the Nature of Exposure

Three categories of exposure can be described based on the amount of blood/fluid involved and the entry port. These categories are intended to help in assessing the severity of the exposure but may not cover all possibilities (Table 50.1).

Assessing the HIV Status of the Source of Exposure

PEP must be initiated as soon as possible, preferably within 2 hours and certainly within 72 hours. A baseline **rapid HIV testing** should be done before starting PEP. Initiation of PEP where indicated should not be delayed while waiting for the results of HIV testing of the source of exposure.

There are two types of regimens:
1. Basic regimen: 2-drug combination
2. Expanded regimen: 3-drug combination

TABLE 50.2: Basic and expanded regimens of post-exposure prophylaxis

Basic regimen
- Zidovudine 300 mg BD for 4 weeks
- Lamivudine 150 mg BD for 4 weeks

Expanded regimen
- Basic regiment + Nelfinavir 750 mg TDS for 4 weeks

The decision to initiate the type of regimen depends on the type of exposure and HIV serostatus of the source person (Table 50.2).

Both risk of infections and possible side effects of drugs should be carefully considered when deciding to prescribe PEP. Exposure with a lower infection risk may not be worth the risk of the side effects associated with the drugs. To know if the exposed HCW has acquired HIV infection following exposure, HIV testing should be done at the time of exposure, and 3 months and 6 months following exposure. If the test at 6 months is negative, no further testing is recommended.

Chapter 51

Overview of Microbiology

Medical Microbiology is the study of living organisms that infect humans. These include viruses, bacteria, fungi and parasites (protozoa and helminths). Comparison of medically important microbial groups is given in Table 51.1. Overview of bacterial and viral infections is given in Figs. 51.1 and 51.2.

Table 51.2 enlists microbes affecting blood cells or haemopoiesis and Table 51.3 enlists the dose of microorganisms required to produce infections in human volunteers.

Strict aerobes

- *Mycobacterium tuberculosis*
- *Pseudomonas aeruginosa*
- *Burkholderia*
- *Bordetella pertussis*

Strict anerobes

- *Clostridium tetani*
- *C. difficile*
- *Bacteroides fragilis*
- *Peptostreptococcus*
- *Anaeroplasma*

Microaerophilic Bacteria

- *Campylobacter*
- *Helicobacter*

Clostridia which can grow in microaerophilic condition

- *Clostridium perfringens*

TABLE 51.1: Comparison of medically important microbial groups

Characteristic	Viruses	Bacteria	Fungi	Protozoa
Diameter	0.02–0.3 µm	0.3–2.0 µm	2–15 µm	2.5–60 µm
Cell type	• Acellular (no cell), no nucleus	Prokaryotic cells; no nuclear membrane	Eukaryotic cells; nucleus with nuclear membrane	
	• Either DNA or RNA	Both DNA and RNA; one chromosome	Both DNA and RNA; more than one chromosome	
	• Obligate intracellular parasites; use host organelles	No membrane-bound organelles	Mitochondria and other membrane-bound organelles	
	• No ribosomes	70S ribosomes (30S + 50S)	80S ribosomes (40S + 60S)	
Cell membrane	No cell membrane; some are enveloped	Cell membrane does not possess sterol except mycoplasmas, which have cholesterol	Membrane ergosterol is major sterol	Sterols such as cholesterol
Cell wall	No cell wall	Peptidoglycan	Complex carbohydrate cell wall: chitin, glucans, or manans	No cell wall
Replication	Make and assemble viral components	Binary fission (asexual)	Cytokinesis with mitosis/meiosis	

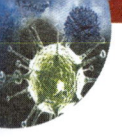

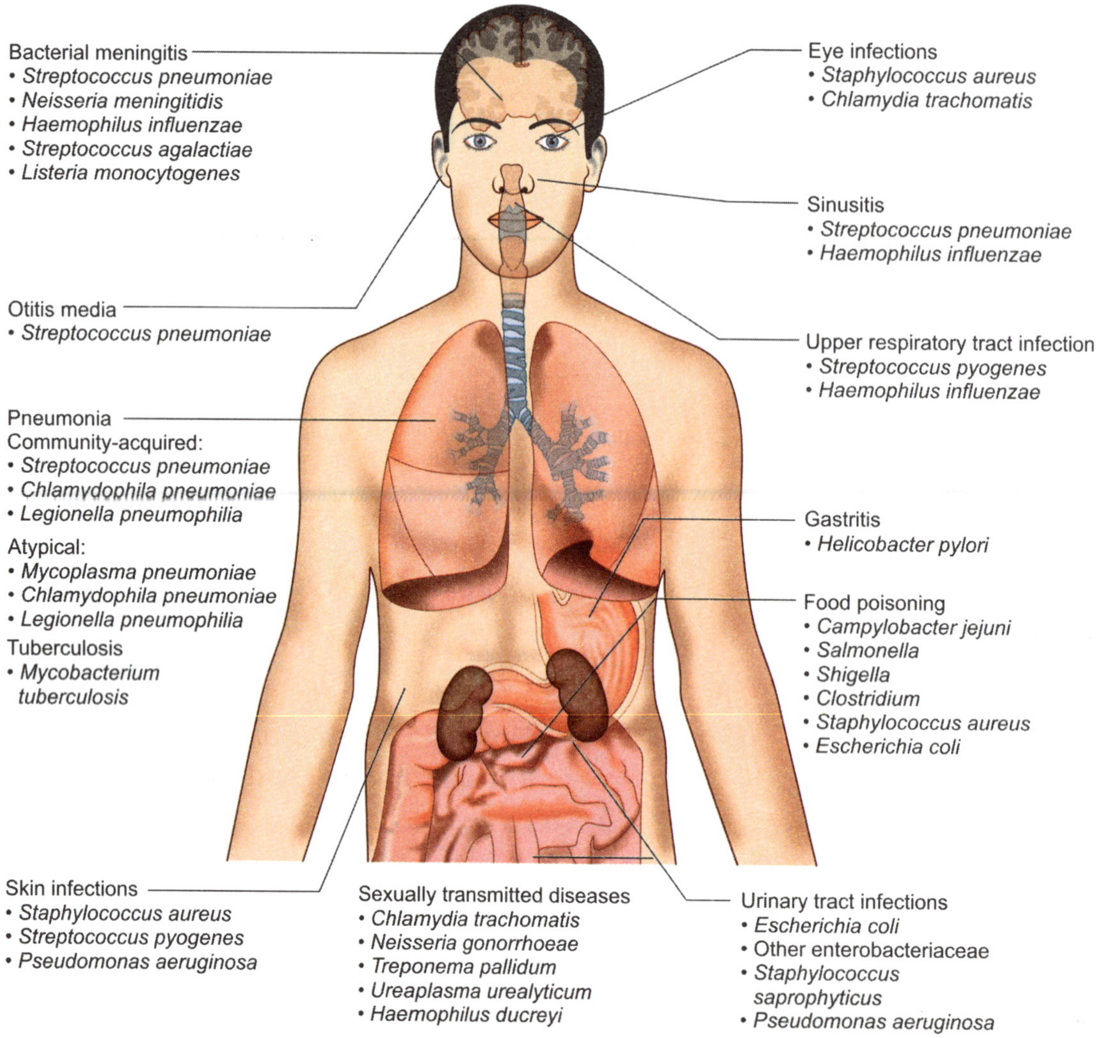

Bacterial meningitis
• *Streptococcus pneumoniae*
• *Neisseria meningitidis*
• *Haemophilus influenzae*
• *Streptococcus agalactiae*
• *Listeria monocytogenes*

Eye infections
• *Staphylococcus aureus*
• *Chlamydia trachomatis*

Sinusitis
• *Streptococcus pneumoniae*
• *Haemophilus influenzae*

Otitis media
• *Streptococcus pneumoniae*

Upper respiratory tract infection
• *Streptococcus pyogenes*
• *Haemophilus influenzae*

Pneumonia
Community-acquired:
• *Streptococcus pneumoniae*
• *Chlamydophila pneumoniae*
• *Legionella pneumophilia*
Atypical:
• *Mycoplasma pneumoniae*
• *Chlamydophila pneumoniae*
• *Legionella pneumophilia*
Tuberculosis
• *Mycobacterium tuberculosis*

Gastritis
• *Helicobacter pylori*

Food poisoning
• *Campylobacter jejuni*
• *Salmonella*
• *Shigella*
• *Clostridium*
• *Staphylococcus aureus*
• *Escherichia coli*

Skin infections
• *Staphylococcus aureus*
• *Streptococcus pyogenes*
• *Pseudomonas aeruginosa*

Sexually transmitted diseases
• *Chlamydia trachomatis*
• *Neisseria gonorrhoeae*
• *Treponema pallidum*
• *Ureaplasma urealyticum*
• *Haemophilus ducreyi*

Urinary tract infections
• *Escherichia coli*
• Other enterobacteriaceae
• *Staphylococcus saprophyticus*
• *Pseudomonas aeruginosa*

Fig. 51.1: Bacterial infections overview

TABLE 51.2: Microbes affecting blood cells or haemopoiesis

Microbe	Disease	Effect
Plasmodium spp.	Malaria	Anaemia
Babesia spp.	Babesiosis	Anaemia
Bartonella bacilliformis	Oroya fever	Anaemia
Ehrlichia spp.	Ehrlichiosis	Leucopenia, thrombocytopenia
Human parvovirus	Erythema infectiosum	Temporary fall in haemoglobin, aplastic crisis
Colorado tick fever virus	Colorado tick fever	Leucopenia, rash
Human T cell lymphotropic (leukaemia) virus (HTLV-1)	Human T cell leukaemia/lymphoma	Malignant transformation of infected cells
Human immunodeficiency virus (HIV)	AIDS	Immunosuppression
Epstein-Barr virus (EBV)	Infectious mononucleosis	Thrombocytopenia, anaemia

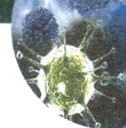

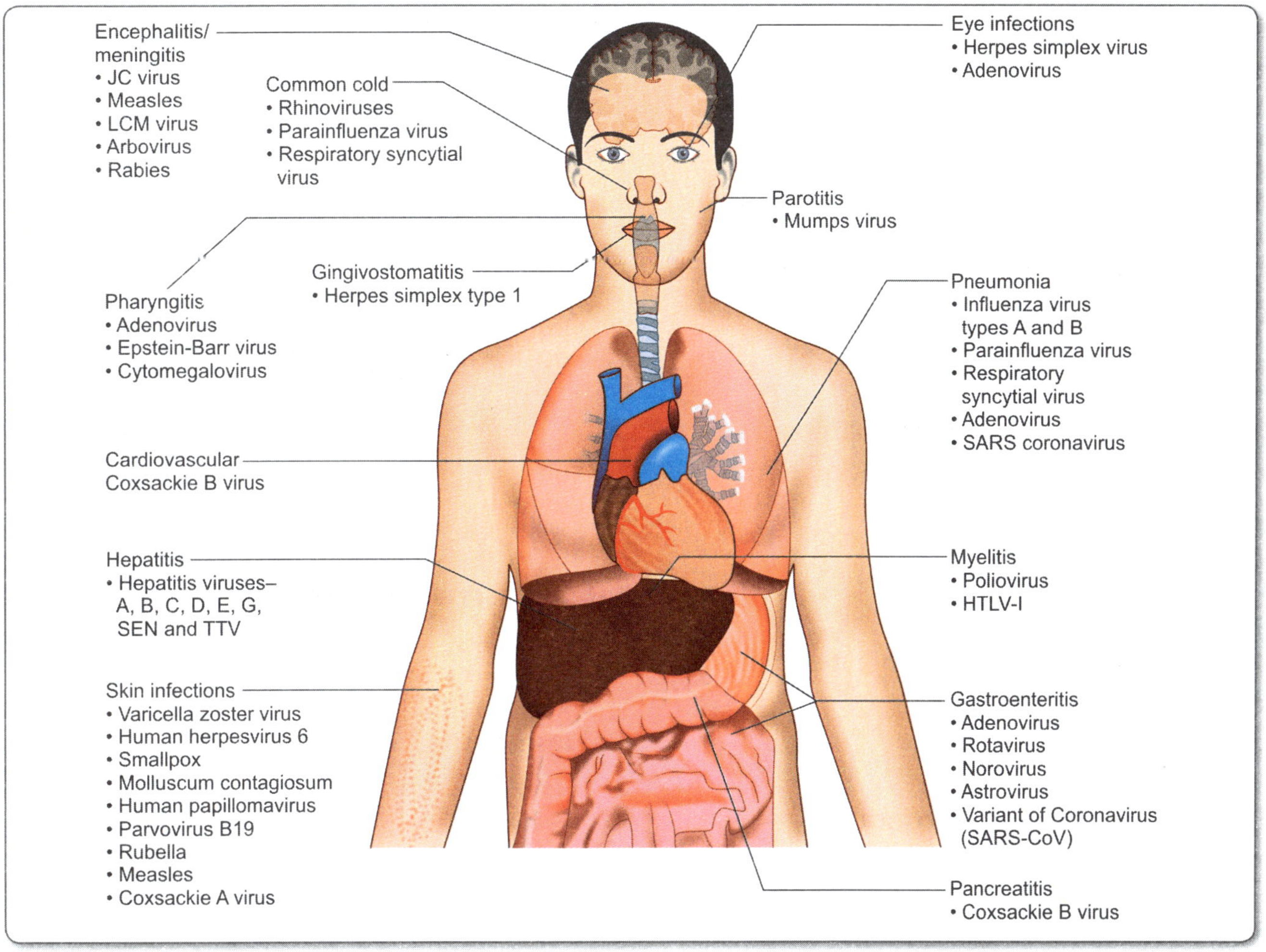

Encephalitis/
meningitis
• JC virus
• Measles
• LCM virus
• Arbovirus
• Rabies

Common cold
• Rhinoviruses
• Parainfluenza virus
• Respiratory syncytial
  virus

Pharyngitis
• Adenovirus
• Epstein-Barr virus
• Cytomegalovirus

Gingivostomatitis
• Herpes simplex type 1

Cardiovascular
Coxsackie B virus

Hepatitis
• Hepatitis viruses–
  A, B, C, D, E, G,
  SEN and TTV

Skin infections
• Varicella zoster virus
• Human herpesvirus 6
• Smallpox
• Molluscum contagiosum
• Human papillomavirus
• Parvovirus B19
• Rubella
• Measles
• Coxsackie A virus

Eye infections
• Herpes simplex virus
• Adenovirus

Parotitis
• Mumps virus

Pneumonia
• Influenza virus
  types A and B
• Parainfluenza virus
• Respiratory
  syncytial virus
• Adenovirus
• SARS coronavirus

Myelitis
• Poliovirus
• HTLV-I

Gastroenteritis
• Adenovirus
• Rotavirus
• Norovirus
• Astrovirus
• Variant of Coronavirus
  (SARS-CoV)

Pancreatitis
• Coxsackie B virus

Fig. 51.2: Viral infections overview

Nonmotile clostridia

- *Clostridium perfringens*
- *C. tetani* type VI

Acid-fast bacteria

- Tubercle bacilli
- Non-tuberculous mycobacteria

- *Mycobacterium leprae*
- *Nocardia*

Microorganisms which cannot be kept back by bacterial filters

- *Mycoplasma*
- Viruses

TABLE 51.3: Dose of microorganisms required to produce infection in human volunteers

Microbe	Route	Disease-producing dose
Rhinovirus	Pharynx	200
Salmonella serotype Typhi	Oral	10^6–10^9
Shigella spp.	Oral	10–100
Vibrio cholerae	Oral	10^8
Mycobacterium tuberculosis	Inhalation	1–10

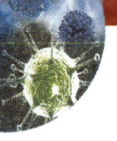

Bacteria that can invade tissues in the absence of physical injury

- *Neisseria meningitidis*
- *Salmonella*
- *Shigella*
- Enteroinvasive *Escherichia coli*

Microorganism which survives pasteurization by holder method

- *Coxiella burnetii*

Insect vectors which transmit pathogens transovarially from one generation of the insects to the next

- Ticks
- Mites

Microorganisms possessing polypeptide capsule

- *Bacillus anthracis*

Bacteria invading both sensory and motor nerves

- *Mycobacterium leprae*

Organisms that can be demonstrated by Quellung reaction

- *Streptococcus pneumoniae*
- *Klebsiella*
- *Haemophilus influenzae*

Microorganisms that normally do not invade the blood stream

- *Clostridium tetani*
- *C. perfringens*
- *Corynebacterium diphtheriae*
- *Shigella* spp.

Microorganisms excreted in milk

- *Mycobacterium leprae*
- Human immunodeficiency virus

Microorganisms which readily undergo antigenic variation

- *Neisseria gonorrhoeae*
- *N. meningitidis*
- *Borrelia recurrentis*
- *B. duttoni*
- *Trypanosoma brucei gambiense*
- Influenza virus
- Human immunodeficiency virus

Lactose-fermenting bacilli

- *Escherichia*
- *Klebsiella*
- *Enterobacter*
- *Citrobacter*
- *Vibrio vulnificus*

Late lactose-fermenters

- *Shigella sonnei*
- *Vibrio cholerae*

Oxidase-positive bacteria

- *Neisseria meningitidis*
- *N. gonorrhoeae*
- *Vibrio*
- *Pseudomonas*
- *Aeromonas*
- *Pleisomonas*
- *Campylobacter*
- *Helicobacter*
- *Alkaligenes*
- *Burkholderia* (except *B. mallei* and *B. maltophila*)
- *Haemophilus influenzae*

Smallest free-living (extracellular) bacteria

- *Mycoplasma*
- *Ureaplasma*

Bacteria unable to grow on cell-free media

- *Rickettsia*
- *Orientia*
- *Ehrlichia*

Bacterial carcinogen

- *Helicobacter pylori* (gastric adenocarcinoma)

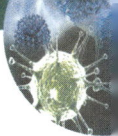

Smallest viruses

- Parvoviruses (about 20 nm in diameter)

Largest viruses

- Poxviruses (about 300 nm in diameter)

Viruses which carry two identical copies of its genome (diploid)

- Retroviruses

Viruses which do not withstand freeze-drying

- Polioviruses

Viruses relatively resistant to chlorination

- Polioviruses
- Hepatitis A virus

Human disease that can be prevented by active immunization after acquisition of infection

- Rabies

Hepatitis viruses causing hepatocellular carcinoma

- Hepatitis B virus
- Hepatitis C virus

Hepatitis viruses transmitted by parenteral and sexual routes

- Hepatitis B virus
- Hepatitis C virus
- Hepatitis D virus
- Hepatitis G virus

Hepatitis viruses with DNA genome

- Hepatitis B virus
- SEN virus
- Transfusion-transmitted virus

Hepatitis viruses transmitted by faecal-oral route

- Hepatitis A virus
- Hepatitis E virus

Viruses transmitted by transfusion and transplantation

- Hepatitis B virus
- Hepatitis C virus
- Hepatitis D virus
- Transfusion-transmitted virus
- Human immunodeficiency virus
- Human T cell lymphotropic (leukaemia) virus-1
- Cytomegalovirus

Culture of microorganisms

- Obligate intracellular pathogens (viruses, *Rickettsia*, *Chlamydia* and *Chlamydophila*):
  - Cell cultures
  - Fertilized hen's eggs
  - Animals
- Facultative intracellular or extracellular organisms:
  - Inert laboratory media (broths and agar)

Spore-forming bacteria

- *Bacillus*
- *Clostridium*

Non-motile Gram-positive rods

- *Corynebacterium diphtheriae*
- *Nocardia*
- *Clostridium perfringens*
- *Bacillus anthracis*

Encapsulated microorganisms

- *Streptococcus pneumoniae*
- *Klebsiella pneumoniae*
- *Haemophilus influenzae*
- *Neisseria meningitidis*
- *N. gonorrhoeae*
- *Bordetella pertussis*
- *Pseudomonas aeruginosa* – slime-producing especially in cystic fibrosis patients' lungs
- *Bacillus anthracis*
- *B. subtilis*
- *Salmonella* serotype Typhi
- *Campylobacteria fetus*
- *Yersinia pestis*
- *Streptococcus pyogenes*
- *S. agalactiae*
- *Staphylococcus aureus*
- *Cryptococcus neoformans*

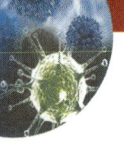

SECTION IX • MISCELLANEOUS

Biofilm producers

- *Staphylococcus epidermidis* (catheter-related infections)
- *Streptococcus mutants* (dental plaque)

Pigment producers

- *Pseudomonas aeruginosa* – blue-green
- *Serratia* – red pigment
- *Staphylococcus aureus* – yellow pigment
- Photochromogenic and scotochromogenic mycobacteria – yellow and orange

Urease-positive organisms

- *Proteus*
- *Klebsiella*
- *Ureaplasma*
- *Helicobacter*
- *Cryptococcus*

Catalase-positive organisms

- *Staphylococcus*
- Enterobacteriaceae (except *Shigella dysenteriae* type 1)
- *Pseudomonas aeruginosa*
- *Candida*
- *Aspergillus*

Coagulase-positive organisms

- *Staphylococcus aureus*
- *Yersinia pestis*

Heat-stable toxins

60°C
- *Staphylococcus aureus* enterotoxin
- ST of *Escherichia coli*
- *Yersinia enterocolitica* toxin

100°C
- Endotoxin

Obligate intracellular parasites

- Bacteria
  - All rickettsiae
  - All Chlamydiaceae
  - *Mycobacterium leprae*
- Viruses
- Protozoa
  - *Plasmodium*
  - *Babesia*
  - *Leishmania*
  - *Trypanosoma cruzi* – amastigote form
  - *Toxoplasma gondii*

Organisms that are found extracellular in the body but cannot be cultured on inert media

- *Treponema pallidum*
- *Pneumocystis jirovecii*

Organisms that cross the placenta (Mnemonic: TORCH)

- T-**T**oxoplasma gondii
- O-**O**ther (*Treponema pallidum*)
- R-**R**ubella
- C-**C**ytomegalovirus
- H-**H**erpes and HIV

Bacteria entering the body by ingestion

- *Salmonella* serotypes
- *Shigella* spp.
- *Yersinia enterocolitica*
- Enterotoxigenic *Escherichia coli*
- *Vibrio* spp.
- *Campylobacter* spp.
- *Clostridium botulinum*
- *Bacillus cereus*
- *Listeria* spp.
- *Brucella* spp.

Bacteria entering the body by inhalation

- *Mycobacterium* spp.
- *Nocardia* spp.
- *Mycoplasma pneumoniae*
- *Legionella* spp.
- *Bordetella* spp.
- *Chlamydophila psittaci*
- *Streptococcus* spp.

Bacteria entering the body following trauma

- *Clostridium tetani*
- *C. perfringens*

Organisms entering the body through needle-stick injury

- Hepatitis B virus
- Hepatitis C virus
- Human immunodeficiency virus
- *Staphylococcus aureus*
- *Pseudomonas* spp.

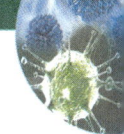

Bacteria transmitted by arthropod bite

- *Rickettsia*
- *Ehrlichia*
- *Francisella*
- *Borrelia* spp.
- *Yersinia pestis*

Sexually-transmitted bacteria

- *Neisseria gonorrhoeae*
- *Treponema pallidum*
- *Chlamydia trachomatis*

Organisms which inhibit fusion of the phagosome with lysosome

- *Mycobacterium tuberculosis*
- *Legionella* spp.

A-B exotoxins

- Cholera toxin
- Heat-labile toxin (LT) of *Escherichia coli*
- Diphtheria toxin
- Pertussis toxin

Organisms resistant to lysosomal enzymes

- *Salmonella* serotype Typhimurium
- *Coxiella* spp.
- *Ehrlichia* spp.
- *Mycobacterium leprae*
- *Leishmania* spp.

NOTES

INDEX

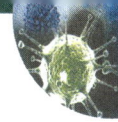

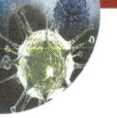

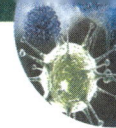

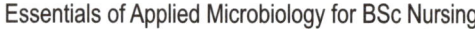

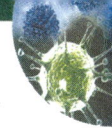

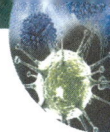

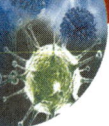

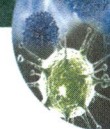

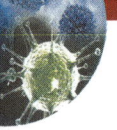